International Classification of Diseases Tenth Revision Procedure Coding System (ICD-10-PCS): An Applied Approach

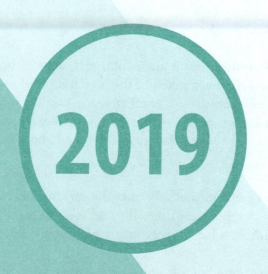

2019

Lynn Kuehn, MS, RHIA, CCS-P, FAHIMA

Therese M. Jorwic, MPH, RHIA, CCS, CCS-P, FAHIMA

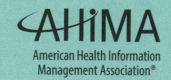

AHIMA

American Health Information
Management Association®

ISBN: 978-1-58426-689-1
AHIMA Product No.: AC201118

AHIMA Press Staff:
Jessica Block, MA, Production Development Editor
Chelsea Brotherton, MA, Assistant Editor
Megan Grennan, Managing Editor

Cover image: ©ALMAGAMI, Shutterstock

For more information, including updates, about AHIMA Press publications, visit **http://www.ahima.org/education/press.**

American Health Information Management Association
233 North Michigan Avenue, 21st Floor
Chicago, Illinois 60601-5809
ahima.org

Table of Contents

How to Use This Book and Online Student Workbook..xiii

About the Authors..xv

Acknowledgments...xvii

Part I	System Definitions and Guidelines	1

Chapter 1	System Structure and Design 3

Background and Rationale for Implementing ICD-10-PCS... 3
Accessing the Code Set... 4
Code Format and Structure 4
Character 1: Section.. 5
Character 2: Body System 6
Character 3: Root Operation 7
Character 4: Body Part 10
Character 5: Approach.. 11
Character 6: Device.. 15
Character 7: Qualifier 19
Code Building Process 19
CMS File Method.. 20
Code Book Method... 27
    Locating the Tables.. 28
    Building the Complete Code 28
    Other Index References.. 29
    Directly Referencing the Code Tables 30
Clinical Documentation and Terminology in ICD-10-PCS... 31
Check Your Understanding 32
    Code Building.. 32

Chapter 2	ICD-10-PCS Coding Guidelines 35

Coding Guidelines... 35
Conventions.. 35
Guidelines for the Medical and Surgical Section 39
    Guidelines for Body System... 39
    Guidelines for Root Operation 40
    Guidelines for Body Part.. 46
    Guidelines for Approach 49
    Guidelines for Device 51
Obstetrics Section Guidelines... 51
New Technology Section 52

Selection of Principal Procedure..52
Applying the Conventions and Guidelines and Researching the Procedure.................53
Check Your Understanding 62
  Case Studies...64

Part II   Introduction to the Medical and Surgical Section   69

Chapter 3   Root Operations that Take Out All/Part or Take Out Solids/Fluids/Gases 71

Character Descriptions...71
Root Operation 71
Group 1: Root Operations that Take Out Some or All of a Body Part............................72
  Excision 72
  Resection..74
  Detachment 77
  Destruction 81
  Extraction..82
Group 2: Root Operations that Take Out Solids/Fluids/Gases from a Body Part..........83
  Drainage...83
  Extirpation...85
  Fragmentation...87
Check Your Understanding 88
  Case Studies...90

Chapter 4   Root Operations that Cut or Separate, Put in or Put Back, or Move Body Parts.........93

Group 3: Root Operations Involving Cutting or Separation Only 93
  Division...93
  Release 94
Group 4: Root Operations that Put in or Put Back or Move Some or All of a Body Part 95
  Transplantation...95
  Reattachment...97
  Transfer 97
  Reposition...99
Check Your Understanding 100
  Case Studies...102

Chapter 5   Root Operations that Alter Diameter or Route of Body Parts, or Involve a Device 105

Group 5: Root Operations that Alter Diameter or Route of a Tubular Body Part..........105
  Restriction 105
  Occlusion...106
  Dilation 107
  Bypass 109
Group 6: Root Operations that Always Involve a Device...113
  Insertion 113
  Removal 115
  Revision 118
  Change..118
  Replacement..118
  Supplement 119

Check Your Understanding 120
    Case Studies... 123

Chapter 6   Root Operations that Involve Examination Only, Other Repairs, or Other Objectives 125

Group 7: Root Operations that Involve Examination Only... 125
    Inspection 125
    Map.. 127
Group 8: Root Operations that Define Other Repairs 127
    Repair.. 127
    Control 127
Group 9: Root Operations that Define Other Objectives.. 129
    Fusion 129
    Alteration 132
    Creation... 133
Check Your Understanding 133
    Case Studies... 135

Chapter 7   Anatomical Regions 139

Anatomical Regions: General, Upper Extremities, and Lower Extremities 139
Organization of the Anatomical Regions 139
    General Anatomical Regions.. 140
    Upper Extremity Region... 141
    Lower Extremity Region 143
Common Root Operations Used in Coding Procedures on the Anatomical Regions 143
Body Parts for the Anatomical Regions 145
Approaches Used for the Anatomical Regions.. 147
Devices Common to the Anatomical Regions.. 148
Qualifiers Used in the Anatomical Regions... 148
Check Your Understanding 153
    Case Studies... 154

Chapter 8   Nervous System 159

Functions of the Nervous System 159
Organization of the Nervous System.. 159
    Central Nervous System.. 159
    Peripheral Nervous System 160
Common Root Operations Used in Coding Procedures Performed on the Nervous System 163
Body Part Values for the Nervous System 164
Approaches Used for the Nervous System.. 166
Devices Common to the Nervous System 167
Qualifiers Used in the Nervous System 167
Check Your Understanding 172
    Case Studies... 173

Chapter 9   Sense Organs 179

Functions of the Sense Organs... 179
Organization of the Sense Organs 179
    Ocular (Eye) System.. 179
    Ear, Nose, and Sinus... 181

Common Root Operations Used in Coding Procedures Performed on the Sense Organs 182
Body Part Values for the Sense Organs 183
Approaches Used for the Sense Organs 185
Devices Common to the Sense Organs 185
Qualifiers Used in the Sense Organs 186
Check Your Understanding 189
    Case Studies 190

Chapter 10   Respiratory System 195

Functions of the Respiratory System 195
Organization of the Mouth, Throat, and Respiratory System 195
    Mouth and Throat 195
    Respiratory System 197
Common Root Operations Used in Coding Procedures on the Mouth, Throat,
and Respiratory System 199
    Bronchoscopy-Based Procedures 199
    Thoracoscopy- or Thoracotomy-Based Procedures 201
Body Part Values for the Mouth, Throat, and Respiratory System 201
Approaches Used in the Mouth, Throat, and Respiratory System 202
Devices Common to the Mouth, Throat, and Respiratory System 203
Qualifiers for the Mouth, Throat, and Respiratory System 204
Check Your Understanding 207
    Case Studies 209

Chapter 11   Circulatory System 213

Functions of the Circulatory System 213
Organization of the Circulatory System 213
    Heart and Great Vessels 213
    Upper and Lower Arteries 216
    Upper and Lower Veins 216
Common Root Operations Used in Coding of Procedures on the Circulatory System 218
    Insertion of Devices 219
    Cardiac Rhythm–Related Devices 219
    Heart Assist Devices 220
    Inferior Vena Cava Filter 220
    Vascular Access Devices 220
    Removal 221
    Revision 221
    Heart Valve Procedures 221
    Creation 222
    Aneurysms 222
    Map and Ablation of Cardiac Mechanism 223
    Heart Transplantation 223
    Cardiac (Heart) Catheterization 223
    Percutaneous Transluminal Coronary Angioplasty (PTCA) 224
    Bypasses 225
    Percutaneous Bypasses 228
    Percutaneous Transluminal Angioplasty of NonCoronary Sites 228

AV Fistulas and Grafts...229
Drainage...229
Laser Revascularization..229
Body Part Values for the Circulatory System...229
Approaches Used for the Circulatory System...232
Devices Common to the Circulatory System...232
Qualifiers Used in the Circulatory System..235
Check Your Understanding 242
Case Studies...243

Chapter 12   Gastrointestinal and Hepatobiliary Systems...249
Functions of the Gastrointestinal System...249
Organization of the Gastrointestinal System 249
Digestive System..249
Hepatobiliary System..252
Common Root Operations Used in Coding of Procedures on the Gastrointestinal System 252
Body Parts for the Gastrointestinal and Hepatobiliary Systems 254
Approaches Used for the Gastrointestinal and Hepatobiliary Systems..................................256
Devices Common to the Gastrointestinal System...256
Qualifiers Used in the Gastrointestinal and Hepatobiliary Systems 258
Check Your Understanding 262
Case Studies...263

Chapter 13   Endocrine and Lymphatic Systems...267
Functions of the Endocrine System 267
Organization of the Endocrine System...267
Common Root Operations Used in Coding Procedures on the Endocrine System.....................268
Body Part Values for the Endocrine System 268
Approaches Used in the Endocrine System...269
Devices Common to the Endocrine System...270
Qualifiers for the Endocrine System...270
Functions of the Lymphatic System...270
Organization of the Lymphatic System 270
Common Root Operations Used in Coding Procedures on the Lymphatic System 271
Body Part Values for the Lymphatic System..272
Approaches Used in the Lymphatic System 273
Devices Common to the Lymphatic System..274
Qualifiers for the Lymphatic System..274
Check Your Understanding 277
Case Studies...279

Chapter 14   Integumentary System..285
Functions of the Integumentary System 285
Organization of the Integumentary System..285
Skin and Breast...285
Subcutaneous Tissue and Fascia...287
Common Root Operations Used in Coding Procedures Performed on the Integumentary System..............287
Mastectomy and Reconstruction Procedures..288

Replacements 288
Reconstruction with a Transfer 288
Breast Implants 289
Body Part Values for the Integumentary System 290
Approaches Used for the Integumentary System 291
Devices Common to the Integumentary System 291
Qualifiers Used in the Integumentary System 293
Check Your Understanding 297
Case Studies 298

Chapter 15   Muscular System: Muscles, Tendons, Bursae, and Ligaments................................303

Functions of the Muscular System... 303
Organization of the Muscular System 303
Muscles.. 303
Tendons.. 305
Bursae and Ligaments 305
Common Root Operations Used in Coding of Procedures on the Muscular System.... 307
Body Parts for the Muscular System... 308
Approaches Used for the Muscular System 309
Devices Common to the Muscular System.. 309
Qualifiers Used in the Muscular System 310
Check Your Understanding 314
Case Studies.. 315

Chapter 16   Skeletal System: Bones and Joints 321

Functions of the Bones and Joints... 321
Organization of the Bones and Joints 321
Bones... 321
Joints 324
Common Root Operations Used in Coding of Procedures on the Bones and Joints.... 324
Replacement of Bones and Joints.. 329
Repair of Joints 331
Body Parts for Bones and Joints.. 331
Approaches Used for the Bones and Joints... 333
Devices Common to the Bones and Joints.. 334
Coding of Spinal Fusion 334
Qualifiers Used for the Bones and Joints 340
Check Your Understanding 346
Case Studies.. 347

Chapter 17   Urinary System 353

Functions of the Urinary System... 353
Organization of the Urinary System 353
Common Root Operations Used in Coding Procedures on the Urinary System........ 355
Body Part Values for the Urinary System.. 356
Approaches Used in the Urinary System 357
Devices Common to the Urinary System... 358

Qualifiers for the Urinary System 359
Check Your Understanding 362
    Case Studies 363

Chapter 18 **Male Reproductive System** 367

Functions of the Male Reproductive System 367
Organization of the Male Reproductive System 367
Common Root Operations Used in Coding Procedures on the Male Reproductive System 369
Body Part Values for the Male Reproductive System 369
Approaches Used in the Male Reproductive System 370
Devices Common to the Male Reproductive System 370
Qualifiers for the Male Reproductive System 371
Check Your Understanding 375
    Case Studies 376

Chapter 19 **Female Reproductive System** 381

Functions of the Female Reproductive System 381
Organization of the Female Reproductive System 381
Common Root Operations Used in Coding Procedures on the Female Reproductive System 382
Body Part Values for the Female Reproductive System 384
Approaches Used in the Female Reproductive System 385
Devices Common to the Female Reproductive System 386
Qualifiers for the Female Reproductive System 386
Check Your Understanding 390
    Case Studies 391

Part III **Medical and Surgical-related Sections**   **397**

Chapter 20 **Obstetrics** 399

Products of Conception 399
Common Root Operations Used in Coding Obstetrics Procedures 400
    Abortion 400
    Delivery and Extraction 401
    Drainage 401
    Other Root Operations 401
    In Vitro Fertilization 402
Body Part Values for Obstetrics 403
Approaches Used in Obstetrics 403
Devices Common to Obstetrics 403
Qualifiers for Obstetrics 404
Check Your Understanding 409
    Case Studies 410

Chapter 21 **Placement, Administration, Measurement, and Monitoring** 415

Types of Procedures Included in these Sections 415
Character Definition for the Placement Section (2) 415
    Common Root Operations Used in the Placement Section 415

Body Regions for Placement..416
Approaches Used for the Placement Section 417
Devices Common to the Placement Section...417
Qualifiers Used in the Placement Section 418

Character Definition for the Administration Section (3)..**418**
Common Root Operations Used in the Administration Section.....................................418
Body Systems and Regions for Administration Section 419
Approaches Used for the Administration Section 419
Substance Values for the Administration Section..419
Qualifiers Used in the Administration Section...422

Character Definition for the Measurement and Monitoring Section (4) **423**
Common Root Operations Used in the Measurement and Monitoring Section 423
Body Systems for the Measurement and Monitoring Section 423
Approaches Used for the Measurement and Monitoring Section 424
Function and Device Values for the Measurement and Monitoring Section................424
Qualifiers Used in the Measurement and Monitoring Section 425

Check Your Understanding **427**
Case Studies..428

Chapter 22   Extracorporeal or Systemic Assistance, Performance, and Therapies...................................**431**

Types of Procedures Included in these Sections 431
Character Definition for the Extracorporeal or Systemic Assistance and Performance Section (5)...............**431**
Common Root Operations Used in the Extracorporeal or Systemic Assistance and Performance Section....431
Body Systems for Extracorporeal or Systemic Assistance and Performance Section 432
Duration Values Used for the Extracorporeal or Systemic Assistance and Performance Section 432
Function Values for the Extracorporeal or Systemic Assistance and Performance Section 433
Qualifiers Used in the Extracorporeal or Systemic Assistance and Performance Section..........................434

Character Definition for the Extracorporeal or Systemic Therapies Section (6) **436**
Common Root Operations Used in the Extracorporeal or Systemic Therapies Section 437
Body Systems for Extracorporeal or Systemic Therapies Section...438
Duration Values Used for the Extracorporeal or Systemic Therapies Section...438
6th Character Qualifier Values for the Extracorporeal or Systemic Therapies Section 438
7th Character Qualifiers Used in the Extracorporeal or Systemic Therapies Section 438

Check Your Understanding **441**
Case Studies..442

Chapter 23   Osteopathic, Other Procedures, and Chiropractic Sections **447**

Types of Procedures Included in these Sections 447
Character Definition for the Osteopathic Section (7)..**447**
Common Root Operations Used in the Osteopathic Section 447
Body Regions for Osteopathic Section..448
Approaches Used for the Osteopathic Section 448
Method Values for the Osteopathic Section..448
Qualifiers Used in the Osteopathic Section 449

Character Definition for the Other Procedures Section (8) **449**
Common Root Operations Used in the Other Procedures Section...............................449
Body Regions for Other Procedures Section 450
Approaches Used for the Other Procedures Section 450

Method Values for the Other Procedures Section 450

Qualifiers Used in the Other Procedures Section 451

Character Definition for the Chiropractic Section (9) 452

Common Root Operations Used in the Chiropractic Section 452

Body Regions for the Chiropractic Section 452

Approaches Used for the Chiropractic Section 453

Method Values for the Chiropractic Section 453

Qualifiers Used in the Chiropractic Section 454

Check Your Understanding 456

Case Studies 457

Part IV   Ancillary Sections   461

Chapter 24   Imaging, Nuclear Medicine, and Radiation Therapy 463

Types of Procedures Included in these Sections 463

Character Definition for the Imaging Section (B) 463

Common Root Types Used in the Imaging Section 464

Body Parts for Imaging Section 465

Contrast Used for the Imaging Section 465

6th Character Qualifiers Common to the Imaging Section 466

7th Character Qualifiers Used in the Imaging Section 466

Character Definition for the Nuclear Medicine Section (C) 467

Common Root Types Used in the Nuclear Medicine Section 467

Body Parts for Nuclear Medicine Section 468

Radionuclides Used for the Nuclear Medicine Section 468

6th and 7th Character Qualifier Values for the Nuclear Medicine Section 469

Character Definition for the Radiation Therapy Section (D) 469

Common Root Types (Modalities) Used in the Radiation Therapy Section 470

Treatment Sites for the Radiation Therapy Section 470

Modality Qualifiers Used for the Radiation Therapy Section 470

Isotope Values for the Radiation Therapy Section 471

Qualifiers Used in the Radiation Therapy Section 472

Check Your Understanding 474

Case Studies 475

Chapter 25   Physical Rehabilitation and Diagnostic Audiology, Mental Health, Substance Abuse Treatment, and New Technology 481

Types of Procedures Included in these Sections 481

Character Definition for the Physical Rehabilitation Section (F) 481

Section Qualifiers Used in the Physical Rehabilitation and Diagnostic Audiology Section 481

Common Root Types Used in the Physical Rehabilitation and Diagnostic Audiology Section 482

Body System and Regions for Physical Rehabilitation and Diagnostic Audiology Section 482

5th Character Type Qualifiers Common to the Physical Rehabilitation and Diagnostic Audiology Section 483

6th Character Equipment Common to the Physical Rehabilitation and Diagnostic Audiology Section 483

Qualifiers Used in the Physical Rehabilitation and Diagnostic Audiology Section 484

Character Definition for the Mental Health Section (G) 484

Common Root Types Used in the Mental Health Section 484

Type Qualifiers Used in the Mental Health Section 485

5th, 6th, and 7th Character Qualifiers Used in the Mental Health Section 487

Character Definition for the Substance Abuse Treatment Section (H) 487

Common Root Types Used in the Substance Abuse Treatment Section 487

Type Qualifiers for the Substance Abuse Treatment Section 488

5th, 6th, and 7th Qualifier Characters Used in the Substance Abuse Treatment Section 489

Character Definition for the New Technology Section (X) 489

Body Systems and Regions for New Technology Section 489

Root Operations for New Technology Section 489

Approach Character for New Technology Section 490

Device/Substance/Technology Character for New Technology Section 490

Qualifiers Used in the New Technology Section 491

Check Your Understanding 493

Case Studies 494

Part V   **Review Exercises and Case Studies**   **499**

Exercises and Case Studies 501

Exercises 501

Case Studies 503

Appendix A Roots and Approaches 541

Appendix B Partial Answer Key 551

References 599

Index 603

Online Resources

Student Workbook
2019 ICD-10-PCS Guidelines
Complete 2019 ICD-10-PCS Code Set
Roots and Approaches Quick Reference Tool

How to Use This Book and Online Student Workbook

This text is designed to provide thorough training in the process of building codes in ICD-10-PCS. Included are a comprehensive review of the structure and conventions of the system as well as an in-depth discussion of the anatomy and code structure by body part for each of the body systems and related sections of ICD-10-PCS.

ICD-10-PCS is the procedural portion of the ICD-10 system and is the code set mandated by the Health Insurance Portability and Accountability Act (HIPAA) for inpatient procedure coding. This text is intended to provide the information and background necessary to use the system to build ICD-10-PCS codes. This includes a thorough discussion of the coding concepts that are unique to ICD-10-PCS as well as a review of the intricacies of anatomy necessary for complete coding. All of these concepts, as well as definitions, conventions, and guidelines, will be illustrated through exercises and case studies.

Icons

 Coding Tip: This icon provides the reader with helpful hints to be used in the coding process. Example: A small nick in the skin does not constitute an open approach. These small nicks in the skin are made to accommodate needles and other small-diameter instruments. When the needle or other instrument reaches all the way to the operative site, the correct approach value is Percutaneous.

 Anatomy Alert: This icon points out important information about how the anatomy is classified in ICD-10-PCS and warns the coder about unique aspects of anatomy in ICD-10-PCS. Example: ICD-10-PCS does not classify regions of the body by the traditional abdominopelvic quadrant divisions. The anatomical regions are defined as general regions, the upper extremity regions, and the lower extremity regions. The inguinal region is defined as part of the Anatomical Regions, Lower Extremities body system in ICD-10-PCS.

 Coding Guideline: This icon displays coding guidelines that directly relate to the area of ICD-10-PCS being discussed in the chapter, including the coding guideline number. Example: B2.1b—Body systems designated as upper and lower contain body parts located above or below the diaphragm, respectively.

 Root Operation or Type: This icon highlights the discussion of a root operation or root type and provides the complete definition at a glance. Example: Excision (B): Cutting out or off, without replacement, a portion of a body part.

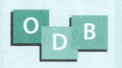 **Code Building:** This icon highlights review activities designed to emphasize important concepts via case exercises that provide step-by-step instructions for use in coding a procedure statement related to the subject being studied. The associated Code Building Exercises guide the reader through the process of evaluating an operative report by providing thought-provoking questions, along with complete in-text answers and rationales.

 Check Your Understanding: This icon signals the end-of-chapter questions and case studies designed to help the reader determine his or her level of understanding of the concepts presented. Answers to the odd-numbered questions are located in appendix B of this book.

Anatomy Illustrations

Labeled anatomy illustrations are found throughout the text to help the reader visualize the body parts being discussed. Identical illustrations without the labels can be found in the online student workbook to allow the reader to test his or her knowledge by labeling the anatomy and testing his or her work against the illustrations in the text.

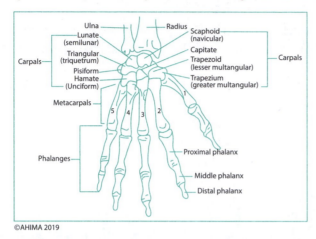

©AHIMA 2019

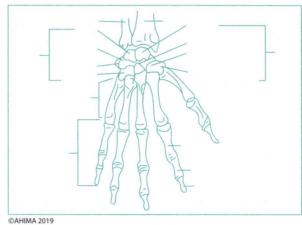

©AHIMA 2019

Tables

The text contains tables that demonstrate the valid values for many of the characters of the ICD-10-PCS code set. These summary tables of character values found in this text are for reference and visualization purposes only. All codes must be chosen from the ICD-10-PCS tables to ensure a valid code assignment.

Unless otherwise stated, all tables are credited to the Centers for Medicare and Medicaid Services (CMS) 2019 ICD-10-PCS at https://www.cms.gov/Medicare/Coding/ICD10/2019-ICD-10-PCS.html.

Online Student Resources

The following material may be found at http://www.ahimapress.org/KuehnJorwic6891/ using the unique code found on the interior front cover of this text:

- Online Student Workbook—Includes code building and other exercises, case studies, anatomy quiz worksheets, and crossword puzzles
- Roots and Approaches Quick Reference Tool
- ICD-10-PCS files from CMS
  * Complete 2019 ICD-10-PCS Code Set
  * 2019 ICD-10-PCS Guidelines

Note to Educators

The ICD-10-PCS codes included in this publication are current as of October 1, 2018. A file containing the most current versions of the codes can be found at https://www.cms.gov/Medicare/Coding/ICD10/2019-ICD-10-PCS.html.

AHIMA provides supplementary materials for educators who use this book in their classes. Materials include PowerPoint slides for lectures, instructor guides, test questions for each chapter, and cases for laboratory activities. A comprehensive answer key for all exercises and case studies and an answer key for the Student Workbook is also included. Visit http://www.ahima.org/education /press for more information about instructor's materials. If you have any questions regarding the instructor materials, contact AHIMA Customer Relations at (800) 335-5535.

Please note: The instructor materials, including answer keys, are only available to approved instructors. For more information about obtaining instructor codes, see http://ahima.org/publications/educators.aspx.

About the Authors

Lynn Kuehn, MS, RHIA, CCS-P, FAHIMA, is president of Kuehn Consulting in Waukesha, Wisconsin. Previously, she has served in health information management and coordination positions in a variety of healthcare settings. In her volunteer role, Kuehn has served as the chair of several national committees. She was a member of the AHIMA Board of Directors from 2005 to 2007 and Chair of the AHIMA Foundation Board of Directors from 2011 to 2012. She has been active as a presenter at numerous meetings and seminars in the field of physician office management, inpatient coding, and reimbursement. Previous AHIMA publications include *CCS-P Exam Preparation*, which she wrote with Anita Hazelwood and Carol Venable, and *Procedural Coding and Reimbursement for Physician Services*. Ms. Kuehn has been the recipient of the AHIMA Educator-Practitioner Award and the Wisconsin Health Information Management Association Distinguished Member Award and Educator Award. She holds an MS in health services administration and a BS in medical record administration, is a certified coding specialist–physician-based, and is a Fellow of AHIMA.

Therese M. Jorwic, MPH, RHIA, CCS, CCS-P, FAHIMA, is a clinical assistant professor in health information management at the University of Illinois at Chicago and an independent consultant. In these roles, Ms. Jorwic has presented numerous workshops and developed educational material for in-class and online courses on ICD-10-CM/PCS, and HCPCS/CPT for hospitals, physicians, and other healthcare providers and associations. Ms. Jorwic is the past president and recipient of the distinguished member award for both the Chicago Area and Illinois Health Information Management Associations. She has served AHIMA as Chairman of the Practice Council on Clinical Terminology and Classification and Council on Coding and Classification. She was the first chairman of the AHIMA Society for Clinical Coding and is a recipient of the AHIMA's Pioneer and Literary Awards. Ms. Jorwic received the Amoco Silver Circle, Excalibur, and Educator of the Year awards for teaching excellence at the University of Illinois at Chicago. Ms. Jorwic holds an MPH with a concentration in health services and administration and received her BS in medical record administration. She is a certified coding specialist, a certified coding specialist–physician-based, and a Fellow of AHIMA.

Lynn Kuehn and Therese Jorwic proudly accepted AHIMA's 2014 Literary Legacy Award for their work on this and other texts during their careers.

Acknowledgments

The authors would like to thank our colleagues who helped us to shape this textbook. In addition to the technical reviewers listed on the copyright page, we would like to especially acknowledge Lou Ann Schraffenberger, MBS, RHIA, CCS, CCS-P, FAHIMA, Pat Shaw, EdD, RHIA, FAHIMA, and Margaret Skurka, MS, RHIA, CCS, FAHIMA, for their assistance in helping us to produce what the authors feel is a comprehensive coverage of the subject of ICD-10-PCS. In addition, the authors would like to recognize Gail Smith, MA, RHIA, CCS-P, for her expert guidance throughout the development and writing of this text. Her thoughtful input helped shape the outline, structure, and content of the book.

We thank Michelle Callahan, Darcy Carter, Karen Feltner, Angela Lee, Mari Petrik, and Rhonda Voelz for their helpful comments.

Finally, we acknowledge our families and friends, especially Jeff Kuehn and Lee Jorwic, who supported us in so many ways throughout this extensive writing and review process. Thank you so much.

———————

AHIMA Press and the authors would like to thank Linda Hyde, RHIA, and Erica Wilson, MHA, RHIA, CPC for their work as technical reviewers of this edition, and Jason Isley for providing medical illustrations.

Part I

System
Definitions
and Guidelines

Chapter 1

System Structure and Design

The International Classification of Diseases, Tenth Revision, Procedure Coding System (ICD-10-PCS) is the procedure classification used for inpatient procedures in the United States. ICD-10-PCS was implemented on October 1, 2015, along with the diagnosis coding system, the International Classification of Diseases, Tenth Revision, Clinical Modification (ICD-10-CM).

Unlike the ICD-10-CM system, which is based on the international ICD-10 system for classifying diagnoses, ICD-10-PCS was developed in the United States specifically for procedure reporting. The Health Insurance Portability and Accountability Act (HIPAA) has established ICD-10-PCS as the mandated code set for reporting inpatient procedures, and ICD-10-CM for diagnoses in all settings. The Official ICD-10-CM and ICD-10-PCS Guidelines for Coding and Reporting for each respective system are also recognized as an official part of the code sets.

Coding Tip

The ICD-10-PCS system was developed for use in the United States. The international ICD-10 system does not include a procedure classification.

Background and Rationale for Implementing ICD-10-PCS

ICD-10-PCS replaced volume 3 of the ICD-9-CM system. Development of ICD-10-PCS began in 1993 when 3M Health Information Systems started to design the system under a contract from the Centers for Medicare and Medicaid Services (CMS), the government agency responsible for the inpatient procedure classification in the United States. The draft of the new system was completed in 1998 and was updated and enhanced on a regular basis throughout the implementation process.

By design, the ICD-10-PCS system is a total departure from the previous procedure classification systems. ICD-10-PCS attempts to address the challenges of earlier versions by constructing a system that is complete, expandable, and multiaxial. Recommendations from the Committee on Vital and Health Statistics as well as clinicians, researchers, and other interested organizations were integrated into the new system.

The system is complete in that a unique code is available for each substantially different procedure. This is reflected in the number of codes in the systems; the ICD-9-CM procedure codes numbered approximately 4,000, whereas the ICD-10-PCS system contains more than 78,000 codes.

ICD-10-PCS is expandable, with a 7-character structure that allows for easy updates. For example, if a new approach is used for surgery in a given body system, that value can be added to the system within the current structure. The ICD-10-PCS system is updated annually, with new codes effective on October 1st of a given year to coincide with the fiscal year of the US government. For example, the fiscal year 2019 ICD-10-PCS and ICD-10-CM codes were effective on October 1, 2018. New code proposals are introduced at the ICD-10 Coordination and Maintenance Committee (C&M), held twice a year in Baltimore, Maryland. The Committee proceedings are also broadcast and recorded. According to CMS, "C&M is a federal interdepartmental committee comprised of representatives from the CMS and the Centers for Disease Control and Prevention's (CDC) National Center for Health Statistics (NCHS)" (CMS 2016a). Although no final decisions are made at the meeting, the committee is responsible for considering "coding changes, developing errata, addenda, and other modifications. Requests for coding changes are submitted to the committee for discussion at either the Spring or Fall C&M meeting" (CMS 2016a).

Another feature of the system is that it is multiaxial. Each of the seven characters is independent and retains its meaning throughout the range of codes whenever possible. For example, in most sections the 3rd character is the root operation, or objective, of the procedure. In some sections, the term changes to root type, as in the Imaging section, but this character still reflects the purpose of the service.

The ICD-10-PCS system attempts to be as specific as possible, with only limited references to "not elsewhere classified" or "NEC." Diagnostic information is not included in the ICD-10-PCS code. Instead of listing descriptions such as "cleft lip repair," the code identifies the specific procedure performed, including the site and approach. Eponyms, or procedures named after persons, are not included in ICD-10-PCS. Rather than listing eponyms such as the Whipple procedure, the individual procedure objectives are coded.

Although the terminology in the ICD-10-PCS system is standardized and there are explicit definitions for terms used in the classification, it is not necessary that the provider document the exact terms as they appear in ICD-10-PCS. It is the coding professional's responsibility to read and analyze the documentation and translate this into the appropriate ICD-10-PCS definition. We will revisit the importance of this translation later in this chapter and in chapter 2 of this text.

Accessing the Code Set

The ICD-10-PCS developers designed the code set to be used as an interactive online system, which is in the public domain and downloadable from the CMS website (CMS 2019). The system includes the ICD-10-PCS Tables, Index, and other resources. Although the online CMS file can be used for code building, a code book may also be used as desired.

We will examine both methods of using the code set, with an emphasis on using the online CMS file, as this is the technique that the system was designed to use. To begin this process, we will take a thorough look at the ICD-10-PCS code format and structure.

Coding Tip

The ICD-10-PCS system is published by CMS and is in the public domain. The entire system is available for download online.

Code Format and Structure

An ICD-10-PCS code always consists of seven characters. Each character has a designated meaning, called a value, represented by a letter or number. Note that the letters O and I are not used in ICD-10-PCS codes to eliminate confusion with the numbers 0 and 1. The remaining 24 letters and the 10 numerals from 0 to 9 provide a maximum of 34 values available for any given character.

All codes must be seven characters in length; a character cannot be left blank. If a value does not exist for a given character, the Z is used as the value such as No Device or No Qualifier. There are no decimal points or other punctuation marks in the codes.

Coding Tip

The letters O and I are not used in the ICD-10-PCS system to eliminate confusion with the numbers 0 and 1. Therefore the 0 in any code should be pronounced "zero" rather than "O."

The seven characters of the ICD-10-PCS code are listed in figure 1.1. Note that the first character indicates the section for that particular code. In this chapter, we will describe the seven characters of the ICD-10-PCS system for the Medical and Surgical section. The meaning of the seven characters is the same throughout the Medical and Surgical section; however, some of the descriptions of the characters differ slightly in other sections of the system. For example, in the Medical and Surgical section, the 6th character is the value for any applicable device placed during the procedure. However, in the Administrative section, the 6th character designates the substance. In the Measurement and Monitoring section, the 6th character is used to indicate the function or device instead of device. The meanings of each character in sections other than Medical and Surgical will be described in detail in the chapters devoted to these sections of ICD-10-PCS; chapters 20 through 25.

Figure 1.1. Components of an ICD-10-PCS code in the Medical and Surgical section

1	2	3	4	5	6	7
Section	Body System	Root Operation	Body Part	Approach	Device	Qualifier

Character 1: Section

The 1st character in the ICD-10-PCS code always represents the section. This character indicates the general type of procedure performed. There are 17 sections in ICD-10-PCS, and the largest is the first one, the Medical and Surgical section. The majority of the codes in the ICD-10-PCS system come from this section, and the codes begin with the character 0.

The next nine sections are considered Medical and Surgical-related, in that they represent procedures performed in conjunction with the Medical and Surgical services. Included here is the Obstetrics section for procedures performed on the products of conception. Coding from this section will be covered in detail in chapter 20 of this text. The other eight Medical and Surgical-related sections are for Placement, Administration, Measurement and Monitoring, Extracorporeal or Systemic Assistance and Performance, Extracorporeal or Systemic Therapies, Osteopathic, Other Procedures, and Chiropractic. These sections will be described in chapters 21 through 23.

There are six sections for Ancillary procedures: Imaging, Nuclear Medicine, Radiation Therapy, Physical Rehabilitation and Diagnostic Audiology, Mental Health, and Substance Abuse. The last section is New Technology. These sections will be described in detail in chapters 24 and 25.

As noted, Medical and Surgical section codes begin with the character 0, with Medical and Surgical-related sections beginning with other numerals. For example, obstetrics codes begin with 1 and placement codes begin with 2. The ancillary sections have alphabetic first characters, beginning with B (for Imaging) and ending with X (for New Technology). A complete list of the sections and their values is found in table 1.1.

Table 1.1. Sections of ICD-10-PCS

Value	Section
0	Medical and Surgical
1	Obstetrics
2	Placement
3	Administration
4	Measurement and Monitoring
5	Extracorporeal or Systemic Assistance and Performance
6	Extracorporeal or Systemic Therapies
7	Osteopathic
8	Other Procedures

(Continued)

Table 1.1. Sections of ICD-10-PCS (continued)

Value	Section
9	Chiropractic
B	Imaging
C	Nuclear Medicine
D	Radiation Therapy
F	Physical Rehabilitation and Diagnostic Audiology
G	Mental Health
H	Substance Abuse Treatment
X	New Technology

Coding Tip

To demonstrate the structure and format of the Medical and Surgical section, refer to the online CMS file or an ICD-10-PCS code book and scan through the code tables in the Medical and Surgical section, starting with the first code table, 001. Note that the code tables have a predictable order: first by the section value 0, then by the body system values beginning with 0 for Central Nervous System and Cranial Nerves and ending with Y for Anatomical Regions, Lower Extremities, followed by the root operations in each body system. The numbers 0–9 appear first, followed by alphabetical characters.

Character 2: Body System

The 2nd character represents the body system, the general anatomical region, or the physiological system involved in the procedure.

There are 31 body systems in the Medical and Surgical section, and they are listed in table 1.2. Some larger body systems are broken into subsystems in the Medical and Surgical section of ICD-10-PCS. For example, the circulatory system has separate body system values for the heart and great vessels, upper arteries, lower arteries, upper veins, and lower veins. The musculoskeletal system is divided into the body systems muscles, tendons, bursae and ligaments, head and facial bones, upper bones, lower bones, upper joints, and lower joints. This allows for increased specificity in the codes. A thorough discussion of each of the body systems, including an anatomy and medical terminology review, will be covered in chapters 7 through 19 of this text.

Table 1.2. Body systems in the Medical and Surgical section

Value	Body System
0	Central Nervous System and Cranial Nerves
1	Peripheral Nervous System
2	Heart and Great Vessels
3	Upper Arteries
4	Lower Arteries
5	Upper Veins
6	Lower Veins
7	Lymphatic and Hemic Systems
8	Eye
9	Ear, Nose and Sinus
B	Respiratory System

(Continued)

Table 1.2.	Body systems in the Medical and Surgical section (continued)
Value	**Body System**
C	Mouth and Throat
D	Gastrointestinal System
F	Hepatobiliary and Pancreas
G	Endocrine
H	Skin and Breast
J	Subcutaneous Tissue and Fascia
K	Muscles
L	Tendons
M	Bursae and Ligaments
N	Head and Facial Bones
P	Upper Bones
Q	Lower Bones
R	Upper Joints
S	Lower Joints
T	Urinary System
U	Female Reproductive System
V	Male Reproductive System
W	Anatomical Regions, General
X	Anatomical Regions, Upper Extremities
Y	Anatomical Regions, Lower Extremities

Character 3: Root Operation

The 3rd character in the Medical and Surgical section ICD-10-PCS code is the root operation. This value describes the objective of the procedure. Analyzing documentation to determine the objective of the procedure is perhaps one of the most important and challenging aspects of learning to use ICD-10-PCS codes. For instance, if the objective is to take out a portion of a body part without replacement, then Excision is the applicable root operation. If the objective is to widen a vessel, then the applicable root operation is Dilation. Thorough review of the medical record documentation is required to determine the objective. Specific guidelines for many root operations have been developed and will be covered in detail in chapter 2 and other applicable chapters of this text.

Understanding these root operations and their definitions is key to the successful use of ICD-10-PCS. There are 31 root operations in the Medical and Surgical section. Other sections include some of these root operations also but may also have root operations specific to that section. For example, the Obstetrics section has a root operation for Delivery, which is not found in the Medical and Surgical section. See table 1.3 for a complete alphabetical list and definitions of the 31 root operations in the Medical and Surgical section. Note that not all 31 root operations are used in each of the body systems. For example, Bypass is a root operation in the central nervous system and cranial nerves body system, but is not found in the peripheral nervous body system.

These root operations are organized into nine groups based on common attributes that describe the intent of the procedure. Understanding these nine groups can be helpful in determining the root operation and familiarizing the coding professional with the definitions. For example, Group 1 includes root operations that have an objective of taking out either part or all of a body part without replacement. This includes Excision, Resection, Detachment, Destruction, and Extraction. Group 7 contains the two root operations that represent the objective

Table 1.3.   Root operations in the Medical and Surgical section

Alteration	Modifying the anatomical structure of a body part without affecting the function of the body part
Bypass	Altering the route of passage of the contents of a tubular body part
Change	Taking out or off a device from a body part and putting back an identical or similar device in or on the same body part without cutting or puncturing the skin or a mucous membrane
Control	Stopping, or attempting to stop, postprocedural or other acute bleeding
Creation	Putting in or on biological or synthetic material to form a new body part that to the extent possible replicates the anatomic structure or function of an absent body part
Destruction	Eradicating all or a portion of a body part by the use of energy, force, or a destructive agent
Detachment	Cutting off all or a portion of an extremity
Dilation	Expanding an orifice or the lumen of a tubular body part
Division	Cutting into a body part, without draining fluids and/or gases from the body part, in order to separate or transect a body part
Drainage	Taking or letting out fluids and/or gases from a body part
Excision	Cutting out or off, without replacement, a portion of a body part
Extirpation	Taking or cutting out solid matter from a body part
Extraction	Pulling or stripping out or off all or a portion of a body part by the use of force
Fragmentation	Breaking solid matter in a body part into pieces
Fusion	Joining together portions of an articular body part rendering the articular body part immobile
Insertion	Putting in a nonbiological device that monitors, assists, performs, or prevents a physiological function but does not physically take the place of a body part
Inspection	Visually and/or manually exploring a body part
Map	Locating the route of passage of electrical impulses and/or locating functional areas in a body part
Occlusion	Completely closing an orifice or the lumen of a tubular body part
Reattachment	Putting back in or on all or a portion of a separated body part to its normal location or other suitable location
Release	Freeing a body part from an abnormal physical constraint by cutting or by use of force
Removal	Taking out or off a device from a body part
Repair	Restoring, to the extent possible, a body part to its normal anatomical structure and function
Replacement	Putting in or on biological or synthetic material that physically takes the place of all or a portion of a body part
Reposition	Moving to its normal location or other suitable location all or a portion of a body part
Resection	Cutting out or off, without replacement, all of a body part
Restriction	Partially closing an orifice or the lumen of a tubular body part
Revision	Correcting, to the extent possible, a portion of a malfunctioning device or the position of a displaced device
Supplement	Putting in or on a biological or synthetic material that physically reinforces and/or augments the function of a portion of a body part
Transfer	Moving, without taking out, all or a portion of a body part to another location to take over the function of all or a portion of a body part
Transplantation	Putting in or on all or a portion of a living body part taken from another individual or animal to physically take the place and/or function of all or a portion of a similar body part

of examination only: Inspection and Mapping. Group 6 includes six root operations that always involve a device: Insertion, Removal, Revision, Change, Replacement, and Supplement.

It is helpful to review the root operations within the groups to learn them more thoroughly in smaller and more related sets. The nine groups of root operations and definitions are presented in tables 1.4 through 1.12. Each of the groups and individual root operations will be discussed in detail in chapters 3 through 6 in this text.

Table 1.4.	Group 1–Root operations that take out some or all of a body part
Excision	Cutting out or off, without replacement, a portion of a body part
Resection	Cutting out or off, without replacement, all of a body part
Detachment	Cutting off all or part of the upper or lower extremities
Destruction	Physical eradication of all or a portion of a body part by the direct use of energy, force, or a destructive agent
Extraction	Pulling or stripping out or off all or a portion of a body part by the use of force

Table 1.5.	Group 2–Root operations that take out solids/fluids/gases from a body part
Drainage	Taking or letting out fluids and/or gases from a body part
Extirpation	Taking or cutting out solid matter from a body part
Fragmentation	Breaking solid matter in a body part into pieces

Table 1.6.	Group 3–Root operations involving cutting or separation only
Division	Cutting into a body part, without draining fluids and/or gases from the body part, in order to separate or transect a body part
Release	Freeing a body part from an abnormal physical constraint by cutting or by use of force

Table 1.7.	Group 4–Root operations that put in/put back or move some/all of a body part
Transplantation	Putting in or on all or a portion of a living body part taken from another individual or animal to physically take the place and/or function of all or a portion of a similar body part
Reattachment	Putting back in or on all or a portion of a separated body part to its normal location or other suitable location
Transfer	Moving, without taking out, all or a portion of a body part to another location to take over the function of all or a portion of a body part
Reposition	Moving to its normal location or other suitable location all or a portion of a body part

Table 1.8.	Group 5–Root operations that alter the diameter/route of a tubular body part
Restriction	Partially closing an orifice or the lumen of a tubular body part
Occlusion	Completely closing an orifice or the lumen of a tubular body part
Dilation	Expanding an orifice or the lumen of a tubular body part
Bypass	Altering the route of passage of the contents of a tubular body part

Table 1.9.	Group 6–Root operations that always involve a device
Insertion	Putting in a nonbiological device that monitors, assists, performs, or prevents a physiological function but does not physically take the place of a body part
Removal	Taking out or off a device from a body part
Revision	Correcting, to the extent possible, a portion of a malfunctioning device or the position of a displaced device
Change	Taking out or off a device from a body part and putting back an identical or similar device in or on the same body part without cutting or puncturing the skin or a mucous membrane
Replacement	Putting in or on biological or synthetic material that physically takes the place of all or a portion of a body part
Supplement	Putting in or on a biological or synthetic material that physically reinforces and/or augments the function of a portion of a body part

Table 1.10.   Group 7–Root operations involving examination only

Inspection	Visually and/or manually exploring a body part
Map	Locating the route of passage of electrical impulses and/or locating functional areas in a body part

Table 1.11.   Group 8–Root operations that define other repairs

Control	Stopping, or attempting to stop, postprocedural or other acute bleeding
Repair	Restoring, to the extent possible, a body part to its normal anatomical structure and function

Table 1.12.   Group 9–Root operations that define other objectives

Fusion	Joining together portions of an articular body part rendering the articular body part immobile
Alteration	Modifying the anatomical structure of a body part without affecting the function of the body part
Creation	Putting in or on biological or synthetic material to form a new body part that to the extent possible replicates the anatomic structure or function of an absent body part

Character 4: Body Part

The 4th character of the ICD-10-PCS code is for the specific body part involved in the procedure. There are up to 34 values available for body parts within a given body system. The body part character is in context with the 2nd character for body system. For example, the liver is a body part in the hepatobiliary and pancreatic body system. The frontal bone is a body part in the head and facial bones body system. There are specific guidelines related to body parts that will be discussed in chapter 2.

Coding Tip

Characters 2 and 4 work together to define the body part. For example, value 0 represents a different body part when used in different body systems. To determine what value 0 represents in character 4, character 2 must be known:

Character 2	Character 4
F, Hepatobiliary System and Pancreas	0, Liver
N, Head and Facial Bones	0, Skull
U, Female Reproductive System	0, Ovary, Right

Also, because there are more than 34 body parts in some specific body systems, body part values may be grouped into more general areas, or the closest proximal branch of the body part that has a specific value in ICD-10-PCS. This particularly is the case with the nerves, vessels, and bones that number many more than the 34 available body part values. ICD-10-PCS includes a body part key, which contains entries that refer a common anatomical term to its corresponding ICD-10-PCS body part value.

For example, a specific body part for the piriformis muscle is not found in the code tables. Instead, the procedure would be classified based on the body part key. The entry for the piriformis muscle directs the coding professional to use the hip muscle on the appropriate side, right or left, for the body part. These entries have also been integrated into the Index and can be located in alphabetical order with a cross-reference to the appropriate value that should be used for that body part.

Character 5: Approach

The 5th character of the ICD-10-PCS code is for the approach. This is the method or technique used to reach the operative site. There are a total of seven different approaches, either through the skin or mucous membranes, via a natural or artificial orifice, or external.

Approaches through the skin or mucous membranes are:

- **Open**—Cutting through the skin or mucous membrane and any other body layers necessary to expose the site of the procedure. This may involve several layers, including the bone. For example, a craniotomy is an open approach through the bones of the skull to reach and expose the brain. Another example is a hysterectomy performed via an incision. The key to this approach is that the operative site must be exposed to the surgeon's eye. See figure 1.2 for an example of an open approach to a cholecystectomy.
- **Percutaneous**—Entry, by puncture or minor incision, of instrumentation through the skin or mucous membrane and any other body layers necessary to reach the site of the procedure. A needle biopsy of the liver is an example of the percutaneous approach. A minor cut or small incision may be necessary to accommodate the instrument, in this case the needle. In the percutaneous approach, the operative site is not directly visualized by the surgeon's eye, though imaging guidance may be used to reach the operative site. Figure 1.3 includes an example of a percutaneous approach using a needle.

Figure 1.2. Percutaneous Endoscopic versus Open approach

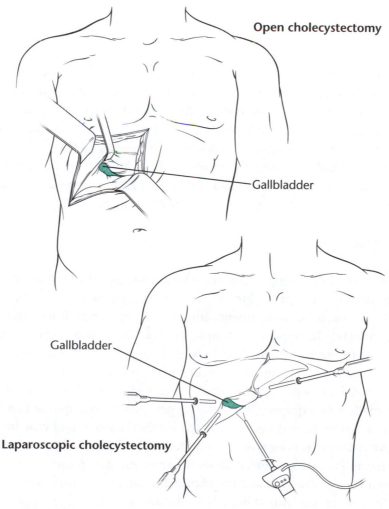

Open cholecystectomy

Gallbladder

Gallbladder

Laparoscopic cholecystectomy

© AHIMA 2019

Figure 1.3. Percutaneous approach

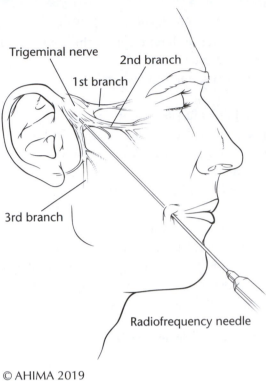

© AHIMA 2019

- **Percutaneous Endoscopic**—Entry, by puncture or minor incision, of instrumentation through the skin or mucous membrane and any other body layers necessary to reach and visualize the site of the procedure. An arthroscopic knee repair and a laparoscopic cholecystectomy are types of percutaneous endoscopic approaches. In this approach, the operative site is visualized via the instrumentation or scope. Figure 1.2 includes a contrast of a percutaneous endoscopic versus an open approach for a cholecystectomy. In the Open approach, the gallbladder is directly exposed and visible to the surgeon's eye. In the Percutaneous Endoscopic approach, small incisions are made in the abdomen and trocars are inserted to accommodate the lighted scope attached to a video camera that guides the surgeon to the operative site for the procedure.

Approaches through an orifice are:

- **Via Natural or Artificial Opening**—Entry of instrumentation through a natural or artificial external opening to reach the site of the procedure. Figure 1.4 exhibits the insertion of an endotracheal tube via the mouth. In this approach, the instruments enter via the opening without any visualization of the site.
- **Via Natural or Artificial Opening Endoscopic**—Entry of instrumentation through a natural or artificial external opening to reach and visualize the site of the procedure. An esophagogastroduodenoscopy with dilation of an esophageal stricture and a bronchoscope used for a bronchial procedure are examples of via Natural or Artificial Opening Endoscopic. For this approach, instruments are placed via the opening along with visualization equipment. Figure 1.5 presents an example of this approach, a cystoscopy. In this procedure, a lighted tube is inserted via the urethra to reach and visualize the bladder.
- **Via Natural or Artificial Opening with Percutaneous Endoscopic Assistance**—Entry of instrumentation through a natural or artificial external opening and entry, by puncture or minor incision, of instrumentation through the skin or mucous membrane and any other body layers necessary to aid in the performance of the procedure. This approach is only available in two body systems: the gastrointestinal system for the Excision and Resection root operations and the female reproductive system for Resection.

See figure 1.6 for an example of this approach in a laparoscopic-assisted vaginal hysterectomy. In this procedure, the laparoscope is used to dissect the uterus, fallopian tubes, and ovaries. These organs, along with the cervix, are removed via the natural opening of the vagina.

- **External** is the 7th approach and includes procedures performed directly on the skin or mucous membrane and procedures performed indirectly by the application of external force through the skin or mucous membrane. For example, a closed reduction of a fracture involves manipulating the broken bone without making an incision. Suture of a laceration of the skin of the forehead is performed on the outside of the body, which means an external approach is used. Also, procedures performed within an orifice or a structure that is visible without the aid of any instrumentation is coded to the External approach. Figure 1.7 illustrates this approach in removing the tonsils, which are directly visualized.

Selecting the approach, along with specific guidelines, will be covered in more detail in chapter 2.

Figure 1.4. Approach Via Natural or Artificial Opening

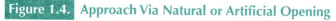
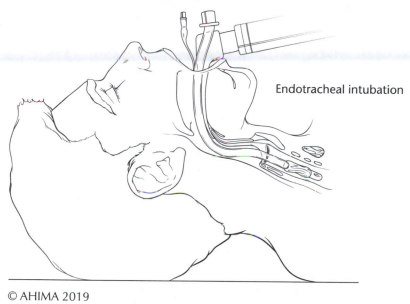

Endotracheal intubation

© AHIMA 2019

Figure 1.5. Approach Via Natural or Artificial Opening, Endoscopic

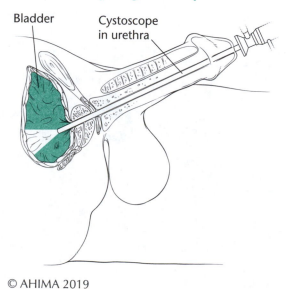

Bladder

Cystoscope in urethra

© AHIMA 2019

Figure 1.6.   Approach Via Natural or Artificial Opening with Percutaneous Endoscopic Assistance

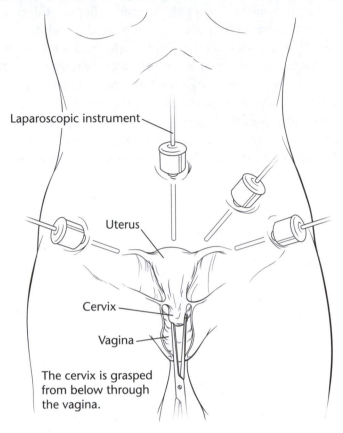

Laparoscopic instrument

Uterus

Cervix

Vagina

The cervix is grasped
from below through
the vagina.

© AHIMA 2019

Figure 1.7.   External approach for tonsillectomy

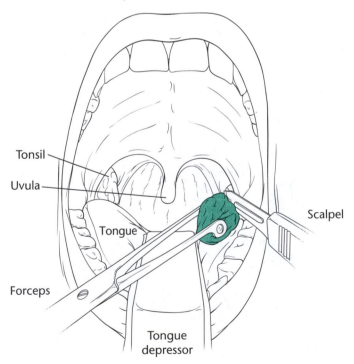

Tonsil

Uvula

Tongue

Forceps

Scalpel

Tongue
depressor

© AHIMA 2019

Character 6: Device

The 6th character in the ICD-10-PCS code is for the device, if applicable. Note that procedures not involving a device have the character Z listed for the value, No Device. Only devices that remain at the conclusion of the procedure are coded as devices. Devices that are used as part of the procedure but removed as the procedure concludes are not coded as devices because they do not remain in the body. For example, the balloon catheter used in an angioplasty procedure is not coded as a device because the catheter is removed when the angioplasty is accomplished. However, if a stent is placed in the vessel to maintain the dilation from the angioplasty, the stent is coded as a device.

The devices reflected in the 6th character may be the reason for a procedure, such as Insertion, in which the device is placed in the body as the objective of the procedure. They can also be previously placed devices that are now being taken out (in a Removal procedure, for example) or altered in some way (as in a Revision procedure). Devices can also be part of a procedure, such as an internal fixation device used in a fracture reduction, or Reposition procedure. However, incidental drains, sutures, or similar items are considered integral to the procedure and are not coded as devices.

Coding Tip

All seven of the characters must be assigned a value. If a device is not applicable for a given procedure, the character Z, No Device, is listed for the device character.

Devices can be classified into four basic groups:

- **Grafts and prostheses**—Biological or synthetic material that takes the place of all or a portion of a body part, for example, a joint prosthesis used in a hip replacement or a tissue substitute that is either autologous or nonautologous, such a skin graft.
- **Implants**—Therapeutic material that is not absorbed, eliminated, or incorporated into a body part. These therapeutic material implants can be removed. An example is a pin placed internally into a fracture site.
  - Another example of an implant is a pessary, a small device that is made of a synthetic substance such as plastic, rubber, or silicone. A therapeutic pessary may be used in a procedure to treat urinary incontinence or uterine prolapse by supporting the bladder, or uterus and vagina. A pessary device is displayed in figure 1.8.
  - A tissue expander is another type of implant. A silicone balloon expander is inserted under the skin or muscle, the balloon is slowly filled with salt water, and the skin is allowed to grow and stretch. This new tissue is then large enough to accept an implant or be used for reconstruction procedures from birth defects, injuries, or surgeries. Figure 1.9 is an illustration of a tissue expander used to prepare for a postmastectomy breast reconstruction.
- **Simple or mechanical appliances**—Biological or synthetic material that assists or prevents a physiological function. For example, see figure 1.10 for a tracheostomy device.
  - Another example of an appliance is an external fixation device. See figure 1.11 for an example of an external fixation device used to treat a tibial fracture.
  - Extraluminal and intraluminal devices, as well as endobronchial valves, are additional examples of appliances that assist in a physiological function. Figure 1.12 depicts a vascular clamp device, an example of an extraluminal, or outside the vessel, device. An intraluminal device is placed within the vessel. Figure 1.13 shows an example of a graft that is inserted within the abdominal aorta.
  - An endobronchial valve is a device that is implanted in the pulmonary system to help a lung compartment to empty itself of air. An example of an endobronchial valve is shown in figure 1.14.

Figure 1.8.   Pessary device

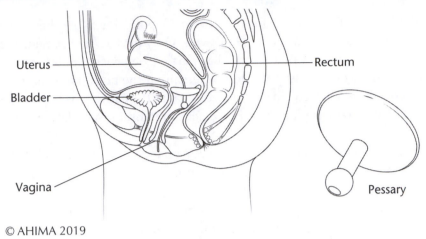

© AHIMA 2019

Figure 1.9.   Tissue expander

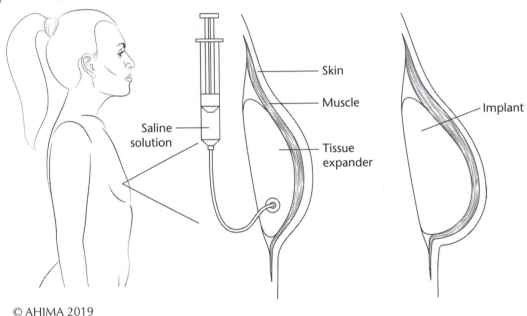

© AHIMA 2019

A tunneled vascular access device (VAD) is another example of an appliance that assists a physiological function. This type of tunneled VAD allows frequent access to a patient's veins without the necessity of a needle stick. Figure 1.15 includes an example of a tunneled VAD.

A device can also serve to prevent a function. For example, an intrauterine device (IUD) prevents pregnancy. See figure 1.16 for an example of an IUD.

- **Electronic appliances**—Assist, take the place of, monitor, or prevent a physiological function. For example, a cochlear implant is an electronic device that provides a sense of sound. See figure 1.17 for an example of a cochlear implant. Another example is a neurostimulator implanted to stimulate the brain in neurological diseases. Figure 1.18 shows an example of a neurostimulator.

To be classified as a device, the material or appliance should be central to the procedural objective and located at the procedure site without an intention of changing the location of the device. Tissue taken from the patient is classified as autologous tissue substitute. In order to be considered an autologous device,

Figure 1.10. Tracheostomy airway device

Tracheostomy
tube in place

Tube for
inflating cuff

© AHIMA 2019

Figure 1.11. External fixation device

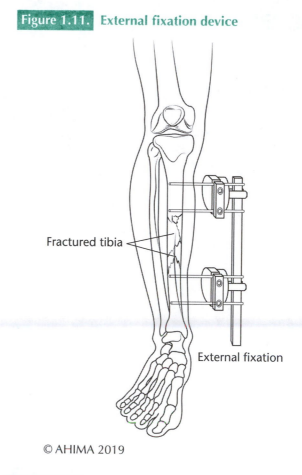

Fractured tibia

External fixation

© AHIMA 2019

Figure 1.12. Extraluminal device

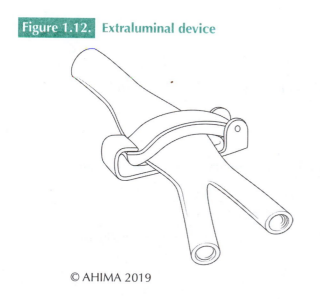

© AHIMA 2019

Figure 1.13. Intraluminal device

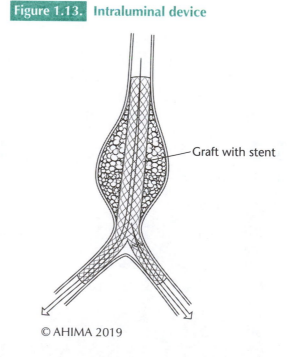

Graft with stent

© AHIMA 2019

the tissue must be completely separated from the patient. For example, a free skin graft is classified as an autologous tissue substitute as it is harvested from a site in the patient's body to be used in a Replacement procedure. A saphenous vein harvested for use in a Bypass procedure is classified as autologous venous tissue. A device should also be capable of being removed. For example, a neurostimulator generator and

Figure 1.14. Endobronchial valve

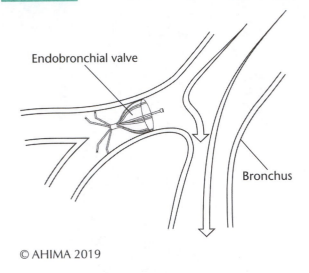

© AHIMA 2019

Figure 1.15. Tunneled vascular access device

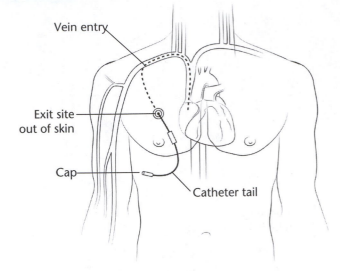

© AHIMA 2019

Figure 1.16. Contraceptive device

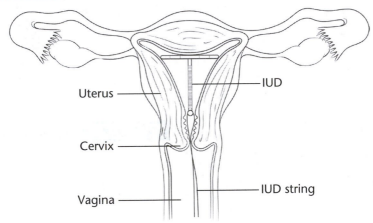

© AHIMA 2019

Figure 1.17. Cochlear implant hearing device

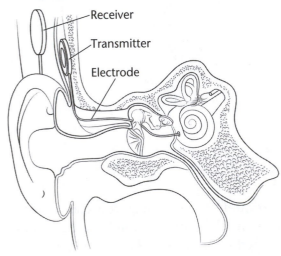

© AHIMA 2019

Figure 1.18. Neurostimulator generator and lead

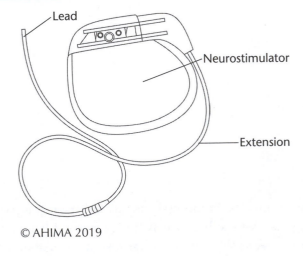

© AHIMA 2019

lead, pictured in figure 1.18, can be removed at a later time, as needed. Devices are distinct from substances and equipment. Substances that are liquid or blood components are different than devices in that they are intended to be absorbed or dispersed within the body without a fixed position. Once absorbed or dispersed, a substance cannot be removed. Equipment is machinery or other aids that reside primarily outside the body and is temporary, only used for the duration of the procedure. Table 1.13 highlights the differences between devices, substances, and equipment.

Table 1.13. Device, substance, and equipment

Item	Procedural Objective	Location	Removability	Example
Device	Material or appliance central to accomplishing a procedure	At the site of procedure, not intended to change location	In most cases capable of being removed from procedure site	Neurostimulator lead insertion
Substance	Liquid or blood components central to accomplishing a procedure	No fixed position, intended to be dispersed or absorbed	Not removable once dispersed or absorbed	Antibiotic injection
Equipment	Machinery or other aid to perform a procedure	Resides primarily outside the body	Temporary, used for duration of procedure only	Mechanical ventilation

Character 7: Qualifier

The 7th character in the ICD-10-PCS code is for the Qualifier. This character provides additional information about a specific attribute of the code. For example, the qualifier X in procedures coded with the root operation Excision, Extraction, or Drainage indicates a diagnostic procedure or a biopsy. There are specific qualifiers to indicate whether there was an anterior or posterior approach as well as an anterior or posterior column involved in a Fusion procedure performed on a vertebral joint. In joint replacement procedures, the qualifier can identify whether cement was used. There are two qualifiers available in select code tables of the Medical and Surgical section that relate to devices: Temporary (J) and Intraoperative (G). These qualifiers indicate devices that are used during the procedure or for a short time during the inpatient stay. The majority of the codes do not have a qualifier indicated. For that reason, many of the codes in the Medical and Surgical section end in the character Z, No Qualifier.

Coding Tip

All seven of the characters must be assigned a value. If a Qualifier is not applicable for a given procedure, the character Z, No Qualifier is listed for the qualifier character.

Code Building Process

Now that we have discussed the seven characters, ICD-10-PCS code building can begin. Code building is based on the first three characters of the code, which identify the code table. Getting to the correct code table is key to the process. This can be accomplished by using either the online CMS file or an ICD-10-PCS code book. Coding software, such as an encoder, can also be used, but one must first have a thorough understanding of the ICD-10-PCS system. A description of both the use of the CMS file and the code book method follows.

The first step in the coding process is to review the medical record documentation to establish the objective of the procedure, which will determine the root operation. This review involves analyzing the operative report and other portions of the medical record. Thorough knowledge of the root operation groups and definitions of the root operations will assist with this process. Also, make note of the specific body system and body part that is the focus of the procedure as well as the approach used to reach the operative site and any devices that are left after the procedure is completed.

CMS File Method

As discussed, the entire ICD-10-PCS system is produced by CMS and can be located and downloaded from the CMS website (see CMS 2019 in the reference list at the end of this book). On the CMS website, first download the ZIP file titled 2019 ICD-10-PCS Code Tables and Index (see figure 1.19). Within that file, open the PDF file called "pcs_2019" (see figure 1.20). This file is the 2019 Tables and Index File. The front page of the file is illustrated in figure 1.21. This file is interactive and serves as a tool for building ICD-10-PCS codes.

Continue with the CMS file method for coding a procedure in the Medical and Surgical section, by clicking the ICD-10-PCS Tables link. (All blue highlighted text in the file is a hyperlink.) A page with a list of the 17 sections of ICD-10-PCS is displayed as shown in figure 1.22. Note that the Medical and Surgical section is listed first, and other sections of ICD-10-PCS can be reached from this section table of content page as well, such as Obstetrics (1) or Imaging (B).

Figure 1.19. Code tables and index file location on CMS 2019 ICD-10-PCS web page

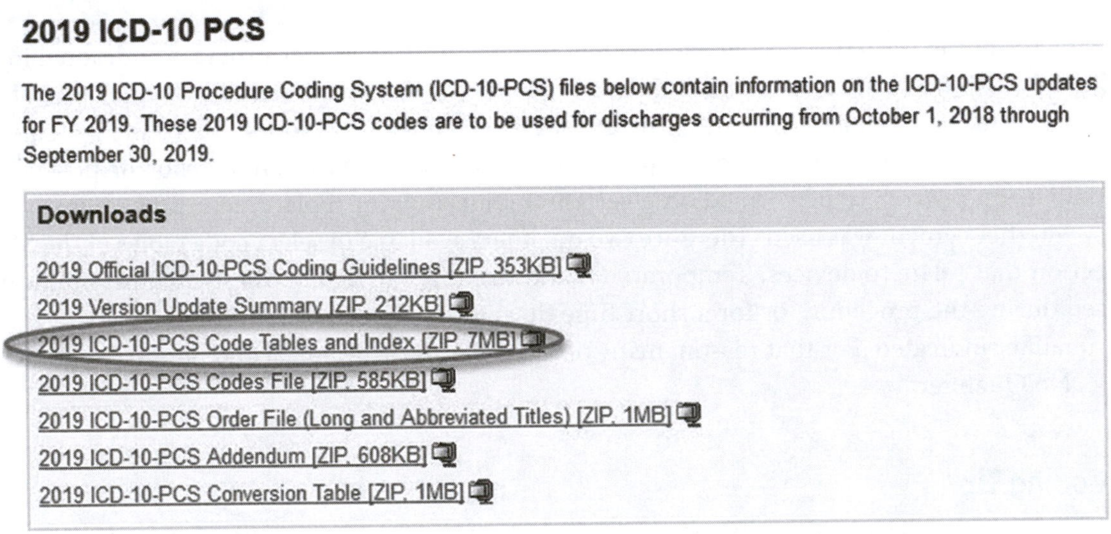

2019 ICD-10 PCS

The 2019 ICD-10 Procedure Coding System (ICD-10-PCS) files below contain information on the ICD-10-PCS updates for FY 2019. These 2019 ICD-10-PCS codes are to be used for discharges occurring from October 1, 2018 through September 30, 2019.

Downloads

2019 Official ICD-10-PCS Coding Guidelines [ZIP, 353KB]

2019 Version Update Summary [ZIP, 212KB]

2019 ICD-10-PCS Code Tables and Index [ZIP, 7MB]

2019 ICD-10-PCS Codes File [ZIP, 585KB]

2019 ICD-10-PCS Order File (Long and Abbreviated Titles) [ZIP, 1MB]

2019 ICD-10-PCS Addendum [ZIP, 608KB]

2019 ICD-10-PCS Conversion Table [ZIP, 1MB]

Source: CMS 2019

Figure 1.20. 2019 ICD-10-PCS code file location within ZIP file

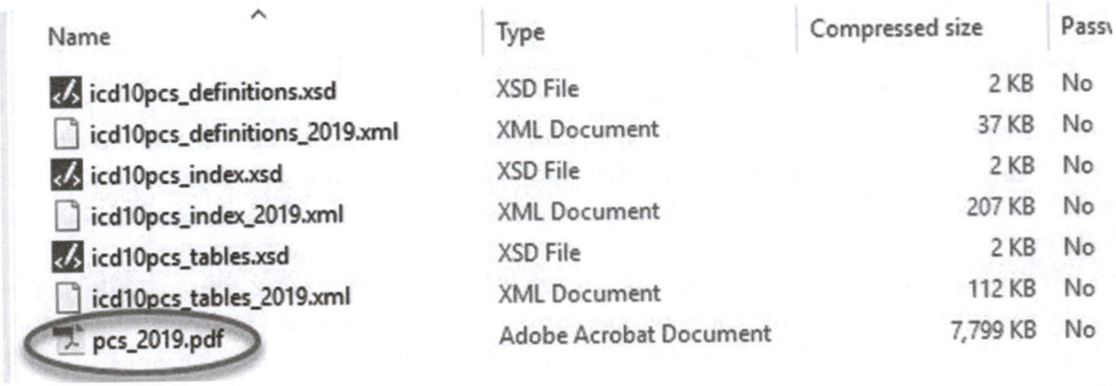

Name	Type	Compressed size	Passv
icd10pcs_definitions.xsd	XSD File	2 KB	No
icd10pcs_definitions_2019.xml	XML Document	37 KB	No
icd10pcs_index.xsd	XSD File	2 KB	No
icd10pcs_index_2019.xml	XML Document	207 KB	No
icd10pcs_tables.xsd	XSD File	2 KB	No
icd10pcs_tables_2019.xml	XML Document	112 KB	No
pcs_2019.pdf	Adobe Acrobat Document	7,799 KB	No

Source: CMS 2019

Figure 1.21.   2019 ICD-10-PCS Tables and Index front page

ICD-10 Procedure Coding System
(ICD-10-PCS)
2019 Tables and Index

Introduction

The **ICD-10-PCS Tables** contains all valid codes in table format. The tables are arranged in alphanumeric order, and organized into separate tables according to the first three characters of the seven-character code.

The **ICD-10-PCS Index** contains entries based on the terms (known as values) used in the ICD-10-PCS Tables, as well as entries based on common procedure terms. Index entries either link directly to a PCS table or refer the user to another index entry.

The **ICD-10-PCS Definitions** contain the official definitions of ICD-10-PCS values in characters 3 through 7 of the seven-character code, and may also provide additional explanation or examples. The definitions are arranged in section order, and designate the section and the character within the section being defined.

The ICD-10-PCS **Body Part Key** contains entries that refer a common anatomical term to its corresponding ICD-10-PCS body part value(s).

The ICD-10-PCS **Device Key** contains entries that refer a common device term or manufacturer's device name to its corresponding ICD-10-PCS device value.

The ICD-10-PCS **Substance Key** contains entries that refer a common substance name or manufacturer's substance name to its corresponding ICD-10-PCS substance value.

The ICD-10-PCS **Device Aggregation Table** contains entries that correlate a specific ICD-10-PCS device value with a general device value to be used in tables containing only general device values.

Source: CMS 2019

Continue by selecting the Medical and Surgical section from this list to get to the second character of the code, body system. Figure 1.23 shows the list of body systems that are included in the Medical and Surgical section.

To get to the code tables, click the applicable body system to display all of the available root operations for that body system. For example, figure 1.24 includes the entries for the Hepatobiliary and Pancreas body system. Code tables are available by clicking on the applicable root operation, as in Resection shown in table 1.14. Note that the coding professional can return to the section table of contents and the front page by progressively selecting Back to Top in the upper right-hand corner of the page.

For example, to construct a code for an open cholecystectomy, removing all of the gallbladder, one must determine the section and body system to get to the correct place in the ICD-10-PCS system. This is a Medical and Surgical procedure, so that section is selected from the front page (see figure 1.22). The gallbladder

Figure 1.22.   Section table of contents page

Return to Introduction

Tables

The ICD-10-PCS section values are listed below. Click on a section to access its list of body systems

0   Medical and Surgical
1   Obstetrics
2   Placement
3   Administration
4   Measurement and Monitoring
5   Extracorporeal or Systemic Assistance and Performance
6   Extracorporeal or Systemic Therapies
7   Osteopathic
8   Other Procedures
9   Chiropractic
B   Imaging
C   Nuclear Medicine
D   Radiation Therapy
F   Physical Rehabilitation and Diagnostic Audiology
G   Mental Health
H   Substance Abuse Treatment
X   New Technology

Source: CMS 2019

is part of the Hepatobiliary System and Pancreas body system in ICD-10-PCS. The classification for the gallbladder can be verified by using the Find feature from the Tables page. Once can access this feature by simultaneously pressing the Control and F keys on the keyboard (on most computers) or by selecting the Edit menu at the top of the PDF and then selecting Find within that menu. In the Find search box, enter the term "gallbladder" and click on next. Note that a code table from the Hepatobiliary System and Pancreas body system appears with the gallbladder as one of the body parts; this verifies that the gallbladder is coded to this body system. Close the Find box and click the Back to Top link in the upper right-hand corner to return to the section table of contents. Select Medical and Surgical and select the Hepatobiliary System and Pancreas 0F, from the body systems list. Note that the list of all root operations applicable to this body system is located on the page. These are all of the available code tables in the Hepatobiliary System and Pancreas body system (see figure 1.24). To continue coding the open cholecystectomy, which is removal of all of the gallbladder, the root operation Resection is selected, as the definition of Resection is cutting out or off, without replacement, all of a body part. The 0FT table is selected (see table 1.14) and used to build the code. Values for characters 4 through 7 are selected from the same row. Using the first row of the 0FT code table, character 4 is selected for the gallbladder body part, 0 for the Open approach, Z for No Device, and Z for No Qualifier for a complete code 0FT40ZZ.

Note that when using tables in the CMS file, it is important to scroll to the end of the table to be sure that the entire table is referenced on a given page. Refer to code table 0DW by selecting Gastrointestinal System from the list of body systems (figure 1.23) and select the 0DW table for Revision. Scroll through this table and note that this code table continues to a second page.

We have noted that all of the pages have a Back to Top option. When clicked, this will bring the coder back to the section table of contents, and the process can be repeated. For example, if the next procedure to be coded was an excision of a cervical lymph node, the coder would select Back to Top, then Medical and Surgical section, 07 for Lymphatic and Hemic system, and then 07B for Excision. The 07B table is then displayed and the complete code can be built. Note that the section table of contents page in figure 1.22 has a Return to Introduction

Figure 1.23. Medical and Surgical Section

Back to top

Medical and Surgical

Medical and Surgical body system values are listed below. Click on a body system to access its list of operations.

00	Central Nervous System and Cranial Nerves
01	Peripheral Nervous System
02	Heart and Great Vessels
03	Upper Arteries
04	Lower Arteries
05	Upper Veins
06	Lower Veins
07	Lymphatic and Hemic Systems
08	Eye
09	Ear, Nose, Sinus
0B	Respiratory System
0C	Mouth and Throat
0D	Gastrointestinal System
0F	Hepatobiliary System and Pancreas
0G	Endocrine System
0H	Skin and Breast
0J	Subcutaneous Tissue and Fascia
0K	Muscles
0L	Tendons
0M	Bursae and Ligaments
0N	Head and Facial Bones
0P	Upper Bones
0Q	Lower Bones
0R	Upper Joints
0S	Lower Joints
0T	Urinary System
0U	Female Reproductive System
0V	Male Reproductive System
0W	Anatomical Regions, General
0X	Anatomical Regions, Upper Extremities
0Y	Anatomical Regions, Lower Extremities

Source: CMS 2019

link at the top of the page. This brings the coder back to the front page shown in figure 1.21, which includes the ICD-10-PCS code table link and links to other resources including the ICD-10-PCS Index.

The Official Coding Guidelines, discussed in chapter 2 of this text, include a guideline that states that it is not necessary to consult the Index, though the code tables must always be referenced to build the code. Use of the Index is an optional, though slower method of getting to the correct code table. The online CMS Index file can be referenced as in a book-based index. From the front page, select the Index. Then, reference the first letter of the procedure to be coded. For example, to code a procedure involving the resection of bladder, the Index could be referenced under the letter R to get the page where the letter begins. To navigate through the Index, the search function can also be used. For example, once under the R entry in the Index, Resection can be entered in the find box. After three clicks of the Next in the find box the beginning of the Resection entries is located. From here, scroll down to find the bladder entry, 0TTC. The 0TT table is viewed for building the code.

Also, note that the front page (see figure 1.21) has several links, including a link to the body part key. This key can be referenced to determine the correct body part to be used when coding a procedure. See table 1.15

Figure 1.24. The Hepatobiliary and Pancreas Body System

Back to top

Medical and Surgical, Hepatobiliary System and Pancreas

ICD-10-PCS operation values in the Hepatobiliary System and Pancreas of the Medical and Surgical section are listed below. Click on an operation to access the corresponding ICD-10-PCS table.

0F1	Bypass
0F2	Change
0F5	Destruction
0F7	Dilation
0F8	Division
0F9	Drainage
0FB	Excision
0FC	Extirpation
0FF	Fragmentation
0FH	Insertion
0FJ	Inspection
0FL	Occlusion
0FM	Reattachment
0FN	Release
0FP	Removal
0FQ	Repair
0FR	Replacement
0FS	Reposition
0FT	Resection
0FU	Supplement
0FV	Restriction
0FW	Revision
0FY	Transplantation

Source: CMS 2019

Table 1.14. 0FT table

Section	0	Medical and Surgical
Body System	F	Hepatobiliary System and Pancreas
Operation	T	Resection: Cutting out or off, without replacement, all of a body part

Body Part	Approach	Device	Qualifier
0 Liver 1 Liver, Right Lobe 2 Liver, Left Lobe 4 Gallbladder G Pancreas	0 Open 4 Percutaneous Endoscopic	Z No Device	Z No Qualifier
5 Hepatic Duct, Right 6 Hepatic Duct, Left 7 Hepatic Duct, Common 8 Cystic Duct 9 Common Bile Duct C Ampulla of Vater D Pancreatic Duct F Pancreatic Duct, Accessory	0 Open 4 Percutaneous Endoscopic 7 Via Natural or Artificial Opening 8 Via Natural or Artificial Opening Endoscopic	Z No Device	Z No Qualifier

Source: CMS 2019

Table 1.15. Body Part key

Body Part Key

Return to Introduction

Term	ICD-10-PCS Value
Abdominal aortic plexus	Use: Abdominal Sympathetic Nerve
Abdominal esophagus	Use: Esophagus, Lower
Abductor hallucis muscle	Use: Foot Muscle, Right Foot Muscle, Left

Source: CMS 2019

for the first three entries. For example, a procedure performed on the abductor hallucis muscle would be coded to the foot muscle, on the right or left side as applicable, because there is not a specific body part assigned to this muscle. The coder can search the body part key alphabetically or use the search function to locate the ICD-10-PCS value for a given term. The entries from the body part key can also be located in the Index. Search the Index under the term abductor hallucis muscle and the same cross-reference is found; *Use* Foot Muscle, Right and *Use* Foot Muscle, Left. Select Back to Top and Return to Introduction to get back to the front page.

The front page includes a link to the Device Key that shows both brand and generic names, where available, for selected devices and the PCS description for the device. Although not comprehensive, the device key can assist in determining the use for devices in procedures. See table 1.16 for an excerpt from the device key. For example, the entry for "acellular hydrated dermis" notes to "*Use* nonautologous tissue substitute." In coding a procedure that used acellular hydrated dermis as a device, the value for nonautologous tissue substitute would be used. The device key is also integrated into the Index, with cross-reference to the type of device to be used.

Table 1.16. Device key

Term	ICD-10-PCS Value
3f (Aortic) Bioprosthesis valve	Use: Zooplastic Tissue in Heart and Great Vessels
AbioCor(R) Total Replacement Heart	Use: Synthetic Substitute
Absolute Pro Vascular (OTW) Self- Expanding Stent System	Use: Intraluminal Device
Acculink (RX) Carotid Stent System	Use: Intraluminal Device
Acellular Hydrated Dermis	Use: Nonautologous Tissue Substitute
Acetabular cup	Use: Liner in Lower Joints
Activa PC neurostimulator	Use: Stimulator Generator, Multiple Array for Insertion in Subcutaneous Tissue and Fascia
Activa AC neurostimulator	Use: Stimulator Generator, Multiple Array Rechargeable for Insertion in Subcutaneous Tissue and Fascia

Source: CMS 2019

Another tool available in the front page is the device aggregation table. This table contains information to correlate a specific device, listed in the first column, used in the root operation and body system, shown in the second and third columns, to the general device term and value, listed in the last column. See table 1.17 for an excerpt from this table. For example, cardiac resynchronization defibrillator pulse generator used in the Insertion root operation in the subcutaneous tissue and fascia body system is coded to value P for cardiac rhythm–related device in the Removal root operation in this body system.

Table 1.17. Device aggregation table

Specific Device	for Operation	in Body System	General Device
Autologous Arterial Tissue	All applicable	Heart and Great Vessels Lower Arteries Upper Arteries Lower Veins Upper Veins	Autologous Tissue Substitute
Autologous Venous Tissue	All applicable	Heart and Great Vessels Lower Arteries Upper Arteries Lower Veins Upper Veins	Autologous Tissue Substitute
Cardiac Lead, Defibrillator	Insertion	Heart and Great Vessels	Cardiac Lead
Cardiac Lead, Pacemaker	Insertion	Heart and Great Vessels	Cardiac Lead
Cardiac Resynchronization Defibrillator Pulse Generator	Insertion	Subcutaneous Tissue and Fascia	Cardiac Rhythm Related Device
Cardiac Resynchronization Pacemaker Pulse Generator	Insertion	Subcutaneous Tissue and Fascia	Cardiac Rhythm Related Device
Contractility Modulation Device	Insertion	Subcutaneous Tissue and Fascia	Cardiac Rhythm Related Device
Defibrillator Generator	Insertion	Subcutaneous Tissue and Fascia	Cardiac Rhythm Related Device
Epiretinal Visual Prosthesis	All applicable	Eye	Synthetic Substitute
External Fixation Device, Hybrid	Insertion	Lower Bones Upper Bones	External Fixation Device

Source: CMS 2019

Also included is a substance key. Like the device key, this is not an all-inclusive list and it has additions and changes with each new version of the system. The substance key lists the substance and how the substance should be classified in ICD-10-PCS. For example, Seprafilm would be classified as an adhesion barrier substance. The substances are also located in the index as cross-references for the type of substance used. See table 1.18 for the complete substance key.

Another valuable resource located on the front page is the link to the definitions, where the official definitions of ICD-10-PCS values in characters 3 through 7 are organized by section order. The definitions contain both the body part and device key in reverse. For example, table 1.15 is an excerpt from the body part key and references the foot muscle for the abductor hallucis muscle. In the definitions for the Medical and Surgical section body parts, a comprehensive list of all body parts assigned to the foot muscle is found, as shown in figure 1.25.

Table 1.18. Substance key

Term	ICD-10-PCS Value
AIGISRx Antibacterial Envelope Antimicrobial envelope	Use: Anti-Infective Envelope
Bone morphogenetic protein 2 (BMP 2)	Use: Recombinant Bone Morphogenetic Protein
Clolar	Use: Clofarabine
Kcentra	Use: 4-Factor Prothrombin Complex Concentrate
Nesiritide	Use: Human B-type Natriuretic Peptide
rhBMP-2	Use: Recombinant Bone Morphogenetic Protein
Seprafilm	Use: Adhesion Barrier
Tissue Plasminogen Activator (tPA)(r-tPA)	Use: Other Thrombolytic
Voraxaze	Use: Glucarpidase
Zyvox	Use: Oxazolidinones

Source: CMS 2019

Figure 1.25. Definitions for Medical and Surgical Body Part—Foot Muscle

Foot Muscle, Left Foot Muscle, Right	Includes: Abductor hallucis muscle Adductor hallucis muscle Extensor digitorum brevis muscle Extensor hallucis brevis muscle Flexor digitorium brevis muscle Flexor hallucis brevis muscle Quadratus plantae muscle

Source: CMS 2019

Code Book Method

The other method for code building is with the use of a code book. Many publishers have taken the online CMS system and formatted the code tables and other resources into a printed book version. If the code book is used, the code tables can be directly referenced as described in the CMS file method without consulting the Index. However, some coders prefer to use the Index to locate the code table needed to build the ICD-10-PCS code and this process is described here.

As in the online CMS file, the index is organized by main terms that appear in boldface type with subterms that follow the main terms in alphabetical order. The Index may be searched under the term for the root operation, with subterms for the anatomical site or body system involved in the surgery. Common procedure names, such as cholecystectomy or colonoscopy, are also included.

Note that all Index entries for common procedure names should be considered only as guidance on possible coding options. These entries should not be followed without first analyzing the documentation to determine the intent of the procedure and translating this intent into the official root operation names. For example, in coding an osteotomy, or an incision into the bone, the Index directs the coder to see Division and Drainage in the head and facial bones and upper and lower bones with the applicable code tables listed. However, if the documentation indicates that the bone was cut in order to change the placement of the bone (for example, to correct a valgus deformity of the femur), this documentation leads to the intent of the root operation Reposition rather than Division or Drainage and the appropriate Reposition code table is consulted to build the code.

The terminology used by the surgeon is interpreted based on the ICD-10-PCS definitions. For example, if an operative report describes an open excision of the entire right kidney, the criteria for the root operation Resection are met because this procedure involves taking out the entire kidney without replacement. The main term Resection is located in the Alphabetic Index, and the subterms Kidney, Right are referenced. Note that only a portion of the code is listed in the Index, 0TT0. The Index entry may list more than three characters, but the first three characters are the key to getting to the code table used to build the code.

Locating the Tables

To locate the tables in an ICD-10-PCS code book, reference the pages that begin immediately after the Index. The tables are arranged in a manner that assists with finding the correct one. For example, within the Medical and Surgical section, the tables are arranged by body system and begin first with the numbers: 001 is the first table, representing the central nervous system and cranial nerves for Bypass procedures. Other tables in the Central Nervous System and Cranial Nerves follow this format. For example, 002 for Change in the central nervous system and cranial nerves, and 005 for Destruction. The last of the Central Nervous System and Cranial Nerves code tables is 00X for the Transfer root operation.

Next come the code tables for the Peripheral Nervous System, which all begin with 01. The first table in this body system is 012 for Change in the peripheral nervous system. This arrangement continues sequentially, ending with the 09 grouping of tables for ear, nose, and sinus. The alphabetic characters follow, starting with the 0B1 for Bypass of the Respiratory System.

Note that not every root operation can be found in every body system because not all root operations can be performed on every body system. For example, the Bypass root operation is not found in the Peripheral Nervous System, while it is found in the Central Nervous System and Cranial Nerves, 001.

Using the example of the open resection of the right kidney, after referencing the Index, the 0TT table (shown in table 1.19) is located by referencing the 0T grouping in the tables for the urinary system and finding the table to represent third character T for the root operation Resection. The table is then used to select the values for the 4th, 5th, 6th, and 7th characters.

Building the Complete Code

Continuing with the example of the Resection of the right kidney, note that the body part character for the right kidney, 0, was listed in the Index. This body part is located in the first row of the code table in the column for body part, character 4. Moving across to the column for approach, the 0 is selected for the approach as the procedure was completed using an open approach. Note that there are only two available approach options for the kidney body part, Open and Percutaneous Endoscopic. There are no device or qualifier values available or appropriate, so the Z value is selected in the columns for device and qualifier, and the complete code is 0TT00ZZ.

Table 1.19.   0TT table

Section	0	Medical and Surgical		
Body System	T	Urinary System		
Operation	T	Resection: Cutting out or off, without replacement, all of a body part		
Body Part	*Approach*		*Device*	*Qualifier*
0 Kidney, Right 1 Kidney, Left 2 Kidneys, Bilateral	0 Open 4 Percutaneous Endoscopic		Z No Device	Z No Qualifier
3 Kidney Pelvis, Right 4 Kidney Pelvis, Left 6 Ureter, Right 7 Ureter, Left B Bladder C Bladder Neck D Urethra	0 Open 4 Percutaneous Endoscopic 7 Via Natural or Artificial Opening 8 Via Natural or Artificial Opening Endoscopic		Z No Device	Z No Qualifier

Source: CMS 2019

Section	Body System	Root Operation	Body Part	Approach	Device	Qualifier
Medical and Surgical	Urinary System	Resection	Kidney, Right	Open	No Device	No Qualifier
0	T	T	0	0	Z	Z

For example, in the 0TT table, the approach value 7 for Via Natural or Artificial Opening or 8 for Via Natural or Artificial Opening Endoscopic found in the column for approach cannot be selected for the body parts right, left, or bilateral kidneys as they are not in the same row as these body parts listed in the body part column.

Coding Tip

When building an ICD-10-PCS code, the same row must be referenced in the columns for the 4th, 5th, 6th, and 7th character selection. It is not permissible to change rows when building the code.

Other Index References

There are cross-references in the Index that may serve as a guide to direct the coder from a composite term, which includes an operation and a site, to a root operation and a body system.

For example, if the clinical documentation shows that the procedure performed was an angiorrhaphy of the left subclavian artery by incision, the main term angiorrhaphy is referenced in the Index. There are three cross-references listed as subterms:

See Repair, Heart and Great Vessels, 02Q
See Repair, Upper Arteries, 03Q
See Repair, Lower Arteries, 04Q

This translates the term "angiorrhaphy" to the root operation Repair and references the three body systems that are applicable to this type of repair procedure. If the coder is unsure of the location of the subclavian artery, the code tables can be referenced to find the body part. Note that the subclavian artery is one of the upper arteries and is found in the 03Q table. This code table, as seen in table 1.20, is used to build the remainder of the code.

There is only one row in the 03Q code table, and the value of 3 for the right subclavian artery is selected from the column for the 4th character body part. The 5th character for approach is open as it was by incision and the 0 value is selected. The Z value is selected for both the 6th character for device and the 7th character for qualifier; no device and no qualifier.

Table 1.20. 03Q table

Section	0	Medical and Surgical
Body System	3	Upper Arteries
Operation	Q	Repair: Restoring, to the extent possible, a body part to its normal anatomic structure and function

Body Part	Approach	Device	Qualifier
0 Internal Mammary Artery, Right **1** Internal Mammary Artery, Left **2** Innominate Artery **3** Subclavian Artery, Right **4** Subclavian Artery, Left **5** Axillary Artery, Right **6** Axillary Artery, Left **7** Brachial Artery, Right **8** Brachial Artery, Left **9** Ulnar Artery, Right **A** Ulnar Artery, Left **B** Radial Artery, Right **C** Radial Artery, Left **D** Hand Artery, Right **F** Hand Artery, Left **G** Intracranial Artery **H** Common Carotid Artery, Right **J** Common Carotid Artery, Left **K** Internal Carotid Artery, Right **L** Internal Carotid Artery, Left **M** External Carotid Artery, Right **N** External Carotid Artery, Left **P** Vertebral Artery, Right **Q** Vertebral Artery, Left **R** Face Artery **S** Temporal Artery, Right **T** Temporal Artery, Left **U** Thyroid Artery, Right **V** Thyroid Artery, Left **Y** Upper Artery	**0** Open **3** Percutaneous **4** Percutaneous Endoscopic	**Z** No Device	**Z** No Qualifier

Source: CMS 2019

The complete code is 03Q30ZZ.

Section	Body System	Root Operation	Body Part	Approach	Device	Qualifier
Medical and Surgical	Upper Arteries	Repair	Subclavian Artery, Right	Open	No Device	No Qualifier
0	3	Q	3	0	Z	Z

Directly Referencing the Code Tables

As the coder becomes more familiar with the ICD-10-PCS system, it may be possible to build codes by going directly to the code tables in the code book without first consulting the Index. As in the CMS file method, this is due to the predictable organization of the system and the code tables by section, body system, and root operation. For example, if the coder knows this is a heart transplant procedure, the 02Y table could be directly consulted. This would assume that the coder knows that this procedure would be found in the Medical and Surgical section, that the 2 value for the body system character includes the heart and great vessels and the Y value is used for Transplantation root operations.

Whether using the CMS file or the code book, it is necessary to have a good understanding of the body systems, body parts, and the root operations groupings and definitions to be proficient in building

ICD-10-PCS codes. Once the coder is more familiar with the coding process, the CMS file method may prove to be the most efficient.

The basic steps to code building in ICD-10-PCS are listed in figure 1.26.

Figure 1.26. Steps in code building in ICD-10-PCS

1. Thoroughly review the medical record documentation, including the operative report and other clinical information.

2. Determine the objective of the procedure based on the documentation review.

3. Review the root operations within their nine groups to help determine the objective of the procedure. Review the specific definitions within the groups to determine the root operation.

4. Consult the code table, either by direct reference in the CMS file or code book or via the Index.

5. Select the appropriate value for the body part, approach, device, and qualifier from the same row in the code table.

6. Continue coding until all aspects of a given operation have been coded.

Clinical Documentation and Terminology in ICD-10-PCS

ICD-10-PCS includes standardized terminology, such as the 31 root operations in the Medical and Surgical section, all of which have very specific definitions. For example, the root operation Resection is defined as cutting out or off, without replacement, all of a body part. All portions of this definition must be applicable to the given operation in order for this root operation to be selected. Therefore, if the body part is removed but is also replaced, then the root operation is not Resection but rather Replacement. If only part of the body part is removed, then the root operation is not Resection but rather Excision.

The Official Guidelines for ICD-10-PCS state that the provider does not have to document the exact terms as they appear in the definitions. Instead, it is the coding professional's responsibility to read and interpret the documentation to determine the objective of the procedure. Based on this analysis, the root operation can be established.

For example, the provider documents the term "removal" of a kidney. There is a Removal root operation, but this refers to taking out or off a device from a body part. Since the kidney is a body part that is taken out, root operations in Group 1 (Excision, Resection, Detachment, Destruction, Extraction) are referenced. (See table 1.4.) After review of the documentation, it is noted that the entire kidney is removed, which translates to the root operation Resection, or cutting out or off, without replacement, all of a body part.

However, in this same scenario, if the kidney is removed as part of a kidney transplant operation the removal of the kidney has a different objective. See Group 4 for root operations that put in/put back or move some or all of a body part (Transplantation, Reattachment, Transfer, and Reposition). (See table 1.7.) In this case, the objective of the procedure meets the definition of the root operation Transplantation: putting in or on all of a living body part taken from another individual to physically take the place and/or function of all or a portion of a body part. In the root operation Transplantation, the removal of the native kidney is considered integral to the procedure.

Using the medical record documentation to determine the correct definitions in code building will also be discussed in detail in chapter 2 of this text, which concentrates on the ICD-10-PCS Coding Guidelines.

Check Your Understanding

1. What does the 1st character of the ICD-10-PCS code indicate?
   a. Body System
   b. Root Operation
   c. Section
   d. Approach

2. What value is used if there is a character that does not apply to a given code?
   a. X
   b. Z
   c. 0
   d. –

3. What does the 5th character of the ICD-10-PCS code indicate?
   a. Body Part
   b. Root Operation
   c. Device
   d. Approach

4. Which of the following was not one of the objectives of the new ICD-10-PCS system?
   a. Multiaxial
   b. Diagnosis-based
   c. Expandable
   d. Complete

5. Which letters are not used in ICD-10-PCS?
   a. I and O
   b. E and T
   c. S and X
   d. O and S

6. Consult the 02W code table. Which of these is an incorrect ICD-10-PCS code?
   a. 02W50JZ
   b. 02WF37Z
   c. 02WY02Z
   d. 02WFX7Z

 Code Building

Use either the CMS files or a code book to complete these exercises.

1. The patient has a partial laparoscopic gastrectomy. Answer the following questions about this procedure:

   1.1. What group of root operations should be referenced to reflect the objective of the procedure?

   _____

   1.2. Reviewing the entries in this group, which root operation is selected?

   _____

   1.3. What code table is referenced?

   _____

1.4. What body part value is selected?

1.5. What approach value is selected?

1.6. What values are assigned for the device and qualifier?

1.7. What is the correct ICD-10-PCS code for this procedure?

2. The patient has an open reduction of a dislocation of the temporomandibular joint on the left side. Answer the following questions about this procedure:

2.1. Referring to either the CMS file or code book index, what is the cross-reference for reduction of a dislocation?

2.2. What body system is the left temporomandibular joint located in?

2.3. What code table is referenced?

2.4. What body part value is selected?

2.5. What approach value is selected?

2.6. What values are assigned for the device and qualifier?

2.7. What is the correct ICD-10-PCS code for this procedure?

2.8. Review of the clinical documentation finds that an internal fixation device was used for this procedure. What is the correct code?

3. The pediatric patient has an open orchiopexy for undescended testicles. Answer the following questions about this procedure:

3.1. Referring to either the CMS file or code book index, what are the cross-references for orchiopexy?

3.2. After review of the definitions for these references, what root operation represents the objective of this orchiopexy?

3.3. What code table is referenced?

3.4. What body part value is selected?

3.5. What approach value is selected?

_____

3.6. What values are assigned for the device and qualifier?

_____

3.7. What is the correct ICD-10-PCS code for this procedure?

_____

4.   The patient has a percutaneous thoracentesis of the pleural cavity on the right side with placement of a drainage tube. Answer the following questions about this procedure:

4.1. Referring to either the CMS file or code book index, what is the cross-reference for thoracentesis?

_____

4.2. What root operation does this procedure represent?

_____

4.3. What code table is referenced?

_____

4.4. What body part value is selected?

_____

4.5. What approach value is selected?

_____

4.6. What values are assigned for the device and qualifier?

_____

4.7. What is the correct ICD-10-PCS code for this procedure?

_____

Chapter 2

ICD-10-PCS Coding Guidelines

The ICD-10-PCS system includes specific guidelines for the procedure system. These guidelines provide instruction on how to use the system and the codes themselves. The applicable guidelines will be discussed in the appropriate part of the text in coming chapters. However, this chapter includes a comprehensive review of the guidelines to assist in the process of learning to use ICD-10-PCS. Much like the "rules of the road," these guidelines provide important information that is necessary when building codes, applying definitions, and interpreting documentation.

Coding Guidelines

As with all official coding guidelines, the ICD-10-PCS guidelines are subject to the unanimous approval of the Cooperating Parties: the American Hospital Association (AHA), American Health Information Management Association (AHIMA), Centers for Medicare and Medicaid Services (CMS), and National Center for Health Statistics (NCHS). The guidelines are an official part of the ICD-10-PCS code set and are updated as needed. The information in this text is based on the guidelines released along with the 2019 version of ICD-10-PCS. The 2019 guidelines can be found online (see CMS 2019 in the reference list at the end of this book). The introduction to the guidelines emphasizes that they complement any instructions found in the classification, and that those rules take precedence over the guidelines. The Health Insurance Portability and Accountability Act (HIPAA) requires adherence to these guidelines for hospital inpatient healthcare settings. The introduction also emphasizes the importance of complete and accurate documentation for accurate coding.

The guidelines are organized into five sections: Conventions, Medical and Surgical Section, Obstetrics Section, New Technology Section, and Selection of the Principal Procedure.

Conventions

There are 11 general guidelines in the Conventions section that provide information on how a code is built in the ICD-10-PCS system. The first four guidelines concern the seven characters of the ICD-10-PCS code and emphasize that the character meaning stays the same in a given group of codes.

A1. ICD-10-PCS codes are composed of seven characters. Each character is an axis of classification that specifies information about the procedure performed. Within a defined code range, a character specifies the same type of information in that axis of classification.

Example: The 5th axis of classification specifies the approach in sections 0 through 4 and 7 through 9 of the system.

This guideline specifies that all ICD-10-PCS codes contain seven characters, each with a different definition. As discussed in chapter 1 of this text, the seven characters for a code from the Medical and Surgical section are as shown in figure 2.1. The information relayed in a given character can change in a given section

Figure 2.1.   Components of an ICD-10-PCS code in the Medical and Surgical section

1	2	3	4	5	6	7
Section	Body System	Root Operation	Body Part	Approach	Device	Qualifier

of ICD-10-PCS. For example, in section 6, Extracorporeal or Systemic Therapies, the 5th character denotes the duration of the procedure.

This organization of the ICD-10-PCS system allows for predictability in translating the codes. For example, in most sections of ICD-10-PCS the 3rd character specifies the root operation or root type: the objective of the procedure.

The next guideline specifies the number of values possible for a given character.

A2. One of 34 possible values can be assigned to each axis of classification in the seven-character code: they are the numbers 0 through 9 and the letters of the alphabet (except I and O because they are easily confused with the numbers 1 and 0). The number of unique values used in an axis of classification differs as needed.

Example: Where the 5th axis of classification specifies the approach, seven different approach values are currently used to specify the approach.

While there are only seven approach values, in other characters many more values are used. For example, in the body part value for the lower veins, there are 24 possible body part values for the root operation Release.

One of the characteristics of the ICD-10-PCS system is that it can be easily expanded. This is noted in guideline A3.

A3. The valid values for an axis of classification can be added to as needed.

Example: If a significantly distinct type of device is used in a new procedure, a new device value can be added to the system.

This guideline was followed in the 2018 release of the system. Device value 6 Synthetic Substitute, Oxidized Zirconium on Polyethylene was added to the 0SR table for replacement of knee and hip procedures to represent this specific type of ceramic bearing surface.

The next two guidelines emphasize that the codes must be translated in context and that this becomes more prevalent as the system expands. The value of one character is dependent on the other characters that make up the code.

A4. As with words in their context, the meaning of any single value is a combination of its axis of classification and any preceding values on which it may be dependent.

Example: The meaning of a body part value in the Medical and Surgical section is always dependent on the body system value. The body part value 0 in the Central Nervous body system specifies Brain, and the body part value 0 in the Peripheral Nervous body system specifies Cervical Plexus.

A5. As the system is expanded to become increasingly detailed, over time more values will depend on preceding values for their meaning.

Example: In the Lower Joints body system, the device value 3 in the root operation Insertion specifies Infusion Device and the device value 3 in the root operation Replacement specifies Ceramic Synthetic Substitute.

These two guidelines mean that the code is built with the consideration of how each character is dependent on each of the other character values. Alternative meanings for character values are found within the device character for different body systems. For example, the value of 4 is used as the device character for a single Drug-Eluting Intraluminal Device for Dilation in the Heart and Great Vessels body system. However, the value 4 is used for Internal Fixation Device in the Head and Facial Bones body system.

The next two guidelines, A6 and A7, emphasize the use of the Index and the code tables in building the ICD-10-PCS code. While in many cases the Index is referenced to begin the coding process, use of the Index is optional. As the coding professional becomes more familiar with the system, it may be possible to go directly to the applicable code table in the code book or the CMS file to build the code. However, the applicable code table must be consulted in every case to select the appropriate values and build the complete code, even if all seven characters are given in the Index entry.

A6. The purpose of the alphabetic index is to locate the appropriate table that contains all information necessary to construct a procedure code. The PCS Tables should always be consulted to find the most appropriate valid code.

A7. It is not required to consult the index first before proceeding to the tables to complete the code. A valid code may be chosen directly from the tables.

The next guideline reinforces the fact that all ICD-10-PCS codes must have seven characters. Blank values are not an option.

A8. All seven characters must contain valid values to be a valid procedure code. If the documentation is incomplete for coding purposes, the physician should be queried for the necessary information.

A thorough review of all documentation is necessary to get to the most accurate ICD-10-PCS code. However, if the review of the documentation does not include enough information to build the complete code, it may be necessary to ask the provider for the appropriate information.

For example, if the procedure to be coded is a revision of a bone growth stimulator of the facial bone, the main term Bone Growth Stimulator is referenced in the Index, followed by the subterms Revision of device from Bone, Facial. The code table referenced would be 0NW (table 2.1). The W can be selected for the 4th character for body part value and the M for the 6th character for device, Bone Growth Stimulator, and Z for the 7th character to indicate No Qualifier. Note, however, that there are four possibilities for the approach character: Open, Percutaneous, Percutaneous Endoscopic, or External. This information should be available by a review of documentation such as in reading the operative report for the procedure. If, after reviewing all available documentation, the approach used to complete this revision is still not clear, the provider should be queried to determine the correct approach.

The next guideline, A9, emphasizes that the code building process has to take place by selecting values from a given row. It is not permissible to pick values for a given character in one row and then select a value from a different row for the next character.

A9. Within a PCS table, valid codes include all combinations of choices in characters 4 through 7 contained in the same row of the table.

For an illustration of this, see table 2.2, the 08W table. If this table were being used to build a code for a revision of a device in the left or right lens, the only two approaches that would be applicable would be 3 for Percutaneous and X for External. These body parts are found only in the third and fourth rows of the table. It would not be possible to use the 0 for Open because this approach is located in the first row for either the left or right eye or the last row for extraocular muscle, right or left.

Table 2.1. 0NW table

Section	0	Medical and Surgical
Body System	N	Head and Facial Bones
Operation	W	Revision: Correcting, to the extent possible, a portion of a malfunctioning device or the position of a displaced device

Body Part	Approach	Device	Qualifier
0 Skull	0 Open	0 Drainage Device 4 Internal Fixation Device 5 External Fixation Device 7 Autologous Tissue Substitute J Synthetic Substitute K Nonautologous Tissue Substitute M Bone Growth Stimulator N Neurostimulator Generator S Hearing Device	Z No Qualifier
0 Skull	3 Percutaneous 4 Percutaneous Endoscopic X External	0 Drainage Device 4 Internal Fixation Device 5 External Fixation Device 7 Autologous Tissue Substitute J Synthetic Substitute K Nonautologous Tissue Substitute M Bone Growth Stimulator S Hearing Device	Z No Qualifier
B Nasal Bone W Facial Bone	0 Open 3 Percutaneous 4 Percutaneous Endoscopic X External	0 Drainage Device 4 Internal Fixation Device 7 Autologous Tissue Substitute J Synthetic Substitute K Nonautologous Tissue Substitute M Bone Growth Stimulator	Z No Qualifier

Source: CMS 2019

Guideline A10 clarifies that the word "and" can be interpreted as "and/or" in the description of codes, with certain exceptions.

A10. "And," when used in a code description, means "and/or," except when used to describe a combination of multiple body parts for which separate values exist for each body part (e.g., Skin and Subcutaneous Tissue used as a qualifier, where there are separate body part values for "Skin" and "Subcutaneous Tissue").

Example: Lower Arm and Wrist Muscle means lower arm and/or wrist muscle.

The final guideline in the Conventions section reinforces the roles of the provider and the coding professional in building an ICD-10-PCS code. It is not necessary for the physician to document the exact terms used in ICD-10-PCS in order for a given value to be selected. Instead, the coding professional thoroughly reviews the documentation and applies the definitions of the ICD-10-PCS character values.

A11. Many of the terms used to construct PCS codes are defined within the system. It is the coder's responsibility to determine what the documentation in the medical record equates to in the PCS definitions. The physician is not expected to use the terms used in PCS code descriptions, nor is the coder required to query the physician when the correlation between the documentation and the defined PCS terms is clear.

Example: When the physician documents "partial resection," the coder can independently correlate "partial resection" to the root operation Excision without querying the physician for clarification.

Table 2.2. 08W table

Section	0	Medical and Surgical
Body System	8	Eye
Operation	W	Revision: Correcting, to the extent possible, a portion of a malfunctioning device or the position of a displaced device

Body Part	Approach	Device	Qualifier
0 Eye, Right 1 Eye, Left	0 Open 3 Percutaneous 7 Via Natural or Artificial Opening 8 Via Natural or Artificial Opening Endoscopic	0 Drainage Device 3 Infusion Device 7 Autologous Tissue Substitute C Extraluminal Device D Intraluminal Device J Synthetic Substitute K Nonautologous Tissue Substitute Y Other Device	Z No Qualifier
0 Eye, Right 1 Eye, Left	X External	0 Drainage Device 3 Infusion Device 7 Autologous Tissue Substitute C Extraluminal Device D Intraluminal Device J Synthetic Substitute K Nonautologous Tissue Substitute	Z No Qualifier
J Lens, Right K Lens, Left	3 Percutaneous	J Synthetic Substitute Y Other Device	Z No Qualifier
J Lens, Right K Lens, Left	X External	J Synthetic Substitute	Z No Qualifier
L Extraocular Muscle, Right M Extraocular Muscle, Left	0 Open 3 Percutaneous	0 Drainage Device 7 Autologous Tissue Substitute J Synthetic Substitute K Nonautologous Tissue Substitute Y Other Device	Z No Qualifier

Source: CMS 2019

It is important that this final Conventions guideline be understood and applied. For example, it is not necessary for a physician to document the term "Extirpation" to describe a thrombectomy. Instead, the coding professional would use the definition of this root operation and the procedure performed to determine that a thrombectomy is a type of extirpation.

Guidelines for the Medical and Surgical Section

The Medical and Surgical section is by far the largest section in the ICD-10-PCS system. The majority of the guidelines refer to this section and its seven characters. Each of these guidelines will be reviewed.

Guidelines for Body System

There are two guidelines that refer to the 2nd character, Body System. The first one, B2.1a, refers to the general anatomical regions body system, 0W, may be applicable for procedures that are not confined to one body system. For example, an episiotomy is coded in the general anatomic regions as a division of the female perineum because more than one layer is separated in the procedure. More information on the anatomical regions is found in chapter 7. The general anatomical region can also be used if there is insufficient information to code more specifically. This should be an uncommon occurrence.

The second guideline, B2.1b, specifies that the diaphragm is the line of demarcation for the upper and lower body parts, when applicable.

B2.1a. The procedure codes in the general anatomical regions body systems can be used when the procedure is performed on an anatomical region rather than a specific body part (e.g., root operations Control and Detachment, Drainage of a body cavity) or on the rare occasion when no information is available to support assignment of a code to a specific body part.

Examples: Control of postoperative hemorrhage is coded to the root operation Control found in the general anatomical regions body systems.

Chest tube drainage of the pleural cavity is coded to the root operation Drainage found in the general anatomical regions body systems. Suture repair of the abdominal wall is coded to the root operation Repair in the general anatomical regions body system.

B2.1b. Where the general body part values "upper" and "lower" are provided as an option in the Upper Arteries, Lower Arteries, Upper Veins, Lower Veins, Muscles and Tendons body systems, "upper" or "lower" specifies body parts located above or below the diaphragm, respectively.

Example: Vein body parts above the diaphragm are found in the Upper Veins body system; vein body parts below the diaphragm are found in the Lower Veins body system.

Guidelines for Root Operation

There are 17 guidelines for the 3rd character, Root Operation, many of which contain more than one part. Some of these guidelines are general to all root operations while several are specific to a particular root operation. The guidelines that are more pertinent to specific root operations or body systems will be covered in more detail in the appropriate chapters in this text.

The first two guidelines are general, referring to the use of the full definition of the root operation and emphasizing that integral parts of a root operation are not coded separately.

B3.1a. In order to determine the appropriate root operation, the full definition of the root operation as contained in the PCS Tables must be applied.

B3.1b. Components of a procedure specified in the root operation definition and explanation are not coded separately. Procedural steps necessary to reach the operative site and close the operative site, including anastomosis of a tubular body part, are also not coded separately.

Examples: Resection of a joint as part of a joint replacement procedure is included in the root operation definition of Replacement and is not coded separately. Laparotomy performed to reach the site of an open liver biopsy is not coded separately. In a resection of sigmoid colon with anastomosis of descending colon to rectum, the anastomosis is not coded separately.

For example, in the operative report shown in figure 2.2, the cystoscope is the approach, or method, to get to the operative site and dilate the urethra. Therefore, a cystoscopy would not be coded separately.

The next guideline, B3.2, has four components and specifies when multiple procedures are coded.

B3.2. During the same operative episode, multiple procedures are coded if:

a. The same root operation is performed on different body parts as defined by distinct values of the body part character.

Examples: Diagnostic excision of liver and pancreas are coded separately. Excision of lesion in the ascending colon and excision of lesion in the transverse colon are coded separately.

b. The same root operation is repeated in multiple body parts, and those body parts are separate and distinct body parts classified to a single ICD-10-PCS body part value.

Examples: Excision of the sartorius muscle and excision of the gracilis muscle are both included in the upper leg muscle body part value, and multiple procedures are coded. Extraction of multiple toenails are coded separately.

c. Multiple root operations with distinct objectives are performed on the same body part.

Example: Destruction of sigmoid lesion and bypass of sigmoid colon are coded separately.

d. The intended root operation is attempted using one approach, but it is converted to a different approach.

Example: Laparoscopic cholecystectomy converted to an open cholecystectomy is coded as percutaneous endoscopic Inspection and open Resection.

Figure 2.2. Operative report

PREOPERATIVE DIAGNOSES:
1. Interstitial cystitis
2. Urethral stenosis

POSTOPERATIVE DIAGNOSES:
1. Interstitial cystitis
2. Urethral stenosis

OPERATIONS PERFORMED:
1. Cystoscopy
2. Urethral dilation and hydrodilation

SURGEON: John Doe, MD

OPERATIVE FINDINGS: Urethra was tight at 26-French and dilated with 32-French. Bladder neck is normal. Ureteral orifice is normal size, shape, and position, effluxing clear bilaterally. Bladder mucosa is normal. Bladder capacity is 700 mL under anesthesia. There is moderate glomerulation consistent with interstitial cystitis at the end of hydrodilation. Residual urine was 150 mL.

INDICATIONS: A patient with severe symptoms.

DESCRIPTION OF OPERATION: The patient was brought to the cystoscopy suite and placed on the table in lithotomy position. The patient was prepped and draped in the usual sterile fashion. A 21 Olympus cystoscope was inserted, and the bladder was viewed with 12- and 70-degree lenses. Bladder was filled by gravity to capacity, emptied, and again cystoscopy was performed with findings as above. Urethra was then calibrated with 32-French. The patient was taken to the recovery room in stable condition.

> The cystoscope is the method used to reach the operative site

In a situation where the procedure has to be stopped before completion, guideline B3.3 applies. Inspection is the root operation selected if another root operation is not performed before the procedure is canceled.

B3.3.   If the intended procedure is discontinued or otherwise not completed, code the procedure to the root operation performed. If a procedure is discontinued before any other root operation is performed, code the root operation Inspection of the body part or anatomical region inspected.

Example: A planned aortic valve replacement procedure is discontinued after the initial thoracotomy and before any incision is made in the heart muscle, when the patient becomes hemodynamically unstable. This procedure is coded as an open Inspection of the mediastinum.

The next guideline is for biopsy procedures. There are two parts to the guideline. The first, B3.4a, lists the three root operations that can be coded as biopsies: Excision, Extraction, and Drainage. Note that in order to be coded as a biopsy, the intent of the procedure must be to analyze the tissue, fluid, and gases that are excised, extracted, or drained. Noting that a sample was sent to Pathology does not constitute a biopsy, as almost all body parts and substances removed from a patient are sent to Pathology. To be considered a biopsy, the intent of the Excision, Extraction, or Drainage must be diagnostic. For these cases the qualifier, represented in the 7th character, is X for Diagnostic. More details on biopsy procedures will be covered in the areas of the text that discuss the Excision, Extraction, and Drainage root operations.

B3.4a. Biopsy procedures are coded using the root operations Excision, Extraction, or Drainage and the qualifier Diagnostic.

Examples: Fine needle aspiration biopsy of fluid in the lung is coded to the root operation Drainage with the qualifier Diagnostic. Biopsy of bone marrow is coded to the root operation Extraction with the qualifier Diagnostic. Lymph node sampling for biopsy is coded to the root operation Excision with the qualifier Diagnostic.

The second part of the guideline states that both a biopsy and a more definitive treatment are coded, as applicable, with an ICD-10-PCS code for each procedure.

B3.4b. If a diagnostic Excision, Extraction, or Drainage procedure (biopsy) is followed by a more definitive procedure, such as Destruction, Excision, or Resection at the same procedure site, both the biopsy and the more definitive treatment are coded.

Example: Biopsy of breast followed by partial mastectomy at the same procedure site, both the biopsy and the partial mastectomy procedure are coded.

The next guideline provides instructions on coding overlapping layers of the musculoskeletal system in a given procedure. Because different body part values are available for each layer, the value for the deepest layer is selected.

The remaining guidelines in the Root Operation section are specific to given root operations. These will be covered in more detail in the chapters of this text applicable to the root operations and body systems, but each of the guidelines will be reviewed in this chapter to assist in understanding how these particular root operations and definitions are applied.

The first guideline concerns the Bypass root operation and has three parts. First, the use of Bypass for non-coronary bypass procedures is discussed. In these procedures, the 4th character designates where the bypass originates, and the 7th character qualifier designates where the bypass terminates.

B3.6a. Bypass procedures are coded by identifying the body part bypassed "from" and the body part bypassed "to." The 4th character body part specifies the body part bypassed from, and the qualifier specifies the body part bypassed to.

Example: In a bypass from stomach to jejunum, the stomach is the body part and jejunum is the qualifier.

The next two guidelines are applicable to coronary artery bypass procedures. These procedures are handled differently from noncoronary bypass operations, with the number of coronary arteries bypassed to represented in the 4th character body part and the 7th character qualifier denoting where the bypass originated. Also, separate codes are assigned for procedures that either use a different device (for example, autologous venous tissue or autologous arterial tissue) or have different vessels bypassed from.

B3.6b. Coronary artery bypass procedures are coded differently than other bypass procedures as described in the previous guideline. Rather than identifying the body part bypassed from, the body part identifies the number of coronary arteries bypassed to, and the qualifier specifies the vessel bypassed from.

Example: Aortocoronary artery bypass of the left anterior descending coronary artery and the obtuse marginal coronary artery is classified in the body part axis of classification as two coronary arteries, and the qualifier specifies the aorta as the body part bypassed from.

B3.6c. If multiple coronary arteries are bypassed, a separate procedure is coded for each coronary artery that uses a different device and/or qualifier.

Example: Aortocoronary artery bypass and internal mammary coronary artery bypass are coded separately.

Table 2.3 summarizes the differences for body part and qualifier values in noncoronary and coronary bypass procedures. These Bypass guidelines will be more specifically covered in chapter 5 of this text as well as in several of the specific body system chapters. Coronary bypass procedures are covered in more detail in chapter 11.

Table 2.3. Bypass procedures

Type of Bypass	Body Part Value	Qualifier Value
Non-coronary	Site Bypassed from	Site Bypassed to
Coronary	Number of Arteries Bypassed to	Vessel Bypassed from

The root operation Control will be covered in more detail in chapter 6. This is a root operation describing the specific purpose of stopping postprocedural or other acute bleeding. The next guideline advises that if a more definitive root operation is performed, that root operation is coded rather than Control.

B3.7. The root operation Control is defined as, "Stopping, or attempting to stop, postprocedural or other acute bleeding." If an attempt to stop postprocedural or other acute bleeding is unsuccessful, and to stop the bleeding requires performing a more definitive root operation, such as Bypass, Detachment, Excision, Extraction, Reposition, Replacement, or Resection, then the more definitive root operation is coded instead of Control.

Example: Resection of spleen to stop bleeding is coded to Resection instead of Control.

Excision and Resection are two root operations that are closely related: Excision is the removal of a portion of a body part, and Resection is the removal of the entire body part. These two root operations will be explored in more detail in chapter 3 of the text. The next guideline goes into more detail as to how the body part values help to determine which root operation is selected.

B3.8. PCS contains specific body parts for anatomical subdivisions of a body part, such as lobes of the lungs or liver and regions of the intestine. Resection of the specific body part is coded whenever all of the body part is cut out or off, rather than coding Excision of a less specific body part.

Example: Left upper lung lobectomy is coded to Resection of Upper Lung Lobe, Left rather than Excision of Lung, Left.

The next guideline specifies that a separate procedure code is necessary for Excisions performed for the purpose of harvesting an autograft. Note that the autograft must be procured via a separate operative site in order to be coded separately.

B3.9. If an autograft is obtained from a different procedure site in order to complete the objective of the procedure, a separate procedure is coded.

Example: Coronary bypass with excision of saphenous vein graft, excision of saphenous vein is coded separately.

Guideline B3.10 provides specific information on fusion procedures of the spine. There are three parts to the guideline, and the first specifies how the body part value is determined for a fusion procedure, which can be either a single vertebral joint or multiple vertebral joints.

B3.10a. The body part coded for spinal vertebral joint(s) rendered immobile by a spinal fusion procedure is classified by the level of the spine (e.g., thoracic). There are distinct body part values for a single vertebral joint and for multiple vertebral joints at each spinal level.

Example: Body part values specify Lumbar Vertebral Joint; Lumbar Vertebral Joints, 2 or More; and Lumbosacral Vertebral Joint.

The next guideline instructs that separate codes are assigned if more than one device or qualifier is applicable. A fusion procedure that involves two vertebral joints, with one utilizing an internal fixation device and the other a synthetic substitute, would require two codes. This also applies for procedures on more than one joint that vary in the approach or column.

B3.10b. If multiple vertebral joints are fused, a separate procedure is coded for each vertebral joint that uses a different device and/or qualifier.

Example: Fusion of lumbar vertebral joint, posterior approach, anterior column and fusion of lumbar vertebral joint, posterior approach, posterior column are coded separately.

The next guideline gives extensive instructions on how to code vertebral joint devices and materials that are used in the fusion procedures when a combination of methods is used.

B3.10c. Combinations of devices and materials are often used on a vertebral joint to render the joint immobile. When combinations of devices are used on the same vertebral joint, the device value coded for the procedure is as follows:

- If an interbody fusion device is used to render the joint immobile (alone or containing other material, like bone graft), the procedure is coded with the device value Interbody Fusion Device.
- If bone graft is the *only* device used to render the joint immobile, the procedure is coded with the device value Nonautologous Tissue Substitute or Autologous Tissue Substitute.
- If a mixture of autologous and nonautologous bone graft (with or without biological or synthetic extenders or binders) is used to render the joint immobile, code the procedure with the device value Autologous Tissue Substitute.

Examples: Fusion of a vertebral joint using a cage-style interbody fusion device containing morselized bone graft is coded to the device Interbody Fusion Device. Fusion of a vertebral joint using a bone dowel interbody fusion device made of cadaver bone and packed with a mixture of local morselized bone and demineralized bone matrix is coded to the device Interbody Fusion Device. Fusion of a vertebral joint using both autologous bone graft and bone bank bone graft is coded to the device Autologous Tissue Substitute.

These guidelines will be more thoroughly covered in chapter 6, which includes the Fusion root operation, with more information and examples in chapter 16.

Guideline B3.11 has three parts and gives specific instructions on the root operation Inspection. The first part of the guideline emphasizes that when Inspection is an integral part of a procedure it is not coded separately.

B3.11a. Inspection of a body part(s) performed to achieve the objective of a procedure is not coded separately.

Example: Fiberoptic bronchoscopy performed for irrigation of the bronchus, only the irrigation procedure is coded.

The next part of the guideline concerns multiple inspections of either tubular or nontubular body parts.

B3.11b. If multiple tubular body parts are inspected, the most distal body part (the body part furthest from the starting point of the inspection) is coded. If multiple non-tubular body parts in a region are inspected, the body part that specifies the entire area inspected is coded.

Examples: Cystoureteroscopy with inspection of bladder and ureters is coded to the ureter body part value. Exploratory laparotomy with general inspection of abdominal contents is coded to the peritoneal cavity body part value.

The last part of the Inspection guideline gives instruction on multiple Inspection procedures on the same body part using different approaches.

 B3.11c. When both an Inspection procedure and another procedure are performed on the same body part during the same episode, if the Inspection procedure is performed using a different approach from the other procedure, the Inspection procedure is coded separately.

Example: Endoscopic Inspection of the duodenum is coded separately when open Excision of the duodenum is performed during the same procedural episode.

Guideline number B3.12 distinguishes between Occlusion and Restriction for vessel embolization procedures. These root operations will be covered in more detail in chapter 5 of the text.

 B3.12. If the objective of an embolization procedure is to completely close a vessel, the root operation Occlusion is coded. If the objective of an embolization procedure is to narrow the lumen of a vessel, the root operation Restriction is coded.

Examples: Tumor embolization is coded to the root operation Occlusion, because the objective of the procedure is to cut off the blood supply to the vessel. Embolization of a cerebral aneurysm is coded to the root operation Restriction, because the objective of the procedure is not to close off the vessel entirely but to narrow the lumen of the vessel at the site of the aneurysm where it is abnormally wide.

Guidelines B3.13 and B3.14 for Root Operations concern Release and Division procedures. These root operations will be discussed in more detail in chapter 4 of the text. The first of these guidelines concerns the designation of the body part for a Release procedure.

 B3.13. In the root operation Release, the body part value coded is the body part being freed and not the tissue being manipulated or cut to free the body part.

Example: Lysis of intestinal adhesions is coded to the specific intestine body part value.

Next, the difference between the two root operations Release and Division (involving cutting only) is highlighted based on the objective of the procedure.

 B3.14. If the sole objective of the procedure is freeing a body part without cutting the body part, the root operation is Release. If the sole objective of the procedure is separating or transecting a body part, the root operation is Division.

Examples: Freeing a nerve root from surrounding scar tissue to relieve pain is coded to the root operation Release. Severing a nerve root to relieve pain is coded to the root operation Division.

Specific guidelines for the root operation Reposition in fracture treatment are included in the 15th guideline for root operations. The Reposition root operation will be covered in more detail in chapter 4 of the text.

B3.15. Reduction of a displaced fracture is coded to the root operation Reposition, and the application of a cast or splint in conjunction with the Reposition procedure is not coded separately. Treatment of a nondisplaced fracture is coded to the procedure performed.

Examples: Casting of a nondisplaced fracture is coded to the root operation Immobilization in the Placement section. Putting a pin in a nondisplaced fracture is coded to the root operation Insertion.

The next guideline distinguishes between Transplantation procedures of living body parts coded in the Medical and Surgical section and transplanted cells, which are coded in the Administration section of ICD-10-PCS.

B3.16. Putting in a mature and functioning living body part taken from another individual or animal is coded to the root operation Transplantation. Putting in autologous or nonautologous cells is coded to the Administration section.

Example: Putting in autologous or nonautologous bone marrow, pancreatic islet cells, or stem cells is coded to the Administration section.

The final guideline in the root operation section specifies the use of the body part and qualifier characters for the Transfer root operation.

B3.17. The root operation Transfer contains qualifiers that can be used to specify when a transfer flap is composed of more than one tissue layer, such as a musculocutaneous flap. For procedures involving transfer of multiple tissue layers including skin, subcutaneous tissue, fascia or muscle, the procedure is coded to the body part value that describes the deepest tissue layer in the flap, and the qualifier can be used to describe the other tissue layer(s) in the transfer flap.

Example: A musculocutaneous flap transfer is coded to the appropriate body part value in the body system Muscles, and the qualifier is used to describe the additional tissue layer(s) in the transfer flap.

Guidelines for Body Part

Along with the body system and root operation guidelines, there are eight guidelines that are specific to the coding of body parts. The first guideline, B4.1, has three components. The first, B4.1a, is general in nature, specifying how to code a portion of a body part that does not have a designated body part value. The second part, B4.1b, gives instruction on coding the site of a procedure stated to be around a given body part. Note that this second part of the guideline is only applied when a more specific body part value is not available for the site of the procedure. The third part, B4.1c, is specific to tubular body parts and procedures that are performed on a continuous section of that body part. In this case, the body part value will be for the farthest site reached in the procedure.

B4.1a. If a procedure is performed on a portion of a body part that does not have a separate body part value, code the body part value corresponding to the whole body part.

Example: A procedure performed on the alveolar process of the mandible is coded to the mandible body part.

B4.1b. If the prefix "peri" is combined with a body part to identify the site of the procedure, and the site of the procedure is not further specified, then the procedure is coded to the body part named. This guideline applies only when a more specific body part value is not available.

Examples: A procedure site identified as perirenal is coded to the kidney body part when the site of the procedure is not further specified. A procedure site described in the documentation as peri-urethral, and the documentation also indicates that is the vulvar tissue and not the urethral tissue that is the site of the procedure, then the procedure is coded to the vulva body part.

B4.1c.   If a procedure is performed on a continuous section of a tubular body part, code the body part value corresponding to the furthest anatomical site from the point of entry.

Example: A procedure performed on a continuous section of artery from the femoral artery to the external iliac artery with the point of entry at the femoral artery is coded to the external iliac body part.

The next guideline deals with branches of body parts. Recall that only a maximum of 34 values are available for a given body part character: 24 letters of the alphabet (excluding O and I) and the 10 numerals 0–9. Since there are many areas of the body that have more than 34 subdivisions, it is often necessary to code a specific body part to its closest anatomical part. The body part key is integrated into the Index and as a stand-alone part of the ICD-10-PCS system, as described in chapter 1. The appropriate body part to reference for coding the procedure can be found using either the Index entry or the body part key. For example, when using a code book, the Index directs the coding professional to the correct body part by stating "*Use* Artery, Internal Iliac, Left" or "*Use* Artery, Internal Iliac, Right" when referencing the term "Obturator Artery." The second part of the guideline is specific to the cardiovascular body systems and reminds the coding professional that the body part branches are in context with the PCS system. Although the bronchial artery is technically a branch of the descending thoracic artery, procedures on this structure are coded in the upper artery body system (03) versus the heart and great vessels (02) using the generic body part upper artery. The body part key instructs that the upper artery is used for the bronchial artery. In the example given, Occlusion of the descending thoracic aorta in the heart and great vessels would not be compatible with maintaining life, while occlusion of a bronchial artery may be performed for a condition such as severe hemoptysis.

B4.2.   Where a specific branch of a body part does not have its own body part value in PCS, the body part is typically coded to the closest proximal branch that has a specific body part value. In the cardiovascular body systems, if a general body part is available in the correct root operation table, and coding to a proximal branch would require assigning a code in a different body system, the procedure is coded using the general body part value.

Examples: A procedure performed on the mandibular branch of the trigeminal nerve is coded to the trigeminal nerve body part value. Occlusion of the bronchial artery is coded to the body part value Upper Artery in the body system Upper Arteries, and not to the body part value Thoracic Aorta, Descending in the body system Heart and Great Vessels.

Bilateral body parts are addressed in the next guideline, which reminds the coding professional that, in some cases, bilateral body part values are available and should be selected when applicable. In cases where a procedure is performed on both sides of the body and a bilateral body part value does not exist, both of the individual body part values are used and two codes are assigned. For example, a Supplement procedure performed on both fallopian tubes should have the bilateral body part value (7); however, a Supplement procedure performed on both eyes requires two codes: one for the right eye (0) and one for the left eye (1) because there is not a bilateral body part value available.

B4.3.   Bilateral body part values are available for a limited number of body parts. If the identical procedure is performed on contralateral body parts, and a bilateral body part value exists for that body part, a single procedure is coded using the bilateral body part value. If no bilateral body part value exists, each procedure is coded separately using the appropriate body part value.

Example: The identical procedure performed on both fallopian tubes is coded once using the body part value Fallopian Tube, Bilateral. The identical procedure performed on both knee joints is coded twice using the body part values Knee Joint, Right and Knee Joint, Left.

The next guideline has specific information on the coronary artery body part, which is considered a single body part, with the procedure codes based on the number of arteries treated. More information on this guideline will be presented in chapters 5 and 11 of this text.

B4.4. The coronary arteries are classified as a single body part that is further specified by number of arteries treated. One procedure code specifying multiple arteries is used when the same procedure is performed, including the same device and qualifier values.

Examples: Angioplasty of two distinct coronary arteries with placement of two stents is coded as Dilation of Coronary Artery, Two Arteries with Two Intraluminal Devices.

Angioplasty of two distinct coronary arteries, one with stent placed and one without, is coded separately as Dilation of Coronary Artery, One Artery with Intraluminal Device, and Dilation of Coronary Artery, One Artery with no device.

The next two guidelines concern procedures involving joints. First, procedures including tendons, ligaments, bursae, and fascia near a joint have a specific guideline pertaining to the objective of the procedure. The next guideline pertains to the skin, subcutaneous tissue, and fascia that overlie a joint and classifies the joint to a given body part. More information on this guideline is included in chapter 15.

B4.5. Procedures performed on tendons, ligaments, bursae, and fascia supporting a joint are coded to the body part in the respective body system that is the focus of the procedure. Procedures performed on joint structures themselves are coded to the body part in the Joint body systems.

Example: Repair of the anterior cruciate ligament of the knee is coded to the knee bursae and ligament body part in the bursae and ligaments body system. Knee arthroscopy with shaving of articular cartilage is coded to the knee joint body part in the Lower Joints body system.

B4.6. If a procedure is performed on the skin, subcutaneous tissue, or fascia overlying a joint, the procedure is coded to the following body parts:

- Shoulder is coded to Upper Arm
- Elbow is coded to Lower Arm
- Wrist is coded to Lower Arm
- Hip is coded to Upper Leg
- Knee is coded to Lower Leg
- Ankle is coded to Foot

The next body part guideline involves the fingers and toes, which are coded to the hand and foot, respectively, if a specific body part is not available.

B4.7. If a body system does not contain a separate body part value for fingers, procedures performed on the fingers are coded to the body part value for the hand. If a body system does not contain a separate body part value for toes, procedures performed on the toes are coded to the body part value for the foot.

Example: Excision of finger muscle is coded to one of the hand muscle body part values in the Muscles body system.

The final body part guideline explains the components of the upper and lower intestinal tract for selected root operations.

B4.8. In the Gastrointestinal body system, the general body part values Upper Intestinal Tract and Lower Intestinal Tract are provided as an option for the root operations Change, Inspection, Removal and Revision. Upper Intestinal Tract includes the portion of the gastrointestinal tract from the esophagus down to and including the duodenum, and Lower Intestinal Tract includes the portion of the gastrointestinal tract from the jejunum down to and including the rectum and anus.

Example: In the root operation Change table, change of a device in the jejunum is coded using the body part Lower Intestinal Tract.

Guidelines for Approach

There are four guidelines that assist in assigning the value for the approach character. The first gives instructions on open approaches that include percutaneous assistance. In this case the open approach supersedes the percutaneous endoscopic assistance.

B5.2. Procedures performed using the open approach with percutaneous endoscopic assistance are coded to the approach Open.

Example: Laparoscopic-assisted sigmoidectomy is coded to the approach Open.

The next two guidelines concern the external approach. The first states that an external approach is designated for surgeries that involve visualization of the operative field via a body orifice. The second clarifies that procedures involving external force exerted through applicable body layers are also coded to the external approach.

B5.3a. Procedures performed within an orifice on structures that are visible without the aid of any instrumentation are coded to the approach External.

Example: Resection of tonsils is coded to the approach External.

B5.3b. Procedures performed indirectly by the application of external force through the intervening body layers are coded to the approach External.

Example: Closed reduction of fracture is coded to the approach External.

The final approach guideline covers the situation where a device is used in a percutaneous procedure.

B5.4. Procedures performed percutaneously via a device placed for the procedure are coded to the approach Percutaneous.

Example: Fragmentation of kidney stone performed via percutaneous nephrostomy is coded to the approach Percutaneous.

When determining the appropriate approach for a given procedure, the approach decision tree depicted in figure 2.3 can be used as a tool. Refer to chapter 1 for the full definition of the seven approaches and the illustrations of the approaches. An approach review exercise is also included at the end of this chapter.

Assigning the approach can be challenging. Review the decision tree as the approaches are discussed. The first question is whether there was an incision through the skin or mucous membranes. For the Open approach, the incision must reach to at least the subcutaneous tissues so that the surgeon is looking directly at the area where the procedure will be performed. This may involve entering a cavity or cutting through several layers and body systems. If these criteria are met and the surgery site is directly exposed, the Open approach is selected. For example, for an open appendectomy, the abdomen is entered directly, and the appendix is visualized for resection by the surgeon.

If the criteria for an Open approach do not apply, the next question is whether there was a puncture or minor incision made in order to reach the procedure site without exposing the surgical site; which constitutes a percutaneous approach. Figure 1.3 shows a percutaneous approach with the needle reaching the nerve that is being treated without exposing the operative site. If there was a puncture or minor incision made, and this approach is not percutaneous, the next question is whether a scope was used to visualize the site. Note that the operative site is not directly exposed as in the open approach, but rather is visualized through the scope and the minor incision or puncture. The operative report may mention trocars or ports that are used to accommodate the visualization equipment. In this case, the percutaneous endoscopic approach is used. Figure 1.2 includes a visual of a laparoscopic cholecystectomy that uses a trocar as a portal for instruments used in the procedure.

Figure 2.3. Approach decision tree

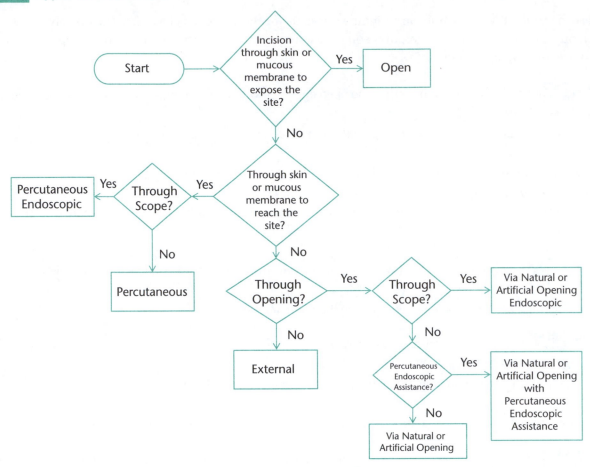

©Kuehn Consulting, LLC. Used with Permission.

This is an example of a percutaneous endoscopic approach because the operative site is reached and visualized without exposing the operative site. In the open approach depicted in figure 1.2, the abdomen is incised and the intervening layers are cut through to expose the gallbladder.

Returning to the decision tree, if the approach has still not been assigned, the next group of questions asks if the procedure was performed through an opening. This might be a natural opening such as throat, anus, or nose or an artificial opening created by a surgical procedure such as a colostomy. See figure 1.4 for an example of an approach made through the natural opening of the throat. If a natural or artificial opening was the approach, the next question is whether a scope was used to visualize the site. Figure 1.5 includes an example of an approach via the natural opening of the urethra with visualization, a cystoscopy. The final approach involving an opening is Via Natural or Artificial Opening with Percutaneous Assistance. Figure 1.6 depicts this approach for a laparoscopically assisted vaginal hysterectomy, where the uterus and other organs such as the fallopian tubes and ovaries, if applicable, are disconnected laparoscopically and the cervix is resected via the vagina with all the organs removed via the vagina. This procedure will be discussed in more detail in chapter 19. The only other application for this approach is in the gastrointestinal system for Excision and Resection in laparoscopic-assisted pull-through procedures.

The final approach that does not involve incisions, punctures, or openings is the External approach. This approach involves procedures performed on the outside of the body such as a closed reduction of a fracture or suture of the skin. Procedures performed within a cavity that are visible without any instrumentation are coded as external approach. Figure 1.7 shows a tonsillectomy. Since the tonsils are visible without any instrumentation, the External approach is selected.

Guidelines for Device

There are two device guidelines. The first guideline has three parts and the first two relate to what can and cannot be coded as devices.

B6.1a. A device is coded only if a device remains after the procedure is completed. If no device remains, the device value No Device is coded. In limited root operations, the classification provides the qualifier values Temporary and Intraoperative, for specific procedures involving clinically significant devices, where the purpose of the device is to be utilized for a brief duration during the procedure or current inpatient stay. If a device that is intended to remain after the procedure is completed requires removal before the end of the operative episode in which it was inserted (for example, the device size is inadequate or a complication occurs), both the insertion and removal of the device should be coded.

B6.1b. Materials such as sutures, ligatures, radiological markers, and temporary postoperative wound drains are considered integral to the performance of a procedure and are not coded as devices.

The last part of the first guideline concerns procedures that are performed on the device versus the body part.

B6.1c. Procedures performed on a device only and not on a body part are specified in the root operations Change, Irrigation, Removal, and Revision and are coded to the procedure performed.

Example: Irrigation of percutaneous nephrostomy tube is coded to the root operation Irrigation of indwelling device in the Administration section.

The second guideline involves procedures with the objective of inserting a drainage device, which is coded to the root operation Drainage.

B6.2. A separate procedure to put in a drainage device is coded to the root operation Drainage with the device value Drainage Device.

An example of applying this guideline is a thoracotomy with drainage and placement of a chest tube drainage device. The drainage device is represented by the value of 0 in the 6th character for device.

Obstetrics Section Guidelines

There are two guidelines that are specific to the second section in ICD-10-PCS: Obstetrics. The first guideline clarifies that this section is only used for procedures performed specifically on the products of conception. The products of conception include the fetus, placenta, amniotic sac, amniotic fluid, and umbilical cord.

C1. Procedures performed on the products of conception are coded to the Obstetrics section. Procedures performed on a pregnant female other than the products of conception are coded to the appropriate root operation in the Medical and Surgical section.

Example: Amniocentesis is coded to the products of conception body part in the Obstetrics section. Repair of obstetric urethral laceration is coded to the urethra body part in the Medical and Surgical section.

The final Obstetrics guideline clarifies the timing of the use of the Obstetrics codes versus the Medical and Surgical section codes. These guidelines will be covered in more detail in chapter 20 of this book.

C2. Procedures performed following a delivery or abortion for curettage of the endometrium or evacuation of retained products of conception are all coded in the Obstetrics section, to the root operation Extraction and the body part Products of Conception, Retained. Diagnostic or therapeutic dilation and curettage performed during times other than the postpartum or postabortion period are all coded in the Medical and Surgical section, to the root operation Extraction and the body part Endometrium.

New Technology Section

A general guideline for the new technology codes includes information on the X codes. More information on this section will be covered in chapter 25 of this text.

D1. Section X codes are standalone codes. They are not supplemental codes. Section X codes fully represent the specific procedure described in the code title, and do not require any additional codes from other sections of ICD-10-PCS. When section X contains a code title that describes a specific new technology procedure, only the X code is reported for the procedure. There is no need to report a broader, nonspecific code in another section of ICD-10-PCS.

Example: XW04321 Introduction of Ceftazidime-Avibactam anti-infective into Central Vein, Percutaneous Approach, New Technology Group 1, can be coded to indicate that Ceftazidime-Avibactam anti-infective was administered via a central vein. A separate code from table 3E0 in the Administration section of ICD-10-PCS is not coded in addition to this code.

A thorough study of the ICD-10-PCS Coding Guidelines will assist in learning to use the codes in the system. These guidelines will be referenced again in applicable chapters in the text.

Selection of Principal Procedure

The instructions for designating the principal procedure are the final portion of the guidelines. If more than one procedure is performed, these guidelines provide instructions on which should be listed first. This can be based on the definitive procedure versus a diagnostic procedure, with the definitive procedure listed first. However, the procedure most related to the principal diagnosis takes precedence. The procedure performed for definitive treatment of a secondary diagnosis is only designated as principal if there are no definitive or diagnostic procedures related to the principal diagnosis.

The following instructions should be applied in the selection of principal procedure and clarification on the importance of the relation to the principal diagnosis when more than one procedure is performed:

1. Procedure performed for definitive treatment of both principal diagnosis and secondary diagnosis
    a. Sequence procedure performed for definitive treatment most related to principal diagnosis as principal procedure

2. Procedure performed for definitive treatment and diagnostic procedures performed for both principal diagnosis and secondary diagnosis
    a. Sequence procedure performed for definitive treatment most related to principal diagnosis as principal procedure

3. A diagnostic procedure was performed for the principal diagnosis and a procedure is performed for definitive treatment of a secondary diagnosis
    a. Sequence diagnostic procedure as principal procedure, since the procedure most related to the principal diagnosis takes precedence

4. No procedures performed that are related to principal diagnosis; procedures performed for definitive treatment and diagnostic procedures were performed for secondary diagnosis

a. Sequence procedure performed for definitive treatment of secondary diagnosis as principal procedure, since there are no procedures (definitive or nondefinitive treatment) related to principal diagnosis

Applying the Conventions and Guidelines and Researching the Procedure

Using the knowledge of the conventions of the system found in chapter 1 and the guidelines covered in this chapter, the process of building an ICD-10-PCS code can begin. Often, additional research is needed to build the ICD-10-PCS code. Careful review of the operative report can be supplemented with internet searches for more information on a procedure to help with deciphering the intent of the procedure, the approach used, and other factors. Using a search engine, the name of the procedure is entered and articles and studies of the cited procedure can be reviewed. Referring to the images tabs can provide some excellent visualization of the site and components of the procedure. Requesting animated images or videos is another method for learning more about the procedure.

To assist in organizing this process, the Dissecting an Operative Report worksheet in figure 2.4 can be used to determine the elements needed to build the code.

Determining the root operation or intent of the procedure is a key component in building the ICD-10-PCS code. In the Medical and Surgical section, there are 31 root operations that represent these intents as listed and defined in chapter 1. These nine groups and the root operations in each group are listed in table 2.4. Full definitions of the root operations can be found in tables 1.3–1.12 in chapter 1 of this book.

The root operations are placed into nine groups based on the purpose or other aspects of the procedure. For example, there are six root operations in group 6 that always involve a device: Insertion, Removal, Revision, Change, Replacement, and Supplement. If the procedure does not include an applicable device that is left in the operative site at the conclusion of the procedure, root operations from this group cannot be used. There are four root operations in group 5 that alter the diameter or route of a tubular body part: Restriction, Occlusion, Dilation, and Bypass. If the site operated on is not a tubular body part, the root operations in this group cannot be selected. Referring to the groups can help to streamline the selection of the root operation.

For example, review the operative report found in figure 2.5. The intent of the procedure is to biopsy the left lobe of the liver, by taking out a small wedge of tissue. Referring to the nine groups of root operations, this procedure fits into the description of group 1, taking out some or all of a body part without replacement. The five root operations in this group are Excision, Resection, Detachment, Destruction, and Extraction. Since only a portion of the left lobe of the liver is removed by cutting, the root operation Excision is selected. The liver is part of the hepatobiliary and pancreas body system, with the left lobe of the liver as the specific body part.

Figure 2.4.   Worksheet: Dissecting an Operative Report

Dissecting an Operative Report

Intent of Procedure:_____

Root Operation:_____ (Index Main Term)

Where:

   Major—(Body System): _____

   Minor—(Body Part):_____ (Index Subterm)

Approach:_____
(See Approach Decision Tree)

Device: _____

       Yes—See Table, No—Z

Qualifier: _____

       Yes—See Table, No—Z

Table 2.4.   Nine groups of Medical and Surgical root operations

Group Description	Root Operations
1. Take out some or all of a body part	Excision
	Resection
	Detachment
	Destruction
	Extraction
2. Take out solids/fluids/gases from a body part	Drainage
	Extirpation
	Fragmentation
3. Involving cutting or separation only	Division
	Release
4. Put in/put back or move some or all of a body part	Transplantation
	Reattachment
	Transfer
	Reposition
5. Alter the diameter/route of a tubular body part	Restriction
	Occlusion
	Dilation
	Bypass
6. Always involve a device	Insertion
	Removal
	Revision
	Change
	Replacement
	Supplement
7. Involve examination only	Inspection
	Map
8. Define other repairs	Control
	Repair
9. Define other objectives	Fusion
	Alteration
	Creation

Referring to the approach decision tree in figure 2.5, the decision on the approach is determined by reviewing the report and noting that the procedure was performed via a midline incision, to expose the operative site, an open approach. There were no devices used. Since the procedure was done as a biopsy, the qualifier of Diagnostic is applicable.

Using the CMS file method to build the code, the Medical and Surgical section is selected, then the hepatobiliary and pancreas body system, and Excision as the root operation. If a code book was used, the code table could be directly referenced by consulting the hepatobiliary and pancreas body system and locating the Excision table. This can also be referenced by looking under the main term Excision in the code book index, subterm Liver, Left Lobe, 0FB2. In either case, the 0FB table is referenced, as in table 2.5. The values for the 4th through 7th characters are selected from the first row of the table, and the complete code is built as 0FB20ZX.

Figure 2.5.   **Exploratory laparotomy and liver biopsy**

Operative Report

Name of Operation: Exploratory Laparotomy and Liver Biopsy

Preoperative Diagnosis: Carcinoma of the Stomach

Postoperative Diagnosis: Carcinoma of the Stomach

Operative Findings

Clinical History: This 74-year-old black male was admitted to the General Surgery Service for a thorough GI workup carried out because of a history of 60 lb. weight loss during the past eight months. GI series demonstrated a large space-occupying lesion in the fundus of the stomach, and the diagnosis of carcinoma of the stomach was established. Chest films, liver scan, and further diagnostic studies did not indicate metastatic spread. Therefore, it was elected to explore this patient; on 03/11 he was taken to the operating room.

Procedure in Detail: Under adequate endotracheal anesthesia, the abdomen was prepped with pHiso-Hex and Betadine and draped for an upper midline incision. A small upper midline incision was made to explore the abdomen. The peritoneum was entered. Manual exploration demonstrated a large, hard, fixed mass on the posterior wall of the fundus of the stomach. There were some tumor studdings in the left lobe of the liver. A portion was selected for biopsy, and a small wedge of tissue was removed. The midline was then closed with interrupted figure-eight sutures of 0-stainless steel wire; retention sutures were utilized to close the same. The skin was closed with 3–0 black silk, and no blood was administered during the surgical procedure. The patient tolerated the procedure well.

Open Approach

Where the procedure was performed

Intent of procedure/ Root Operation

The worksheet would be completed as follows:

Dissecting an Operative Report

Intent of Procedure: _Biopsy Liver Tumor_

Root Operation: _Excision_   (Index Main Term)

Where:

   Major—(Body System): _Hepatobiliary and Pancreas_

   Minor—(Body Part): _Liver, Left Lobe_   (Index Subterm)

Approach: _Open (mid-line incision)_

(See Approach Decision Tree)

Device: _None_

      Yes—See Table, No—Z

Qualifier: _Diagnostic_

      Yes—See Table, No—Z

Figure 2.6 includes an additional operative report to analyze and build the ICD-10-PCS code. This case is for a neuroblastoma of the adrenal gland. Research will show that this is a type of adrenal cancer found in the developing nerve cells of the adrenal gland. The adrenal gland is an endocrine gland that produces hormones including adrenaline, aldosterone, and cortisol.

After reviewing the operative report, the intent of the procedure was to remove the neuroblastoma of the adrenal gland. This procedure also fits into the first group of root operations, taking out some or all of a body part. A biopsy was not performed, as the type of tumor was already established. The root operation Excision is selected as a portion of the right adrenal gland is removed to excise the tumor. Using the CMS file method, the Medical and Surgical section is referenced, with the Endocrine body system and the Excision root operation selected. If a code book is used, the code table can be directly referenced in the Endocrine body system, Excision

Table 2.5.   0FB table

Section	0	Medical and Surgical		
Body System	F	Hepatobiliary System and Pancreas		
Operation	B	Excision: Cutting out or off, without replacement, a portion of a body part		
Body Part	Approach		Device	Qualifier
0 Liver 1 Liver, Right Lobe 2 Liver, Left Lobe	0 Open 3 Percutaneous 4 Percutaneous Endoscopic		Z No Device	X Diagnostic Z No Qualifier
4 Gallbladder G Pancreas	0 Open 3 Percutaneous 4 Percutaneous Endoscopic 8 Via Natural or Artificial Opening Endoscopic		Z No Device	X Diagnostic Z No Qualifier
5 Hepatic Duct, Right 6 Hepatic Duct, Left 7 Hepatic Duct, Common 8 Cystic Duct 9 Common Bile Duct C Ampulla of Vater D Pancreatic Duct F Pancreatic Duct, Accessory	0 Open 3 Percutaneous 4 Percutaneous Endoscopic 7 Via Natural or Artificial Opening 8 Via Natural or Artificial Opening Endoscopic		Z No Device	X Diagnostic Z No Qualifier

Source: CMS 2019

root operation. This can also be located in the index under the main term Excision, subterms Adrenal, Right, with the first four characters given; 0GB3. In either case, the 0GB table is referenced, as in table 2.6. The 3 is verified as the body part for the right adrenal gland. Since the report states the incision was reopened and extended medially and laterally, and the peritoneal cavity was entered, the approach is Open and the 0 is selected. There is no device and no qualifier. The complete code is 0GB30ZZ.

Figure 2.6.   Excision of neuroblastoma

PREOPERATIVE DIAGNOSIS:	Neuroblastoma right adrenal gland
POSTOPERATIVE DIAGNOSIS:	Neuroblastoma right adrenal gland
PROCEDURE PERFORMED:	Excision of neuroblastoma
ANESTHESIA:	General

Approach is via incision = Open

Body part = right adrenal gland, Endocrine body system

Intent of the procedure—removal of the neuroblastoma = Excision—cutting out or off, without replacement, a portion of the body part.

PROCEDURE: The child was brought to the operating room, and general anesthesia induced. The right upper quadrant and right flank were prepped and draped in the usual sterile fashion. The previous right upper quadrant incision was reopened, and extended medially and laterally, until the peritoneal cavity was entered. The liver was retracted superiorly, and the kidney inferiorly revealing a 4 to 5 cm firm mass in the right adrenal gland. Using electrocautery, the peritoneum overlying the mass was opened, and all attachments of the mass to the liver and peritoneum, and kidney were taken down using electrocautery. Medially, the adrenal vein was clamped at its entrance point to the vena cava. The vein was then divided, and the specimen removed from the field. 3-0 Prolene suture was used to suture ligate the adrenal vein. No bleeding was seen from that site at the conclusion of the case. The right upper quadrant was copiously irrigated, and the lymph nodes were found to biopsy in the area. The abdomen was closed in layers using 2-0 Vicryl suture for the deep layers, and 5-0 Monocryl suture for the skin. Steri-Strips and a sterile dressing were applied. Sponge, needle, and instrument counts were reported to be correct at the conclusion of the procedure. The child was awakened and taken to the recovery room in satisfactory condition.

Figure 2.7 includes another example of an operative report for analysis.

After reviewing the operative report, the objective of the procedure is noted to be an excisional biopsy. The behavior of the lesion was not known, so it was sent to pathology for analysis. This procedure is once

Table 2.6. 0GB table

Section	0	Medical and Surgical
Body System	G	Endocrine System
Operation	B	Excision: Cutting out or off, without replacement, a portion of a body part

Body Part	Approach	Device	Qualifier
0 Pituitary Gland 1 Pineal Body 2 Adrenal Gland, Left 3 Adrenal Gland, Right 4 Adrenal Glands, Bilateral 6 Carotid Body, Left 7 Carotid Body, Right 8 Carotid Bodies, Bilateral 9 Para-aortic Body B Coccygeal Glomus C Glomus Jugulare D Aortic Body F Paraganglion Extremity G Thyroid Gland Lobe, Left H Thyroid Gland Lobe, Right J Thyroid Gland Isthmus L Superior Parathyroid Gland, Right M Superior Parathyroid Gland, Left N Inferior Parathyroid Gland, Right P Inferior Parathyroid Gland, Left Q Parathyroid Glands, Multiple R Parathyroid Gland	0 Open 3 Percutaneous 4 Percutaneous Endoscopic	Z No Device	X Diagnostic Z No Qualifier

Source: CMS 2019

again found in the first group of root operations, taking out some or all of a body part, and is coded as an Excision, with a qualifier for diagnostic. Note that this procedure was performed on both the right index finger and the left hand. Following the guideline for multiple procedures B3.2a, if the same root operation is performed on different body parts as defined by distinct values of the body part character, multiple procedures are coded.

B3.2 During the same operative episode, multiple procedures are coded if:

a. The same root operation is performed on different body parts as defined by distinct values of the body part character.

Examples: Diagnostic excision of liver and pancreas are coded separately. Excision of lesion in the ascending colon and excision of lesion in the transverse colon are coded separately.

b. The same root operation is repeated in multiple body parts, and those body parts are separate and distinct body parts classified to a single ICD-10-PCS body part value.

Examples: Excision of the sartorius muscle and excision of the gracilis muscle are both included in the upper leg muscle body part value, and multiple procedures are coded.
Extraction of multiple toenails are coded separately.

Laparoscopic cholecystectomy converted to an open cholecystectomy is coded as percutaneous endoscopic Inspection and open Resection.

Since the operative report described this procedure as to the level of the subcutaneous tissue and fat, the subcutaneous tissue and fascia body system is chosen. This follows the direction of coding guideline B3.5, coding the deepest layer for the body part.

Figure 2.7.   Excision of lesion

PREOPERATIVE DIAGNOSES:

1. SUSPICIOUS LESION, RIGHT INDEX FINGER
2. SUSPICIOUS LESION, LEFT DORSAL HAND

POSTOPERATIVE DIAGNOSES:

1. SUSPICIOUS LESION, RIGHT INDEX FINGER
2. SUSPICIOUS LESION, LEFT DORSAL HAND

PROCEDURES:

1. EXCISION OF RIGHT INDEX FINGER LESION WITH EXCISED DIAMETER TOTALING 0.7 CM AND SIMPLE CLOSURE
2. EXCISION OF LEFT DORSAL HAND LESION WITH EXCISED DIAMETER TOTALING 0.9 CM AND SIMPLE CLOSURE

ASSISTANT: NONE

ANESTHESIA: LOCAL

ESTIMATED BLOOD LOSS: MINIMAL

COMPLICATIONS: NONE

INDICATIONS FOR PROCEDURE:

The patient is a 73-year-old female with a history of skin cancers who presented with scaly, nonhealing lesions on her right index finger and dorsum of her left hand. She requires excisional biopsy given the suspicious nature.

DESCRIPTION OF PROCEDURE:

Informed consent was obtained from the patient. The risks of surgery including bleeding, infection, scarring, injury to neurovascular structures, delayed wound healing, unexpected pathology or positive margins requiring re-excision were discussed. The patient expressed understanding and wished to proceed. The patient was taken to the procedure room, properly identified and placed in the supine position. Bilateral hands were prepped and draped sterilely. The procedure began on the right index finger. Using loupe magnification, the affected area was marked. A longitudinal ellipse was then drawn encompassing the lesion. The area was then infiltrated with approximately 2 mL of 1% lidocaine without epinephrine. The digit was then manually exsanguinated and a 1/4-inch Penrose drain was used as a digital tourniquet. An incision was made and the lesion was then excised at the level of the subcutaneous fat and sent to Pathology for analysis with a short suture proximal and a long suture radial. The skin was then reapproximated with interrupted 4-0 nylon horizontal mattress sutures. The wound was then dressed with bacitracin, Xeroform, Kling and loosely wrapped with Coban.

Next, attention was turned to the left hand. Using loupe magnification, the affected area was marked. An ellipse encompassing this area was then drawn. The area was infiltrated with 1% lidocaine. The ellipse was then incised and the lesion was taken to the level of the subcutaneous fat. It was marked with a short suture proximal and a long suture radial and sent to Pathology for analysis. The skin was then reapproximated with interrupted 4-0 nylon horizontal mattress sutures. The skin was then dressed with bacitracin, Xeroform, 4 × 4 and a Coban.

Objective of the procedure excisional biopsy

Body part

By incision = open approach to the level of the subcutaneous fat = subcutaneous tissue and fascia body system

Sent to Pathology for analysis = biopsy

This was the stated objective of the procedure

Second body part. Guideline B3.2a.

This is a separate and distinct body part.

B3.5.   If the root operations Excision, Repair, or Inspection are performed on overlapping layers of the musculoskeletal system, the body part specifying the deepest layer is coded.

Example: Excisional debridement that includes skin and subcutaneous tissue and muscle is coded to the muscle body part.

This procedure is performed on the right index finger and the dorsum of the left hand.

To code the Excision of the lesion of the right index finger using the code book method, refer to the index entry for Excision, subcutaneous tissue and fascia, and note that there is not an entry for finger. Guideline B4.7 is followed, using the hand for the body part.

B4.7. If a body system does not contain a separate body part value for fingers, procedures performed on the fingers are coded to the body part value for the hand. If a body system does not contain a separate body part value for toes, procedures performed on the toes are coded to the body part value for the foot.

The Index entry for Excision, Subcutaneous Tissue and Fascia, Hand, Right is referenced with the first four characters of the code noted: 0JBJ. Using the CMS file method, the Medical and Surgical section is selected, with the Subcutaneous Tissue and Fascia body system and Excision root operation. The 0JB code table (see table 2.7) is

Table 2.7. 0JB table

Section	0	Medical and Surgical		
Body System	J	Subcutaneous Tissue and Fascia		
Operation	B	Excision: Cutting out or off, without replacement, a portion of a body part		

Body Part	Approach	Device	Qualifier
0 Subcutaneous Tissue and Fascia, Scalp **1** Subcutaneous Tissue and Fascia, Face **4** Subcutaneous Tissue and Fascia, Right Neck **5** Subcutaneous Tissue and Fascia, Left Neck **6** Subcutaneous Tissue and Fascia, Chest **7** Subcutaneous Tissue and Fascia, Back **8** Subcutaneous Tissue and Fascia, Abdomen **9** Subcutaneous Tissue and Fascia, Buttock **B** Subcutaneous Tissue and Fascia, Perineum **C** Subcutaneous Tissue and Fascia, Pelvic Region **D** Subcutaneous Tissue and Fascia, Right Upper Arm **F** Subcutaneous Tissue and Fascia, Left Upper Arm **G** Subcutaneous Tissue and Fascia, Right Lower Arm **H** Subcutaneous Tissue and Fascia, Left Lower Arm **J** Subcutaneous Tissue and Fascia, Right Hand **K** Subcutaneous Tissue and Fascia, Left Hand **L** Subcutaneous Tissue and Fascia, Right Upper Leg **M** Subcutaneous Tissue and Fascia, Left Upper Leg **N** Subcutaneous Tissue and Fascia, Right Lower Leg **P** Subcutaneous Tissue and Fascia, Left Lower Leg **Q** Subcutaneous Tissue and Fascia, Right Foot **R** Subcutaneous Tissue and Fascia, Left Foot	**0** Open **3** Percutaneous	**Z** No Device	**X** Diagnostic **Z** No Qualifier

Source: CMS 2019

referenced to build the code. The first code for the right index finger is built by using J for the value of right hand. The approach was by incision, so the 0 is selected for Open. There is no device. This was a biopsy, so the X is selected for Diagnostic. The complete code is 0JBJ0ZX. The same steps are followed for the left hand, using the body part character of K for the subcutaneous tissue and fascia of the left hand: 0JBK0ZX.

Figure 2.8 includes another operative report for placement of an IVC filter. The imaging guidance will not be coded. Note that there is a device involved in this procedure that is left in place at the conclusion of the procedure. Review table 2.4 to determine which group of root operations this procedure fits into. Because there is a device involved, the group of root operations that always involves a device is selected. Because the device is put in, Insertion is selected as the root operation. Note that research shows an inferior vena cava filter is an intraluminal device that is implanted in the large vein that receives blood from the lower extremities, pelvis, and abdomen and delivers it to the right atrium. The inferior vena cava is in the lower veins body system.

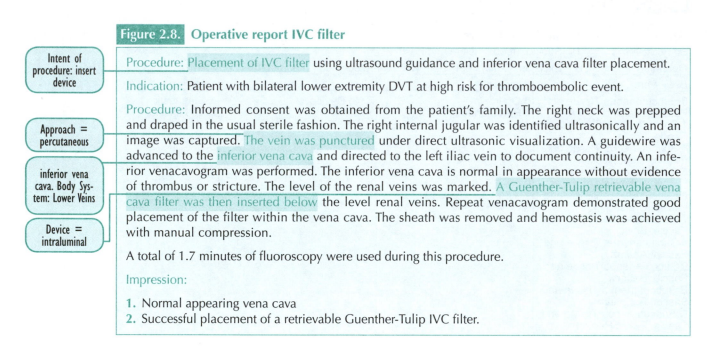

Figure 2.8. Operative report IVC filter

Intent of procedure: insert device

Procedure: Placement of IVC filter using ultrasound guidance and inferior vena cava filter placement.

Indication: Patient with bilateral lower extremity DVT at high risk for thromboembolic event.

Approach = percutaneous

Procedure: Informed consent was obtained from the patient's family. The right neck was prepped and draped in the usual sterile fashion. The right internal jugular was identified ultrasonically and an image was captured. The vein was punctured under direct ultrasonic visualization. A guidewire was advanced to the inferior vena cava and directed to the left iliac vein to document continuity. An inferior venacavogram was performed. The inferior vena cava is normal in appearance without evidence of thrombus or stricture. The level of the renal veins was marked. A Guenther-Tulip retrievable vena cava filter was then inserted below the level renal veins. Repeat venacavogram demonstrated good placement of the filter within the vena cava. The sheath was removed and hemostasis was achieved with manual compression.

inferior vena cava. Body System: Lower Veins

Device = intraluminal

A total of 1.7 minutes of fluoroscopy were used during this procedure.

Impression:

1. Normal appearing vena cava
2. Successful placement of a retrievable Guenther-Tulip IVC filter.

Using the CMS file method, the Medical and Surgical section and Lower Veins body system, the Insertion root operation is selected. Using the code book method and referring to the Index under the main term Insertion of device in, subterm vena cava, inferior, the first four characters of the code are given: 06H0. In both cases the 06H table is referenced; see table 2.8.

The body part for inferior vena cava has the value of 0. Note that the operative report states the right internal jugular was identified and punctured, and the guidewire was advanced to the inferior vena cava. Referring to the approach decision tree in figure 2.5, note that an incision was not made to expose the site of the surgery, but the skin was punctured to reach the vein that provided access for the procedure, insertion of the IVC filter. Therefore, the approach is Percutaneous, via the jugular vein, for a value of 3. The filter is placed within the inferior vena cava, so the value of D is selected for the device, and there is no qualifier, Z. The complete code is 06H03DZ.

Table 2.8. 06H table

Section	0	Medical and Surgical		
Body System	6	Lower Veins		
Operation	H	Insertion: Putting in a nonbiological appliance that monitors, assists, performs, or prevents a physiological function but does not physically take the place of a body part		

Body Part	Approach	Device	Qualifier
0 Inferior Vena Cava	0 Open 3 Percutaneous	3 Infusion Device	T Via Umbilical Vein Z No Qualifier
0 Inferior Vena Cava	0 Open 3 Percutaneous	D Intraluminal Device	Z No Qualifier
0 Inferior Vena Cava	4 Percutaneous Endoscopic	3 Infusion Device D Intraluminal Device	Z No Qualifier
1 Splenic Vein 2 Gastric Vein 3 Esophageal Vein 4 Hepatic Vein 5 Superior Mesenteric Vein 6 Inferior Mesenteric Vein 7 Colic Vein 8 Portal Vein 9 Renal Vein, Right B Renal Vein, Left C Common Iliac Vein, Right D Common Iliac Vein, Left F External Iliac Vein, Right G External Iliac Vein, Left H Hypogastric Vein, Right J Hypogastric Vein, Left M Femoral Vein, Right N Femoral Vein, Left P Saphenous Vein, Right Q Saphenous Vein, Left T Foot Vein, Right V Foot Vein, Left	0 Open 3 Percutaneous 4 Percutaneous Endoscopic	3 Infusion Device D Intraluminal Device	Z No Qualifier
Y Lower Vein	0 Open 3 Percutaneous 4 Percutaneous Endoscopic	2 Monitoring Device 3 Infusion Device D Intraluminal Device Y Other Device	Z No Qualifier

Source: CMS 2019

Code Building: Approach Review

Practice determining the approach for a procedure. Match the procedure description to the approach. Use the approach decision tree in figure 2.3 as a guide. Answers are located in appendix B.

Descriptions

_____ 1. A burr hole was made in the skull and the drainage tube was inserted

_____ 2. An arthroscopic debridement of the right knee joint was performed

_____ 3. Laceration of the skin of the right arm was repaired with dissolvable sutures

_____ 4. A cervical cerclage suture was placed in the vagina for cervical incompetence

_____ 5. A craniectomy was performed with a removal of a benign brain tumor

_____ 6. Using trocars and a video camera, a portion of the diseased descending and sigmoid colon was dissected. A circular incision was made in the rectum and the colon was removed via the anus

_____ 7. This patient has a tracheobronchoscopy with a biopsy of the right main bronchus

Approaches

a. Open
b. Percutaneous
c. Percutaneous Endoscopic
d. Via Natural or Artificial Opening
e. Via Natural or Artificial Opening, Endoscopic
f. Via Natural or Artificial Opening with Percutaneous Endoscopic Assistance
g. External

 Check Your Understanding

For each of the following, select the correct answer and cite the guideline that applies.

1. This procedure is performed by visualizing the operative field via an orifice, without using instrumentation. Which approach is correct?
    a. Open
    b. Percutaneous Endoscopic
    c. External
    d. Via Natural or Artificial Opening

    Guideline _____

2. Which of the following is false regarding methods used to build the ICD-10-PCS codes?
    a. The Index must always be consulted.
    b. All seven characters must have values associated with them.
    c. The code tables must always be referenced.
    d. Values can have different meanings in a given body system.

    Guideline _____

3. The patient has a biopsy of the colon followed by a hemicolectomy. Which procedure(s) is(are) coded?
    a. The hemicolectomy only
    b. The biopsy only
    c. Both the biopsy and the hemicolectomy
    d. It depends on the results of the biopsy

    Guideline _____

4. The patient has a cerebral aneurysm that is treated with an endovascular coil to narrow the lumen. What root operation is used for this procedure?
    a. Insertion
    b. Restriction
    c. Bypass
    d. Occlusion

    Guideline _____

5. Refer to the 0CQ table that follows. Which of the following codes would be considered invalid?
    a. 0CQ3XZZ
    b. 0CQ80ZZ
    c. 0CQ9XZZ
    d. 0CQWXZ2

    Guideline _____

Section	0 Medical and Surgical
Body System	C Mouth and Throat
Operation	Q Repair: Restoring, to the extent possible, a body part to its normal anatomic structure and function

Body Part	Approach	Device	Qualifier
0 Upper Lip 1 Lower Lip 2 Hard Palate 3 Soft Palate 4 Buccal Mucosa 5 Upper Gingiva 6 Lower Gingiva 7 Tongue N Uvula P Tonsils Q Adenoids	0 Open 3 Percutaneous X External	Z No Device	Z No Qualifier
8 Parotid Gland, Right 9 Parotid Gland, Left B Parotid Duct, Right C Parotid Duct, Left D Sublingual Gland, Right F Sublingual Gland, Left G Submaxillary Gland, Right H Submaxillary Gland, Left J Minor Salivary Gland	0 Open 3 Percutaneous	Z No Device	Z No Qualifier
M Pharynx R Epiglottis S Larynx T Vocal Cord, Right V Vocal Cord, Left	0 Open 3 Percutaneous 4 Percutaneous Endoscopic 7 Via Natural or Artificial Opening 8 Via Natural or Artificial Opening Endoscopic	Z No Device	Z No Qualifier
W Upper Tooth X Lower Tooth	0 Open X External	Z No Device	0 Single 1 Multiple 2 All

6. The patient was scheduled for a laparoscopic excision of her appendix. Due to excessive abdominal adhesions, this was converted to an open removal of the appendix. How is the appendectomy coded?
   a. As an open excision of the appendix
   b. As an open resection of the appendix
   c. As an open resection and percutaneous endoscopic inspection of the appendix
   d. As a percutaneous endoscopic resection of the appendix

   Guideline _____

(Continued)

7. The patient has a vertebral joint fusion with both autologous and nonautologous bone graft material. Which value is used for the device?
    a. Both autologous and nonautologous tissue substitute
    b. Only the autologous tissue substitute
    c. Only the nonautologous tissue substitute
    d. No device value is assigned

    Guideline _____

8. Which of the following body part designations is incorrect for procedures performed on the skin overlying a joint?
    a. Ankle is coded to Foot
    b. Shoulder is coded to Upper Arm
    c. Knee is coded to Upper Leg
    d. Elbow is coded to Lower Arm

    Guideline _____

9. What body part is the line of demarcation for the upper and lower body parts in the muscles body system?
    a. Stomach
    b. Kidneys
    c. Diaphragm
    d. Umbilicus

    Guideline _____

10. The patient has a percutaneous transluminal angioplasty of three coronary arteries, with one of the arteries treated with two drug-eluting stents, one with a bare metal stent, and one without a stent. Which of the following is the correct coding for this case?
    a. Three codes, one with the two drug-eluting stents, one with intraluminal device placed, and one without a stent
    b. One code because these are all coronary arteries
    c. Two codes, one to represent the arteries with stents, and the other for the artery without a stent
    d. Two codes, both with stent placement, because these are all coronary arteries

    Guideline _____

Case Studies

The following operative reports are being used for ICD-10-PCS coding. Review each document and answer the questions that follow.

1. Operative Report

PREOPERATIVE DIAGNOSIS: Biliary colic

POSTOPERATIVE DIAGNOSIS: Biliary colic

OPERATIVE PROCEDURE: 1. Laparoscopic Cholecystectomy with intraoperative cholangiogram
2. Tru-Cut liver biopsy

ANESTHESIA:	General
DRAINS:	None
COMPLICATIONS:	None
ESTIMATED BLOOD LOSS:	Minimal

DETAILS: After the induction of general anesthesia, the patient's abdomen was prepped and draped sterilely. A small supraumbilical incision was created. The abdomen was entered. The peritoneal cavity was cannulated with a Veress needle. Position was confirmed with the drop test. The abdomen was insufflated to 250 mmHg with CO_2 gas. A 5-mm trocar was placed under laparoscopic visualization. The laparoscope was introduced. Two 5-mm trocars were placed in the right flank. The patient was placed in reverse Trendelenburg position and rotated to the left. A 10-mm trocar was placed in the epigastrium. The fundus of the gallbladder was then grasped and retracted superolaterally. There were some adhesions in the midbody of the gallbladder that were mobilized away from the gallbladder. The infundibulum of the gallbladder was then grasped and retracted inferolaterally. The peritoneum overlying the cystic duct and cystic artery was then mobilized. The cystic duct and cystic artery were each isolated. Calot triangle was bluntly visualized. The artery was clipped proximally and distally. The duct was clipped to the level of the gallbladder and incised. This was then cannulated with the cholangiocatheter brought in through a separate port for the angiocath. A cholangiogram was obtained in real-time fluoroscopically and demonstrated normal biliary anatomy with free flow in the duodenum and no intraluminal filling defects. The catheter was then removed. The duct was clipped proximally and divided. The artery was divided. The gallbladder was then elevated from the gallbladder fossa with electrocautery. All bleeding points were controlled with electrocautery. There was excellent hemostasis. When the gallbladder dissection was completed, it was placed in an EndoCatch bag and removed through the epigastric trocar site. This was then sent to pathology for evaluation. The trocar was replaced in the right upper quadrant, and it was copiously irrigated until the effluent was clear. The trocars were then removed under laparoscopic visualization. There was excellent hemostasis.

We then took four passes of the Tru-Cut needle to obtain a sample of the liver under direct laparoscopic visualization. The site was then cauterized with good hemostasis. The specimen was placed in formalin and sent for pathologic evaluation. The abdomen was irrigated. There was excellent hemostasis. The trocars were removed under laparoscopic visualization. Hemostasis was excellent. The abdomen was allowed to desufflate. The wounds were infiltrated with local anesthetic and closed with 4-0 Monocryl subcuticular sutures. Benzoin and Steri-strips were applied. A gauze and tape dressing was applied. The patient was then awakened and taken to the postanesthesia care unit in good condition having tolerated the procedure well.

1. a. Based on the documentation, what is the root operation for the gallbladder operation?

    _____

    b. In addition to the intraoperative cholangiogram, how many procedure codes are needed to completely code this case?

    _____

    c. What are the codes for the procedures other than the intraoperative cholangiogram?

    _____

2. Operative Report

PREOPERATIVE DIAGNOSIS: Gangrene left foot

POSTOPERATIVE DIAGNOSIS: Gangrene left foot

OPERATION: Amputation of left 2nd, 3rd, and 4th toes with excisional debridement of left foot

ANESTHESIA: LMA

DESCRIPTION OF OPERATIVE TECHNIQUE: The patient was brought to the operative suite where general LMA anesthesia was induced. The lower leg and foot were widely prepped and draped in sterile fashion. The patient had an extensive area of gangrene involving the dorsum of the left foot. The 3rd and 4th toes were completely gangrenous, and the skin above and on the plantar aspect of the 2nd toe was gangrenous as well. A sharp incision was used to remove all dead tissue at the line of demarcation of what was alive and what was not. The underlying 2nd, 3rd, and 4th metatarsals were involved. The infection was transected somewhat proximally, necessitating complete removal of the 2nd, 3rd, and 4th toes. A portion of the skin of the plantar aspect of the foot was debrided, because the skin was also nonviable. Fortunately, there was good bleeding at the margins of the wound once the necrotic tissue was fully debrided. This was controlled with electrocautery and 1–0 Vicryl LigaSure. The wound was copiously irrigated. Our intention was to treat this initially with a wound vac, but because there was bleeding that was worsened with application of wound vac, this was abandoned, and the patient was treated with Surgicel followed by sterile gauze fluff dressings and an Ace wrap. Throughout the procedure, estimated blood loss was approximately 150 mL. She was transported to the recovery room in overall stable condition and tolerated the procedure well.

2. a.   How many ICD-10-PCS codes are necessary for complete coding of this case?

    _____

    b.   What is (are) the code(s)?

    _____

    c.   Are any guidelines pertinent to the coding of this case?

    _____

    _____

3. Operative Report

PREOPERATIVE DIAGNOSIS: Chronic laryngitis with polypoid disease

POSTOPERATIVE DIAGNOSIS: Same

PROCEDURE: Laryngoscopy with removal of polyps

After adequate premedication, the 60-year-old female patient was taken to the operating room and placed in supine position. The patient was given a general oral endotracheal anesthetic with a small endotracheal tube. The Jako laryngoscope was then inserted. Large polyps were noted on both vocal cords, essentially obstructing the glottic airway when the tube was in place. The polyps appeared larger on the right cord. Using the straight-cup forceps, the polyps were removed from the left cord first. The polyps were removed from the right cord up to the anterior commissure. Very minimal bleeding was noted. This opened up the airway extremely well. The patient was extubated and sent to recovery in good condition.

3. a. How many ICD-10-PCS codes are necessary for complete coding of this case?

    _____

    b. What is (are) the code(s)?

    _____

    c. Are any guidelines pertinent to the coding of this case?

    _____

    _____

Part II

Introduction to the Medical and Surgical Section

Root Operations that Take Out All/Part or Take Out Solids/Fluids/Gases

The ICD-10-PCS system is used to code hospital inpatient procedures, and the majority of codes assigned to these procedures are found in the first section of the system—the Medical and Surgical section. Because codes from this section are so widely used, a great deal of this text concentrates on the Medical and Surgical section. Beginning with this chapter and continuing through chapter 19, the body systems, root operations, and body parts that relate to the Medical and Surgical section will be discussed.

The 1st character of all codes in the Medical and Surgical section of ICD-10-PCS is 0. The Medical and Surgical section of the PCS system is the largest of the 17 sections, with more than 650 code tables. There are just over 300 code tables for all of the other 16 sections of the PCS system.

Coding Tip

The letters O and I are not used in the PCS system, making this 1st character for the Medical and Surgical section a zero, not a letter O. Practicing the pronunciation of the word "zero" for the 0 character instead of "oh" will help minimize substitution errors.

Character Descriptions

As with all PCS codes, the Medical and Surgical section codes have seven characters. In this section, the characters represent the section, body system, root operation, body part, approach, device, and qualifier. See chapter 1 of this text for an extensive review of each of these characters as they relate to all of the sections of ICD-10-PCS.

For the 2nd character, the Medical and Surgical section has a total of 31 body systems. Some of these body systems are those that are typically regarded as a body system. For example, the Respiratory System is one of the 31 body systems, as is the Endocrine System. However, some of the systems are subdivided into smaller components. For example, what is generally thought of as the Circulatory System in total is broken down into five body systems: the Heart and Great Vessels, Upper Arteries, Lower Arteries, Upper Veins, and Lower Veins. See table 1.2 for a comprehensive list of the body systems in the Medical and Surgical section.

While the body system is reflected in the 2nd character of the PCS code, the specific body part is designated in the 4th character. The body part character is always in context with the body system. For example, in the Upper Arteries body system, the 0 value indicates the right internal mammary artery, while in the Upper Veins body system, the 0 indicates the azygos vein.

Extensive information on each of the body systems and their corresponding body parts is found in chapters 7 through 19 of this text.

Root Operation

The character that comes between the body system and body part is the root operation. This 3rd character for root operation designates the objective of the procedure.

To correctly build an ICD-10-PCS code, the coding professional must first select the correct root operation to arrive at the correct code table. Along with 0 for the Medical and Surgical section, and the second character for the body system, the third character for the root operation completes the first three characters of the code, which determines the code table. The coding professional begins by reviewing and analyzing clinical documentation to translate the operation performed into the applicable root operation designation. The remainder of the ICD-10-PCS code is built from the code table by analyzing the clinical information to determine the values for the 4th character, the body part; the 5th character, the approach used to complete the procedure; and any applicable devices and qualifiers used for the 6th and 7th character.

There are 31 root operations in the Medical and Surgical section, and the system places these root operations into nine groups based on their common attributes. See tables 1.4 through 1.12 for a complete listing of the nine groups and root operations. This text emphasizes learning the root operations within these groups and applying the definitions in selecting the appropriate root operation. For example, to select a root operation in the group that involves devices from group 6 (Insertion, Removal, Revision, Change, Replacement, and Supplement), the procedure must involve a device. If a device is not a part of the procedure, no root operation from this group may be selected.

It is important to learn and apply the complete definition of each of the root operations. As described in chapter 2 on the ICD-10-PCS Coding Guidelines, the entire definition of the root operation must be applied.

B3.1a. In order to determine the appropriate root operation, the full definition of the root operation as contained in the PCS tables must be applied.

Root operations for the Medical and Surgical section will be thoroughly discussed within their groups in chapters 3 through 6 of this text. Discussion of root operations for other sections of ICD-10-PCS can be found in chapters 20 through 25.

The first two groups of root operations in the Medical and Surgical section both involve a process of taking out: either the body part itself or other matter. These two groups are group 1, Root Operations that Take Out Some or All of a Body Part and group 2, Root Operations that Take Out Solids, Fluids, or Gases from a Body Part.

Group 1: Root Operations that Take Out Some or All of a Body Part

There are five root operations that involve taking out either some or all of a body part: Excision, Resection, Detachment, Destruction, and Extraction. The body part is the focus of the procedure in this group. The five root operations describe the method used to take out some or all of the body part. The differences between the root operations may be the amount of body part that is taken out, for example, all or a portion of a body part, or how the removal is accomplished, for example, by cutting, eradicating, or pulling out the body part. These root operations do not involve replacement of the body part. If there is replacement of all or a portion of the body part then the appropriate root operation, for example Replacement, would be selected. See chapter 5 for further discussion of the root operation Replacement.

Coding Tip

For root operations in Group 1: Excision, Resection, Detachment, Destruction and Extraction that take out some or all of the body part, no replacement of the body part is allowed. If there is a replacement along with the removal, then these root operations do not apply.

Excision

Root Operation

Excision (B): Cutting out or off, without replacement, a portion of a body part.

The first procedure in the group of root operations that take out some or all of a body part is Excision—defined as cutting out or off, without replacement, a portion of a body part. The value of B is used for the Excision root operation in the 3rd character of the ICD-10-PCS code. A key distinction in the Excision root operation is that only a portion of a body part is removed. If the entire body part is removed then Resection is the appropriate root operation, not Excision. Examples of Excision procedures include partial gastrectomy, removal of cysts, and excision of lesions. A cyst or a lesion is a portion of the body part that has transformed in some aberrant way. Removing the lesion or cyst is cutting out or off a portion of the body part; an Excision. Tumors, moles, polyps, and the like are other examples of abnormal parts of an organ or structure that are removed, and these are also coded as Excision procedures.

Excision is the root operation used for excisional biopsies of tissue. If a portion of a body part is cut out or off specifically for diagnostic purposes, this is indicated by using the qualifier value of X in the 7th character. Extraction is the root operation used for endometrial and bone marrow biopsies rather than Excision. This is due to the method used to remove the tissue, which is by pulling or stripping. The Extraction root operation also uses the X qualifier for Diagnostic. These procedures will be discussed under the Extraction root operation later in this chapter.

Excising a portion of the peroneal nerve percutaneously for biopsy would be coded as an Excision with a Diagnostic qualifier. The peroneal nerve is part of the peripheral nervous system and code table 01B is referenced with the H value for the body part and the 3 value for the percutaneous approach. There is no device value available in the table and the X is used for the biopsy; code 01BH3ZX.

Section	Body System	Root Operation	Body Part	Approach	Device	Qualifier
Medical and Surgical	Peripheral Nervous System	Excision	Peroneal Nerve	Percutaneous	No Device	Diagnostic
0	1	B	H	3	Z	X

The X qualifier is only used for procedures such as biopsies, where the intent of the procedure is to remove a portion of the body part for the purpose of analysis. Documentation stating that the tissue was removed and sent to pathology does not indicate that this removal is for diagnostic purposes, as all removed tissue is forwarded to pathology. Either the term "biopsy" should be stated, or the purpose of the removal of a portion of the body part for diagnostic analysis should be specifically noted in the documentation.

Coding Tip

The X qualifier is used in the Excision root operation when the procedure is stated to be a biopsy or if the purpose of the procedure was diagnostic. Documentation that the specimen was sent to Pathology does not equate to a diagnostic intent as this is standard procedure for all removed tissue.

The Excision procedure can be for therapeutic purposes. If, for example, there was a lesion of the peroneal nerve that was excised by incision, the diagnostic qualifier is not used, and the code is 01BH0ZZ, with 0 for the Open approach at the 5th character and Z for the 7th qualifier value for No Qualifier.

Section	Body System	Root Operation	Body Part	Approach	Device	Qualifier
Medical and Surgical	Peripheral Nervous System	Excision	Peroneal Nerve	Open	No Device	No Qualifier
0	1	B	H	0	Z	Z

The X qualifier is used for biopsies that are Excisions, Extractions and Drainage procedures. The Extraction and Drainage root operations are discussed later in this chapter. Coding guideline B3.4a specifies the root operations that can be coded as biopsies.

B3.4a. Biopsy procedures are coded using the root operations Excision, Extraction, or Drainage and the qualifier Diagnostic.

Example: Fine needle aspiration biopsy of fluid in the lung is coded to the root operation Drainage with the qualifier Diagnostic.

Biopsy of bone marrow is coded to the root operation Extraction with the qualifier Diagnostic. Lymph node sampling for biopsy is coded to the root operation Excision with the qualifier Diagnostic.

If the biopsy is followed by another more definitive procedure, then both the biopsy and the subsequent, definitive, procedure are coded. If the percutaneous peroneal biopsy is followed by a complete removal of this same nerve, then both codes the Excision with the X qualifier and the Resection codes are assigned. This is noted in coding guideline B3.4b.

B3.4b. If a diagnostic Excision, Extraction, or Drainage procedure (biopsy) is followed by a more definitive procedure, such as Destruction, Excision, or Resection at the same procedure site, both the biopsy and the more definitive treatment are coded.

Example: For a biopsy of the breast followed by partial mastectomy at the same procedure site, both the biopsy and the partial mastectomy are coded.

An excision may be performed in conjunction with another procedure. For example, the harvesting of an autograft from a different procedure site is an excision of that body part and is coded as a separate procedure. This harvesting code is reported along with the code for the other procedure. For example, the excision of a portion of the iliac bone to be used as bone graft material in a spinal fusion would have a separate Excision code assigned as this harvesting is accomplished from a separate procedural site. However, if a portion of the vertebrae was used for this bone graft in the spinal fusion, the Excision would not be coded because the bone is harvested from the same operative site as the fusion procedure. This is noted in coding guideline B3.9.

B3.9. If an autograft is obtained from a different procedure site in order to complete the objective of the procedure, a separate procedure is coded.

Example: Coronary bypass with excision of saphenous vein graft, excision of saphenous vein is coded separately.

Excisional debridement is coded to the Excision root operation, while nonexcisional debridement is coded as an Extraction, discussed later in this chapter. Specific documentation of excisional debridement is critical as there is no default root operation for debridement. The use of particular instruments does not qualify the procedure as excisional debridement. If more than one layer of the body is involved in the excisional debridement, the deepest layer is used for the body system. This is noted in Coding Guideline B3.5.

B3.5. If the root operations Excision, Repair or Inspection are performed on overlapping layers of the musculoskeletal system, the body part specifying the deepest layer is coded.

Example: Excisional debridement that includes skin and subcutaneous tissue and muscle is coded to the muscle body part.

Resection

Root Operation

Resection (T): Cutting out or off, without replacement, all of a body part.

The next root operation in group 1 is Resection, which is defined as cutting out or off, without replacement, all of a body part. Examples of the root operation Resection are a total mastectomy, lobectomy of the lung, and appendectomy. This is in contrast to Excision, where only a portion of the body part is taken out. The Resection root operation has the value of T in the 3rd character.

The term "body part" in the root operation definition refers to an individual body part (4th character) named within a particular body system (2nd character) in ICD-10-PCS. Many body part names are those commonly thought of as body parts in anatomy. Other body parts are subdivided into more detailed body part names within the ICD-10-PCS system. For example, the lung is generally thought of as a body part. However, in ICD-10-PCS, the Respiratory System has nine possible body part values for unique areas of the lung, including one for each lung, one for bilateral lung body part, and six for specific sites in either the right or left lung as follows:

C   Upper Lung Lobe, Right
D   Middle Lung Lobe, Right
F   Lower Lung Lobe, Right
G   Upper Lung Lobe, Left
H   Lung Lingula
J   Lower Lung Lobe, Left
K   Lung, Right
L   Lung, Left
M   Lungs, Bilateral

These body part values must be taken in context when selecting the appropriate root operation. If the entire body part is removed, this is a Resection. If only a portion of the body part is removed, Excision is the appropriate root operation. This is emphasized in the Coding Guideline B3.8.

B3.8.   PCS contains specific body parts for anatomical subdivisions of a body part, such as lobes of the lungs or liver and regions of the intestine. Resection of the specific body part is coded whenever all of the body part is cut out or off, rather than coding Excision of a less specific body part.

Example: Left upper lung lobectomy is coded to Resection of Upper Lung Lobe, Left rather than to Excision of Lung, Left.

Using the respiratory system and the lung as an example, removal of the left lower lobe of the lung is coded as a Resection, as the left lower lobe of the lung has its own body part value. However, if only part of the lobe was removed, Excision is the appropriate root operation.

For an open removal of the left lower lobe of the lung the code is 0BTJ0ZZ.

Section	Body System	Root Operation	Body Part	Approach	Device	Qualifier
Medical and Surgical	Respiratory System	Resection	Lower Lung Lobe, Left	Open	No Device	No Qualifier
0	B	T	J	0	Z	Z

However, if only a part of the left lower lung lobe is excised via incision, Excision is the root operation, and the code is 0BBJ0ZZ.

Section	Body System	Root Operation	Body Part	Approach	Device	Qualifier
Medical and Surgical	Respiratory System	Excision	Lower Lung Lobe, Left	Open	No Device	No Qualifier
0	B	B	J	0	Z	Z

If the Excision or Resection was preceded by a biopsy of the tissue of the left lower lobe, performed via bronchoscopy, the code is 0BBJ8ZX. Note that the qualifier X is not an available value for Resection procedures as the entire body part would not be removed to perform a biopsy or for other diagnostic purposes. The intent of Resection is therapeutic.

Section	Body System	Root Operation	Body Part	Approach	Device	Qualifier
Medical and Surgical	Respiratory System	Excision	Lower Lung Lobe, Left	Via Natural or Artificial Opening, Endoscopic	No Device	Diagnostic
0	B	B	J	8	Z	X

In the Lymphatic and Hemic Systems body system there are body part values for lymph nodes for both Excision and Resection root operations. For example, value 5 for right axillary lymphatic. The entire lymph node chain is considered a body part. Level is another term used for chain. Therefore, if an entire lymph node chain or level is removed, Resection is the root operation because the entire body part is removed. However, when only some of the lymph nodes in the chain are removed, as in a sentinel node sampling, the appropriate root operation is Excision. If the documentation states that there is a "radical" resection, it must be clear that this refers to the lymph node chain or level to code resection of the lymph node body part. A query may be necessary.

For example, if the entire lymph node chain in the right axillary area is removed via incision, the correct code is 07T50ZZ.

Section	Body System	Root Operation	Body Part	Approach	Device	Qualifier
Medical and Surgical	Lymphatic and Hemic System	Resection	Right Axillary	Open	No Device	No Qualifier
0	7	T	5	0	Z	Z

However, if several of the lymph nodes in the axillary area are removed by incision, but the entire chain is not excised, the correct code is 07B50ZZ.

Section	Body System	Root Operation	Body Part	Approach	Device	Qualifier
Medical and Surgical	Lymphatic and Hemic System	Excision	Right Axillary	Open	No Device	No Qualifier
0	7	B	5	0	Z	Z

Coding Tip

When an entire lymph node chain is cut out, the appropriate root operation is Resection. When only some of the lymph nodes are cut out, the root operation is Excision. Physicians may refer to a lymph node chain as a lymph node level. Level and chain are synonymous.

The definitions for the root operations Excision and Resection are identical, other than Excision stating a portion and Resection stating all of a body part is being cut out or off without replacement. The distinguishing factor is whether the entire body part or only a portion is being removed. This is in context with the body parts. For example, in the gastrointestinal system there are body parts for the large intestine, large intestine right and left, as well as the cecum, ascending, descending and sigmoid colon and rectum. If any of these body parts are taken out in their entirety a Resection is coded, while removal of only a portion of the body part would be an Excision. Reviewing the Resection table for a given body system will help in determining whether the Excision or Resection root operation is applicable; if the body part is listed in the Resection table it by definition has its own body part and its complete removal would be a Resection. Review the 0DT table and note the body parts listed.

Detachment

Root Operation

Detachment (6): Cutting off all or part of the upper or lower extremities.

The next root operation in group 1 is Detachment—defined as cutting off all or a part of the upper or lower extremities. Amputations, such as disarticulations of the shoulder and above-the-knee amputations, are coded with the value of 6 for Detachment procedures. Because the Detachment procedure only refers to the upper and lower extremities, codes for Detachment are found in two body systems; X for Anatomical Regions, Upper Extremities and Y for Anatomical Regions, Lower Extremities. The amputations are performed across overlapping body layers rather than only through the bones or muscles. Therefore, the body system for the Anatomical Regions of the applicable extremity is more appropriate than individual, specific body systems.

Coding Tip

Anatomical Regions Upper Extremities and Anatomical Regions Lower Extremities body systems are applicable for Detachment procedures. Code tables 0X6 for upper extremities or 0Y6 for lower extremities are the only code tables available for building Detachment procedure codes.

The body part character for Detachment procedures is selected depending on the site of the amputation. For example, refer to table 3.1, the 0X6 table. If the upper portion of the right arm is detached, the value of 8 is selected for the body part, making the first four characters of the code 0X68. Refer to table 3.2, the 0Y6 table. If the left foot is detached, the value of N is selected for the body part, making the first four

Table 3.1. 0X6 table

Section	0	Medical and Surgical		
Body System	X	Anatomical Regions, Upper Extremities		
Operation	6	Detachment: Cutting off all or a portion of the upper or lower extremities		

Body Part	Approach	Device	Qualifier
0 Forequarter, Right 1 Forequarter, Left 2 Shoulder Region, Right 3 Shoulder Region, Left B Elbow Region, Right C Elbow Region, Left	0 Open	Z No Device	Z No Qualifier
8 Upper Arm, Right 9 Upper Arm, Left D Lower Arm, Right F Lower Arm, Left	0 Open	Z No Device	1 High 2 Mid 3 Low
J Hand, Right K Hand, Left	0 Open	Z No Device	0 Complete 4 Complete 1st Ray 5 Complete 2nd Ray 6 Complete 3rd Ray 7 Complete 4th Ray 8 Complete 5th Ray 9 Partial 1st Ray B Partial 2nd Ray C Partial 3rd Ray D Partial 4th Ray F Partial 5th Ray
L Thumb, Right M Thumb, Left N Index Finger, Right P Index Finger, Left Q Middle Finger, Right R Middle Finger, Left S Ring Finger, Right T Ring Finger, Left V Little Finger, Right W Little Finger, Left	0 Open	Z No Device	0 Complete 1 High 2 Mid 3 Low

Source: CMS 2019

Table 3.2. 0Y6 table

Section	0	Medical and Surgical		
Body System	Y	Anatomical Regions, Lower Extremities		
Operation	6	Detachment: Cutting off all or a portion of the upper or lower extremities		
Body Part		**Approach**	**Device**	**Qualifier**
2 Hindquarter, Right 3 Hindquarter, Left 4 Hindquarter, Bilateral 7 Femoral Region, Right 8 Femoral Region, Left F Knee Region, Right G Knee Region, Left		0 Open	Z No Device	Z No Qualifier
C Upper Leg, Right D Upper Leg, Left H Lower Leg, Right J Lower Leg, Left		0 Open	Z No Device	1 High 2 Mid 3 Low
M Foot, Right N Foot, Left		0 Open	Z No Device	0 Complete 4 Complete 1st Ray 5 Complete 2nd Ray 6 Complete 3rd Ray 7 Complete 4th Ray 8 Complete 5th Ray 9 Partial 1st Ray B Partial 2nd Ray C Partial 3rd Ray D Partial 4th Ray F Partial 5th Ray
P 1st Toe, Right Q 1st Toe, Left R 2nd Toe, Right S 2nd Toe, Left T 3rd Toe, Right U 3rd Toe, Left V 4th Toe, Right W 4th Toe, Left X 5th Toe, Right Y 5th Toe, Left		0 Open	Z No Device	0 Complete 1 High 2 Mid 3 Low

Source: CMS 2019

characters of the code 0Y6N. The only possible approach for Detachment procedures is Open, with the value of 0. The device character is not applicable; therefore, the Z is the value for the 6th character. Assigning the 7th character qualifier for the Detachment root operation requires specific definitions because the qualifier indicates the portion of the body part that is amputated. In some cases, the qualifier is not defined and the Z value is selected because the entire body part is amputated.

Refer to the first row of the 0X6 and 0Y6 tables. Note that in the 0X6 code table, the body parts forequarter right and left are listed. This describes the entire upper limb as well as the scapula and clavicle. The shoulder and elbow regions for each side describe amputations that take place at that joint level of the extremity. In the first row of code table 0Y6 the hindquarter body parts right and left are listed and describe the entire lower limb, including all of the pelvic girdle and the buttock. Also listed is the right and left femoral regions, where amputation is at the very top of the femur as well as the right and left knee regions and which includes removal of all of the lower leg at the knee joint. Amputations at these levels are rare, and since the body parts described are completely removed, no qualifier is applicable and only Z for No Qualifier is available in this first row.

Review the second row in each of the detachment tables in code tables 0X6 and 0Y6. Note that the upper and lower arm, right and left, is in the 0X6 table and right and left upper and lower leg in the 0Y6 table. Qualifiers available for these rows are high, mid, or low. These qualifiers are defined as

- **High**—Amputation at the proximal portion of the shaft of the humerus, lower arm, femur, or lower leg
- **Mid**—Amputation at the middle portion of the shaft of the humerus, lower arm, femur, or lower leg
- **Low**—Amputation at the distal portion of the shaft of the humerus, lower arm, femur, or lower leg

In our example of amputation of the upper portion of the right arm, if this detachment was made in the distal portion of the humerus the complete code is 0X680Z3 as the detachment qualifies as low.

The third row of the tables is for the hands in 0X6 and feet in 0Y6. Qualifier value 0 is for Complete Detachment is defined as follows:

- **Complete**—Amputation through the carpometacarpal joint of the hand, or through the tarsometatarsal joint of the foot

A carpometacarpal joint amputation of the right hand, for example, would be coded as 0X6J0Z0 because the definition of complete includes the carpometacarpal joint.

Section	Body System	Root Operation	Body Part	Approach	Device	Qualifier
Medical and Surgical	Anatomical Regions, Upper Extremities	Detachment	Hand, Right	Open	No Device	Complete
0	X	6	J	0	Z	0

Some terms may need further study to determine the correct code. For example, a mid-foot or Lisfranc joint amputation is documented. Research shows that the Lisfranc joint is the tarsometatarsal joint and, therefore, detachment took place at the tarsometatarsal joint. Note that the definition of complete amputation of the foot is defined as being at the level of the tarsal-metatarsal joint, which is included in this description. If a mid-foot, or Lisfranc, amputation was completed on the right side, it would be coded as 0Y6M0Z0 because this is a tarsometatarsal amputation.

Section	Body System	Root Operation	Body Part	Approach	Device	Qualifier
Medical and Surgical	Anatomical Regions, Lower Extremities	Detachment	Foot, Right	Open	No Device	Complete
0	Y	6	M	0	Z	0

A partial amputation of a hand or foot is defined as amputation anywhere along the shaft or head of the metacarpal bone of the hand or of the metatarsal bone of the foot. In the third row of the detachment tables, note the qualifiers for the hands and feet, with partial amputation defined based on the individual rays and whether amputation was complete or partial:

- Qualifier 0 Complete
- Qualifier 4 Complete 1st Ray
- Qualifier 5 Complete 2nd Ray
- Qualifier 6 Complete 3rd Ray
- Qualifier 7 Complete 4th Ray
- Qualifier 8 Complete 5th Ray
- Qualifier 9 Partial 1st Ray
- Qualifier B Partial 2nd Ray
- Qualifier C Partial 3rd Ray
- Qualifier D Partial 4th Ray
- Qualifier F Partial 5th Ray

The term "ray" is used to designate the fingers and associated metacarpals and toes and associated metatarsals. A ray of the hand consists of the continuous grouping of a metacarpal and phalanx associated with one finger. Chapter 7 of this text includes additional information on the detachment procedure, and figure 7.3

depicts the rays of the hand, including the metacarpals and phalanges. A ray of the foot consists of the continuous grouping of a metatarsal and phalanx associated with one toe. Figure 3.1 depicts the rays of the foot, including the metatarsals and phalanges.

Figure 3.1. Rays of the foot

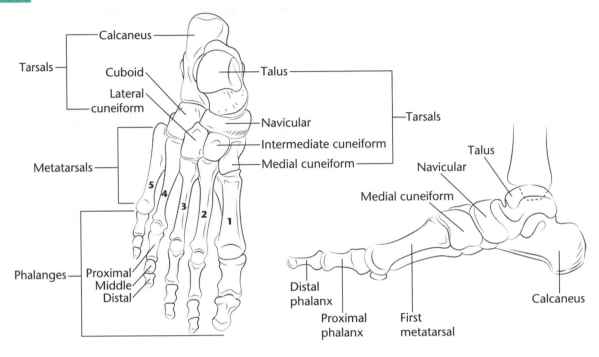

© AHIMA 2019

The first ray consists of the thumb and first metacarpal in the hand or the great toe and first metatarsal in the foot. The same designation is made for the second ray, index finger and associated metacarpal of the hand and second toe and metatarsal of the foot; third ray, middle finger and associated metacarpal of the hand and third toe and metatarsal of the foot; fourth ray, ring finger and associated metacarpal of the hand and fourth toe and metatarsal of the foot; and fifth ray, little finger and associated metacarpal of the hand and little toe and metatarsal of the foot.

If the entire metacarpal and finger of the hand or metatarsal and toe are amputated, this is considered a complete ray. For example, a complete detachment of the ring finger and associated metacarpal of the left hand constitutes a complete 4th ray detachment and would be coded 0X6K0Z7. If the detachment took place anywhere along the shaft or head of the metacarpal bone of the ring finger, this would be considered a partial 4th ray detachment and the qualifier value would be D in code 0X6K0ZD.

Section	Body System	Root Operation	Body Part	Approach	Device	Qualifier
Medical and Surgical	Anatomical Regions, Upper Extremities	Detachment	Hand, Left	Open	No Device	Complete 4th Ray
0	X	6	K	0	Z	7

The last row of the detachment tables is for the thumbs and fingers in the 0X6 table and toes in the 0Y6 table. The qualifiers for the thumb, finger, or toe are defined as:

- **Qualifier 0—Complete:** Amputation at the metacarpophalangeal/metatarsal-phalangeal joint
- **Qualifier 1—High:** Amputation anywhere along the proximal phalanx

- **Qualifier 2—Mid:** Amputation through the proximal interphalangeal joint or anywhere along the middle phalanx
- **Qualifier 3—Low:** Amputation through the distal interphalangeal joint or anywhere along the distal phalanx

Using these qualifiers, if the amputation was of the left third or middle finger at the metacarpophalangeal joint, this would be considered a complete detachment of the finger and the 0 value would be selected for the qualifier for the complete code 0X6R0Z0. If, instead, this amputation was made through the distal phalanx of the left third finger, this would be a low amputation and the qualifier value would be 3 for the complete code 0X6R0Z3. If more than one finger was amputated, an additional code would be listed for that body part and qualifier.

As with all coding in ICD-10-PCS, it is important to carefully review the complete documentation and apply the definitions of the system when building a code. For example, if the surgeon uses the word "toe" to describe the amputation, but the operative report says the amputation extends to the midshaft of the 5th metatarsal, the qualifier selected would be partial 5th ray, as the definition for partial amputation is anywhere along the shaft or head of the metatarsal bone of the foot. Careful review of the operative report is necessary to determine the correct qualifier. Be sure to research any procedure that is unfamiliar to assure correct coding. A query may be necessary if the specific site of detachment cannot be determined. More information about detachment procedures is provided in chapter 7 of this text.

Destruction

Root Operation

Destruction (5): Physical eradication of all or a portion of a body part by the direct use of energy, force, or a destructive agent

The next root operation in group 1 is Destruction, defined as physical eradication of all or a portion of a body part by the direct use of energy, force, or a destructive agent. The value of 5 is used for Destruction procedures. This root operation represents a wide range of procedures performed at a variety of body sites. Included here are destruction of aberrant tissue such as warts, polyps, varices, and other lesions. Recall that this aberrant tissue is considered to be a portion of the body part.

None of the body part is cut out in Destruction root operations, though in some cases a small amount of tissue may be left in instruments used to complete the destruction procedure. Either the complete body part or a portion is obliterated via the procedure. Terms such as coagulation, cryotherapy, or fulguration may be used to describe destruction procedures.

Another term used for destruction is coblation. Coblation uses radiofrequency power to disintegrate the aberrant portions of the body part while minimizing the damage to surrounding tissue. All of these terms are coded as Destruction in ICD-10-PCS (DeNoon 2005).

For example, a Destruction root operation is coded for radiofrequency needle ablation of endometrial fibroids. Research on the term Ablation indicates that this is a type of destruction. Using the CMS file method, the body system for female reproductive system is selected, followed by selection of the root operation of Destruction. If using a code book and referring to the Index, the main term Ablation has a cross-reference to "See Destruction." Under the main term Destruction, subterm Endometrium, the 0U5B characters are given. In either method the 0U5 table is selected, with the B for the endometrium body part is located in the second row of the table. Note that in this table there are no values for Device or Qualifier. The approach is the only other character that requires definition. Because this was a Destruction procedure performed via a needle there was a puncture made to reach the operative site, and the Percutaneous approach is selected. The code for this procedure is 0U5B3ZZ.

Section	Body System	Root Operation	Body Part	Approach	Device	Qualifier
Medical and Surgical	Female Reproductive System	Destruction	Endometrium	Percutaneous	No Device	No Qualifier
0	U	5	B	3	Z	Z

Coding Tip

A small nick in the skin, for example, to accommodate a radiofrequency needle for a Destruction procedure, does not constitute an open approach. Because the needle is advanced all the way to the operative site, the correct approach value is Percutaneous.

Extraction

Root Operation

Extraction (D): Pulling or stripping out or off all or a portion of a body part by use of force.

The final root operation in group 1 is Extraction, pulling or stripping out or off all or a portion of a body part by the use of force. The value of D is used as the 3rd character value for Extraction.

In contrast to the Destruction root operation, which eradicates the body part or a portion of the body part that has aberrant tissue or lesions, the Extraction root operation uses force to complete the objective of the procedure, which is to pull or strip out all or a portion of the body part. This is also distinguished from Excision and Resection, where cutting is used to remove all or a portion of the body part, though minor cutting may be necessary to reach the site of the Extraction operation.

Coding Tip

Minor cutting, such as that used in vein-stripping procedures, is included in Extraction if the objective of the procedure is met by pulling or stripping. The approach character includes any cutting used to get to the operative site.

Examples of Extraction procedures include liposuction for medical purposes or dilation and curettage (D&C). In the D&C procedure, the dilation of the cervix is not the objective of the procedure but rather the method used to gain access to the procedural site. The curettage is the objective, in which scraping and suction is used to remove tissue for therapeutic or diagnostic purposes. Tooth extraction is another example of the Extraction root operation. Cataract surgery involves stripping the lens of the eye, which is an Extraction procedure. Note that only cataract surgery that does not involve the insertion of an intraocular lens (IOL) prosthesis is coded as an Extraction procedure. If the IOL is inserted, this is a device and the procedure meets the definition of a Replacement procedure and the Extraction becomes integral to the procedure. See chapter 5 for a discussion of Replacement procedures. Nonexcisional debridement is coded as an Extraction, while excisional debridement is coded as an Excision because the tissue is surgically cut and removed. In contrast, nonexcisional debridement involves pulling or stripping away the devitalized or contaminated tissue. This nonexcisional debridement may be accomplished by use of equipment such as a Versajet and may be described as waterjet, hydrosurgery, wet-to-dry dressing changes, or mechanical debridement. Note that the nonexcisional debridement should be coded to the deepest layer involved. Extraction code tables are available in many of the body systems, including the Lymphatic and Hemic Systems (07D), Respiratory System (0BD), Gastrointestinal System (0DD), Hepatobiliary System and Pancreas (0FD), skin and Breast Body System (0HD), Subcutaneous Tissue and Fascia (0JD), Muscles (0KD), Tendons (0LD), Bursae And ligaments (0MD), Head and Facial Bones (0ND), Upper Bones (0PD), and Lower Bones (0QD).

Bone marrow and endometrial biopsies involve removal of the tissue by pulling or stripping and therefore this removal meets the definition of Extraction rather than Excision. Since the intent of the Extraction is for diagnostic purposes, a biopsy, the X is used for the qualifier. For example, a D&C with biopsy of the endometrium would be coded 0UDB7ZX.

Section	Body System	Root Operation	Body Part	Approach	Device	Qualifier
Medical and Surgical	Female Reproductive System	Extraction	Endometrium	Via Natural or Artificial Opening	No Device	Diagnostic
0	U	D	B	7	Z	X

Note that not all Extraction tables have an X qualifier available. For example, reference code table 00D for Extraction in the Central Nervous System and Cranial Nerves. Only the Z for No Qualifier is available.

Coding Tip

Bone marrow and endometrial biopsies remove tissue by pulling or stripping and are coded as Extraction root operations with the Diagnostic qualifier rather than as an Excision with a Diagnostic qualifier.

Group 2: Root Operations that Take Out Solids/Fluids/Gases from a Body Part

There are three root operations in group 2 that are involved in taking out solids, fluids, or gases from a body part: Drainage, Extirpation, and Fragmentation. All three of these root operations are performed within the body part and involve either taking or letting out fluids, gases, or solid matter or breaking this solid matter into pieces. In these root operations the focus is not on the body part, as was the case with Excision, Resection, Detachment, Destruction, and Extraction. Instead the focus is on something that should not be present, such as a foreign body, clot, excess fluid, or solid matter.

Coding Tip

The focus of the root operations in Group 2; Drainage, Extirpation and Fragmentation is not the body part, but rather something around the body part that should not be present, such as fluid or a blood clot.

Drainage

Root Operation

Drainage (9): Taking or letting out fluids and/or gases from a body part.

The first root operation in group 2 is Drainage, which is taking or letting out fluids and/or gases from a body part. The value of 9 is used for Drainage. In these procedures, the emphasis is not on the body part itself, but rather the fluids or gases within the body part. Examples are incision and drainage of an abscess, chest tube insertion for removal of pleural effusion, and arthrotomy for fluid drainage.

Drainage procedures can be diagnostic biopsies. Just as with the Excisional biopsies and Extractions for biopsy purposes, the qualifier value of X is assigned for Diagnostic to indicate that the Drainage procedure is performed as a diagnostic biopsy. A thoracentesis with removal of fluid in the right pleural cavity, with the fluid sent to pathology to test for metastasis of a cancerous tumor, would be coded as a diagnostic Drainage. Using the CMS file or the code book index, the main term Thoracentesis has a cross reference to "See Drainage, Anatomical Regions, General, 0W9." The General Anatomical Region is selected because the pleural cavity is the body cavity rather than a more specific body part. Use of the General Anatomical Region body systems is outlined in Coding Guideline B2.1a.

B2.1.a. The procedure codes in the general anatomical regions body systems can be used when the procedure is performed on an anatomical region rather than a specific body part (e.g., root operations Control and Detachment, Drainage of a body cavity) or on the rare occasion when no information is available to support assignment of a code to a specific body part.

Example: Control of postoperative hemorrhage is coded to the root operation Control found in the general anatomical regions body systems. Chest tube drainage of the pleural cavity is coded to the root operation Drainage found in the general anatomical regions body systems. Suture repair of the abdominal wall is coded to the root operation Repair in the general anatomical regions body system.

The body part value for the pleural cavity is either the right or the left side; a general pleural cavity value or an unspecified selection is not available. If the information on the specific side was not immediately available, the documentation is carefully reviewed to determine the side of the body involved. If this review still does not provide the information, the provider should be queried. The importance of the complete code is emphasized in Coding Guideline A8.

A8. All seven characters must contain valid values to be a valid procedure code. If the documentation is incomplete for coding purposes, the physician should be queried for the necessary information.

If the right pleural cavity was specified for the thoracentesis, the value of 9 is selected for the body part. Because the procedure is performed via a needle, the percutaneous approach is selected. There is no device, and the Diagnostic qualifier is selected to indicate that this is a biopsy. The code is 0W993ZX.

Section	Body System	Root Operation	Body Part	Approach	Device	Qualifier
Medical and Surgical	Anatomical Regions, General	Drainage	Pleural Cavity, Right	Percutaneous	No Device	Diagnostic
0	W	9	9	3	Z	X

Another type of diagnostic drainage is a lumbar puncture or tap to test the fluid for any abnormalities or infection, such as meningitis. In this procedure, the fluid is drained from the spinal canal using a needle. The cerebrospinal fluid is not body part per se, but fluid around the body part, so Drainage is the correct root operation. Since this is a diagnostic procedure, the X is used for the qualifier. The code would be 009U3ZX.

Note that the term biopsy must be further studied to determine the correct root operation. If fluid is aspirated, this is from around the body part and Drainage is the correct root operation with the qualifier X for diagnostic. However, if tissue is involved, this is a portion of the body part that is being removed and studied. Therefore, Excision is the correct root operation with the qualifier X.

Coding Tip

The only three root operations that can have an X as a qualifier for Diagnostic are Excision, Extraction, and Drainage, all for biopsy procedures.

The drainage procedure can also be performed for therapeutic purposes. When the drainage is accomplished by putting in a tube that remains in the patient after the procedure is completed, the value of 0 for Drainage Device is selected for the 6th character. Note that a drainage procedure that includes a drainage device cannot be coded as diagnostic because there is not an X qualifier available in that row. Reference the 009 table for Drainage of the Central Nervous System and Cranial Nerves Body System and locate the two rows available, one with a 0 for device and only the Z value available for the qualifier and the other with a Z for No Device and the two options of X for Diagnostic and Z for No Qualifier for the 7th character. Drainage procedures with a drainage device left in place are therapeutic rather than diagnostic.

For example, percutaneous drainage of peritoneal ascites with a drainage tube that is left in place. Using the CMS file method, the term peritoneal cavity can be searched in the file, with the body system of Anatomical Regions, General located, and the root operation Drainage referenced. Using the index in a code book, the main term Drainage with a subterm of peritoneal cavity is located and the characters of 0W9G are listed. In either case the 0W9 table is referenced. See table 3.3. The value of 3 is selected for the percutaneous approach and the value of 0 is used for the drainage device. The value of Z is used for the qualifier as this is a therapeutic procedure versus a diagnostic Drainage procedure. The code is 0W9G30Z. Because the procedure includes a drainage device that is left in place, the code is built from the first row of the 0W9 table that includes the drainage device in the 6th character. In this row the only value available for the qualifier is Z for No Qualifier.

Section	Body System	Root Operation	Body Part	Approach	Device	Qualifier
Medical and Surgical	Anatomical Regions, General	Drainage	Peritoneal Cavity	Percutaneous	Drainage Device	No Qualifier
0	W	9	G	3	0	Z

Table 3.3. 0W9 table—first row

Section	0	Medical and Surgical		
Body System	W	Anatomical Regions, General		
Operation	9	Drainage: Taking or letting out fluids and/or gases from a body part		

Body Part	Approach	Device	Qualifier
0 Head 1 Cranial Cavity 2 Face 3 Oral Cavity and Throat 4 Upper Jaw 5 Lower Jaw 6 Neck 8 Chest Wall 9 Pleural Cavity, Right B Pleural Cavity, Left C Mediastinum D Pericardial Cavity F Abdominal Wall G Peritoneal Cavity H Retroperitoneum J Pelvic Cavity K Upper Back L Lower Back M Perineum, Male N Perineum, Female	0 Open 3 Percutaneous 4 Percutaneous Endoscopic	0 Drainage Device	Z No Qualifier

Source: CMS 2019

Extirpation

Root Operation

Extirpation (C): Taking or cutting out solid matter from a body part.

The next root operation in group 2 is Extirpation, taking or cutting out solid matter from a body part. The value of C is used for Extirpation. The solid matter that is taken out of the body part may be an abnormal by-product of a biological function, for example, a blood clot, hematoma, or thrombus. It may also be a foreign body, for example, pieces of glass. It may be embedded in a body part or the lumen of a tubular body part, such as a piece of shrapnel implanted in the subcutaneous tissue of the upper arm or a plaque deposit in an artery. In any of these cases, the solid matter is not body part itself, but rather the solid material from the body part.

In Extirpation procedures, the body part itself is not the focus of the procedure; instead, the objective of the root operation is to remove the solid material from the body part. The solid matter may or may not have been previously broken into pieces or fragmented. For example, a kidney stone that was fragmented via lithotripsy that is now extirpated via a stone basket is coded only as an Extirpation. Removal of a cerclage suture is another example of an extirpation because the suture is not a device, but a foreign body that is removed from the cervix.

Extirpation is not a term that is often used by providers. Instead, the composite terms for the procedure, such as thrombectomy, extraction of kidney stone, or endarterectomy, will more likely be found in the documentation. Recall that the provider is not required to use the exact ICD-10-PCS term. Instead, it is the responsibility of the coder to translate the clinical documentation to reflect the ICD-10-PCS terms. This is emphasized in Coding Guideline A11.

A11. Many of the terms used to construct PCS codes are defined within the system. It is the coder's responsibility to determine what the documentation in the medical record equates to in the PCS definitions. The physician is not expected to use the terms used in PCS code descriptions, nor is the coder required to query the physician when the correlation between the documentation and the defined PCS terms is clear.

Example: When the physician documents "partial resection," the coder can independently correlate "partial resection" to the root operation Excision without querying the physician for clarification.

It is not necessary for the provider to document the term "extirpation" to describe a thrombectomy. Instead, the coder would use the definition of this root operation and the procedure performed to determine that a thrombectomy is a type of Extirpation.

For example, to code a percutaneous thrombectomy of the left radial artery using the CMS file, the upper arteries body system is selected from the Medical and Surgical section as the radial artery is in the upper part of the body. The Extirpation root operation is referenced. If using a code book, the extirpation code table could be directly located in the Upper Artery body system. In either case. code table 03C is referenced, with the body part value of C for the left radial artery. Since the approach is percutaneous, the 3 value is selected from the 03C table, with no Device and no Qualifier. The complete code is 03CC3ZZ.

Section	Body System	Root Operation	Body Part	Approach	Device	Qualifier
Medical and Surgical	Upper Arteries	Extirpation	Radial Artery, Left	Percutaneous	No Device	No Qualifier
0	3	C	C	3	Z	Z

Removal of foreign bodies from a body part is included in the root operation Extirpation. For example, a patient who swallowed a needle has a laparoscopic removal of the needle from the distal ileum under general anesthesia. In this case, it is necessary to know the objective of the procedure meets the definition of Extirpation, taking out solid matter from a body part. The root operation Removal is not the correct code table, as a removal always involves a device. In this case the needle is a foreign body and it is extirpated, or taken out of the body part. The body part itself is not the focus of the procedure. There are no device values available in any of the Extirpation code tables in the Medical and Surgical section. If a device is involved, Extirpation cannot be the correct root operation. Qualifier 7 for Stent Retriever is available in the 03C table for extirpation of intracranial carotid and vertebral arteries. This stent is not coded as a device because it does not remain in the patient's body after the procedure; rather, it is used in the extirpation procedure to assist in removing matter such as a blood clot.

If using the CMS file, the gastrointestinal body system is referenced for the ileum and the Extirpation root operation is selected. Using a code book and referring to the main term Extirpation and the subterm ileum, the characters of 0DCB are given. In either case, the 0DC code table is referenced to build the code. The approach was laparoscopic, so the value of 4 is used for the approach, percutaneous endoscopic. There is no device and no qualifier. The complete code is 0DCB4ZZ.

Section	Body System	Root Operation	Body Part	Approach	Device	Qualifier
Medical and Surgical	Gastrointestinal	Extirpation	Ileum	Percutaneous Endoscopic	No Device	No Qualifier
0	D	C	B	4	Z	Z

Note that removal of solid matter is Extirpation, while removal of liquid material is Drainage. If both solid and liquid materials are removed only Extirpation is used. Extirpation is only used for taking or cutting out solid matter, not body part. A statement such as "extirpation of lung mass" would be coded as an Excision as a part of the lung is being removed, not solid matter that is around the body part.

Fragmentation

Root Operation

Fragmentation (F): Breaking solid matter in a body part into pieces.

The final root operation in group 2 is Fragmentation, breaking solid matter in a body part into pieces. The value of F is used for Fragmentation.

In Fragmentation procedures, a physical force is used either directly or indirectly to break the solid matter into pieces. Indirect methods are also known as extracorporeal procedures, such as shockwave lithotripsy. This fragmentation can be accomplished by ultrasonic, manual, or other methods. As with the Extirpation root operation, the solid matter involved in Fragmentation procedures may be an abnormal by-product of a biological function or a foreign body. In Fragmentation procedures, however, the material is not removed or taken out. If fragmented material is taken out of the body, the root operation Extirpation is used. The fragmentation is not coded separately as the explanation of the root operation Extirpation states that the material may have been broken into pieces.

For example, a staghorn calculus of the left renal pelvis is treated by electrohydraulic lithotripsy via a percutaneous nephrostomy track. Using the CMS file, the urinary system is selected with the root operation Fragmentation. Using a code book index the main term Lithotripsy has a cross reference to see Fragmentation. Under this main term, subterm Kidney Pelvis, Left, 0TF4 is given. In either case code table 0TF is used to build the code.

As the approach is via a percutaneous nephrostomy, the percutaneous approach is used. Coding Guideline B5.4 provides information on the use of procedures performed percutaneously via a device. There is no device used to perform the procedure, as the nephrostomy was already in place. There is also no qualifier. The complete code is 0TF43ZZ.

Section	Body System	Root Operation	Body Part	Approach	Device	Qualifier
Medical and Surgical	Urinary System	Fragmentation	Kidney Pelvis, Left	Percutaneous	No Device	No Qualifier
0	T	F	4	3	Z	Z

B5.4. Procedures performed percutaneously via a device placed for the procedure are coded to the approach Percutaneous.

Example: Fragmentation of kidney stone performed via percutaneous nephrostomy is coded to the approach Percutaneous.

Root operations in groups 1 and 2 have been reviewed. Group 1 includes the five root operations that involve taking out some or all of a body part, with the emphasis on the body part itself. These are the Excision, Resection, Detachment, Destruction, and Extraction root operations. Group 2 includes three root operations that also involve taking out, but in this case, it is material that should not be present, such as a blood clot, excess fluid, or a calcified stone. The focus of the procedure is not the body part, but rather taking out the material that should not be there. These root operations are Drainage, Extirpation, and Fragmentation.

The next chapter reviews the next two groups—group 3, root operations that involve cutting or separation only, and group 4, root operations that or put in, put back, or move body parts.

 Check Your Understanding

General Questions

1. Which of the following root operations involves eradication of all or a portion of a body part?
   a. Detachment
   b. Destruction
   c. Resection
   d. Excision

2. Detachment of the third finger of the left hand at the proximal phalanx would be coded with which qualifier?
   a. 0—Complete
   b. 1—High
   c. 2—Mid
   d. 3—Low

3. Which root operation cannot include an X for Diagnostic in the qualifier character?
   a. Excision
   b. Extraction
   c. Resection
   d. Drainage

4. Which of the following is the root operation that involves pulling out some or all of a body part using force?
   a. Detachment
   b. Extraction
   c. Fragmentation
   d. Destruction

5. In a Destruction procedure, a small incision is made into the skin to allow a needle to be advanced to the operative site for delivery of cryotherapy. What approach is selected?
   a. Open
   b. Percutaneous
   c. Percutaneous Endoscopic
   d. External

6. Which type of biopsy is not coded as an Excision?
   a. Percutaneous biopsy of the left deltoid muscle
   b. Esophageal biopsy by EGD
   c. Endometrial biopsy via D&C
   d. Needle core biopsy of the left breast

7. Removal of a blood clot in the right leg that had been treated by thrombolysis is coded to which root operation(s)?
   a. Fragmentation
   b. Destruction
   c. Fragmentation and Extirpation
   d. Extirpation

8. This patient had an ablation of the peritoneal cavity as an adjunct to a radical pelvic debulking. What root operation is used for the ablation?
   a. Excision
   b. Resection
   c. Destruction
   d. Extraction

Which Root Operation Is It?

For each of the following descriptions, identify the root operation and the complete ICD-10-PCS code.

1. The patient was admitted for an open removal of the left lobe of the liver due to metastasis from a colon carcinoma.

   Root Operation _____

   ICD-10-PCS Code _____

2. The inpatient is being evaluated for septic arthritis of the knee. A diagnostic needle arthrocentesis was performed on the left side, and the fluid was evaluated in pathology.

   Root Operation _____

   ICD-10-PCS Code _____

3. A staghorn calculus of the left renal pelvis was treated by lithotripsy and is now removed via a percutaneous nephrostomy tube.

   Root Operation _____

   ICD-10-PCS Code _____

4. This patient has a craniectomy with removal of a malignant brain tumor of the cerebral hemisphere.

   Root Operation _____

   ICD-10-PCS Code _____

5. The four-year-old, admitted for workup for potential leukemia, has a bone marrow biopsy with the sample taken percutaneously from the right hip bone.

   ICD-10-PCS Code _____

6. A 49-year-old morbidly obese patient is admitted for a vertical sleeve gastrectomy for weight loss. The greater curvature of the stomach is removed laparoscopically.

   Root Operation _____

   ICD-10-PCS Code _____

(*Continued*)

7. A 22-year-old long-distance bike rider had a pudendal nerve entrapment that was unresponsive to physical therapy and medication. A percutaneous pulsed radiofrequency ablation of the pudendal nerve is accomplished.

    Root Operation _____

    ICD-10-PCS Code _____

8. The patient sustained an injury working on his farm, using a hay baler. Due to the unsustainability of the limb, an amputation of the left arm is performed at the midshaft of the humerus.

    Root Operation _____

    ICD-10-PCS Code _____

9. The patient undergoes cystoscopy and laser lithotripsy for calculus of the left ureter.

    Root Operation _____

    ICD-10-PCS Code _____

10. A patient with thyroid carcinoma has an open removal of the thyroid gland. Samples of lymph nodes on the right side of the neck are removed for biopsy.

    Root Operation _____

    ICD-10-PCS Code _____

11. A patient has a non-excisional debridement of an open wound of his abdomen on the left side, with debridement completed with jet lavage of the muscle.

    Root Operation _____

    ICD-10-PCS Code _____

12. A patient has an open biopsy of the axillary sentinel node on the right side.

    Root Operation _____

    ICD-10-PCS Code _____

Case Studies

Review the documentation in each case to determine the root operation and body system. Refer to the index to find the code table for building the code, selecting the body part, approach, device, and qualifier.

1. Operative Report

PREOPERATIVE DIAGNOSIS:	Left adrenal tumor
POSTOPERATIVE DIAGNOSIS:	Left adrenal tumor
PROCEDURE PERFORMED:	Laparoscopic left adrenalectomy

The patient was seen in the office multiple times with a tumor of the left adrenal, with a size close to 4 cm. The endocrine workup was negative for functional tumor. Because of the size of the tumor and the patient continuing to have pain on the left side, it was recommended to remove the tumor. I discussed with the patient the options and we decided on a laparoscopic adrenalectomy.

The patient was taken to surgery. Under general anesthesia, with the patient in the lateral position with the kidney rest to elevate the space between the iliac crest and the costal margin. A pneumoperitoneum using Veress needle by placing the needle in the anterior axillary line up to a pressure of 15 was obtained. A cannula was inserted first on that site which could not be used to visualize because of adhesions. So, another incision was made medial to the midclavicular line and the 10 mm cannula was inserted. Visualization revealed adhesions in the area of the left upper quadrant, so another cannula was inserted close to the midline through which a scope was inserted. Using the Harmonic scalpel the adhesions were lysed. After lysing the adhesions, the colosplenic ligament (splenocolic ligament) was dissected with the Harmonic scalpel. The left colon and splenic flexure were retracted down. After mobilizing the ligament, the lateral attachment of the spleen was divided using the Harmonic scalpel and with gravity the spleen tilted towards the right side. The kidney was identified. The fascia was opened above and medial to the kidney. The pancreas was visualized. Above the pancreas the adrenal gland was palpated. The fat was dissected off the adrenal gland. The adrenal surface anteriorly was visualized. Dissection started around the adrenal gland laterally, superiorly and medially. The area of the splenic vein was identified inferiorly, it was surrounded by fatty tissue, so this was transected and stapled close to the adrenal gland using the Endo-GIA vascular stapler. After that was done, the adrenal gland was placed in an Endobag and retrieved through the cannula site, Hemostasis secured. Irrigation was done. After that the cannula was removed and pneumoperitoneum evacuated. The trocar site where the tumor was removed was closed with 0-Vicryl and the skin was closed with 4-0 Vicryl and Steri-Strips.

2. Operative Report

PREOPERATIVE DIAGNOSIS: Diabetic foot infection, gangrenous right third toe

POSTOPERATIVE DIAGNOSIS: Diabetic foot infection, gangrenous right third toe

PROCEDURE: Right third toe amputation

HISTORY: This 83-year-old white female patient with diabetes was admitted with gangrenous discoloration and purulent drainage from the right third toe.

PROCEDURE DESCRIPTION: The patient was taken to the operating room, monitored and sedated per anesthesia. 35 cc of 0.25% Marcaine plain was infiltrated into the skin and subcutaneous tissues over the forefoot and ankle, and at the base of third toe for a regional block anesthesia. The foot was prepped and draped in a sterile fashion.

An elliptical incision at the base of the toe was then made with a scalpel. The incision was extended through the subcutaneous tissue. The anterior and posterior tendons were divided. The joint was disarticulated. The toe was completely removed and sent as a surgical specimen. The wound was irrigated with copious amounts of saline. The subcutaneous tissue and tendinous tissue was then approximated over the bone using interrupted sutures of 2-0 Vicryl and the skin was closed with interrupted mattress sutures of 3-0 Prolene. A sterile dressing was applied.

The patient tolerated the procedure well.

ESTIMATED BLOOD LOSS: 5 cc

4

Root Operations that Cut or Separate, Put in or Put Back, or Move Body Parts

The next two groups of root operations involve Cutting or Separating, Putting In or Back, or Moving Body Parts. There are a total of six root operations in these two groups.

Group 3: Root Operations Involving Cutting or Separation Only

Group 3 contains two root operations that involve cutting or separation only. These root operations are Division and Release. The definitions of these root operations contrast with the root operations from group 1; Excision, Resection, and Detachment described in chapter 3 in that the group 1 root operations involve cutting but also take out or off some or all of a body part. Division and Release only involve cutting and separation without taking any body part or other material out.

Division

 Root Operation

Division (8): Cutting into a body part without drawing fluids and/or gases from the body part in order to separate or transect a body part.

The first of these root operations is Division, which is cutting into a body part without drawing fluids and/or gases from the body part in order to separate or transect a body part. The value of 8 is used for this root operation.

The key term in this definition is "separate." In the root operation Division, all or a portion of the body part is separated into two or more portions. This is in contrast with the root operation Release, which will be discussed next. In Release procedures, cutting relieves some abnormal constraint, but the body part is not separated.

Division can also be contrasted with the root operation Drainage, in which there may be some cutting in order to let out fluids or gases, which is the objective of the procedure. This cutting is an integral part of the Drainage procedure. In the Division procedure, the objective is to cut in order to separate, and cutting is the only action. Osteotomy, or cutting a bone to reshape and realign, is coded as a Reposition rather than a Division procedure; the cutting is integral to the realignment of the bone. This procedure is discussed later in this chapter and in chapter 16.

There are limited examples of procedures with the objective of Division. One example of is an episiotomy, a separation of the perineum, the skin and muscles between the vaginal opening and anus, to facilitate childbirth and prevent obstetrical lacerations. Another example is a rhizotomy, in which selected spinal nerve roots are severed or separated before they enter the spinal cord. This may be performed for conditions such as neck pain due to arthritis of facet joints. It can also be performed to treat spasticity that has not responded to more conservative treatment.

Release

Root Operation

Release (N): Freeing a body part from an abnormal physical constraint by cutting or by the use of force.

Release is the other root operation in the group that involves cutting or separating only. Release is freeing a body part from an abnormal physical constraint by cutting or by the use of force. The value of N is used for Release procedures. Lysis of adhesions and release of scar contracture are examples of Release procedures.

"Freeing" is the key word in this definition. In Release procedures, some of the tissue that is restraining the body part may be taken out; however, none of the body part itself may be removed. If the body part or a portion of the body part is taken out, then the objective of the procedure is not Release, but rather Extraction (pulling or stripping out or off all or a portion of a body part by the use of force), or Excision (cutting out or off a portion of a body part). See chapter 3 for more information about the root operation Extraction.

The body part value for the Release procedure is the body part being freed. If another body part is cut to accomplish the Release, the body part that is being released is still the value coded for the 4th character body part rather than the body part that is cut. For example, in a carpal tunnel release procedure, the carpal tunnel is visualized, and carpal ligament is cut, but the objective of the procedure is freeing the median nerve. The body part for the carpal tunnel release procedure is the median nerve. This is emphasized in Coding Guideline B3.13.

B3.13. In the root operation Release, the body part value coded is the body part being freed and not the tissue being manipulated or cut to free the body part.

Example: Lysis of intestinal adhesions is coded to the specific intestine body part value.

The Release procedure can be performed on the area around the body part, on the attachments to a body part, or between subdivisions of a body part that are causing the abnormal constraint. In a procedure to release adhesions around a recently replaced knee, the intent of the procedure is to lyse the adhesions that are restricting the knee joint from full range of motion, and the applicable knee joint is the body part selected for the Release procedure.

A capsulotomy to release a contracture or a fasciotomy to treat compartment syndrome are examples of Release procedures because these procedures free a constrained body part. For the fasciotomy example, the body part value is based on what is freed. The cutting of the fascia is often part of the approach to get to the constrained area. In compartment syndrome, pressure builds to dangerous levels within the groupings, or compartments, of the muscles. This is often a result of an injury and may require immediate surgery to release the muscle and avoid damage or amputation of the affected area. Since the body part value for the release code is based on the area that is freed, multiple codes may be assigned. For example, an open fasciotomy of both the anterior and posterior compartments of the muscles of the right lower arm would have the code 0KN90ZZ listed twice.

Coding for lysis of adhesions is dependent on the circumstances of the procedure. If this is the intent of the procedure—for example, if the adhesions are causing an intestinal obstruction that is now being treated—then the Release procedure is coded. Lysis of adhesions necessary to reach an operative site is considered integral to the surgery and part of the approach. The inclusion of the diagnosis of adhesions and documentation of the lysis is not sufficient to add the code for the release procedure.

Coding Tip

Separating is the key word in the definition for Division, which seeks to separate or transect a body part, while freeing is the key word in the definition for Release, which involves an abnormal physical constraint.

The differences between the Division and Release procedures are highlighted in the root operations Coding Guideline B3.14.

B3.14. If the sole objective of the procedure is freeing a body part without cutting the body part, the root operation is Release. If the sole objective of the procedure is separating or transecting a body part, the root operation is Division.

Examples: Freeing a nerve root from surrounding scar tissue to relieve pain is coded to the root operation Release. Severing a nerve root to relieve pain is coded to the root operation Division.

Decompressive laminectomy is another example of a Release procedure. In this operation the lamina are removed as an approach to the operative site, but the intent is to free the nerve or nerve roots that have been constrained; the laminectomy is inherent in the procedure and is not coded separately. A decompressive lumbar laminectomy using an open approach to treat spinal stenosis that compresses the lumbar nerve is coded as 01NB0ZZ.

Section	Body System	Root Operation	Body Part	Approach	Device	Qualifier
Medical and Surgical	Peripheral Nervous System	Release	Lumbar Nerve	Open	No Device	No Qualifier
0	1	N	B	0	Z	Z

Group 4: Root Operations that Put in or Put Back or Move Some or All of a Body Part

The root operations in group 4 involve putting in or back or moving some or all of a body part. These root operations are Transplantation, Reattachment, Transfer, and Reposition. These procedures focus on the body part that is being put in, put back, or moved, rather than a device. There may be a device involved in the procedure, but this is not the objective of the procedure. In a Reposition procedure for a fractured bone, an internal or external fixation device may be used, but the intent of the procedure is to move all or a part of the body part to reduce the fracture, rather than only inserting a device.

Transplantation

Root Operation

Transplantation (Y): Putting in or on all or a portion of a living body part taken from another individual or animal to physically take the place and/or function of all or a portion of a similar body part.

Transplantation is the putting in or on either a portion or all of a living body part taken from another human or animal. The transplant takes the place and functions of the entire body part or the portion of the body part that is replaced. The value of Y is used for Transplantation.

There are a limited number of procedures available for transplantation procedures, and these are only applicable to describe body parts that are currently being transplanted: for example, heart, pancreas, liver, and kidney transplants. Using a code book, refer to the index under the main term Transplantation. The terms listed are the only body parts that can currently be coded as Transplantation, for example, esophagus, lung, pancreas, thymus and uterus. Other examples are transplantation of the face and hand. As new transplantation procedures are added to general medical practice, the values will be added as appropriate. This is in accordance with Coding Guideline A3.

A3. The valid values for an axis of classification can be added to as needed.

Example: If a significantly distinct type of device is used in a new procedure, a new device value can be added to the system.

The Transplantation procedures have a 7th character qualifier character that has one of three values. The types of transplants are allogeneic, or from the same species; syngeneic, or from an identical twin; and zooplastic, or from an animal. See table 4.1 for a complete list of these qualifiers.

Table 4.1. Transplantation qualifier characters

Type of Transplant	Qualifier Character	Definition
Allogeneic	0	Taken from different individuals of the same species
Syngeneic	1	Having to do with individuals or tissues that have identical genes, such as identical twins
Zooplastic	2	Tissue from an animal to a human

Often, Transplantation procedures are for complex organs such as the heart or large intestine as well as the thymus and kidney. The term transplant may be used by the provider to refer to other types of procedures that do not meet the criteria for transplant. The provider might document "cornea transplant from a cadaver donor." Refer to the CMS file under the body system 08 for the Eye Body System and note that a code table for Transplantation is not found. There is no code available for Transplantation of the cornea as this is not a living body part but rather a layer of tissue in a portion of a body part. A cornea transplant does not meet the ICD-10-PCS definition of Transplantation. Instead, the cornea transplant procedure would be coded as a Replacement from the 08R code table, which is putting in or on a biological or synthetic material that physically takes the place or function of all or a portion of a body part. Another example is a heart valve replacement, which may be listed by the surgeon as a transplant. As with the corneal transplant, this would be coded as a Replacement rather than a Transplantation. The root operation of Replacement will be discussed in chapter 5 of this text. Recall that the provider does not have to use the exact terms found in ICD-10-PCS, but rather, a coding professional translates these terms to apply the ICD-10-PCS definitions. This is in accordance with Coding Guideline A11.

A11. Many of the terms used to construct PCS codes are defined within the system. It is the coder's responsibility to determine what the documentation in the medical record equates to in the PCS definitions. The physician is not expected to use the terms used in PCS code descriptions, nor is the coder required to query the physician when the correlation between the documentation and the defined PCS terms is clear.

Example: When the physician documents "partial resection," the coder can independently correlate "partial resection" to the root operation Excision without querying the physician for clarification.

Bone marrow transplants are not coded as Transplantation in the Medical and Surgical section but rather in the Administration section of ICD-10-PCS under the root operation Transfusion. This is also true of stem cells and pancreatic islet cells. This is noted in Coding Guideline B3.16.

B3.16. Putting in a mature and functioning living body part taken from another individual or animal is coded to the root operation Transplantation. Putting in autologous or nonautologous cells is coded to the Administration section.

Example: Putting in autologous or nonautologous bone marrow, pancreatic islet cells, or stem cells is coded to the Administration section.

The Administration section will be covered in chapter 21 of this text.

Reattachment

Root Operation

Reattachment (M): Putting back in or on all or a portion of a separated body part to its normal location or other suitable location.

The next root operation is group 4 is Reattachment. Reattachment is putting back in or on all or a portion of a separated body part to its normal location or other suitable location. The value of M is used for Reattachment.

In Reattachment procedures, a body part that has been cut off or avulsed is reattached to the body. The blood supply is restored, and the nerve supply may or may not be restored based on the circumstances of the case. Examples are reattachment of an avulsed kidney or a finger. Note that only completely severed body parts are reattached. The root operation of Repair, covered in chapter 6, would be assigned for procedures involving the reconnection of partially separated body parts, such as a partially severed ear.

Transfer

Root Operation

Transfer (X): Moving, without taking out, all or a portion of a body part to another location to take over the function of all or a portion of a body part.

The next root operation in group 4 is Transfer, or moving all or a portion of a body part to another location to take over the function of all or a portion of a body part. The value of X is used for Transfer. Examples of Transfer procedures are flap closures of open wounds using skin, tendon transfers, and nerve transfers. Note that many body systems do not have the root operation Transfer included in the tables as the operation would not be performed. For example, there are no Transfer procedures performed in the Heart and Great Vessels or Ear, Nose and Sinus body systems, while the procedure is performed in the gastrointestinal and peripheral nervous system and skin and breast. The Transfer root operation is available in code table 0VX for one body part, the prepuce, when the foreskin is used to correct genital malformations. Devices are not involved in a Transfer procedure, so the device value is always Z for No Device.

Key to this root operation is that the body part or portion of the body part that is transferred is not taken out. In other words, the blood vessels and nerves stay attached. An example of a Transfer procedure is a skin pedicle transfer or a transfer of a ligament of the hand. The term "pedicle" is key as this indicates that the graft is still attached to the body via a stem or stalk of tissue. In contrast, a free graft is a skin graft that is harvested from one area of the body, removed, and applied to another area. A free graft is not classified as a Transfer, because the blood vessels and nerves are severed in the harvesting procedure. Instead, this is coded as a Replacement, which is putting in or on a biological or synthetic material that physically takes the place and/or function of all or a portion of a body part. In the Replacement root operation the free skin graft becomes a device and is coded in the 6th character as an autologous tissue substitute.

In Transfer procedures that involve more than one layer, such as the subcutaneous tissue, fascia, and muscle body systems, the body part value represents the deepest tissue layer in the flap. If other tissue layers are involved, the qualifier character indicates this layer or layers. For example, if a Transfer procedure involved a flap from the right shoulder muscle, the Muscles body system would be used with the appropriate body part as this is the deepest layer. If the skin or subcutaneous layers are also involved in the flap this is coded in the qualifier character to account for this portion of the transfer. For an open procedure involving the muscles of the right shoulder as well as the subcutaneous tissue and skin, the code would be 0KX50Z2. (See the 0KX table in table 4.2.) This is emphasized in Coding Guideline B3.17.

B3.17. The root operation Transfer contains qualifiers that can be used to specify when a transfer flap is composed of more than one tissue layer, such as a musculocutaneous flap. For procedures involving transfer of multiple tissue layers including skin, subcutaneous tissue, fascia or muscle, the procedure is coded to the body part value that describes the deepest tissue layer in the flap, and the qualifier can be used to describe the other tissue layer(s) in the transfer flap.

Example: A musculocutaneous flap transfer is coded to the appropriate body part value in the body system Muscles, and the qualifier is used to describe the additional tissue layer(s) in the transfer flap.

Table 4.2. 0KX table

Section	0	Medical and Surgical	
Body System	K	Muscles	
Operation	X	Transfer: Moving, without taking out, all or a portion of a body part to another location to take over the function of all or a portion of a body part	

Body Part	Approach	Device	Qualifier
0 Head Muscle **1** Facial Muscle **2** Neck Muscle, Right **3** Neck Muscle, Left **4** Tongue, Palate, Pharynx Muscle **5** Shoulder Muscle, Right **6** Shoulder Muscle, Left **7** Upper Arm Muscle, Right **8** Upper Arm Muscle, Left **9** Lower Arm and Wrist Muscle, Right **B** Lower Arm and Wrist Muscle, Left **C** Hand Muscle, Right **D** Hand Muscle, Left **H** Thorax Muscle, Right **J** Thorax Muscle, Left **M** Perineum Muscle **N** Hip Muscle, Right **P** Hip Muscle, Left **Q** Upper Leg Muscle, Right **R** Upper Leg Muscle, Left **S** Lower Leg Muscle, Right **T** Lower Leg Muscle, Left **V** Foot Muscle, Right **W** Foot Muscle, Left	**0** Open **4** Percutaneous Endoscopic	**Z** No Device	**0** Skin **1** Subcutaneous Tissue **2** Skin and Subcutaneous Tissue **Z** No Qualifier
F Trunk Muscle, Right **G** Trunk Muscle, Left	**0** Open **4** Percutaneous Endoscopic	**Z** No Device	**0** Skin **1** Subcutaneous Tissue **2** Skin and Subcutaneous Tissue **5** Latissimus Dorsi Myocutaneous Flap **7** Deep Inferior Epigastric Artery Perforator Flap **8** Superficial Inferior Epigastric Artery Flap **9** Gluteal Artery Perforator Flap **Z** No Qualifier

Source: CMS 2019

The Transfer root operation is also found in the Central Nervous System and Cranial Nerves and Peripheral Nervous System body systems, where a nerve branch is moved locally to take over the function of a damaged nerve. In these body systems, the body part value represents where the transfer begins, while the qualifier is where the transfer ends.

Reposition

Root Operation

Reposition (S): Moving to its normal location or other suitable location all or a portion of a body part.

The last root operation in group 4 is Reposition, or moving to its normal location or other suitable location all or a portion of a body part. The value of S is used for Reposition.

In Reposition procedures, the body part can be resituated from an abnormal location or from its normal location where it is not functioning properly. The objective of the move is to restore or establish normal function. For example, moving the anterior cruciate ligament (ACL) of the knee that has slipped is a type of Reposition procedure. Repair of an intussusception or volvulus of the gastrointestinal tract is another example of a Reposition because the body part is moved back to its correct or other suitable location.

A prime example of a Reposition procedure is a fracture reduction. In this procedure, the portions of the bone that have been misplaced during a fracture are restored to their proper location. A device may be used as a part of the procedure and is represented in the 6th character. These can be internal or external fixation devices. See figure 1.11 for an example of an external fixation device.

Reposition is an example of the ICD-10-PCS term differing from the most likely documentation for the root operation, reduction. The provider is not required to state "Reposition" in order to assign this value for the root operation; the coding professional must translate the intent of the reduction of the fracture to the root operation Reposition.

Only displaced (not nondisplaced) fractures are treated using Reposition procedures, as by definition a displaced fracture involves the bone breaking into two or more parts, causing the bones to be out of alignment or position. In contrast, a nondisplaced fracture involves a crack in the bone without movement or misalignment. A nondisplaced fracture would not be treated with a Reposition procedure as the bone is not moved. Guideline B3.15 emphasizes this distinction and specifies that a cast or splint is included in the Reposition procedure.

B3.15. Reduction of a displaced fracture is coded to the root operation Reposition, and the application of a cast or splint in conjunction with the Reposition procedure is not coded separately. Treatment of a nondisplaced fracture is coded to the procedure performed.

Example: Putting a pin in a nondisplaced fracture is coded to the root operation Insertion. Casting a nondisplaced fracture is coded to the root operation Immobilization in the Placement section.

Another example of a Reposition procedure is a rectopexy, performed to treat a prolapsed rectum. It should be noted that in Reposition procedures the body part or portion of the body part may or may not be removed to be relocated to the new location.

An osteotomy is another example of a Reposition procedure. An osteotomy involves cutting, reshaping and realigning the bone. For example, in an arthritic knee, the tibia may be cut and realigned to shift weight from the portion of the joint that has arthritic damage. The objective is to move or reposition the bone and hold the bone in place with an internal fixation device. The Index entry for Osteotomy is Division or Drain for the various bone body systems; however, the objective of the procedure meets the definition of Reposition. Recall that according to Coding Guideline A7, it is not mandatory to use the Index before consulting the code tables. The code assigned for an open osteotomy of the right tibia with internal fixation is 0QSG0ZZ.

A7. It is not required to consult the index first before proceeding to the tables to complete the code. A valid code may be chosen directly from the tables.

Check Your Understanding

General Questions

1. The key word is "freeing" in the definition for which root operation?
   a. Division
   b. Release
   c. Extraction
   d. Transfer

2. Which of the following would be coded as a Transplant?
   a. Heart
   b. Cornea
   c. Bone marrow
   d. Mitral valve

3. Patient with spinal stenosis and compression of the lumbar nerve root has a laminectomy at L4–L5. What root operation is used?
   a. Release
   b. Excision
   c. Division
   d. Repair

4. True or false? Only a limited number of transplants have codes available in ICD-10-PCS. _____

5. Which root operation involves a procedure in which the blood and nerve supply remains intact?
   a. Transplant
   b. Reattachment
   c. Transfer
   d. Reposition

6. This Release procedure involves cutting a ligament en route to releasing a constricted nerve. How is this coded?
   a. Release of the nerve
   b. Release of the ligament
   c. Release of both the nerve and the ligament
   d. Release of the nerve and excision of the ligament

7. Which of the following procedures is not an example of the root operation Reposition?
   a. Closed reduction of a displaced fracture of the femur
   b. Arthroscopic repair of a displaced patellar ligament
   c. Closed treatment of a nondisplaced fracture of the humerus
   d. Repair of an undescended testicle

8. If a body part has been separated from its normal location and an operation is performed to return the body part to its normal location, which of the following root operations applies?
   a. Transplant
   b. Reattachment
   c. Transfer
   d. Reposition

9. A patient has a reduction of an intestinal volvulus. What root operation is coded?
   a. Repair
   b. Reattachment
   c. Transfer
   d. Reposition

Which Root Operation Is It?

For each of the following descriptions, identify the root operation and the complete ICD-10-PCS code.

1. A patient is being treated for a cumulative injury resulting in a frozen right shoulder. The patient has been unresponsive to exercise and medication. An arthroscopic manipulation is performed to release the frozen shoulder.

   Root Operation _____

   ICD-10-PCS Code _____

2. A 19-year-old patient with cystic fibrosis is admitted for a double lung transplant from a cadaver donor.

   Root Operation _____

   ICD-10-PCS Code _____

3. A 17-year-old soccer goal keeper is admitted with diabetes in coma, causing a fall and trauma to the right shoulder. A dislocation is diagnosed and an open reduction is performed to repair the shoulder.

   Root Operation _____

   ICD-10-PCS Code _____

4. A patient has bilateral flexion contractures of the knees at 40 degrees. Posterior capsulotomy via incision is performed on both sides to free the contractures of the knees.

   Root Operation _____

   ICD-10-PCS Code _____

5. A patient who sustained a left hand injury undergoes nerve surgery to prevent a residual claw-hand injury. The anterior interosseous to ulnar nerve graft is accomplished via incision using an operative microscope, and the interosseous and ulnar nerve are brought together without dissection.

   Root Operation _____

   ICD-10-PCS Code _____

6. A patient was involved in a farm injury, and his right arm was severed directly below the elbow. The arm is now reconnected, with full revascularization and nerve attachment.

   Root Operation _____

   ICD-10-PCS Code _____

7. This patient was treated with a percutaneous rhizotomy of the cervical nerve to treat chronic pain.

   Root Operation _____

   ICD-10-PCS Code _____

(Continued)

8. A patient who sustained multiple injuries in a motor vehicle accident has open reduction with intramedullary fixation device of the femoral shaft on the left side and open reduction and monoplanar external fixation of the right tibia.

   Root Operation _____

   ICD-10-PCS Code _____

9. A patient with end-stage renal disease undergoes a donor-matched kidney transplant on the right side.

   Root Operation _____

   ICD-10-PCS Code _____

10. A patient who had a mastectomy on the right side now presents for an open reconstruction procedure involving a pedicle flap of the transverse rectus muscle to the mastectomy site.

   Root Operation _____

   ICD-10-PCS Code _____

Case Studies

Review the documentation in each case to determine the root operation and body system. Refer to the Index to find the code table for building the code, selecting the Body Part, Approach, Device, and Qualifier.

1. Operative Report

PREOPERATIVE DIAGNOSES:	1. Nasal tip defect 2.5 × 2.5 cm status post excision of cutaneous carcinoma 2. Facial pain
POSTOPERATIVE DIAGNOSES:	1. Nasal tip defect 2.5 × 2.5 cm status post excision of cutaneous carcinoma 2. Facial pain
PROCEDURES:	Reconstruction of the nasal tip defect with axial pattern forehead paramedian flap
ANESTHESIA:	General
ESTIMATED BLOOD LOSS:	5 mL
COMPLICATIONS:	None

PREOPERATIVE HISTORY: Patient is a pleasant 63-year-old female with history of large cutaneous carcinoma of the nasal tip. This was recently excised via Mohs surgery. The resultant defect was approximately 2.5 × 2.5 cm in size. Several options were discussed with the patient and her family for reconstruction including healing by secondary intention, use of skin graft, local rotational flap or axial pattern paramedian forehead flap. Due to the optimal cosmesis provided by the forehead flap, the patient elected to undergo reconstruction with this option. The risks, benefits, alternatives and limitations were explained. Risks included (but were not limited to) bleeding, infection, scarring, cosmetic deformity, facial asymmetry, facial numbness either temporary or permanent, failure of the flap possibly requiring secondary procedure, cosmetic deformities, nasal obstruction and the risks associated with anesthesia. Patient understood these risks and consented to surgery as described above.

OPERATIVE REPORT: The patient was taken to the operating room and placed on the operating table in supine position. An LMA tube was placed. Patient was induced with general anesthesia without incidence. The table was turned to 90 degrees. Patient was then prepped and draped in the usual sterile fashion. Next, marking pen was used to draw a paramedian forehead flap centered around the left vascular bundle. Flap was designed to fit into the nasal defect. Local anesthetic consisting of 50/50 mixture of 1% lidocaine with 1:100,000 parts of epinephrine mixed with 0.5% Marcaine was infiltrated around the nose and the forehead. After waiting approximately 10 minutes for the local anesthetic to take effect, a #15 blade was used to make incision around the previously marked forehead flap of the skin and subcutaneous tissue. The flap was elevated above the galea in the superior portion. In the mid forehead region, a subperiosteal dissection was performed in order to preserve the vascular pedicle. Flap was then rotated into the defect and secured into the defect by closing the deep aspect of the wound with 4-0 Vicryl suture. Cutaneous aspect of the wound was closed with 5-0 Prolene suture. Forehead donor site was closed by wide undermining and then closure of the wound by closing the deep aspect of wound with 3-0 Vicryl suture. Cutaneous aspect of wound was closed again with 5-0 Prolene suture. Antibiotic ointment was applied over the wounds and a dressing was applied. The patient was then turned back towards Anesthesia, subsequently extubated and transferred to the recovery room in stable condition. She tolerated the procedure well. She will be observed in the hospital overnight for pain control and to evaluate for viability of the flap. All postoperative instructions were provided to the responsible party. Patient will be evaluated on postoperative day #1.

2. Operative Report

PREOPERATIVE DIAGNOSIS:	Right femoral shaft fracture
POSTOPERATIVE DIAGNOSIS:	Right femoral shaft fracture
PROCEDURE PERFORMED:	Right femoral IM nail
ANESTHESIA:	General endotracheal anesthesia
FINDINGS:	Comminuted right femoral shaft fracture with anterolateral butterfly piece
IMPLANTS:	Stryker T2 gamma intramedullary nail with two proximal locking screws and two distal locking screws
INTRAVENOUS FLUIDS:	1L of LR plus 2 units of packed red blood cells
ESTIMATED BLOOD LOSS:	100 mL
URINE OUTPUT:	Not applicable
SPECIMENS:	None

DISPOSITON: The patient remained intubated as the oral maxillofacial surgeons were going to perform their surgery for her facial fractures.

SURGICAL INDICATIONS: The patient is an 18-year-old female who was involved in an MVA. She sustained multiple injuries including multiple facial fractures, a comminuted right femur fracture and left acetabular fracture. We discussed with her family the need for surgical intervention for her right femur, which would involve an intramedullary rodding. We discussed with her the risks and benefits of surgery. The risks include but are not limited to bleeding, infection, damage to underlying nerves and vessels, scarring and additional surgery. The patient acknowledged understanding of the risks and benefits and consented to the procedure.

SURGICAL PROCEDURE: The patient's right leg was marked in the preoperative holding area. She was taken back to the operating room, during which she was placed in a normal supine position. There, a timeout was performed during which the patient, the site, and the procedure were all confirmed by the entire operating room staff. She was placed under general anesthesia. She was placed on the fracture table with both legs secured. She was given 600 mg of Cleocin. All bony prominences were padded accordingly and SCD and TED hose were placed on the contralateral left leg. Preoperative x-rays were taken under fluoro, which showed the femur fracture with a significant anterior lateral butterfly piece and the fracture subluxed posteriorly and laterally.

The leg was prepped and draped in normal sterile fashion. We utilized a 4 cm incision approximately 5 cm proximal to the greater tuberosity. We made an incision through skin and then through fascia to the greater trochanter. Guidewire was placed down the greater trochanter. This was verified on AP and lateral fluoro that is was in the center position heading straight down the femoral shaft. Once this was complete, we then utilized entry reamer to open up the canal. A guidewire was placed down the entire length of the femur. We utilized a crutch as well as lateral to medial directed force to reduce the fracture. We were able to place the guidewire from the proximal fragment to the distal fragment. With lateral we were able to maintain a reduction. We then reamed starting with a 9 and reamed to a 12.5. We measured the rod to be at 340 mm. We placed an 11 × 340 mm rod down the femoral shaft. The femoral shaft reduced nicely both on the AP and vaginal films. Once this was completed, we then placed our targeting guide for the proximal screws, a 40 and 42.5 mm locking screws in the static holes on the proximal aspect of the nail. We then went distal using perfect circles with the fluoroscopy; we placed two distal locking screws in the static locking holes 50 and 45. Once this was completed, we then took final x-rays. We took an AP lateral of the fracture site. Once this was completed, all wounds were irrigated out copiously with normal saline. The fascia proximally was closed with #0 Vicryl and a figure-of-eight stitch and the subcutaneous tissues were closed with 2-0 Vicryl in a simple interrupted buried stitch and the skin was closed with staples followed by Xeroform, 4 × 4s and Tegaderm. The legs were removed from the arms of the fracture table. At this point the patient was prepped for the oral maxillofacial surgery.

Chapter 5

Root Operations that Alter Diameter or Route of Body Parts, or Involve a Device

This chapter will concentrate on two of the root operation groups—those that alter the diameter or route of tubular body parts and those that always involve a device. There are a total of 10 root operations in these two groups.

Group 5: Root Operations that Alter Diameter or Route of a Tubular Body Part

Group 5 includes four root operations that involve procedures to alter the diameter or route of a tubular body part: Restriction, Occlusion, Dilation, and Bypass. Tubular body parts are those that are hollow and allow for passage of solids, liquids, or gases. Examples of tubular body parts are the vessels of the cardiovascular system and the tubular portions of the genitourinary, respiratory, gastrointestinal, and biliary tracts. Each of these root operations has an objective of changing these tubular body parts in some way.

The tubular body parts are unique. They are typically not transferred as other body parts may be. Instead, the contents of the tubular body part are rerouted, as in a Bypass procedure; the diameter of the body parts is made smaller, as in Restriction; cut off, as in Occlusion; or the orifice or lumen of the body part may be made larger, as in Dilation. Tubular body parts are generally not divided, and any cutting the wall of a tubular body part does not constitute a Division root operation, because the objective of this cutting is an initial action to dilate the body part to make it larger. When a procedure involves a tubular body part, careful review of the intent of the procedure is important, and the first step is to determine if one of the four root operations in this group may apply.

Coding Tip

Many procedures performed on tubular body parts will fit into one of the four root operations in group 5 (Restriction, Occlusion, Dilation, or Bypass) though other root operations may apply. Remember to consider this group first if the procedure involves a change to the size or route of the tubular body part.

Restriction

Root Operation

Restriction (V): Partially closing an orifice or the lumen of a tubular body part.

The first root operation in group 5 is Restriction, or partially closing an orifice or the lumen of a tubular body part. The value of V is used for Restriction.

The objective of a Restriction procedure is to partially narrow the diameter of the tubular body part or orifice. If the procedure is performed on an orifice or opening, this can be a natural orifice, such as the vagina, or an artificially formed opening, such as a colostomy. The procedure could include either intraluminal devices, such as a stent, or extraluminal devices, such as a lap band that restricts the stomach in a bariatric procedure.

These devices are integral to the procedure and to accomplishing the applicable widening or narrowing effect. Other examples of Restriction include clipping of a cerebral aneurysm or cerclage of the cervix. See figure 1.12 in chapter 1 for an example of an extraluminal device.

A Restriction procedure narrows the orifice or lumen without total obstruction. The applicable liquids, solids, or gases can still travel through the orifice or lumen, but at a lesser rate. In the example of a cervical cerclage procedure, a suture is used to obstruct the opening to prevent premature delivery, but the opening is not totally blocked.

Occlusion

Root Operation

Occlusion (L): Completely closing an orifice or the lumen of a tubular body part.

In contrast to Restriction, the next root operation in group 5, Occlusion, involves totally closing an orifice or lumen of a tubular body part. The value of L is used for Occlusion.

Occlusion has the objective of complete closure. As with Restriction, an Occlusion procedure can involve a natural or artificial opening for procedures on orifices. Both intraluminal and extraluminal methods for closing the body part are included. If there is any division of the body part prior to the Occlusion, this is included and considered integral to the procedure. Examples of Occlusion procedures are ligation of fallopian tubes and tying off hemorrhoids. Placement of an intraluminal device to close off or occlude the left atrial appendage is an example of using a device to perform the occlusion. This procedure is performed to minimize blood clot formation in atrial fibrillation.

Coding Tip

Both the root operations Restriction and Occlusion involve closing an orifice or lumen. The key word for this closure is partial for Restriction and total for Occlusion.

Embolization, or the intentional introduction of clotting material to close or narrow a vessel, can be either the root operation Restriction or the root operation Occlusion, depending on the intent of the procedure. The difference between Restriction and Occlusion specific to embolization of vessels is addressed in Coding Guideline B3.12.

B3.12. If the objective of an embolization procedure is to completely close a vessel, the root operation Occlusion is coded. If the objective of an embolization procedure is to narrow the lumen of a vessel, the root operation Restriction is coded.

Example: Tumor embolization is coded to the root operation Occlusion, because the objective of the procedure is to cut off the blood supply to the vessel.

In most cases, embolization of a cerebral aneurysm is coded to the root operation Restriction because the objective of the procedure is not to close off the vessel entirely but to narrow the lumen of the vessel at the site of the aneurysm where it is abnormally wide.

The objective of total closure can be accomplished as described earlier using intraluminal or extraluminal devices to occlude the lumen or orifice. Another method of Occlusion is ligation of a body part using sutures to totally close off the body part. The Occlusion may also involve excision of a portion of the body part as a component of the procedure, but the intent of the procedure still is to completely close the orifice or lumen. For example, in a vasectomy, the vas deferens is ligated to occlude the body part and a portion of the body part may be excised as a part of the procedure. This remains an Occlusion, because the intent of the surgery is to close off the vas deferens. If the Occlusion is accomplished using eradication methods such as cauterization, electrocoagulation, or ablation, this is still coded to Occlusion rather than Destruction, because the intent of the procedure is to close off the tubular body part. For ligation of the fallopian tube, an extraluminal device may be used, such as a Falope ring, or the fallopian tubes may be ligated and stitched. In either case, the objective of the Occlusion is met because the tube is totally blocked.

Coding Tip

Intraluminal or extraluminal devices can be used in Occlusion procedures. If the closure of the tubular body part is accomplished by eradicating the body part or by removal of a portion of the body part, the root operation Occlusion is used as the intent of the procedure is to completely close the orifice or lumen of the tubular body part.

Dilation

Root Operation

Dilation (7): Expanding an orifice or the lumen of a tubular body part.

Dilation, or expanding an orifice or the lumen of a tubular body part, is the next root operation in group 5. The value of 7 is used for Dilation.

The objective of Dilation procedures is opposite that of Restriction or Occlusion procedures. A Dilation root operation involves making the orifice or lumen larger, rather than smaller. As is true of Restriction and Occlusion procedures, Dilation includes both intraluminal and extraluminal methods to accomplish the enlargement. Intraluminal pressure can be used to stretch the tubular body and, thus, make it larger. The Dilation can also be achieved by cutting part of the opening or wall of the body part. Examples of Dilation procedures include esophageal dilations for obstruction and a valvotomy performed for dilation of the annulus of a stenotic pulmonary valve.

Note that the dilation or stretching of the tubular body part is the objective of this root operation. If dilation is the approach to a procedure and the true objective is not the dilation, then the objective of the procedure is the root operation. For example, in a Dilation and Curettage (D&C) procedure, the dilation is the method used to access the endometrium, which is then extracted for diagnostic or therapeutic purposes. Therefore, the Extraction is the root operation for a nonobstetrical D&C. See chapter 3 for a description of the Extraction root operation.

Many Dilation procedures involve the use of a device that is left in place after the procedure to maintain the expansion of the tubular body part. The device is represented with the 6th character of the code and is an integral part of the procedure. In this operation, inserting the device is not the objective of the procedure; rather the Dilation is the intent. For example, a ureteral stent may be inserted as part of a Dilation procedure. The stent is represented by the value D for intraluminal device. Even though the surgeon may state "insertion of a ureteral stent" the objective of the procedure is to expand the lumen of the ureter and therefore Dilation is the root operation rather than Insertion. Another example of a Dilation procedure is a percutaneous transluminal coronary angioplasty (PTCA), used to open up coronary arteries that have been blocked, most likely by arteriosclerotic plaque. The artery is stretched via a balloon catheter that is placed into the vessel via a guide wire. At the blockage site the balloon is inflated to compress the obstruction. Once the blockage is clear, the balloon is deflated and the blood can flow freely through the vessel and to the heart muscle. The procedure may also involve placing a stent within the coronary artery to keep the vessel open.

In ICD-10-PCS coding, Dilation of the coronary arteries is approached differently than Dilation of other vessels. The first difference concerns the body part value. The coronary arteries are considered as one body part and the body part value is based on the number of coronary arteries that are treated; one, two, three, or four or more arteries.

Also, the device character for these codes has values for drug-eluting intraluminal device, intraluminal device also known as bare-metal stent, radioactive intraluminal device, and no device. Within the drug-eluting intraluminal and intraluminal device values, there are choices for a single, two, three, or four or more stents. If multiple arteries are treated with different devices, a separate code is assigned for each procedure that uses a different device. These distinctions are emphasized in Coding Guideline B4.4.

B4.4. The coronary arteries are classified as a single body part that is further specified by number of arteries treated. One procedure code specifying multiple arteries is used when the same procedure is performed, including the same device and qualifier values.

Examples: Angioplasty of two distinct coronary arteries with placement of two stents is coded as Dilation of Coronary Artery, Two Arteries with Two Intraluminal Devices. Angioplasty of two distinct coronary arteries, one with stent placed and one without, is coded separately as Dilation of Coronary Artery, One Artery with Intraluminal Device, and Dilation of Coronary Artery, One Artery with no device.

Code building for Dilation of the coronary arteries can be demonstrated using the 027 table, table 5.1. Using the second example from Coding Guideline B4.4, if there were two distinct coronary arteries treated, one using an intraluminal device, such as a stent, and one without a device, two codes would be required: 02703DZ for the procedure that includes the stent and 02703ZZ for the PTCA without the device.

Table 5.1.   027 table

Section	0	Medical and Surgical		
Body System	2	Heart and Great Vessels		
Operation	7	Dilation: Expanding an orifice or the lumen of a tubular body part		
Body Part	**Approach**		**Device**	**Qualifier**
0 Coronary Artery, One Artery **1** Coronary Artery, Two Arteries **2** Coronary Artery, Three Arteries **3** Coronary Artery, Four or More Arteries	**0** Open **3** Percutaneous **4** Percutaneous Endoscopic		**4** Intraluminal Device, Drug-eluting **5** Intraluminal Device, Drug-eluting, Two **6** Intraluminal Device, Drug-eluting, Three **7** Intraluminal Device, Drug-eluting, Four or More **D** Intraluminal Device **E** Intraluminal Device, Two **F** Intraluminal Device, Three **G** Intraluminal Device, Four or More **T** Intraluminal Device, Radioactive **Z** No Device	**6** Bifurcation **Z** No Qualifier
F Aortic Valve **G** Mitral Valve **H** Pulmonary Valve **J** Tricuspid Valve **K** Ventricle, Right **L** Ventricle, Left **P** Pulmonary Trunk **Q** Pulmonary Artery, Right **S** Pulmonary Vein, Right **T** Pulmonary Vein, Left **V** Superior Vena Cava **W** Thoracic Aorta, Descending **X** Thoracic Aorta, Ascending/Arch	**0** Open **3** Percutaneous **4** Percutaneous Endoscopic		**4** Intraluminal Device, Drug-eluting **D** Intraluminal Device **Z** No Device	**Z** No Qualifier
R Pulmonary Artery, Left	**0** Open **3** Percutaneous **4** Percutaneous Endoscopic		**4** Intraluminal Device, Drug-eluting **D** Intraluminal Device **Z** No Device	**T** Ductus Arteriosus **Z** No Qualifier

Source: CMS 2019

Section	Body System	Root Operation	Body Part	Approach	Device	Qualifier
Medical and Surgical	Heart and Great Vessels	Dilation	Coronary Artery, One Artery	Percutaneous	Intraluminal Device	No Qualifier
0	2	7	0	3	D	Z

Section	Body System	Root Operation	Body Part	Approach	Device	Qualifier
Medical and Surgical	Heart and Great Vessels	Dilation	Coronary Artery, One Artery	Percutaneous	No Device	No Qualifier
0	2	7	0	3	Z	Z

Note that angioplasty of two distinct coronary arteries with three stents, one bare metal and two drug-eluting, would require two codes, one with the device value for intraluminal device and one with the device value for intraluminal device, drug-eluting, two.

Selected rows of code tables for Dilation of the upper arteries, lower arteries, and lower veins have the qualifier option of 1 for Drug-Coated Balloon. These balloons are not coded as devices as they do not remain in the patient's body at the conclusion of the procedure. Instead, the balloon catheter used in the Dilation procedure is coated with a drug that inhibits the restenosis of the vessel and the drug attaches to the vessel wall as the balloon is inflated during the procedure, after which the balloon is removed.

Bypass

Root Operation

Bypass (1): Altering the route of passage of the contents of a tubular body part.

The last root operation in group 5, root operations that alter the diameter or route of a tubular body part is Bypass, value 1. Bypass procedures represent rerouting procedures. This can involve rerouting contents of a body part to a downstream route or to a similar body part and route. For example, a femoropopliteal bypass procedure reroutes blood around blocked areas of the femoral artery to the popliteal artery, which is located in the knee area.

Other types of Bypass procedures reroute contents to an abnormal route and different body parts. For example, excess cerebrospinal fluid from the spinal canal may be rerouted to the atrium of the heart.

Bypass procedures include any anastomoses or surgical union of the tubular parts that are separated in the bypass procedure. Also included are any devices used in the Bypass procedure. Bypass procedures are subdivided into those involving the coronary arteries and any other Bypass not including the coronary arteries.

For noncoronary artery Bypass, the body part value indicates where the bypass originates, or comes from, and the qualifier character denotes where the bypass goes to or terminates. See table 5.2 for an example of a code table involving a Bypass procedure. If, for example, a patient had a Bypass of the cerebral ventricles to the peritoneal cavity to relieve the excess cerebrospinal fluid in hydrocephalus, the origin of the Bypass is the cerebral ventricle, and the termination is the peritoneal cavity. If this Bypass included a ventriculoperitoneal shunt inserted via an open procedure, the code would be 00160J6.

Section	Body System	Root Operation	Body Part	Approach	Device	Qualifier
Medical and Surgical	Central Nervous System and Cranial Nerves	Bypass	Cerebral Ventricle	Open	Synthetic Substitute	Peritoneal Cavity
0	0	1	6	0	J	6

Coding Guideline B3.6a emphasizes this designation of the portions of the Bypass procedure for noncoronary Bypass procedures.

Table 5.2.   001 table

Section	0	Medical and Surgical		
Body System	0	Central Nervous System and Cranial Nerves		
Operation	1	Bypass: Altering the route of passage of the contents of a tubular body part		
Body Part	Approach		Device	Qualifier
6 Cerebral Ventricle	0 Open 3 Percutaneous 4 Percutaneous Endoscopic		7 Autologous Tissue Substitute J Synthetic Substitute K Nonautologous Tissue Substitute	0 Nasopharynx 1 Mastoid Sinus 2 Atrium 3 Blood Vessel 4 Pleural Cavity 5 Intestine 6 Peritoneal Cavity 7 Urinary Tract 8 Bone Marrow B Cerebral Cisterns
6 Cerebral Ventricle	0 Open 3 Percutaneous 4 Percutaneous Endoscopic		Z No Device	B Cerebral Cisterns
U Spinal Canal	0 Open 3 Percutaneous 4 Percutaneous Endoscopic		7 Autologous Tissue Substitute J Synthetic Substitute K Nonautologous Tissue Substitute	2 Atrium 4 Pleural Cavity 6 Peritoneal Cavity 7 Urinary Tract 9 Fallopian Tube

Source: CMS 2019

B3.6a. Bypass procedures are coded by identifying the body part bypassed from and the body part bypassed to. The fourth character, body part, specifies the body part bypassed from, and the qualifier specifies the body part bypassed to.

Example: In a bypass from the stomach to the jejunum, stomach is the body part and jejunum is the qualifier.

If the Bypass procedure involves the coronary arteries, different conventions apply. As with the Dilation procedures, the body part value for the coronary arteries is based on the number of distinct coronary arteries treated. In the case of Bypass procedures, the coronary artery body part value is selected based on the number of arteries bypassed to. The qualifier value is selected based on the vessel bypassed from or the source of the blood flow, for example, the aorta in an aortocoronary bypass. Note that there are seven available qualifier values for bypass of coronary arteries listed in table 5.3 and in code table 021, a portion of which is exhibited in table 5.5.

The device character in the Bypass root operation code tables for the coronary artery has eight choices, as shown in table 5.4. The device includes graft material used to accomplish the Bypass procedure. For Bypass

Table 5.3.   Qualifiers for coronary artery sites—bypass

Value	Bypass Qualifiers
3	Coronary Artery
4	Coronary Vein
8	Internal Mammary, Right
9	Internal Mammary, Left
C	Thoracic Artery
F	Abdominal Artery
W	Aorta

Table 5.4.   Devices for coronary artery bypass

Value	Devices
4	Drug-eluting Intraluminal Device
8	Zooplastic Tissue
9	Autologous Venous Tissue
A	Autologous Arterial Tissue
D	Intraluminal Device
J	Synthetic Substitute
K	Nonautologous Tissue Substitute
Z	No Device

Table 5.5. Portion of 021 table coronary artery bypass

Section	0	Medical and Surgical
Body System	2	Heart and Great Vessels
Operation	1	Bypass: Altering the route of passage of the contents of a tubular body part

Body Part	Approach	Device	Qualifier
0 Coronary Artery, One Site **1** Coronary Artery, Two Sites **2** Coronary Artery, Three Sites **3** Coronary Artery, Four or More Sites	**0** Open	**9** Autologous Venous Tissue **A** Autologous Arterial Tissue **J** Synthetic Substitute **K** Nonautologous Tissue Substitute	**3** Coronary Artery **8** Internal Mammary, Right **9** Internal Mammary, Left **C** Thoracic Artery **F** Abdominal Artery **W** Aorta
0 Coronary Artery, One Site **1** Coronary Artery, Two Sites **2** Coronary Artery, Three Sites **3** Coronary Artery, Four or More Sites	**0** Open	**Z** No Device	**3** Coronary Artery **8** Internal Mammary, Right **9** Internal Mammary, Left **C** Thoracic Artery **F** Abdominal Artery
0 Coronary Artery, One Site **1** Coronary Artery, Two Sites **2** Coronary Artery, Three Sites **3** Coronary Artery, Four or More Sites	**3** Percutaneous	**4** Intraluminal Device, Drug-eluting **D** Intraluminal Device	**4** Coronary Vein
0 Coronary Artery, One Site **1** Coronary Artery, Two Sites **2** Coronary Artery, Three Sites **3** Coronary Artery, Four or More Sites	**4** Percutaneous Endoscopic	**4** Intraluminal Device, Drug-eluting **D** Intraluminal Device	**4** Coronary Vein
0 Coronary Artery, One Site **1** Coronary Artery, Two Sites **2** Coronary Artery, Three Sites **3** Coronary Artery, Four or More Sites	**4** Percutaneous Endoscopic	**9** Autologous Venous Tissue **A** Autologous Arterial Tissue **J** Synthetic Substitute **K** Nonautologous Tissue Substitute	**3** Coronary Artery **8** Internal Mammary, Right **9** Internal Mammary, Left **C** Thoracic Artery **F** Abdominal Artery **W** Aorta
0 Coronary Artery, One Site **1** Coronary Artery, Two Sites **2** Coronary Artery, Three Sites **3** Coronary Artery, Four or More Sites	**4** Percutaneous Endoscopic	**Z** No Device	**3** Coronary Artery **8** Internal Mammary, Right **9** Internal Mammary, Left **C** Thoracic Artery **F** Abdominal Artery
6 Atrium, Right	**0** Open **4** Percutaneous Endoscopic	**9** Autologous Venous Tissue **A** Autologous Arterial Tissue **J** Synthetic Substitute **K** Nonautologous Tissue Substitute	**P** Pulmonary Trunk **Q** Pulmonary Artery, Right **R** Pulmonary Artery, Left

Source: CMS 2019

procedures that receive blood flow from the coronary vein, the device values for Intraluminal (D) and Drug-eluting Intraluminal (4) are available. These two device values are not for grafts, but rather are devices used to keep the vessels open.

If the Bypass procedure involves a graft, the device value choices include grafts taken from the patient or autologous tissue, either a vein graft (9) or an artery graft (A); a synthetic substitute (J); a nonautologous tissue substitute that is not taken from the patient but from another source (K); or a zooplastic device (8), taken from an animal. For example, a saphenous vein graft taken from the patient would be represented by the device value 9, Autologous Venous Tissue. A radial artery graft harvested from the patient would be coded as device value A, Autologous Arterial Tissue.

To be considered a graft, the graft material needs to be separated from its original source and brought into the Bypass procedure, as in the example of a saphenous vein graft. This is key in considering the internal mammary arteries often used in coronary artery bypass procedures. In almost all circumstances, these vessels are not cut out and used as grafts, but rather, they are loosened from one side and brought around to supply blood flow to the blockage area in the coronary artery. Because these are not considered free grafts, the internal mammary arteries are not coded as devices, as in the example of the saphenous vein. Instead, this Bypass would have the device value of Z, No Device. In this procedure, the internal mammary artery is the source of the blood flow and, therefore, is reflected in the qualifier character.

The conventions for coronary artery Bypass procedures body part, qualifier, and device are emphasized in Coding Guideline B3.6b.

B3.6b. Coronary artery bypass procedures are coded differently than other bypass procedures as described in the previous guideline. Rather than identifying the body part bypassed from, the body part identifies the number of coronary arteries bypassed to, and the qualifier specifies the vessel bypassed from.

Example: Aortocoronary artery bypass of the left anterior descending coronary artery and the obtuse marginal coronary artery is classified in the body part axis of classification as two coronary arteries, and the qualifier specifies the aorta as the body part bypassed from.

As with the Dilation root operations involving coronary arteries, if more than one coronary artery is involved in a Bypass procedure and a different device is used, separate codes are assigned to represent each of the devices. This is also the case with procedures involving different qualifiers indicating the source of the Bypass. This is noted in Coding Guideline B3.6c.

 B3.6c. If multiple coronary arteries are bypassed, a separate procedure is coded for each coronary artery that uses a different device and/or qualifier.

Example: Aortocoronary artery bypass and internal mammary coronary artery bypass are coded separately.

Taking all of these conventions together in a coding example, if the procedure to be coded is a coronary artery bypass of two arteries, one from the left internal mammary artery to the left anterior descending artery, and the other using a left saphenous vein graft to the circumflex artery, two codes would be required to reflect the bypass. One of the codes represents the bypass from the left internal mammary to the left anterior descending artery, 02100Z9. The second represents the aortocoronary bypass to the circumflex using the saphenous vein graft, 021009W.

Section	Body System	Root Operation	Body Part	Approach	Device	Qualifier
Medical and Surgical	Heart and Great Vessels	Bypass	Coronary Artery, One Artery	Open	No Device	Internal Mammary, Left
0	2	1	0	0	Z	9

Section	Body System	Root Operation	Body Part	Approach	Device	Qualifier
Medical and Surgical	Heart and Great Vessels	Bypass	Coronary Artery, One Artery	Open	Autologous Venous Tissue	Aorta
0	2	1	0	0	9	W

Also, note that the procedure to harvest any graft material from a different operative site is coded separately using the Excision root operation. This is noted in Coding Guideline B3.9.

 B3.9. If an autograft is obtained from a different procedure site in order to complete the objective of the procedure, a separate procedure is coded.

Example: Coronary bypass with excision of saphenous vein graft, excision of saphenous vein is coded separately

For the procedure example above, an additional code for the harvest of the vein graft would be required. If this vein graft is on the left side, with a percutaneous endoscopic excision of a portion of the greater saphenous vein, the code would be 06BQ4ZZ.

Section	Body System	Root Operation	Body Part	Approach	Device	Qualifier
Medical and Surgical	Lower Veins	Excision	Saphenous Vein, Left	Percutaneous Endoscopic	No Device	No Qualifier
0	6	B	Q	4	Z	Z

More information about Bypass of the coronary arteries will be covered in chapter 11 of this text.

Group 6: Root Operations that Always Involve a Device

Group 6 includes the six root operations that always involve a device. These root operations are Insertion, Removal, Revision, Change, Replacement, and Supplement. These root operations put in, take out, correct, exchange, or use a device to take the place of or reinforce a body part. Key to each of the root operations is the device, which is the focus of the procedure. Other root operations may involve a device, but the device is not the objective of the procedure. For example, as discussed in the root operations that alter the diameter or route of a tubular body part, using the example of Dilation, devices such as bare metal or drug-eluting stents may be left in the vessel at the conclusion of the procedure to expand the lumen of the tubular body part. These intraluminal devices help to maintain the dilation. Placement of the stent was not the objective of the procedure. In any circumstance, if the procedure does not involve a device, then none of these root operations in this group would apply. All code tables for these root operations require the designation of a device; the Z for No Device is not available.

Insertion

Root Operation

Insertion (H): Putting in a nonbiological device that monitors, assists, performs, or prevents a physiological function but does not physically take the place of a body part.

The first root operation in group 6 is Insertion, which is putting in a nonbiological device. The device may monitor, assist, perform, or prevent a function; however, for Insertion procedures the device does not physically take the place of the body part. The value of H is used for Insertion.

In these procedures, the singular objective of the procedure is to put the device into the body part without performing any other procedure. If the objective of the procedure goes beyond inserting the device, then that procedure is coded instead of Insertion, and the device is noted in the device character. For example, as discussed earlier in this chapter, a partial closure of a vessel that involves introduction of embolization coils would be coded to Restriction rather than Insertion, and the embolization coil would be designated as the device in the 6th character of the code. A stent may be inserted as a part of a Dilation procedure, for example, in a percutaneous transluminal angioplasty. In this case, the intent of the procedure is not to insert the stent, but rather to dilate the vessel. The stent helps to maintain the dilation.

Examples of Insertion procedures include putting in a bone growth stimulator, inserting a cardiac pacemaker, or inserting a vascular access device. See figure 1.15 for an example of a tunneled vascular access device and 1.16 for an example of a contraceptive device.

Multiple insertion codes may be required. For example, if a traditional pacemaker is inserted, there are two components of the device, the generator and the lead or leads. A pocket is created in the subcutaneous tissue of the chest and the generator is inserted. See code table 0JH, table 5.6 for Insertion of devices into the subcutaneous tissue and fascia. In the example of a dual-chamber cardiac pacemaker, the code for the insertion of the generator into the subcutaneous tissue and fascia of the chest would be coded as 0JH606Z. The approach is Open because the surgeon makes an incision through the skin and into the subcutaneous tissue to visualize the site for placement of the generator.

Table 5.6. Portion of 0JH table

Section	0	Medical and Surgical
Body System	J	Subcutaneous Tissue and Fascia
Operation	H	Insertion: Putting in a nonbiological appliance that monitors, assists, performs, or prevents a physiological function but does not physically take the place of a body part

Body Part	Approach	Device	Qualifier
6 Subcutaneous Tissue and Fascia, Chest 8 Subcutaneous Tissue and Fascia, Abdomen	0 Open 3 Percutaneous	0 Monitoring Device, Hemodynamic 2 Monitoring Device 4 Pacemaker, Single Chamber 5 Pacemaker, Single Chamber Rate Responsive 6 Pacemaker, Dual Chamber 7 Cardiac Resynchronization Pacemaker Pulse Generator 8 Defibrillator Generator 9 Cardiac Resynchronization Defibrillator Pulse Generator A Contractility Modulation Device B Stimulator Generator, Single Array C Stimulator Generator, Single Array Rechargeable D Stimulator Generator, Multiple Array E Stimulator Generator, Multiple Array Rechargeable H Contraceptive Device M Stimulator Generator N Tissue Expander P Cardiac Rhythm Related Device V Infusion Device, Pump W Vascular Access Device, Totally Implantable X Vascular Access Device, Tunneled	Z No Qualifier

Source: CMS 2019

Section	Body System	Root Operation	Body Part	Approach	Device	Qualifier
Medical and Surgical	Subcutaneous Tissue and Fascia	Insertion	Subcutaneous Tissue and Fascia, Chest	Open	Pacemaker, Dual Chamber	No Qualifier
0	J	H	6	0	6	Z

The lead or leads that come from the pacemaker generator are inserted into the heart. In the example of the dual-chamber pacemaker, two leads are inserted; one into the right atrium and one into the right ventricle. These leads transfer the electrical impulses from the pacemaker generator to the right atrium and ventricle to stimulate contractions and regulate the heart's rhythm. The insertion of cardiac leads into the atrium and ventricle would be coded separately using the 02H table. The leads are percutaneously inserted as they are threaded through the veins of the chest. As reflected in table 5.7, the codes for the Insertion of the leads into the right atrium and right ventricle would be 02H63JZ and 02HK3JZ, respectively.

Section	Body System	Root Operation	Body Part	Approach	Device	Qualifier
Medical and Surgical	Heart and Great Vessels	Insertion	Atrium, Right	Percutaneous	Cardiac Lead, Pacemaker	No Qualifier
0	2	H	6	3	J	Z

Section	Body System	Root Operation	Body Part	Approach	Device	Qualifier
Medical and Surgical	Heart and Great Vessels	Insertion	Ventricle, Right	Percutaneous	Cardiac Lead, Pacemaker	No Qualifier
0	2	H	K	3	J	Z

Table 5.7. 02H table

Section	0	Medical and Surgical		
Body System	2	Heart and Great Vessels		
Operation	H	Insertion: Putting in a nonbiological appliance that monitors, assists, performs, or prevents a physiological function but does not physically take the place of a body part		

Body Part	Approach	Device	Qualifier
4 Coronary Vein **6** Atrium, Right **7** Atrium, Left **K** Ventricle, Right **L** Ventricle, Left	**0** Open **3** Percutaneous **4** Percutaneous Endoscopic	**0** Monitoring Device, Pressure Sensor **2** Monitoring Device **3** Infusion Device **D** Intraluminal Device **J** Cardiac Lead, Pacemaker **K** Cardiac Lead, Defibrillator **M** Cardiac Lead **N** Intracardiac Pacemaker **Y** Other Device	**Z** No Qualifier
A Heart	**0** Open **3** Percutaneous **4** Percutaneous Endoscopic	**Q** Implantable Heart Assist System **Y** Other Device	**Z** No Qualifier
A Heart	**0** Open **3** Percutaneous **4** Percutaneous Endoscopic	**R** Short-term External Heart Assist System	**J** Intraoperative **S** Biventricular **Z** No Qualifier
N Pericardium	**0** Open **3** Percutaneous **4** Percutaneous Endoscopic	**0** Monitoring Device, Pressure Sensor **2** Monitoring Device **J** Cardiac Lead, Pacemaker **K** Cardiac Lead, Defibrillator **M** Cardiac Lead **Y** Other Device	**Z** No Qualifier
P Pulmonary Trunk **Q** Pulmonary Artery, Right **R** Pulmonary Artery, Left **S** Pulmonary Vein, Right **T** Pulmonary Vein, Left **V** Superior Vena Cava **W** Thoracic Aorta, Descending	**0** Open **3** Percutaneous **4** Percutaneous Endoscopic	**0** Monitoring Device, Pressure Sensor **2** Monitoring Device **3** Infusion Device **D** Intraluminal Device **Y** Other Device	**Z** No Qualifier
X Thoracic Aorta, Ascending/Arch	**0** Open **3** Percutaneous **4** Percutaneous Endoscopic	**0** Monitoring Device, Pressure Sensor **2** Monitoring Device **3** Infusion Device **D** Intraluminal Device	**Z** No Qualifier

Source: CMS 2019

Removal

Root Operation

Removal (P): Taking out or off a device from a body part.

The next root operation in the grouping of procedures that always involve a device is Removal, which is taking out a device from a body part. The value of P is used for Removal procedures.

While Insertion procedures involve putting in a device as the objective of the procedure, Removal is taking out the device. A wide range of procedures are included in the Removal root operation, which involves taking out any device in a variety of body parts. Examples of these procedures include Removal of an infusion pump from the spinal canal, Removal of an internal fixation device from a joint, or Removal of a drainage device. In each case, the objective of the procedure is to take out or remove the device.

The device values may be more general than those found for the Insertion procedures. For example, for Removal procedures in the Subcutaneous Tissue and Fascia body system code table (0JP) there is one value for stimulator generator, M. For the Insertion code table in the Subcutaneous Tissue and Fascia code table (0JH) there is a value of M for stimulator generator. Also available are more specific device descriptions: stimulator generator, single array (B); stimulator generator, single array rechargeable (C); stimulator generator, multiple array (D); stimulator, multiple array rechargeable (E) (refer to table 5.6).

There is no restriction on the type of approach used for the Removal procedure. Code tables may list the approaches of open, percutaneous, percutaneous endoscopic, via natural or artificial opening, via natural or artificial opening endoscopic or external as appropriate. For example, the Removal of a bone growth stimulator from a lower bone such as the femur could be accomplished using an Open, Percutaneous, Percutaneous Endoscopic, or External approach as in code table 0QP. If this removal were done percutaneously the code would be 0QPY3MZ (see table 5.8).

Section	Body System	Root Operation	Body Part	Approach	Device	Qualifier
Medical and Surgical	Lower Bones	Removal	Lower Bone	Percutaneous	Bone Growth Stimulator	No Qualifier
0	Q	P	Y	3	M	Z

For a procedure to qualify as a Removal, a device—such as a drainage device, external fixation device, or intraluminal device—must be involved. The term "removal" may be used in clinical documentation to refer to a body part, such as removal of an ovary. However, because this is not a device, but rather a body part, it would be coded as a Resection if the entire ovary was removed or as an Excision if only part of the ovary was removed, as in the case of an ovarian cyst. The same principle would apply for removal of a kidney stone. Because this is not a device and not a body part but solid matter that results from an abnormal biological function, the root operation would be Extirpation if the stone is removed.

Devices are only coded if the device is to remain at the conclusion of the procedure. In limited cases, a qualifier value is available for Temporary or Intraoperative to indicate that a device is used for a short period of time either during the surgery or the hospitalization period. The qualifier of Intraoperative is found in the 02H table for use of a short-term External Heart Assist System. See table 5.9 for a portion of this table.

There are limited circumstances when a device is inserted and removed during the same operative episode. In this case, both an Insertion and a Removal procedure is coded. Coding Guideline B6.1a outlines the criteria for device coding and the limited instances of using the Temporary and Intraoperative qualifiers, as well as when both an Insertion and a Removal is coded.

B6.1a. A device is coded only if a device remains after the procedure is completed. If no device remains, the device value No Device is coded. In limited root operations, the classification provides the qualifier values Temporary and Intraoperative for specific procedures involving clinically significant devices, in which the purpose of the device is to be utilized for a brief duration during the procedure or current inpatient stay. If a device that is intended to remain after the procedure is completed requires removal before the end of the operative episode in which it was inserted (for example, the device size is inadequate or a complication occurs), both the insertion and removal of the device should be coded.

Table 5.8. Portion of 0QP table

Section	0	Medical and Surgical
Body System	Q	Lower Bones
Operation	P	Removal: Taking out or off a device from a body part

Body Part	Approach	Device	Qualifier
0 Lumbar Vertebra 1 Sacrum 4 Acetabulum, Right 5 Acetabulum, Left S Coccyx	0 Open 3 Percutaneous 4 Percutaneous Endoscopic	4 Internal Fixation Device 7 Autologous Tissue Substitute J Synthetic Substitute K Nonautologous Tissue Substitute	Z No Qualifier
0 Lumbar Vertebra 1 Sacrum 4 Acetabulum, Right 5 Acetabulum, Left S Coccyx	X External	4 Internal Fixation Device	Z No Qualifier
2 Pelvic Bone, Right 3 Pelvic Bone, Left 6 Upper Femur, Right 7 Upper Femur, Left 8 Femoral Shaft, Right 9 Femoral Shaft, Left B Lower Femur, Right C Lower Femur, Left D Patella, Right F Patella, Left G Tibia, Right H Tibia, Left J Fibula, Right K Fibula, Left L Tarsal, Right M Tarsal, Left N Metatarsal, Right P Metatarsal, Left Q Toe Phalanx, Right R Toe Phalanx, Left	0 Open 3 Percutaneous 4 Percutaneous Endoscopic	4 Internal Fixation Device 5 External Fixation Device 7 Autologous Tissue Substitute J Synthetic Substitute K Nonautologous Tissue Substitute	Z No Qualifier

Source: CMS 2019

Table 5.9. Portion of 02H table

Section	0	Medical and Surgical
Body System	2	Heart and Great Vessels
Operation	H	Insertion: Putting in a nonbiological appliance that monitors, assists, performs, or prevents a physiological function but does not physically take the place of a body part

Body Part	Approach	Device	Qualifier
4 Coronary Vein 6 Atrium, Right 7 Atrium, Left K Ventricle, Right L Ventricle, Left	0 Open 3 Percutaneous 4 Percutaneous Endoscopic	0 Monitoring Device, Pressure Sensor 2 Monitoring Device 3 Infusion Device D Intraluminal Device J Cardiac Lead, Pacemaker K Cardiac Lead, Defibrillator M Cardiac Lead N Intracardiac Pacemaker Y Other Device	Z No Qualifier
A Heart	0 Open 3 Percutaneous 4 Percutaneous Endoscopic	Q Implantable Heart Assist System Y Other Device	Z No Qualifier
A Heart	0 Open 3 Percutaneous 4 Percutaneous Endoscopic	R Short-term External Heart Assist System	J Intraoperative S Biventricular Z No Qualifier

Source: CMS 2019

Revision

Root Operation

Revision (W): Correcting, to the extent possible, a portion of a malfunctioning device or the position of a displaced device.

The next root operation in group 6 that involves a device is Revision, or correcting a faulty or displaced device. The value of W is used for this root operation.

In a Revision procedure, the objective is to fix a device that is not working correctly or that has moved out of its proper place. If the entire device is removed, this is not a Revision, but rather a Removal or other procedure. However, a portion of the device may be taken out or put back in order to accomplish the Revision. In Revision procedures, the device is the focus of the operation. For example, if a leak develops within a graft that was inserted to treat an aneurysm, the procedure to repair the leak is a Revision. Replacing only a portion of a device, such as a cracked polyethylene liner in the tibial surface of a total knee prosthesis is coded as a Revision. Other examples of Revision procedures include adjustments to cardiac pacemaker leads, Revision of a joint spacer, and Revision of a Sheffield ring external fixator on the tibia.

Again, recall that a device must be involved to be a Revision procedure. If a procedure is performed on a body part rather than a device, the Revision procedure cannot apply. For example, if a patient has a bypass procedure performed, directly rerouting the femoral artery to the popliteal artery, and a thrombus forms in the femoral artery, this is coded as an Extirpation procedure because material is removed from a body part. However, if this bypass was accomplished using a synthetic graft, and the graft became blocked by a thrombus, Revision would be coded for the removal of the thrombus because the device was the focus of the procedure.

Coding Tip

General body part values are used for the root operations Removal and Revision when the specific body part value is not found in the table.

Change

Root Operation

Change (2): Taking out or off a device from a body part and putting back an identical or similar device in or on the same body part without cutting or puncturing the skin or a mucous membrane.

The next root operation that involves a device is Change, which is taking out and putting back a device without cutting or puncturing. This is represented by the value of 2 in the ICD-10-PCS code.

To qualify as a Change procedure, the same or comparable type of device is put back in the body part after removing the original device. All of this must be done without making an incision or perforation in the skin or mucous membranes. These are often termed as exchange procedures. The only applicable approach for Change procedures is External. Examples of Change procedures are devices that are frequently exchanged, like drainage devices, such as chest catheters and feeding tubes. If a device is taken out without an exchange, the root operation is Removal.

Replacement

Root Operation

Replacement (R): Putting in or on biological or synthetic material that physically takes the place and/or function of all or a portion of a body part.

The next root operation in group 6, Replacement, involves putting in either a biological or synthetic material that takes the place and/or function of either an entire body part or a portion of a body part. The value of R is used for Replacement.

In Replacement procedures the original body part may be taken out before the Replacement is complete. It could also be destroyed before the Replacement, or made nonfunctional in some other way. Any of these methods to remove or disable the original body part are included in the Replacement procedure for the original replacement as they are inherent in the Replacement procedure. If, however, the Replacement is a repeat of an earlier Replacement procedure, removing the device placed during an earlier procedure is coded separately as a Removal. The subsequent Replacement is also coded.

An example of a Replacement procedure is a total hip replacement. If this is a first-time Replacement, then the removal of the native hip joint is included in the procedure as integral to the Replacement procedure. If, however, this is a worn-out hip prosthesis that is being replaced with a new total hip, then the Removal of the first prosthesis is coded as well as the Replacement procedure. Knee replacements can be total or partial; with the device value indicating whether the replacement is partial, or unicondylar. For example, a partial left knee replacement involving the medial condyle with cement is coded as 0SRD0L9. Another example of a Replacement procedure is using the big toe to replace a thumb that has been lost, for example in an industrial accident. Since the operation involves multiple body layers, the anatomical regions, upper extremities body system is used, with the autologous tissue substitute as the device. The body part that is being replaced is the thumb, and this is reflected in the body part value, with the toe as the 7th character qualifier. If the procedure was completed with an Open approach and the right thumb was replaced by the left toe, the code would be 0XRL07P.

Coding Tip

In Replacement procedures, removal, eradication, or disabling the native body part is included if this is the first Replacement for that particular body part. Any subsequent Replacement procedures would require separate codes for the Removal of the replaced body part and for the Replacement procedure.

A free skin graft is an example of a Replacement procedure. If this skin graft is from the patient, it is represented as an autologous tissue substitute. To qualify as a device, the skin graft must be completely separated from the body. Skin that remains attached, such as a pedicle graft, is coded as a Transfer. A cadaver skin donor is coded as nonautologous tissue substitute. Another example is an insertion of an intraocular lens as part of a cataract procedure. Because the intraocular lens takes the place of the lens removed in the cataract surgery, Replacement is the correct root operation, and the removal of the lens that included the cataract is not coded separately. Recall that a cataract removal without an insertion of an intraocular lens is coded as an Extraction. See chapter 3 of this text for a discussion of Extraction.

Supplement

Root Operation

Supplement (U): Putting in or on biologic or synthetic material that physically reinforces and/or augments the function of a portion of a body part.

The final root operation in group 6 is Supplement, which involves reinforcing and/or augmenting a portion of a body part using biological or synthetic material. Supplement procedures have the value of U.

The Supplement root operation includes putting in a device that supports or strengthens a body part or a portion of a body part. An example of a Supplement procedure is a hernia repair using mesh. The mesh is used to enhance the procedure. If the hernia is repaired without mesh, the root operation is Repair. This root operation will be covered in chapter 6 of this text.

Another example of a Supplement procedure is the reinforcement done as part of a carotid endarterectomy. After the thrombus is removed, a Dacron patch is used to reinforce the weakened portion of the vessel in the site of the thrombus. This augments the body part. Both the thrombectomy, represented as an Extirpation, and the Supplement are assigned codes because there are two separate objectives.

Supplement procedures augment the body part without replacing it. While in a Replacement procedure, some or all of the body part is replaced by the device, in a Supplement procedure, the device is added to the body to augment or reinforce the body part. For example, a penile prosthesis is inserted to augment or reinforce the function of the body part, the penis is not replaced. Supplement procedures can also be contrasted with Repair procedures, covered in chapter 6, in that a device is always involved for a Supplement procedure and not in Repair. For example, if a mitral valve is repaired using an annuloplasty ring, the ring is a device that reinforces the valve and the root operation is Supplement.

 ### Coding Tip

Supplement procedures always include a device that reinforces a body part without replacing it. The device may be biological material, such as a nerve graft, or synthetic material, such as mesh.

 ## Check Your Understanding

General Questions

1. A procedure that attempts to obstruct the blood flow to a malignant tumor would be coded to which root operation?
   a. Restriction
   b. Bypass
   c. Occlusion
   d. Dilation

2. A PTCA involved the left anterior descending (LAD) coronary artery and the right coronary artery (RCA). The LAD sites were treated with two drug-eluting stents inserted, and the RCA site had a bare metal stent. How many ICD-10-PCS codes will be needed to completely code this procedure?
   a. Four
   b. Three
   c. Two
   d. One

3. This procedure involves exchange of a percutaneous endoscopic gastrostomy tube. This is coded as which root operation?
   a. Removal
   b. Revision
   c. Change
   d. Replacement

4. A tubal ligation for sterility would be coded to which root operation?
   a. Occlusion
   b. Restriction
   c. Repair
   d. Destruction

5. For a procedure that involves a colostomy formation from the descending colon to the outside of the body via the skin, the colon is represented in which character of the ICD-10-PCS code?
   a. Body system
   b. Body part
   c. Device
   d. Qualifier

6. For Dilation procedures performed on the coronary arteries, what is represented in the body part value?
   a. Number of sites treated
   b. Number of stents or other devices inserted
   c. Number of arteries treated
   d. Number of bifurcations involved

7. True or false? In Replacement procedures, the removal of the native body part is coded as a separate procedure as the root operation Removal.
   a. True
   b. False

8. In which root operation is the objective to put in a device that augments a body part, without taking the body part out during the procedure?
   a. Replacement
   b. Revision
   c. Change
   d. Supplement

Which Root Operation Is It?

For each of the following descriptions, identify the root operation and the complete ICD-10-PCS code.

1. This patient is seen for follow up of a right tibial plateau fracture treatment with removal of a Sheffield ring by incision.

   Root Operation _____

   ICD-10-PCS Code _____

2. Newborn with pyloric stenosis was treated with a laparoscopic pyloromyotomy to relieve the stenosis.

   Root Operation _____

   ICD-10-PCS Code _____

3. A patient who has been on a long-term warfarin regimen for atrial fibrillation now presents for a Watchman Left Atrial Appendage closure insertion that is accomplished via cardiac catheterization.

   Root Operation _____

   ICD-10-PCS Code _____

(Continued)

4. A patient who has a history of compartment syndrome has a tissue expander inserted in the subcutaneous tissue of the left lower leg by incision in preparation for further surgery.

    Root Operation _____

    ICD-10-PCS Code _____

5. A patient with osteoarthritis of both knees is admitted for a cemented medial unicondylar knee replacements.

    Root Operation _____

    ICD-10-PCS Code _____

6. A newborn is treated for pulmonary valve stenosis; stretching of the valve opening is accomplished via a percutaneous balloon pulmonary valvuloplasty.

    Root Operation _____

    ICD-10-PCS Code _____

7. During surgery, a patient has a temporary closure of a portion of the descending thoracic aorta via an intraluminal device placed percutaneously.

    Root Operation _____

    ICD-10-PCS Code _____

8. A patient undergoes cystoscopy and repair of a malfunctioning artificial bladder sphincter.

    Root Operation _____

    ICD-10-PCS Code _____

9. Transfemoral transcatheter aortic valve implantation using the balloon expandable SAPIEN transcatheter heart valve device.

    Root Operation _____

    ICD-10-PCS Code _____

10. A patient had an open gastric bypass with Roux-en-Y limb to jejunum to treat morbid obesity.

    Root Operation _____

    ICD-10-PCS Code _____

11. A patient undergoes open coronary artery bypass graft surgery: left internal mammary artery to LAD, left radial artery (LRA) graft from the aorta to the posterior descending artery (PDA), and left saphenous vein graft from the aorta sequential to the diagonal to the obtuse marginal. Both the saphenous and radial artery grafts are harvested in separate incisions using a percutaneous endoscopic approach.

    a. How many codes are required to represent this procedure?

        _____

    b. What are the root operations?

        _____

    c. What are the codes?

        _____

Case Studies

Review the documentation in each case to determine the root operation and body system. Refer to the Index to find the code table for building the code, selecting the body part, approach, device, and qualifier.

1. Operative Report

This is an 86-year-old lady with left bundle, intermittent complete heart block, first-degree AV block and syncope. For the above reasons, she is undergoing implantation of a permanent pacemaker.

PROCEDURE: The patient was brought to the EP laboratory in a fasting state. Her left chest was prepped and draped in the usual sterile fashion. After local anesthesia, an incision was made on the left deltopectoral groove. The cephalic vein was isolated. The distal end was tied off. A venotomy was made and a Medtronic model 5076-52 lead was placed percutaneously into the right ventricular apex. In its final position, it was sutured in place with 2-0 Ethibond sutures. Final thresholds were for R waves of 18. Pacing threshold of 0.5 msec and lead impedance of 950.

An 18-gauge needle was easily placed into the left subclavian vein. Through that needle, a wire was advanced under fluoroscopic guidance into the IVC. Over this wire, a 7-French sheath was advanced and through this sheath, a Medtronic model 5076-52 lead was placed percutaneously in the high right atrium. In its final position, it was sutured in place with 2-0 Ethibond sutures. Final thresholds were for P waves of 18, Pacing threshold of 2 V and pacing impedance was 586.

Pacing was done at 10V and there was no diaphragmatic stimulation from either lead. Pacing threshold with deep breathing and coughing failed to result in loss of capture.

A pocket was made inferomedial to the incision. This was in the prepectoral space. The pocket was examined for bleeding and clots and none were evident. It was irrigated with antibiotic solutions. The leads were attached to a Medtronic model VEDR01. This was placed in the pocket with excess lead posterior to it and was sutured into place. The pocket was closed with interrupted 2-0 Vicryl, reinforced with running 3-0 Vicryl. The skin was closed with subcuticular 4-0 Dexon, and reinforced with Steri-strips. The patient tolerated the procedure well and was transferred back to her room in stable condition.

IMPRESSION: Successful implantation of Medtronic dual-chamber pacemaker.

2. Operative Report

PREOPERATIVE DIAGNOSIS:	Infected Broviac central venous catheter
POSTOPERATIVE DIAGNOSIS:	Infected Broviac central venous catheter
PROCEDURE PERFORMED:	Removal of infected central venous catheter
ANESTHESIA:	General

PROCEDURE: The child was brought to the operating room, and general anesthesia induced. A double-lumen Broviac catheter was identified exiting through an anterior chest wall incision. Local anesthetic was infiltrated at the exit site, and the subcutaneous tissue attached to the catheter was spread and percutaneously divided sharply until the central venous catheter was free and removed from the superior vena cava, and the tunneled catheter was removed from the subcutaneous layer of the chest. Pressure was used for hemostasis, and a sterile dressing applied to the exit site. Sponge, needle and instrument counts were reported to be correct at the conclusion of the procedure. The child was awakened and taken to the recovery room in satisfactory condition.

6

Root Operations that Involve Examination Only, Other Repairs, or Other Objectives

The last three groups of root operations in the Medical and Surgical section are those that involve examination only, that define other repairs, and that define other objectives. There are a total of seven root operations in these three groups, representing root operations that can be either very specific or very general in nature.

Group 7: Root Operations that Involve Examination Only

Group 7 includes two root operations: Inspection and Map.

Inspection

Root Operation

Inspection (J): Visually and/or manually exploring a body part.

Inspection includes exploring a body part visually, manually, or both. The value of J is used for this root operation. Bronchoscopy, colonoscopy, and arthrotomy are all examples of Inspections.

If this is a visual Inspection, optical instrumentation, such as endoscopes, may be used. If it is a manual exploration, this can be accomplished directly or via intervening body layers. When the exploration expands into multiple body layers, the deepest layer is the body part that is coded. This is noted in Coding Guideline B3.5 for Inspection as well as for Excision and Repair root operations.

B3.5. If the root operations Excision, Repair, or Inspection are performed on overlapping layers of the musculoskeletal system, the body part specifying the deepest layer is coded.

Example: Excisional debridement that includes skin and subcutaneous tissue and muscle is coded to the muscle body part.

Inspection procedures have the objective of looking rather than doing. The Inspection could be the objective to begin with, or it could be a procedure that started as another planned root operation but was canceled because of unforeseen circumstances. This is emphasized in Coding Guideline B3.3.

B3.3. If the intended procedure is discontinued or otherwise not completed, code the procedure to the root operation performed. If a procedure is discontinued before any other root operation is performed, code the root operation Inspection of the body part or anatomical region inspected.

Example: A planned aortic valve replacement procedure is discontinued after the initial thoracotomy and before any incision is made in the heart muscle, when the patient becomes hemodynamically unstable. This procedure is coded as an open Inspection of the mediastinum.

If, however, the inspection is merely the method used to get to the operative site in order to reach the objective of another root operation, then the inspection is not coded as it is considered an integral part of the procedure. For example, the use of an arthroscope to perform a procedure on the knee is covered in the Approach character and not coded separately. This is noted in Coding Guideline B3.11a.

B3.11a. Inspection of a body part(s) performed in order to achieve the objective of a procedure is not coded separately.

Example: In a fiberoptic bronchoscopy performed for irrigation of the bronchus, only the irrigation procedure is coded.

On the other hand, the Inspection procedure could be part of a procedure that requires multiple codes. This occurs when the Inspection is accomplished using one approach and another root operation is performed on the same body part using a different approach. This is clarified in Coding Guideline B3.11c.

B3.11c. When both an Inspection procedure and another procedure are performed on the same body part during the same episode, if the Inspection procedure is performed using a different approach than the other procedure, the Inspection procedure is coded separately.

Example: Endoscopic Inspection of the duodenum is coded separately when open Excision of the duodenum is performed during the same procedural episode.

Inspections of multiple tubular body parts in the same body system do not have an Inspection code for each area explored, but rather, the most distal area is coded as the body part. For example, an endoscopy that begins with the throat and ends with the bronchus would be coded to the appropriate bronchus body part as this is the furthest body part explored. If there is an exploration of multiple body parts that are not tubular, the body part value that represents the entire area inspected is selected. Coding Guideline B3.11b covers these situations.

B3.11b. If multiple tubular body parts are inspected, the most distal body part (the body part farthest from the starting point of the inspection) is coded. If multiple non-tubular body parts in a region are inspected, the body part that specifies the entire area inspected is coded.

Example: Cystoureteroscopy with inspection of bladder and ureters is coded to the ureter body part value. Exploratory laparotomy with general inspection of abdominal contents is coded to the peritoneal cavity body part value.

Coding Tip

Inspection involves looking at, rather than doing something to, a body part. If another root operation with a specific objective is completed on the Inspected body part, the Inspection becomes integral to the root operation that is performed.

Inspection may be coded separately if the procedure is changed to a different approach during the course of the operation. For example, a left inguinal hernia repair is attempted as a laparoscopic procedure, but changed to an open repair. In this case there would be two codes: an endoscopic Inspection and an open Repair of the inguinal area. This applies a portion of the multiple procedure guideline, B3.2d.

B3.2d. During the same operative episode, multiple procedures are coded if: The intended root operation is attempted using one approach, but is converted to a different approach.

Example: Laparoscopic cholecystectomy converted to an open cholecystectomy is coded as percutaneous endoscopic Inspection and open Resection.

Map

Root Operation

Map (K): Locating the route of passage of electrical impulses and/or locating functional areas in a body part.

The other root operation that includes only examination is Map, which is locating the route of passage of electrical impulses and/or locating functional areas in a body part. The value of K is used for this root operation.

The root operation Map is only used for the central nervous system and the cardiac conduction mechanism. This is a very small group of codes that encompasses only two code tables, 00K and 02K. Examples of Map procedures are intraoperative brain mapping and cardiac mapping, which are performed via catheterization or during an open-heart surgery.

Group 8: Root Operations that Define Other Repairs

The next two root operations in group 8 include a very general procedure, Repair, and a more specific one, Control.

Repair

Root Operation

Repair (Q): Restoring, to the extent possible, a body part to its normal anatomical structure and function.

The root operation Repair involves restoring a body part to its normal place and function. The value of Q is used to indicate a Repair procedure.

It should be noted that Repair procedures are only selected if no other root operation applies. If the objective of the procedure is reflected in an alternate root operation, then that root operation is selected. For example, if an anterior cruciate ligament repair is accomplished by repositioning the ligament to its correct place in the body, then the root operation Reposition is used rather than the less specific Repair root operation.

Recall that ICD-10-PCS has specificity as one of the goals of the system. Therefore, the codes, characters, and values are as precise as possible. However, the Repair root operation is essentially the Not Elsewhere Classified (NEC) value for ICD-10-PCS root operations, meaning that the procedure cannot be classified elsewhere in the system. Repair is the root operation selected if none of the others apply. Repair procedures include a wide variety of procedures, such as suturing lacerations of the skin or internal organs and herniorrhaphy procedures that do not include mesh.

Repair procedures do not include a device of any sort. If a device is left in place at the conclusion of the procedure, the Repair root operation cannot be applicable. Repair using a device is coded as a Supplement procedure. Refer to the repair decision tree in figure 6.1.

Coding Tip

Repair is the "NEC" or Not Elsewhere Classified root operation, and it is only used if the objective of the procedure is not described in another root operation. Supplement is the root operation used when the repair is accomplished using a device.

Control

Root Operation

Control (3): Stopping, or attempting to stop, postprocedural bleeding or other acute bleeding.

Figure 6.1. **Repair decision tree**

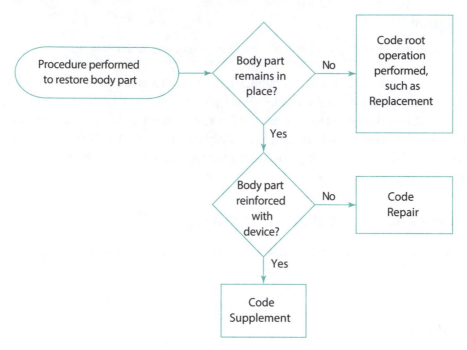

The root operation Control includes a limited range of procedures that attempt to stop postprocedural bleeding or other acute bleeding. The Control root operation is represented by the value of 3 for the 3rd character of the ICD-10-PCS code. Examples of Control procedures include postoperative ligation of bleeding arteries and drainage of postoperative hemorrhage.

Only four body systems are used in Control procedures: Ear. Nose and Sinus, 093, Anatomical Regions, General, 0W3; Anatomical Regions, Upper Extremities, 0X3; or Anatomical Regions, Lower Extremities, 0Y3. The body part is a general body part name, such as nasal mucosa and soft tissue, head, pleural cavity, or gastro-intestinal tract. For example, control of postprocedural or other acute bleeding in the chest wall would be coded to the General Anatomical Regions, the knee region would be coded to the Lower Extremities Region, and the arm would be coded to the Upper Extremities Region.

Coding Tip

Only four code tables are available for Control procedures: 093, 0W3, 0X3, and 0Y3.

Control procedures include preparing the operative site using irrigation and removing any hematomas that may be present. However, if the attempts to control the bleeding are unsuccessful and a more definitive root operations such as Bypass, Detachment, Excision, Extraction, Reposition, Replacement, or Resection is performed, this more definitive root operation is coded and not Control. This is emphasized in Coding Guideline B3.7.

B3.7. The root operation Control is defined as, "Stopping, or attempting to stop, postprocedural or other acute bleeding." If an attempt to stop postprocedural or other acute bleeding is unsuccessful, and to stop the bleeding requires performing a more definitive root operation, such as Bypass, Detachment, Excision, Extraction, Reposition, Replacement, or Resection, then the more definitive root operation is coded instead of Control.

Example: Resection of spleen to stop bleeding is coded to Resection instead of Control.

Group 9: Root Operations that Define Other Objectives

The last grouping of root operations includes a disparate group of three procedures: Fusion, Alteration, and Creation. These are all procedures that define other objectives, though the procedures are not related to one another.

Fusion

Root Operation

Fusion (G): Joining together portions of an articular body part, thereby rendering the articular body part immobile.

Fusion, or joining articular body parts together to make the body part immobile, is represented by the value of G for the root operation character. By definition, these procedures can only be performed on joint structures. The objective of the procedure is to make the joint immobile by fusing the articular parts. Examples of fusion procedures are spinal fusions and fusion of the joints of the hands or feet.

Coding Tip

Fusion root operations are only performed on joints with the objective of making them immobile. Therefore, the only code tables available for Fusion procedures are in the joint body systems—the upper joints, or 0RG, and the lower joints, or 0SG.

Fusion of spinal joints is coded using the 0RG code table for occipito-cervical, cervical, thoracic, or thoracolumbar joints, or the 0SG code table for lumbar, lumbosacral, sacrococcygeal, and sacroiliac joints. When building codes for spinal fusion, these tables are consulted based on the level of the spine involved in the Fusion procedure. The factor used to designate the number of body parts is based on the joint, however, and not the vertebrae. For example, when a Fusion procedure is performed at C1 to C2, this is one joint. In contrast, if the procedure is performed on C1 to C3, there are two joints involved—C1 to C2 and C2 to C3. This is noted in Coding Guideline B3.10a.

B3.10a. The body part coded for a spinal vertebral joint(s) rendered immobile by a spinal fusion procedure is classified by the level of the spine (e.g., thoracic). There are distinct body part values for a single vertebral joint and for multiple vertebral joints at each spinal level.

Example: Body part values specify Lumbar Vertebral Joint; Lumbar Vertebral Joints, 2 or More; and Lumbosacral Vertebral Joint.

When selecting the body part value for Fusion procedures, the device and qualifier designation must also be considered. See tables 6.1 and 6.2 for the 0RG and 0SG tables and refer to the device and qualifier columns for the vertebral joint body parts in each table. If more than one device or qualifier is used for the Fusion procedure, each is represented by a separate procedure code. Note that the qualifier character for spinal fusion indicates the approach to the spinal column, from the front or the back and the applicable side of the spinal column. There are three options in the first row of the 0RG and 0SG tables:

- Anterior approach, anterior column, coming from the front and working on the front of the spinal column
- Posterior approach, posterior column, coming from the back and working on the back of the spinal column
- Posterior approach, anterior column, coming from the back and working on the front of the spinal column

Table 6.1. Portion of 0RG table

Section	0	Medical and Surgical
Body System	R	Upper Joints
Operation	G	Fusion: Joining together portions of an articular body part rendering the articular body part immobile

Body Part	Approach	Device	Qualifier
0 Occipital-cervical Joint **1** Cervical Vertebral Joint **2** Cervical Vertebral Joints, 2 or more **4** Cervicothoracic Vertebral Joint **6** Thoracic Vertebral Joint **7** Thoracic Vertebral Joints, 2 to 7 **8** Thoracic Vertebral Joints, 8 or more **A** Thoracolumbar Vertebral Joint	**0** Open **3** Percutaneous **4** Percutaneous Endoscopic	**7** Autologous Tissue Substitute **J** Synthetic Substitute **K** Nonautologous Tissue Substitute	**0** Anterior Approach, Anterior Column **1** Posterior Approach, Posterior Column **J** Posterior Approach, Anterior Column
0 Occipital-cervical Joint **1** Cervical Vertebral Joint **2** Cervical Vertebral Joints, 2 or more **4** Cervicothoracic Vertebral Joint **6** Thoracic Vertebral Joint **7** Thoracic Vertebral Joints, 2 to 7 **8** Thoracic Vertebral Joints, 8 or more **A** Thoracolumbar Vertebral Joint	**0** Open **3** Percutaneous **4** Percutaneous Endoscopic	**A** Interbody Fusion Device	**0** Anterior Approach, Anterior Column **J** Posterior Approach, Anterior Column
C Temporomandibular Joint, Right **D** Temporomandibular Joint, Left **E** Sternoclavicular Joint, Right **F** Sternoclavicular Joint, Left **G** Acromioclavicular Joint, Right **H** Acromioclavicular Joint, Left **J** Shoulder Joint, Right **K** Shoulder Joint, Left	**0** Open **3** Percutaneous **4** Percutaneous Endoscopic	**4** Internal Fixation Device **7** Autologous Tissue Substitute **J** Synthetic Substitute **K** Nonautologous Tissue Substitute	**Z** No Qualifier

Source: CMS 2019

The 5th character of the code continues to represent the approach to the body, such as the Open or Percutaneous approach.

If combinations of devices and materials are used within the vertebral joint in the Fusion procedure, there are specific rules regarding how the device character is assigned. In the instance where an Interbody Fusion Device is used either alone or in combination with other materials, such as bone graft, the Interbody Fusion Device, value A, is selected for the device character. If the Interbody Fusion Device is not applicable, and bone graft is the device used for the Fusion procedure, either as the sole device or in combination with biological or nonbiological additions, then the bone graft is the device selected. If the bone graft is a combination of autologous and nonautologous material, the autologous tissue substitute is the value selected for the device value.

Subparts b and c of Coding Guideline B3.10 emphasize how to handle these multiple and combination circumstances when coding Fusion of the vertebral joints.

Table 6.2.   0SG table

Section	0	Medical and Surgical		
Body System	S	Lower Joints		
Operation	G	Fusion: Joining together portions of an articular body part rendering the articular body part immobile		

Body Part	Approach	Device	Qualifier
0 Lumbar Vertebral Joint **1** Lumbar Vertebral Joints, 2 or more **3** Lumbosacral Joint	**0** Open **3** Percutaneous **4** Percutaneous Endoscopic	**7** Autologous Tissue Substitute **J** Synthetic Substitute **K** Nonautologous Tissue Substitute	**0** Anterior Approach, Anterior Column **1** Posterior Approach, Posterior Column **J** Posterior Approach, Anterior Column
0 Lumbar Vertebral Joint **1** Lumbar Vertebral Joints, 2 or more **3** Lumbosacral Joint	**0** Open **3** Percutaneous **4** Percutaneous Endoscopic	**A** Interbody Fusion Device	**0** Anterior Approach, Anterior Column **J** Posterior Approach, Anterior Column
5 Sacrococcygeal Joint **6** Coccygeal Joint **7** Sacroiliac Joint, Right **8** Sacroiliac Joint, Left	**0** Open **3** Percutaneous **4** Percutaneous Endoscopic	**4** Internal Fixation Device **7** Autologous Tissue Substitute **J** Synthetic Substitute **K** Nonautologous Tissue Substitute	**Z** No Qualifier
9 Hip Joint, Right **B** Hip Joint, Left **C** Knee Joint, Right **D** Knee Joint, Left **F** Ankle Joint, Right **G** Ankle Joint, Left **H** Tarsal Joint, Right **J** Tarsal Joint, Left **K** Tarsometatarsal Joint, Right **L** Tarsometatarsal Joint, Left **M** Metatarsal-Phalangeal Joint, Right **N** Metatarsal-Phalangeal Joint, Left **P** Toe Phalangeal Joint, Right **Q** Toe Phalangeal Joint, Left	**0** Open **3** Percutaneous **4** Percutaneous Endoscopic	**4** Internal Fixation Device **5** External Fixation Device **7** Autologous Tissue Substitute **J** Synthetic Substitute **K** Nonautologous Tissue Substitute	**Z** No Qualifier

Source: CMS 2019

B3.10b. If multiple vertebral joints are fused, a separate procedure is coded for each vertebral joint that uses a different device and/or qualifier.

Example: Fusion of the lumbar vertebral joint, posterior approach, anterior column and fusion of the lumbar vertebral joint, posterior approach, posterior column are coded separately.

B3.10c. Combinations of devices and materials are often used on a vertebral joint to render the joint immobile. When combinations of devices are used on the same vertebral joint, the device value coded for the procedure is as follows:

- If an interbody fusion device is used to render the joint immobile (alone or containing other material like bone graft), the procedure is coded with the device value Interbody Fusion Device.
- If bone graft is the *only* device used to render the joint immobile, the procedure is coded with the device value Nonautologous Tissue Substitute or Autologous Tissue Substitute.
- If a mixture of autologous and nonautologous bone graft (with or without biological or synthetic extenders or binders) is used to render the joint immobile, code the procedure with the device value Autologous Tissue Substitute.

> **Example:** Fusion of a vertebral joint using a cage-style interbody fusion device containing morselized bone graft is coded to the device Interbody Fusion Device. Fusion of a vertebral joint using a bone dowel interbody fusion device made of cadaver bone and packed with a mixture of local morselized bone and demineralized bone matrix is coded to the device Interbody Fusion Device. Fusion of a vertebral joint using both autologous bone graft and bone bank bone graft is coded to the device Autologous Tissue Substitute.

For example, if the procedure performed was an anterior approach to the anterior column for interbody fusion C5 to C6 utilizing Bengal cage and bone graft, the code selected would be 0RG10A0.

Section	Body System	Root Operation	Body Part	Approach	Device	Qualifier
Medical and Surgical	Upper Joints	Fusion	Cervical Vertebral Joint	Open	Interbody Infusion Device	Anterior Approach, Anterior Column
0	R	G	1	0	A	0

As noted in Coding Guideline B3.9, a bone graft harvest procedure from a different procedure site is assigned a code as an Excision procedure. Excision of local bone for use in the fusion procedure is not coded separately.

B3.9. If an autograft is obtained from a different procedure site in order to complete the objective of the procedure, a separate procedure is coded.

Example: Coronary bypass with excision of saphenous vein graft, excision of saphenous vein is coded separately.

Note that, anatomically, an interbody fusion device can only be placed on the anterior column. As the second row of the 0RG and 0SG tables in tables 6.1 and 6.2 show, the only approaches available using the device value of A for interbody fusion device are for procedures on the anterior column; either the anterior approach (0) or posterior approach to the anterior column (J). The Fusion root operation will be described in more detail in chapter 16.

Alteration

Root Operation

Alteration (0): Modifying the natural anatomical structure of a body part without affecting the function of the body part.

The next root operation, Alteration, is for modifying a body part without affecting its function. This root operation is always designated with the value of 0.

Alteration procedures are those that are performed for cosmetic purposes, that is, only to improve appearance. Included would be procedures such as eyebrow lifts, breast augmentation, and otoplasty. Because there are some procedures that can either be performed to alter appearance or for medical purposes, the reason for the surgery must be noted and analyzed. For example, an eyelid lift or blepharoplasty can be performed for medical reasons and coded as a Repair, Replacement, Supplement, or Reposition. If the eyelid sags to the degree that it interferes with vision, for instance as a result of myasthenia gravis, a Reposition procedure may be the appropriate root operation as the body part is moved back to its normal location. However, if this procedure is done solely for appearance, the Alteration root operation would be used. Using the reason for the surgery in Alteration is the only instance where diagnostic information affects ICD-10-PCS coding.

Creation

Root Operation

Creation (4): Putting in or on biological or synthetic material to form a new body part that to the extent possible replicates the anatomic structure or function of an absent body part.

The last root operation, Creation, is designated by the value of 4. There are two main purposes for this root operation, the first of which is gender reassignment operations. There is only one code table available (0W4), for changing genital structures from male to female or female to male. The body part value in the code describes the structure present at the start of the procedure, and the qualifier value describes the structure created, or found, at the conclusion of the procedure. There are three choices in the device character: Autologous, Synthetic, and Nonautologous tissue substitute. Recall that if an autograft is used in the procedure, the harvesting of this tissue from a different procedure site is coded separately.

The second use of the Creation root operation is in the Heart and Great Vessels body system. Here, Creation represents creating a body part with a device to serve as a body part that is absent in the patient. Code table 024, shown in table 6.3, represents these procedures for the aortic, mitral, and tricuspid valves.

Table 6.3. 024 table

Section	0	Medical and Surgical		
Body System	2	Heart and Great Vessels		
Operation	4	Creation: Putting in or on biological or synthetic material to form a new body part that to the extent possible replicates the anatomic structure or function of an absent body part		

Body Part	Approach	Device	Qualifier
F Aortic Valve	0 Open	7 Autologous Tissue Substitute 8 Zooplastic Tissue J Synthetic Substitute K Nonautologous Tissue Substitute	J Truncal Valve
G Mitral Valve J Tricuspid Valve	0 Open	7 Autologous Tissue Substitute 8 Zooplastic Tissue J Synthetic Substitute K Nonautologous Tissue Substitute	2 Common Atrioventricular Valve

Source: CMS 2019

 Check Your Understanding

General Questions

1. A patient is scheduled for a laparoscopic hysterectomy, but this is converted to an abdominal total hysterectomy after the laparoscope is introduced. How is this coded?
    a. Endoscopic Inspection of the uterus
    b. Endoscopic Resection of the uterus and cervix
    c. Endoscopic Inspection of the uterus and open Resection of the uterus and cervix
    d. Open Resection of the uterus and cervix

(Continued)

2. The Map root operation is only used for the cardiac system and what other system?
   a. Peripheral Nervous System
   b. Respiratory System
   c. Arterial and Venous System
   d. Central Nervous System and Cranial Nerves

3. Which of the following statements is false about the root operation Control?
   a. Only three body systems are applicable to Control.
   b. It refers to postprocedural and other acute bleeding.
   c. Irrigation of hematoma(s) is coded separately.
   d. If another more definitive root operation is performed, then Control is not coded.

4. A patient has a colonoscopy followed by removal of two polyps. How is this coded?
   a. Inspection of the colon
   b. Excision of the colon
   c. Inspection and Excision of the colon
   d. Inspection and Resection of the colon

5. Which root operation is considered the NEC procedure in ICD-10-PCS?
   a. Repair
   b. Control
   c. Creation
   d. Alteration

6. A patient has a spinal fusion that includes a bone graft consisting of both autologous and nonautologous material. How is this graft coded?
   a. With both the autologous and nonautologous grafts
   b. With only the autologous graft
   c. With only the nonautologous graft
   d. With synthetic substitute

7. A patient has a bilateral breast reduction surgery and lift. The documentation states that the patient is experiencing severe back and neck strain due to pendulous breasts. This surgery would be coded to which root operation?
   a. Alteration
   b. Repair
   c. Excision
   d. Reposition

Which Root Operation Is It?

For each of the following descriptions, identify the root operation and the complete ICD-10-PCS code.

1. A patient presents for surgical repair of a rotator cuff tear of the left shoulder and undergoes arthroscopic investigation and repair of the glenohumeral joint.

   Root Operation _____

   ICD-10-PCS Code _____

2. A patient with a blunt injury to the chest undergoes thoracotomy and repair of cardiac rupture.

   Root Operation _____

   ICD-10-PCS Code _____

3. A patient is returned to the operating room after open heart surgery to investigate postoperative hemorrhage. An incision is made at the original operative site without opening the sternum and the source of the bleeding is identified and corrected.

   Root Operation _____

   ICD-10-PCS Code _____

4. An 86-year-old patient is seen after a syncope incident and is suspected to be suffering from bowel ischemia. An exploratory laparotomy is performed with no evidence of transmural ischemia or necrosis of the gastrointestinal tract.

   Root Operation _____

   ICD-10-PCS Code _____

5. The patient has an open posterior spinal fusion of the posterior column, L4 to L5 and L5 to S1, using allograft bone.

   Root Operation _____

   ICD-10-PCS Code _____

6. A patient presents for a cosmetic rhinoplasty in which a Gore-Tex implant is placed by incision.

   Root Operation _____

   ICD-10-PCS Code _____

7. A patient undergoes male to female gender-reassignment surgery in which a vagina is formed using donor tissue.

   Root Operation _____

   ICD-10-PCS Code _____

8. A patient undergoes a female to male gender reassignment operation in which a penis is created using autografts that were previously harvested from both arms and saved in a tissue bank.

   Root Operation _____

   ICD-10-PCS Code _____

9. A patient has an open arthrodesis of the carpometacarpal joint of the right thumb using a cannulated screw and threaded washer.

   Root Operation _____

   ICD-10-PCS Code _____

10. A patient undergoes exploratory arthroscopy of the left shoulder.

   Root Operation _____

   ICD-10-PCS Code _____

Case Studies

Review the documentation in each case to determine the root operation and body system. Refer to the index to find the code table for building the code, selecting the body part, approach, device, and qualifier.

1. Operative Report

PREOPERATIVE DIAGNOSIS:	Incarcerated right inguinal hernia
POSTOPERATIVE DIAGNOSIS:	Strangulated right femoral hernia
PROCEDURE PERFORMED:	1. Small bowel resection
	2. Repair of strangulated right femoral hernia
ANESTHESIA:	General anesthesia
ESTIMATED BLOOD LOSS:	15–20 mL

HISTORY: This patient is an 85-year-old female that apparently has had a painful rock hard bulge in the right groin for at least 3 days. This has been associated with increased pain and vomiting. Exam in the ER revealed a rock hard, tender, irreducible right groin mass consistent with an incarcerated hernia. I was concerned that it perhaps strangulated based on her symptomatology and the length of her symptoms and thus I explained to the patient as well as her daughter at bedside that we might have to resect bowel as well as repair the hernia. The procedure for this and the chance of postop complications were all discussed with the patient and her daughter and they agreed to surgery.

WHAT WAS DONE: With the patient in supine position, she was anesthetized and the abdomen was prepped and draped in the usual fashion. A right groin oblique incision was made and sharp dissection was done and in fact, I found that she had a strangulated femoral hernia, coming out from beneath the inguinal ligament. Through the femoral canal was a tight irreducible fairly thick sac containing what appeared to be ischemic bowel. In order to manipulate this and open it up, I did split the external abdominal oblique fascia, and worked on this hernia from both above and below. I opened up the inguinal ligament a little bit to facilitate opening up the neck of this hernia, so that I could manipulate the bowel. I opened the hernia sac and sure enough found a knuckle of small intestine, probably about 3–4 inches in length was present and appeared ischemic, if not showing early gangrene. I did not feel that this bowel would fly. Thus, the neck of the femoral defect was made a little bit bigger by gently stretching and then I mobilized bowel both proximal and distal to the bowel in question. Once I got an adequate length of intestine out, I fired a GIA stapler both proximally and distally to the bowel that appeared to be ischemic, took down the mesentery with clamps and tied if off with silk and chromic and sent the pieces of intestine as a specimen. I then took the side of the cut end of the distal bowel and did a hand-sewn 2 layer anastomosis. A posterior seromuscular layer of silks was placed followed by making an enterotomy into each bowel limb, followed by a posterior mucosal layer of chromics and anterior mucosal layer of silks. The resulting anastomosis had a good 2 fingerbreadth lumen. No twisting. No tension and it had good color. There was no real mesenteric rent that I could see that was left after I closed this anastomosis. I then gently reduced the anastomosed bowel back into the abdominal cavity through the femoral hernia defect. The femoral hernia defect was then closed with interrupted silk sutures, taking the iliopubic tract down to Cooper's ligament. This was done under direct visualization. Starting at the pubic tubercle and going out laterally and I went just up to the femoral vessels and nerve staying well away from them and yet still closing the defect. A total of 4 sutures were placed and again the iliopubic tract was brought down to Cooper's ligament and the defect was closed and no undue pressure was laced on the femoral nerve and vessels. Copious irrigation was then used throughout the wound and it returned clear. I then reapproximated part of the inguinal ligament with interrupted chromic sutures. I approximated the split external abdominal oblique fascia with interrupted chromic sutures and running chromic sutures. The subcu and fascia were then closed with chromic, followed by staples to the skin. The patient had the wound dressed. She tolerated the procedure well and left the operating room for recovery in stable condition.

2. Operative Report

PREOPERATIVE DIAGNOSES:	1. Spasticity of cerebral and spinal origin 2. Status post successful lumbar puncture for intrathecal baclofen trial
POSTOPERATIVE DIAGNOSES:	1. Spasticity of cerebral and spinal origin 2. Status post successful lumbar puncture for intrathecal baclofen trial
PROCEDURE PERFORMED:	Attempted baclofen pump placement with a lumbar puncture for intra-thecal catheter aborted
ANESTHESIA:	General
PREP:	Standard
SPECIAL CONSIDERATIONS:	Obesity

INDICATIONS: This is a 44-year-old gentleman with longstanding spasticity of both cerebral and spinal origin. He had a successful baclofen trial 2 weeks earlier. He was brought in for placement of baclofen pump. The patient had multiple operations in the low back including fusion previously. After discussion of risks and benefits with the patient and his family, they agreed to proceed with surgery.

FINDINGS: Ancef antibiotic was given within 30 minutes of skin incision and discontinued within 24 hours. Venous thromboembolic precautions were taken prior to surgery and discontinued postop.

ESTIMATED BLOOD LOSS FOR THIS PROCEDURE:	Minimal
SPECIMENS TO PATHOLOGY:	None
INSTRUMENTATION:	None
MONITORING:	None

OPERATION: The patient was identified in the preoperative holding area and taken to the operative suite at which time general anesthesia was induced. He was then placed in the left lateral decubitus position with the right side up, padding pressure points and prepped and draped in standard fashion for placement of baclofen pump. After appropriate time-out to identify the patient, correct location and operation, the operation commenced. A 1% lidocaine with 1:200,000 epinephrine was instilled in previous incision in the low back at approximately the level of L4-L5. Intraoperative fluoroscopy was used to help confirm this level. A Tuohy needle was used to attempt a lumbar puncture. Because of the patient's previous surgery and also the body habitus, it was difficult to attain CSF after three attempts. A second neurosurgeon also tried to access with a longer needle with no success. After multiple attempts at CSF access, it was recommended to abort the procedure and bring the patient back for an open procedure to see if access to the thecal space could be accomplished in that manner. The wound was then copiously irrigated and closed using 3-0 Vicryl interrupted sutures and staples for the skin. The sterile dressing was applied. The patient was extubated in the operating room and taken to post-anesthesia care unit in stable and unchanged condition. Plan was for him to be returning back to the operating room in 1 week.

Chapter 7

Anatomical Regions

ICD-10-PCS includes body systems called Anatomical Regions, which describe general locations of the body. These general locations are for use in coding when procedures are performed on multiple body parts and through various types of structures, such as skin, muscles, arteries, nerves, and bone, all within one area of the body. This facilitates coding of procedures that involve all of these structures and can reduce the number of codes required to correctly describe complex procedures performed in these areas. For example, amputation of the right arm at midshaft, below the elbow, is coded with one code—0X6D0Z2—rather than multiple codes from several body systems, such as the skin, musculoskeletal system, nervous system, and circulatory system.

Anatomical Regions: General, Upper Extremities, and Lower Extremities

When these types of procedures are performed on individual body parts, the procedures are coded based on the root operation performed on a specific body part within the specific body system section and not in the anatomical regions. The 2nd character values for the Anatomical Region body systems are:

W—Anatomical Regions, General
X—Anatomical Regions, Upper Extremities
Y—Anatomical Regions, Lower Extremities

Coding Tip

When procedures are performed on individual body parts, those procedures are coded based on the root operation performed on the specific body part within the specific body system section, not the anatomical region.

Organization of the Anatomical Regions

The anatomical regions include the general regions, the upper extremity regions, and the lower extremity regions. The major body cavities are included in the general regions body system, as well as other larger body areas. The upper extremity regions and lower extremity regions encompass the remainder of the articular skeleton and all of their associated body parts.

Coding Tip

When a specific site within another body system is documented, code the most specific body part value within that system. If a specific site cannot be located within any other body system, evaluate whether ICD-10-PCS has assigned the body part to the Anatomical Regions, General as the normal location.

Anatomy Alert

ICD-10-PCS does not classify regions of the body by the traditional abdominopelvic quadrant divisions. The anatomical regions are defined as the general regions, the upper extremity regions, and the lower extremity regions. The inguinal region is defined as part of the Anatomical Regions, Lower Extremities body system in ICD-10-PCS.

General Anatomical Regions

The general regions include the traditional body cavities. Body cavities are spaces within the body that contain organs and other structures. The body cavities are the cranial cavity; oral cavity and throat; pleural cavity; mediastinum, including the pericardial cavity; peritoneal cavity; retroperitoneum; and pelvic cavity. These cavities include the following organs and structures:

- Cranial cavity
  - Central nervous system structures, including the brain and cranial meninges, above the level of the foramen magnum
- Oral cavity and throat
  - Teeth and gingiva, hard and soft palate, pharynx, tongue, uvula, tonsils, adenoids, larynx and vocal cords
- Mediastinum
  - Thymus, heart (inside the pericardial cavity), great vessels, trachea, upper 2/3 of esophagus, thoracic duct, lymph nodes
- Peritoneal cavity
  - Liver, gallbladder with biliary tract, stomach, tail of pancreas, first part of the duodenum, spleen, omentum, mesentery, small intestines, cecum with appendix, and transverse colon
- Retroperitoneum (retroperitoneal cavity)
  - Adrenal glands, abdominal aorta, inferior vena cava, lower 1/3 of esophagus, parts two through four of the duodenum, pancreas (except tail), ascending colon, descending colon, kidneys, ureters and rectum
- Pelvic cavity
  - Reproductive organs, urinary bladder and sigmoid colon

Also included in the general regions are the larger surface areas of the body such as the head, neck, chest wall, abdominal wall, and upper and lower back. The three main tubular tracts of the body, the gastrointestinal tract, the respiratory tract, and the genitourinary tract, are also included here.

When coding procedures performed on large body areas or cavities, these body parts are categorized in the Anatomical Regions, General section of ICD-10-PCS. For example, Coding Guideline B3.11b states that an exploratory laparotomy (open incision into the abdomen to view the contents) is coded to the peritoneal cavity body part value in this section. Procedures performed on the cavities themselves are also coded within the Anatomical Regions, General body system.

Coding Tip

Procedures performed on the pleural cavity, rather than the pleura itself, are classified in the Anatomical Regions, General body system in ICD-10-PCS. See chapter 10 on the Mouth, Throat, and Respiratory System for the discussion on procedures performed on the pleura.

B3.11b. If multiple tubular body parts are inspected, the most distal body part (the body part farthest from the starting point of the inspection) inspected is coded. If multiple non-tubular body parts in a region are inspected, the body part that specifies the entire area inspected is coded.

Example: Cystoureteroscopy with inspection of bladder and ureters is coded to the ureter body part value. Exploratory laparotomy with general inspection of abdominal contents is coded to the peritoneal cavity body part value.

Figure 7.1 shows the body cavities. Not pictured is the pericardial cavity in the middle chest, which contains the heart and the retroperitoneum, which is behind the peritoneal cavity (Applegate 2011, 247). Figure 7.2 provides a thorough orientation to the anatomical regions of the body, although not all of these regions are used in code assignment. However, they are commonly used as descriptive terms in operative reports. For example, a physician may describe the palmar region in a report but ICD-10-PCS refers to this as the hand for coding purposes.

Upper Extremity Region

The upper extremity region contains body parts that are found above the central dividing line of the diaphragm. Both of the axilla are defined as part of the Anatomical Regions, Upper Extremities body system in ICD-10-PCS. Body part values in this system are used to describe the level of amputation in the root operation of Detachment. A ray of the hand consists of the continuous grouping of a metacarpal and phalanx associated with one finger. The body part Forequarter describes the entire upper limb plus the scapula and clavicle. Figure 7.3 displays the rays of the hand, including the metacarpals and phalanges.

Figure 7.1. Body cavities

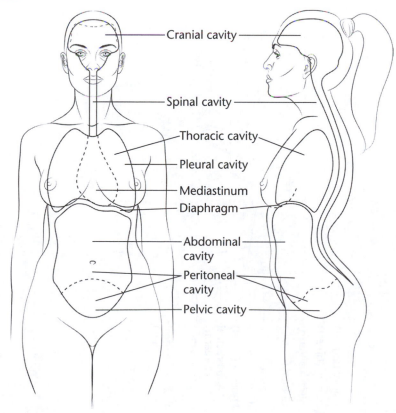

© AHIMA 2019

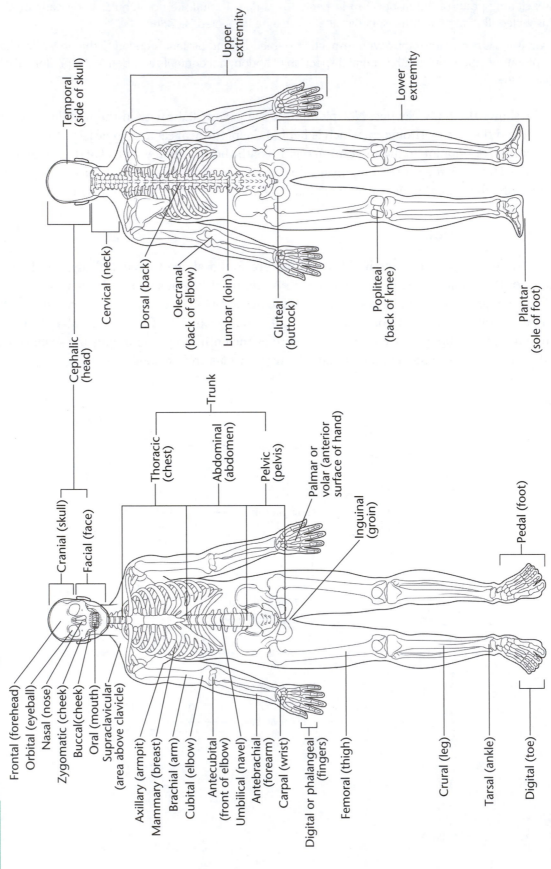

Figure 7.2.   General anatomical regions

© AHIMA 2019

Figure 7.3.   Rays of the hand

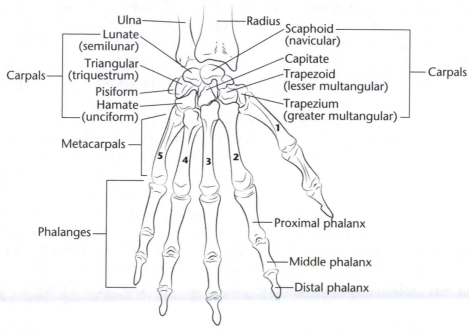

© AHIMA 2019

B2.1b. Where the general body part values "upper" and "lower" are provided as an option in the Upper Arteries, Lower Arteries, Upper Veins, Lower Veins, Muscles and Tendons body systems, "upper" or "lower" specifies body parts located above or below the diaphragm respectively.

Example: Vein body parts above the diaphragm are found in the Upper Veins body system; vein body parts below the diaphragm are found in the Lower Veins body system.

Lower Extremity Region

The lower extremity region contains body parts that are found below the central dividing line of the diaphragm. The inguinal region of the body is defined as part of the Anatomical Regions, Lower Extremities body system in ICD-10-PCS.

Body part values in this system are used to describe the level of amputation in Detachment. A ray of the foot consists of the continuous grouping of a metatarsal and phalanx associated with one toe. The body part Hindquarter describes the entire lower limb, including the associated pelvic girdle and the buttock. The rays of the foot, including the metatarsals and phalanges, are displayed in chapter 3 as figure 3.1.

Common Root Operations Used in Coding Procedures on the Anatomical Regions

The Anatomical Regions body systems are where the root operation value of 3, Control, is commonly found. When postoperative hemorrhage or other acute bleeding is controlled, it is coded to the appropriate anatomical region where the hemorrhage originates. If a definitive root operation such as Bypass, Detachment, Excision, Extraction, Reposition, Replacement, or Resection is performed to stop the acute bleeding, then the root operation of Control is not coded separately. In this case, the procedure is coded to the actual procedure performed and the associated body part value. When cautery is used to control acute bleeding, it is coded to the root operation Control, not to the root operation Destruction. Destruction and Repair are common techniques used to stop the acute bleeding and are coded to the root operation of Control. The root operation Control is also found in the Ear, Nose, and Sinus body system where control of nasal hemorrhage is coded.

B3.7. The root operation Control is defined as "Stopping, or attempting to stop, postprocedural or other acute bleeding." If an attempt to stop postprocedural or other acute bleeding is unsuccessful, and to stop the bleeding requires performing a more definitive root operations, such as Bypass, Detachment, Excision, Extraction, Reposition, Replacement, or Resection, then the more definitive root operation is coded instead of Control.

Example: Resection of the spleen to stop bleeding is coded to Resection instead of Control.

Procedures performed on the cavities of the body are coded in the Anatomical Regions, General body system. Some of the more common procedures are those performed on the left and right pleural cavities, the space between the parietal and visceral pleura within the thorax. These procedures include thoracentesis to percutaneously drain the pleura cavity, placement of a chest tube to drain the pleura cavity with a drainage device, and mechanical pleurodesis to cause adhesions between the two layers of pleura and seal off the cavity.

The root operation Division in the Anatomical Regions, General body system is used to describe the single procedure of episiotomy, or the division of the female perineum, normally performed at the time of the delivery. This is coded in the 0W8 table because the division of the perineum involves multiple tissue layers within a general body area. An episiorrhaphy, the root operation Repair, is not coded separately based on Guideline B3.1b, which states that procedural steps necessary to reach the operative site and close the operative site are not coded separately. However, if a perineal laceration takes place during the delivery or an episiotomy tears further, the root operation Repair is used to code the repair of the laceration after the delivery is complete. See chapter 20 for a complete discussion of perineal laceration repair.

Anatomy Alert

Supernumerary digits do not have unique body part values in ICD-10-PCS. If the supernumerary digit contains bone and soft tissue, the root operation of Detachment is used, with a body part value describing which finger (index, thumb, and such) and the qualifier indicating Complete, High, Mid, or Low for the amputation level. If the supernumerary digit contains only soft tissue and no bone, the root operation of Excision is selected.

The root operation Creation has two purposes. In the general anatomical regions body system, the purpose of this procedure is to describe the process of gender reassignment. In this procedure, the 4th character—the body part value—describes the body part at the beginning of the procedure, and the 7th character—the qualifier—describes the body part at the conclusion of the procedure. The root operation Creation has different meanings in other body systems, such as the circulatory system, which will be discussed in chapter 11.

The root operation Transplantation is assigned in the anatomical regions in two cases. A face transplant is coded in the anatomical regions, general body system because this is a large area, through all the layers of the body part. A hand transplant is coded in the anatomical regions, upper extremities body system when the entire donor hand is transplanted onto the recipient. As with other transplants, the qualifier identifies the source of the organ being transplanted.

To treat a condition called pectus excavatum, a surgeon can reinforce the chest wall with a specially shaped metal support bar called a Nuss bar. The Nuss procedure is performed using the percutaneous endoscopic approach and is coded to the root operation of Supplement with the bar as a synthetic substitute, code 0WU84JZ.

The root operation Detachment is only found in the body systems of the upper and lower extremity regions. The root operation Alteration is used to describe cosmetic procedures that change a large body area that is identified by a body part value within one of the three anatomical regions body systems.

Be sure to research any procedure that is unfamiliar to assure correct coding. If the documentation includes an eponym (procedure named for a person) and the intent of the procedure is unclear, query the physician for specifics.

Coding Tip

The root operation Drainage is coded for both diagnostic and therapeutic drainage procedures. When drainage is accomplished by putting in a catheter, the device value Drainage Device is coded in the 6th character.

Body Parts for the Anatomical Regions

The root operation Detachment is coded within the Anatomical Regions, Upper Extremities and Anatomical Regions, Lower Extremities body systems. A discussion of the subject of toe, ray, and foot detachment can be found in chapter 3. This section will cover the remainder of the body parts in these body systems. The lower extremities body parts are described here and similar definitions apply to the corresponding portions of the upper extremity body parts.

The body part values in the general anatomical regions body system should only be used when more specific body part values are not available within other systems or when the procedure involves multiple body parts and various tissue types, such as an entire forequarter. In table 7.1, the 0Y6 table, the body part value Hindquarter describes the entire lower limb, including all of the pelvic girdle and the buttock. Similarly, in the 0X6 table, the body part Forequarter describes the entire upper limb plus the scapula and clavicle. Interthoracoscapular amputation is coded to the root operation Detachment of the body part Forequarter (AMA 2017, 136). Interpelviabdominal amputation is coded to the root operation Detachment of the body part Hindquarter (AMA 2017, 154).

Table 7.1.   0Y6 table

Section	0	Medical and Surgical		
Body System	Y	Anatomical Regions, Lower Extremities		
Operation	6	Detachment: Cutting off all or a portion of the upper or lower extremities		
Body Part	Approach		Device	Qualifier
2 Hindquarter, Right 3 Hindquarter, Left 4 Hindquarter, Bilateral 7 Femoral Region, Right 8 Femoral Region, Left F Knee Region, Right G Knee Region, Left	0 Open		Z No Device	Z No Qualifier
C Upper Leg, Right D Upper Leg, Left H Lower Leg, Right J Lower Leg, Left	0 Open		Z No Device	1 High 2 Mid 3 Low
M Foot, Right N Foot, Left	0 Open		Z No Device	0 Complete 4 Complete 1st Ray 5 Complete 2nd Ray 6 Complete 3rd Ray 7 Complete 4th Ray 8 Complete 5th Ray 9 Partial 1st Ray B Partial 2nd Ray C Partial 3rd Ray D Partial 4th Ray F Partial 5th Ray
P 1st Toe, Right Q 1st Toe, Left R 2nd Toe, Right S 2nd Toe, Left T 3rd Toe, Right U 3rd Toe, Left V 4th Toe, Right W 4th Toe, Left X 5th Toe, Right Y 5th Toe, Left	0 Open		Z No Device	0 Complete 1 High 2 Mid 3 Low

Source: CMS 2019

The femoral region body part is assigned when the entire lower extremity is disarticulated at the hip, described as the femoral region. The knee region body part is assigned when the entire lower leg is disarticulated at the knee, described as the knee region. When Detachment takes place anywhere along the femur, the upper leg body part value is assigned, along with the appropriate qualifier to describe the level of the Detachment. When Detachment takes place anywhere along the lower leg (tibia and fibula), the lower leg body part is assigned, along with the appropriate qualifier to describe the level of the Detachment.

For example, a left above-the-knee amputation completed just above the knee joint is coded as 0Y6D0Z3 (upper leg body part with a qualifier of 3 for low) and a right below-the-knee amputation, completed mid shaft is coded as 0Y6H0Z2 (lower leg body part with a qualifier of 2 for mid).

Table 7.2 presents the body part values for the general, upper extremity, and lower extremity regions. If the documentation includes specific body part names that are not included in these lists, refer to the body part key for other body part synonyms and alternative terms.

Table 7.2. Body part values for the anatomical regions

Body Part Value	Body Parts—Anatomical Regions, General (W)	Body Part Value	Body Parts—Anatomical Regions, Upper Extremities (X)	Body Part Value	Body Parts—Anatomical Regions, Lower Extremities (Y)
0	Head	0	Forequarter, right	0	Buttock, right
1	Cranial cavity	1	Forequarter, left	1	Buttock, left
2	Face	2	Shoulder region, right	2	Hindquarter, right
3	Oral cavity and throat	3	Shoulder region, left	3	Hindquarter, left
4	Upper jaw	4	Axilla, right	4	Hindquarter, bilateral
5	Lower jaw	5	Axilla, left	5	Inguinal region, right
6	Neck	6	Upper extremity, right	6	Inguinal region, left
8	Chest wall	7	Upper extremity, left	7	Femoral region, right
9	Pleural cavity, right	8	Upper arm, right	8	Femoral region, left
B	Pleural cavity, left	9	Upper arm, left	9	Lower extremity, right
C	Mediastinum	B	Elbow region, right	A	Inguinal region, bilateral
D	Pericardial cavity	C	Elbow region, left	B	Lower extremity, left
F	Abdominal wall	D	Lower arm, right	C	Upper leg, right
G	Peritoneal cavity	F	Lower arm, left	D	Upper leg, left
H	Retroperitoneum	G	Wrist region, right	E	Femoral region, bilateral
J	Pelvic cavity	H	Wrist region, left	F	Knee region, right
K	Upper back	J	Hand, right	G	Knee region, left
L	Lower back	K	Hand, left	H	Lower leg, right
M	Perineum, male	L	Thumb, right	J	Lower leg, left
N	Perineum, female	M	Thumb, left	K	Ankle region, right
P	Gastrointestinal tract	N	Index finger, right	L	Ankle region, left
Q	Respiratory tract	P	Index finger, left	M	Foot, right
R	Genitourinary tract	Q	Middle finger, right	N	Foot, left
		R	Middle finger, left	P	1st toe, right

(Continued)   (Continued)

Table 7.2. Body part values for the anatomical regions (continued)

Body Part Value	Body Parts— Anatomical Regions, Upper Extremities (X)	Body Part Value	Body Parts— Anatomical Regions, Lower Extremities (Y)
S	Ring finger, right	Q	1st toe, left
T	Ring finger, left	R	2nd toe, right
V	Little finger, right	S	2nd toe, left
W	Little finger, left	T	3rd toe, right
		U	3rd toe, left
		V	4th toe, right
		W	4th toe, left
		X	5th toe, right
		Y	5th toe, left

B2.1a. The procedure codes in the general anatomical regions body systems can be used when the procedure is performed on an anatomical region rather than a specific body part (e.g., root operations Control and Detachment, Drainage of a body cavity) or on the rare occasion when no information is available to support assignment of a code to a specific body part.

Example: Control of postoperative hemorrhage is coded to the root operation Control found in the general anatomical regions body systems. Chest tube drainage of the pleural cavity is coded to the root operation Drainage found in the General Anatomical Regions body systems. Suture repair of the abdominal wall is coded to the root operation Repair in the General Anatomical Regions body system.

Coding Tip

The root operation Control includes irrigation or evacuation of hematoma done at the operative site. Both irrigation and evacuation may be necessary to clear the operative field and effectively stop the bleeding.

Approaches Used for the Anatomical Regions

The general anatomical regions include body part values for the three main tubular tracts of the body: the gastrointestinal tract, the respiratory tract, and the genitourinary tract. The approach to these tubular tracts is normally through a natural or artificial orifice, and therefore, approach values of 7, Via Natural or Artificial Opening, and 8, Via Natural or Artificial Opening Endoscopic, are assigned in the general anatomical regions but are not assigned in the upper and lower extremity regions.

As you begin to code operative reports in the body system chapters of this text, remember that the open approach means that an incision is made through the skin or mucous membranes and that the surgeon exposes the site of the procedure. This means that they can see the body part that they are working on directly. The percutaneous and percutaneous endoscopic approaches mean that instruments enter through the skin or mucous membrane. Percutaneous can involve the use of imaging guidance and percutaneous endoscopic involves the use of a scope to visualize the site. The approaches dealing with natural or artificial openings mean that the opening was there previously, either as a natural opening or as an opening that was surgically created during a past procedure. If necessary, refer to information in chapter 2 as you code.

Devices Common to the Anatomical Regions

Device values for the anatomical regions involve those used for drainage, infusion, grafts, and treatment by radioactive implant. Device value Y is available to describe other or new devices that remain at the conclusion of the procedure. The devices that are defined for coding procedures performed on the anatomical regions are displayed in table 7.3.

Table 7.3. Devices for the anatomical regions	
Device Value	**Devices—All Anatomical Regions (W, X, and Y)**
0	Drainage device
1	Radioactive element
3	Infusion device
7	Autologous tissue substitute
J	Synthetic substitute
K	Nonautologous tissue substitute
Y	Other device
Z	No device

B6.2. A separate procedure to put in a drainage device is coded to the root operation Drainage with the device value Drainage Device.

Qualifiers Used in the Anatomical Regions

The qualifier values for the general anatomical regions describe tissues used to describe a bypass and identify the body part bypassed "to." The qualifiers used in the upper and lower extremities body systems define the level of amputation for the Detachment root operation. The definitions for High, Mid, and Low are consistent across all root operations.

- **High amputation**—Amputation at the proximal portion of the shaft of the humerus, lower arm, femur, or lower leg or amputation anywhere along the proximal phalanx
- **Mid amputation**—Amputation at the middle portion of the shaft of those body parts, through the proximal interphalangeal joint, or anywhere along the middle phalanx
- **Low amputation**—Amputation at the distal portion of the shaft of those body parts, through the distal interphalangeal joint, or anywhere along the distal phalanx (AHA 2017, 3)

The terms "Complete" and "Partial" are used in the qualifier values to describe amputations of the rays of the hands and feet. Refer to figure 7.3 for a picture of the rays of the hand and figure 3.1 in chapter 3 for a picture of the rays of the foot, respectively. The first ray is the thumb or great toe. The second ray is the index finger or second toe. The third ray is the middle finger or third toe. The fourth ray is the ring finger or fourth toe, and the fifth ray is the little finger or the little toe.

Complete and partial are defined as follows:

- **Complete amputation**—Amputation through the carpometacarpal joint of the hand or through the tarsal-metatarsal joint of the foot.

- **Partial amputation**—Amputation anywhere along the shaft or head of the metacarpal bone of the hand or the metatarsal bone of the foot (AHA 2017, 3)

Unlike the root operation Detachment, the root operation Reattachment does not use qualifiers to describe the level of the reattachment. A unique qualifier value of 2, Stoma is provided in the 0WB and 0WQ tables for use when an excision, including biopsy, or a repair are performed on an artificial opening (stoma) of the neck or abdominal wall. This qualifier would be associated with a tracheostomy or with one of the many artificial openings that could be created in the abdominal wall, such as a colostomy or ileostomy when excision or repair of the stoma itself is required. Closure of an ostomy site is coded to the root operation of Repair using an open approach and the qualifier of 2, Stoma is not assigned. Table 7.4 displays the qualifiers associated with the anatomical regions.

Coding Tip

When a surgeon uses the word "toe" to describe an amputation, but the operative report states that the amputation extends to the midshaft of the metatarsal of the foot, such as the 5th metatarsal, the qualifier is Partial 5th Ray of the foot.

Table 7.4.   Qualifiers for the anatomical regions

Qualifier Value	Qualifiers—Anatomical Regions, General (W)	Qualifier Value	Qualifiers—Anatomical Regions, Upper Extremities (X)	Qualifier Value	Qualifiers—Anatomical Regions, Lower Extremities (Y)
0	Vagina				
0	Allogeneic	0	Complete	0	Complete
1	Penis	0	Allogeneic	1	High
1	Syngeneic	1	High	2	Mid
2	Stoma	1	Syngeneic	3	Low
4	Cutaneous	2	Mid	4	Complete 1st ray
9	Pleural cavity, right	3	Low	5	Complete 2nd ray
B	Pleural cavity, left	4	Complete 1st ray	6	Complete 3rd ray
G	Peritoneal cavity	5	Complete 2nd ray	7	Complete 4th ray
J	Pelvic cavity	6	Complete 3rd ray	8	Complete 5th ray
W	Upper vein	7	Complete 4th ray	9	Partial 1st ray
X	Diagnostic	8	Complete 5th ray	B	Partial 2nd ray
Y	Lower vein	9	Partial 1st ray	C	Partial 3rd ray
Z	No qualifier	B	Partial 2nd ray	D	Partial 4th ray
		C	Partial 3rd ray	F	Partial 5th ray
		D	Partial 4th ray	X	Diagnostic
		F	Partial 5th ray	Z	No qualifier
		L	Thumb, right		
		M	Thumb, left		
		N	Toe, right		
		P	Toe, left		
		X	Diagnostic		
		Z	No qualifier		

Code Building

Case #1:

PROCEDURE STATEMENT: Reattachment of severed right hand

ADDITIONAL INFORMATION: The patient suffered a severed right hand in an accident in a home workshop. The hand was detached through the carpals of the right wrist.

ROOT AND INDEX ENTRIES FOR THE STATEMENT: Reattachment is the root operation performed in this procedure; it is defined as putting back in or on all or a portion of a separated body part to its normal location or other suitable location. The Index entry is:

Reattachment

    Hand

        Left   0XMK0ZZ

        Right   0XMJ0ZZ

Code Characters:

Section	Body System	Root Operation	Body Part	Approach	Device	Qualifier
Medical and Surgical	Anatomical Regions, Upper Extremities	Reattachment	Hand, Right	Open	No Device	No Qualifier
0	X	M	J	0	Z	Z

RATIONALE FOR THE ANSWER: The index provides the entire code for this procedure because there are no other possible variations to the code. Reattachment of the upper and lower extremities is always an open procedure that does not involve devices or qualifiers. The correct code assignment is 0XMJ0ZZ.

Case #2:

PROCEDURE STATEMENT: Cystoscopic cauterization of postoperative hemorrhage from incision line in the bladder

ADDITIONAL INFORMATION: The patient is seen 2 days after a bladder resection for tumor.

ROOT AND INDEX ENTRIES FOR THE STATEMENT: Control is the root operation performed in this procedure, which is defined as stopping, or attempting to stop, postprocedural or other acute bleeding. The Index entry is
Control bleeding in

        Genitourinary tract   0W3R

Code Characters:

Section	Body System	Root Operation	Body Part	Approach	Device	Qualifier
Medical and Surgical	Anatomical Regions, General	Control	Genitourinary Tract	Via Natural or Artificial Opening, Endoscopic	No Device	No Qualifier
0	W	3	R	8	Z	Z

RATIONALE FOR THE ANSWER: Even though destruction is the method used (cauterization), the root operation Control is coded because it is acute bleeding, and a definitive root operation is not used to stop the bleeding. The approach is endoscopic through the urethra, into the bladder. This approach is value 8, Via Natural or Artificial Opening Endoscopic. No device or qualifier values are appropriate. The correct code assignment is 0W3R8ZZ.

Case #3:

PROCEDURE STATEMENT:	Laparoscopic inguinal hernia repair, left
ADDITIONAL INFORMATION:	The repair is completed without the use of mesh.

ROOT AND INDEX ENTRIES FOR THE STATEMENT: Repair is the root operation performed in this procedure, which is defined as restoring, to the extent possible, a body part to its normal anatomical structure and function. The Index entry is:

Repair

    Inguinal region

      Bilateral   0YQA

      Left   0YQ6

      Right   0YQ5

Code Characters:

Section	Body System	Root Operation	Body Part	Approach	Device	Qualifier
Medical and Surgical	Anatomical Regions, Lower Extremities	Repair	Inguinal Region, Left	Percutaneous Endoscopic	No Device	No Qualifier
0	Y	Q	6	4	Z	Z

RATIONALE FOR THE ANSWER: The hernia is repaired without the use of mesh; therefore, the root operation Repair is assigned. If mesh had been implanted, the root operation Supplement would have been assigned. The inguinal area of the body is categorized to the Anatomical Regions, Lower Extremities in ICD-10-PCS. The laparoscopic approach is 4, Percutaneous Endoscopic in ICD-10-PCS. No device was inserted and no qualifier is appropriate. The correct code assignment is 0YQ64ZZ.

Code Building Exercises

Starting with chapter 7 and continuing through chapter 20, these Code Building Exercises are provided to give you guided practice in dissecting operative reports. Work through each case and check your answers using the answer key in appendix B of the textbook before going on to the Check Your Understanding questions that follow.

Exercise 1:

PRE- AND POSTOPERATIVE DIAGNOSIS: Right lower extremity peripheral vascular disease with non-healing chronic wound

PROCEDURE PERFORMED: Right transfemoral amputation

DESCRIPTION OF PROCEDURE: The patient's right leg was prepped and draped in sterile fashion. I performed a fishmouth-type incision in the area about 3 cm above the knee and exposed the patient's distal femoral diaphysis. I made the bone cut about 3 cm above the fishmouth opening using an oscillating saw. I cut the remainder of the soft tissue attachments using an amputation knife and passed the leg off the field. Once hemostasis was achieved, I irrigated and closed the flaps using 0 Vicryl, followed by 2-0 Vicryl for the subcutaneous tissue and 3-0 Nylon for the skin.

Questions:

1.1. What clues are found in the Operative Report about the body part that is involved in this case?

_____

1.2. The surgeon always cuts the bone slightly higher than the incision made on the outside of the extremity. This places the amputation in the lower third of the femur. What qualifier would you assign?

_____

1.3. What code(s) would be assigned?

_____

Exercise 2:

PRE- AND POSTOPERATIVE DIAGNOSIS: Abscess, left leg

PROCEDURE: Incision and drainage of leg abscess

DETAILS: The patient was brought to the operating room where the leg was prepped and draped in the usual sterile fashion. An incision was made over the abscess and carried down to the abscess cavity where the hematoma and purulent fluid were encountered, evacuated and sent for analysis. The wound was irrigated and packed with saline gauze in wet-to-dry fashion. The patient tolerated the procedure well and was taken to PACU in stable condition.

Questions:

2.1. Can you assign a more specific body system than Anatomical Regions, Lower Extremities for this procedure?

_____

2.2. When the documentation states "Incision and Drainage", which approach is identified? Can this be supported in the procedure details?

_____

2.3. What code(s) would be assigned?

_____

✓ Check Your Understanding

Coding Knowledge Check

1. The forequarter includes the entire _____ limb, _____, and _____.

2. The surgeon repairs a complete traumatic right thumb amputation. How is this coded?
   a. 0RSW0ZZ
   b. 0RRW07Z
   c. 0XML0ZZ
   d. 0XQM0ZZ

3. Amputation of the 3rd ray at the most proximal portion of the metatarsal is coded to the qualifier of
   a. 0, Complete
   b. 1, High
   c. 3, Low
   d. 6, Complete 3rd ray

4. Pleurocentesis for cytology to assess recurrent left-sided pleural effusion is coded as _____.
   a. 0W9B30Z
   b. 0W9B3ZX
   c. 0W9930Z, 0W9B30Z
   d. 0W9B4ZX

5. True or false? The repair of a ventral hernia is coded to the body part value of 8, Chest Wall. _____.

Procedure Statement Coding

Assign ICD-10-PCS codes to the following procedure statements and scenarios. List the root operation selected and the code assigned.

1. Open bilateral "butt" lift for cosmetic reasons.

2. The patient's right leg was prepped and draped. Using a fishmouth incision, the distal aspect of the upper leg was entered. Using the scalpel, the skin and subcutaneous tissue were incised. The muscle groups were separated and the vessels were secured and doubly ligated using free ties of 0-Vicryl. The femoral nerve was secured. The femur was transected using a saw, and the edges were rasped smooth. Hemostasis was achieved, and the muscle groups, the hamstrings, and the quadriceps were approximated. The subcutaneous tissue was then reapproximated, and the skin was closed with staples. Sterile dressings were applied and covered with a stump cap to hold them in place.

3. Diagnosis: Lower abdominal adipose excess, skin excess, and abdominal wall laxity with adipose excess of the hips following excessive weight loss. Procedure: (1) Tumescent liposuction, bilateral hips; (2) Full abdominoplasty.

4. EGD with placement of an endoclip on a bleeding duodenal ulcer.

(Continued)

5. Amputation of a supernumerary digit next to the little finger of the left hand. The digit contains a phalanx bone and nail.

   _____

6. Right index finger to thumb transfer after traumatic amputation of right thumb.

   _____

7. Repair of torn tracheostomy opening using an external approach.

   _____

8. Placement of a peritoneal dialysis infusion catheter into the peritoneal cavity, percutaneous approach.

   _____

9. Gender reassignment surgery from male to female using autologous tissue grafts.

   _____

10. Episiotomy in preparation for vaginal delivery.

   _____

Case Studies

Assign ICD-10-PCS codes to the following case studies.

1. Operative Report

PREOPERATIVE DIAGNOSIS:	Pleural effusion, right side
POSTOPERATIVE DIAGNOSIS:	Metastatic carcinoma of pleura
OPERATION:	Tube thoracostomy—chest tube insertion

HISTORY: A 67-year-old woman with a history of squamous cell carcinoma of the cervix presents with a right pleural effusion that was drained via thoracentesis 3 days earlier, and the culture revealed metastatic carcinoma of pleura. Fluid is re-accumulating, giving the patient symptoms of dyspnea. Chest x-ray reveals a significant pleural effusion up to the midlung region.

PROCEDURE: The patient was taken to the OR and was prepared and draped in the usual fashion. She was then anesthetized using 1 percent lidocaine above the 10th rib. An incision was made in the skin. The subcutaneous fascia was then opened and the pleura penetrated. The pleural cavity was visualized. There was no unusual hemorrhage, and immediately serosanguineous fluid came forth from the opening. A 36-size chest tube was then inserted after palpation of the diaphragm, which was localized just below the entrance to the pleura. The chest tube was inserted posteriorly, extending up to the superior aspects of the right pleural space, and tacked in place; the incision was closed in layers around the tube. The patient tolerated the procedure well. There were no complications. Immediately postop, she was stable. Approximately 400 cc of fluid were drained from the right chest.

2. Operative Report

PREOPERATIVE DIAGNOSIS:	Osteomyelitis, 5th metatarsal, left
POSTOPERATIVE DIAGNOSIS:	Same
PROCEDURE:	Amputation of toe

The patient was brought to the operating room and placed in a supine position. After adequate general anesthesia was obtained, the left foot was scrubbed, prepped, and draped in the usual manner. No tourniquet was utilized. A skin incision was made along the entire lateral border of the 5th metatarsal and carried down to the subcutaneous tissue in line with the skin incision. Bleeders were clamped and electrocoagulated. Dissection was carried down to the base of the 5th metatarsal where a capsulotomy was made at the base. The bone was then delivered from the wound and sent to the pathology department. There was erosion of the head of the 5th metatarsal consistent with osteomyelitis. The entire toe and metatarsal were amputated down to the tarsal space, and all of the specimen was sent to the pathology department. All of the tissues were debrided. The wound was irrigated and hemostasis ensured. The subcutaneous tissue was very loosely reapproximated utilizing 4-0 Vicryl suture. The skin was not closed and was allowed to drain. A sterile dressing was applied to the wound.

3. Operative Report

PREOPERATIVE DIAGNOSIS:	Left inguinal hernia
POSTOPERATIVE DIAGNOSIS:	Same
PROCEDURE:	Left inguinal hernia repair with mesh

INDICATIONS: The patient is a 23-year-old man who presented with several weeks' history of pain in his left groin associated with a bulge. Examination revealed that his left groin did indeed have a bulge and his right groin was normal. We discussed the procedure and the choice of anesthesia.

OPERATIVE SUMMARY: After preoperative evaluation and clearance, the patient was brought into the operating suite and placed in a comfortable supine position on the operating room table. Monitoring equipment was attached, and general anesthesia was induced. His left groin was prepped and draped sterilely and an inguinal incision made. This was carried down through the subcutaneous tissues until the external oblique fascia was reached. This was split in a direction parallel with its fibers, and the medial aspect of the opening included the external ring. The ilioinguinal nerve was identified, and care was taken to retract this inferiorly out of the way. The cord structures were encircled and the cremasteric muscle fibers divided. At this point, we examined the floor of the inguinal canal, and the patient did appear to have a weakness here. We then explored the cord. There was no evidence of an indirect hernia. A piece of 3 × 5 mesh was obtained and trimmed to fit. It was placed in the inguinal canal and tacked to the pubic tubercle. It was then run inferiorly along the pelvic shelving edge until it was lateral to the internal ring and then tacked down superiorly using interrupted sutures of 0-Prolene. A single stitch was placed lateral to the cord to re-create the internal ring. Details of the mesh were tucked underneath the external oblique fascia. The cord and the nerve were allowed to drop back into the wound, and the wound was infiltrated with 30 cc of 0.5 percent Marcaine. The external oblique fascia was then closed with a running suture of 0-Vicryl. Subcutaneous tissues were approximated with interrupted sutures of 3-0 Vicryl. The skin was closed with a running subcuticular suture of 4-0 Vicryl.

4. Operative Report

PREOPERATIVE DIAGNOSIS: Abscess, left buttock

POSTOPERATIVE DIAGNOSIS: Abscess, left buttock

OPERATIONS: Incision, drainage, and anoscopy

FINDINGS: The patient presented with an abscess overlying his left buttock. The patient was prepped and draped in the jackknife position under general endotracheal anesthesia. A bivalve anoscope was placed, and there was no apparent fistula. An 18-gauge needle was placed in the area of induration on the buttock. Purulent material was obtained. An elliptical incision was made, excising a segment of skin. The abscess cavity was bluntly opened, drained, and digitally explored to break up loculations. It was then irrigated and packed with Iodoform gauze. The patient tolerated the procedure satisfactorily and returned to the recovery room in good improvement and good condition. Estimated blood loss was less than 5 mL.

5. Operative Report

PREOPERATIVE DIAGNOSIS: Post-tonsillectomy bleeding

POSTOPERATIVE DIAGNOSIS: Post-tonsillectomy bleeding

OPERATIVE PROCEDURE: Operative control of postoperative bleeding

FINDINGS: The patient had an arterial bleeder from her right tonsillar fossa.

DESCRIPTION OF PROCEDURE: The patient was taken to the operating room, and general anesthesia was administered. A Crowe-Davis mouth gag was placed, and clots were suctioned from the pharynx. An arterial bleeder was noted and was controlled with suction cautery. The stomach was then suctioned and about 200–300 mL of blood was noted. The patient was then awakened, extubated, and transported to the recovery room in stable condition.

6. Operative Report

PREOPERATIVE DIAGNOSIS: Umbilical hernia

POSTOPERATIVE DIAGNOSIS: Umbilical hernia

OPERATION: Umbilical hernia repair

INDICATIONS: An obese woman has an increasing umbilical hernia at the site of a laparoscopic cholecystectomy trocar wound.

FINDINGS: Moderately sized fascial defect

PROCEDURE: The patient was placed supine on the operating room table and induced with a general anesthetic. The abdomen was sterilely prepped and draped, and her previous surgical incision was opened. Sharp dissection led to identification of the hernia, which was dissected free of surrounding tissues. The contents were reduced into the abdominal cavity. The fascial edges were cleaned and reapproximated with interrupted Ethibond suture. Subcutaneous was closed with 3-0 Vicryl, and the skin was closed with 4-0 Vicryl subcuticular suture, Benzoin, and Steri-Strips. Sterile dressings were applied. There were no complications and no blood loss. All counts were correct. She was returned extubated and in stable condition to the recovery room.

Nervous System

The nervous system is a communication network within the body. It controls, coordinates, and regulates the other systems of the body. The system is made up of nerves of various sizes, which are bundles of tissue that send impulses to and from the brain. The second character values for the nervous system are:

> 0—Central Nervous System and Cranial Nerves
> 1—Peripheral Nervous System

Functions of the Nervous System

The main function of the nervous system is to send impulses from one cell to another and from one part of the body to another. The system performs this function through a complex network of neurons and synapses. Neurons are fibrous cells that transmit impulses. Synapses are the connections between the neurons.

Organization of the Nervous System

The nervous system contains two main parts: the central nervous system, or CNS, and the peripheral nervous system, or PNS. The central nervous system is the control center for the entire body. The peripheral nervous system connects the sensory receptors in the nervous system, the muscles, and the glands of the body (Rizzo 2016, 234).

Central Nervous System

The central nervous system is made up of the brain and the brain meninges, the cranial nerves, and the spinal cord. The brain and spinal cord are vital organs of the body and are therefore encased in bone for protection, the brain in the cranial cavity and the spinal cord in the vertebral column (Applegate 2011, 171). The structures of the brain and proximal spinal cord are displayed in figure 8.1.

The coverings of the brain are the pia mater, which is closest to the surface of the brain; the middle arachnoid layer; and the dura mater, which is farthest away from the brain and closest to the skull. There are spaces between the brain, these different layers of covering, and the skull:

- Subarachnoid space—Above the pia mater and below the arachnoid
- Subdural space—Above the arachnoid and below the dura mater
- Epidural space—Above the dura mater and below the skull

In the event of a brain injury, these spaces can collect fluid and blood. Figure 8.2 displays the cerebral meninges and the intracranial spaces between the layers of covering.

Figure 8.1.   Right hemisphere of the central nervous system

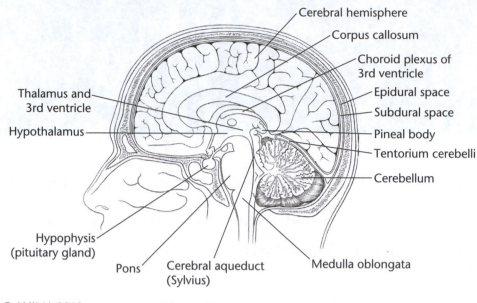

© AHIMA 2019

Figure 8.2.   Cerebral meninges

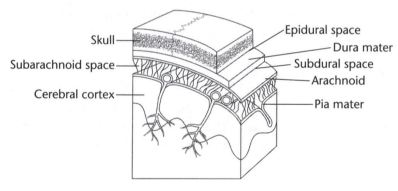

© AHIMA 2019

Basal ganglia are nuclei inside the brain that control complex functions, such as voluntary muscular movements, eye movements, and cognition. The largest basal ganglia is the corpus striatum, which includes the caudate nucleus, putamen, globus pallidus, substantia nigra, and subthalamic nucleus.

Anatomy textbooks classify the cranial nerves as part of the peripheral nervous system, but ICD-10-PCS classifies these nerves in the central nervous system. Figure 8.3 displays the cranial nerves and their origins inside the brain. Cranial nerves 1 and 2 emerge directly from the cerebrum. Cranial nerves 3 through 12 emerge from various locations within the brain stem.

Peripheral Nervous System

The peripheral nervous system consists of nerves and ganglia. Nerves are bundles of nerve fibers. Ganglia are collections, or small knots, of nerve cells found outside of the central nervous system (Applegate 2011, 171). The peripheral system has both sensory and motor functions. Sensory nerves send impulses to the brain, and motor nerves send pulses away from the brain.

The peripheral nervous system is divided into two main systems: the somatic and the autonomic nerves. The somatic nervous system sends impulses from the brain and spinal cord to skeletal muscle (Rizzo 2016, 234).

These nerves are named for the muscles of the body they serve, such as the cervical nerve or the peroneal nerve. Some nerves are large and are known by different names along their length. For example, the sciatic nerve is a combination of the tibial nerve and the peroneal nerve, depending upon the exact location that is being referenced. These peripheral nerves exit the spinal cord through a nerve root, or junction with the spinal cord. Once the nerves exit the spinal cord, they may form complex networks with surrounding nerves. A complex network like this is called a plexus.

The autonomic nervous system conducts impulses from the brain and spinal cord to smooth muscle tissues, such as the digestive system and the cardiopulmonary system. In ICD-10-PCS, body parts are assigned to the sympathetic divisions of these nerves, based on the body regions of head and neck, thoracic, abdominal, lumbar, and sacral regions.

The same layers of meninges cover the spinal cord as are found surrounding the brain. The spaces between the meningeal layers are minimal around the spinal cord, but an epidural space is found between the dura and the vertebra to act as a cushion between the two structures. Figures 8.4 and 8.5 identify the body parts of the peripheral nervous system. Figure 8.4 displays the spinal meninges. Figure 8.5 displays the relationship among the spinal column, the spinal nerves, and the four plexuses of the spine: the cervical plexus, the brachial plexus, the lumbar plexus, and the sacral plexus.

Anatomy Alert

Dura mater is body part value 2 for the cranial dura mater. Dura mater surrounding the spinal cord is classified to the spinal meninges, body part value T. All of the spaces between the spinal meninges (epidural space, subdural space, and subarachnoid space) are classified to the spinal canal, body part value U. These same spaces, when found around the brain, are classified to "intracranial" and their individual body part values in the table.

Figure 8.3. Cranial nerves

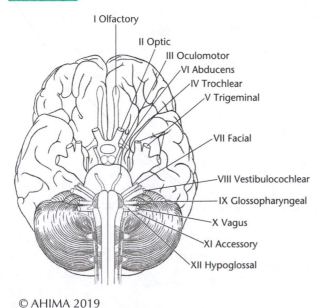

I Olfactory
II Optic
III Oculomotor
VI Abducens
IV Trochlear
V Trigeminal
VII Facial
VIII Vestibulocochlear
IX Glossopharyngeal
X Vagus
XI Accessory
XII Hypoglossal

© AHIMA 2019

Figure 8.4. Spinal meninges

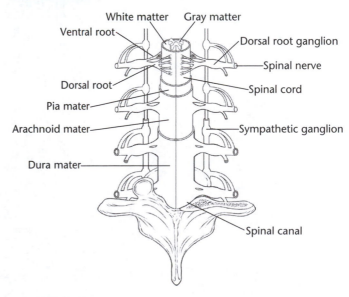

White matter   Gray matter
Ventral root
Dorsal root ganglion
Spinal nerve
Dorsal root
Spinal cord
Pia mater
Arachnoid mater
Sympathetic ganglion
Dura mater
Spinal canal

© AHIMA 2019

Figure 8.5.   Nerves and plexuses of the peripheral nervous system

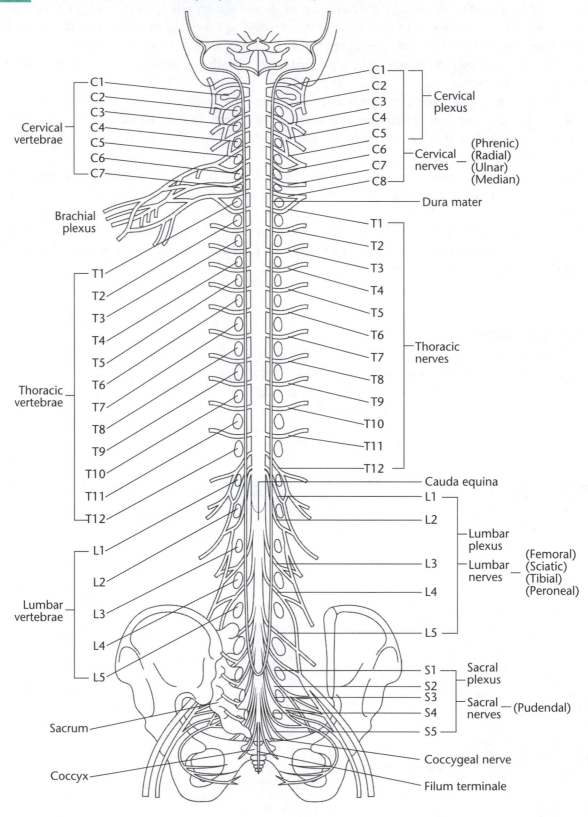

© AHIMA 2019

Common Root Operations Used in Coding Procedures Performed on the Nervous System

Of the 31 root operations, 22 are significant in code selection for the central nervous system and 17 for the peripheral nervous system. Documentation frequently states the procedure name as craniectomy or craniotomy. These procedure names typically define the approach for the procedure, not the actual procedure being performed. The root operation should be assigned based on the intent of the procedure. For example, if the patient has a subdural hemorrhage, and the hemorrhage is drained, the root operation Drainage is assigned. If the craniotomy is performed to insert a pressure-monitoring device or a neurostimulator lead, the root operation Insertion is selected and the appropriate device value is assigned. In all these cases, the craniectomy or craniotomy is the approach and not the procedure.

Neuroplasty is decompression of an intact nerve from scar tissue (AMA 2018, 440) or other constraint and is coded with the root operation Release. Another name for neuroplasty is neurolysis. A neurorrhaphy is "a surgical procedure to suture a severed nerve" (Mosby's 2017, 1228) and is coded with the root operation Repair. Radiofrequency ablation can be used to destroy a nerve for either pain control or to stop nerve spasms. Figure 1.3 in chapter 1 displays the radiofrequency ablation of a branch of the trigeminal nerve.

Central nervous system injury often occurs when the patient has a depressed skull fracture. The elevation of the depressed skull fragments is coded separately (as the root operation Reposition), in addition to the procedures performed to repair any intracranial injury caused by the bone fragments.

Craniosynostosis is the premature fusing of one or more sutures of a baby's head leading to an abnormally shaped head and increased intracranial pressure. The goals of surgery are to relieve any pressure on the brain and allow the skull to grow normally. Therefore, the root operation assigned to this procedure is Release. The body part being released is 0, Brain. Open craniosynostosis surgery involves release of the brain as well as various reposition procedures to remodel the skull. In addition, the orbital bones may also require repositioning.

Endoscopic craniosynostosis surgery is described as "surgery [that] requires making small incisions on the scalp. A small camera (endoscope) is used that is registered to the patient's radiologic images (CT) to ensure precise removal of the pathologic suture and release of the other bones to permit normal bone growth" (Cincinnati Children's Hospital Medical Center 2015). With this surgery, repositioning of bone is not typically necessary, and Release is the only procedure performed.

A ventriculoperitoneal (VP) shunt is used to reroute fluid accumulation in the cerebral ventricles, commonly due to hydrocephalus. The shunting process is a Bypass procedure because the fluid is rerouted from the ventricle to the peritoneal cavity rather than through the normal route through the ventricle and its valve down the spinal canal. The shunt can also be routed to other locations such as the atrium of the heart or the pleural cavity.

The shunt consists of three parts: the cerebral portion, the control valve, and the peritoneal portion. The cerebral portion is a synthetic tube that starts in the cerebral ventricle and connects to the control valve, which is placed in the subcutaneous layer of the head or neck. The third portion is the synthetic tubing that starts at the control valve and terminates in the peritoneal cavity.

The code for the creation of the VP shunt bypass is 00160J6. The approach is open because the valve is placed in a pocket that is directly visualized by the surgeon. These shunts can become blocked or infected, requiring replacement or revision. If the entire shunt device is removed (all three parts) and replaced, the root operations are Removal and Bypass because complete re-dos are coded to the original root operation. When only one or two parts require replacement, the root operation of Revision is assigned because the malfunctioning device needs correction. In other words, "part of a part" needs to be fixed. The code is assigned based on the portion of the shunt that is revised. For example, if the cerebral portion needs to be replaced, the code is 00W60JZ because the synthetic tubing is replaced and connected to the valve. Because this is a "part of a part," the root operation is Revision. If the valve is malfunctioning, the valve is replaced and the code is 0JWS0JZ because the device is located in the subcutaneous layer of the head and neck. If the peritoneal portion is blocked or infected, that portion is replaced. It is coded to Revision, as 0WWG0JZ, because the device is located in the peritoneal cavity.

The spinal cord can also be bypassed for a condition called spinal syrinx. A syrinx is a fluid-filled cavity within the spinal cord, also called a syringomyelia. The syrinx forms when cerebrospinal fluid collects in a small area of the spinal cord and forms a cyst-like structure. Continued enlargement of the cyst causes increasing damage to the cord. To prevent this, the cystic structure is bypassed from the spinal canal to the atrium, pleural cavity, peritoneal cavity, urinary tract or fallopian tube.

Be sure to research any procedure that is unfamiliar to assure correct coding. If the documentation includes an eponym (procedure named for a person) and the intent of the procedure is unclear, query the physician for specifics.

Body Part Values for the Nervous System

The structures of the nervous system affecting procedure code assignment are listed in table 8.1. Note that body part value Y, Peripheral Nerve, is to be used when the code does not require the specification of the individual peripheral nerve, such as in the root operations of Change, Insertion, Inspection, Removal, and Revision. Dura mater is body part value 2, for the cranial dura mater. Dura mater surrounding the spinal cord is classified to the spinal meninges, body part value T. All of the spaces between the spinal meninges (epidural space, subdural space, and subarachnoid space) are classified to the spinal canal, body part value U. These same spaces, when found around the brain, are classified to their individual body part values in the table. Lumbar puncture procedures are performed on the spinal canal to percutaneously drain cerebrospinal fluid. If the lumbar puncture is unsuccessful, the root operation of Inspection is assigned for this incomplete procedure, based on Guideline B3.3 on Discontinued or Incomplete Procedures.

Table 8.1. Body parts in the nervous system

Body Part Value	Body Parts—Central Nervous System and Cranial Nerves (0)	Body Part Value	Body Parts—Peripheral Nervous System (1)
0	Brain	0	Cervical Plexus
1	Cerebral Meninges	1	Cervical Nerve
2	Dura Mater	2	Phrenic Nerve
3	Epidural Space, Intracranial	3	Brachial Plexus
4	Subdural Space, Intracranial	4	Ulnar Nerve
5	Subarachnoid Space, Intracranial	5	Median Nerve
6	Cerebral Ventricle	6	Radial Nerve
7	Cerebral Hemisphere	8	Thoracic Nerve
8	Basal Ganglia	9	Lumbar Plexus
9	Thalamus	A	Lumbosacral Plexus
A	Hypothalamus	B	Lumbar Nerve
B	Pons	C	Pudendal Nerve
C	Cerebellum	D	Femoral Nerve
D	Medulla Oblongata	F	Sciatic Nerve
E	Cranial Nerve (I–XII)	G	Tibial Nerve
F	Olfactory Nerve (I)	H	Peroneal Nerve
G	Optic Nerve (II)	K	Head and Neck Sympathetic Nerve
H	Oculomotor Nerve (III)	L	Thoracic Sympathetic Nerve
J	Trochlear Nerve (IV)	M	Abdominal Sympathetic Nerve

(Continued)   *(Continued)*

Table 8.1. Body parts in the nervous system (continued)

Body Part Value	Body Parts—Central Nervous System and Cranial Nerves (0)	Body Part Value	Body Parts—Peripheral Nervous System (1)
K	Trigeminal Nerve (V)	N	Lumbar Sympathetic Nerve
L	Abducens Nerve (VI)	P	Sacral Sympathetic Nerve
M	Facial Nerve (VII)	Q	Sacral Plexus
N	Acoustic Nerve (VIII)	R	Sacral Nerve
P	Glossopharyngeal Nerve (IX)	Y	Peripheral Nerve
Q	Vagus Nerve (X)		
R	Accessory Nerve (XI)		
S	Hypoglossal Nerve (XII)		
T	Spinal Meninges		
U	Spinal Canal		
V	Spinal Cord		
W	Cervical Spinal Cord		
X	Thoracic Spinal Cord		
Y	Lumbar Spinal Cord		

It can be challenging to select the correct body part value for excision of spinal cord tumors. The surgeon uses the descriptive terms of intra- and extra-dural and intra- and extramedullary to describe the location and tissue involved in the tumor. Extradural tumors are inside the spinal canal but are outside the spinal dura. The location must be determined and may be the vertebral bone or the subcutaneous tissue that lines the spinal canal. If the documentation states "extraosseous," the tumor is of the subcutaneous tissue and fascia of the back. An intradural tumor is inside the spinal dura and can be further identified as intramedullary (inside the spinal cord) or extramedullary (outside the spinal cord). Intramedullary tumors of the spinal cord as coded to the body part of the spinal cord based on their specific region of the spine and extramedullary tumors are coded to the body part value of spinal meninges. Figure 8.6 displays the decision-making process used in coding spinal tumors.

If the documentation includes specific body part names that are not included in these lists, refer to the body part key for other body part synonyms and alternative terms.

B4.2. Where a specific branch of a body part does not have its own body part value in PCS, the body part is typically coded to the closest proximal branch that has a specific body part value. In the cardiovascular body systems, if a general body part is available in the correct root operation table, and coding to a proximal branch would require assigning a code in a different body system, the procedure is coded using the general body part value.

Example: A procedure performed on the mandibular branch of the trigeminal nerve is coded to the trigeminal nerve body part value.

Occlusion of the bronchial artery is coded to the body part value Upper Artery in the body system Upper Arteries, and not to the body part value Thoracic Aorta, Descending in the body system Heart and Great Vessels.

Figure 8.6. Spinal tumor coding

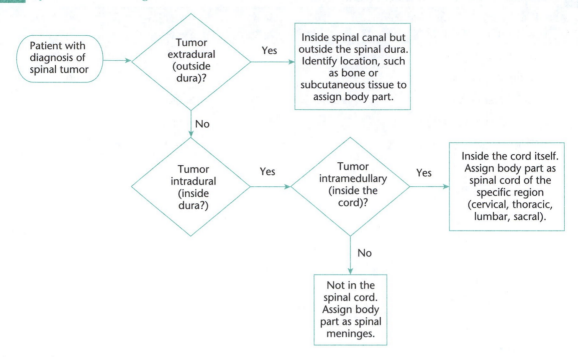

©Kuehn Consulting, LLC. Used with permission.

Coding Tip

Body part value Y, Peripheral nerve, is identified in the Peripheral Nervous System to be used when the code does not require the specification of the individual peripheral nerve, such as in the root operations of Change, Insertion, Inspection, Removal, and Revision. There is no similar body part value in the Central Nervous System.

Anatomy Alert

The peripheral nervous system of ICD-10-PCS classifies the somatic nerves based on the muscles they serve (i.e., ulnar nerve or femoral nerve) and the sympathetic nerves by the body regions they serve (thoracic sympathetic nerve or abdominal sympathetic nerve). Sympathetic nerves send impulses to the smooth muscles of the body organs, not structural muscles.

Approaches Used for the Nervous System

Coding of procedures performed on the nervous system uses only four approaches for both the central and peripheral nervous systems. Approaches that involve the use of a natural or artificial opening are not appropriate in this system, as there are no natural openings to the nervous system.

Coding Tip

A small nick in the skin does not constitute an Open approach. These small nicks in the skin are made to accommodate needles and other small-diameter instruments. When the needle or other instrument reaches all the way to the operative site but the site is not exposed or visualized, the correct approach value is Percutaneous.

Devices Common to the Nervous System

Device values for the nervous system involve those used for stimulation, monitoring, infusion, or drainage. Neurostimulator leads are placed as part of a TENS (transcutaneous electrical nerve stimulation) system to prevent pain messages from being sent to the brain, therefore breaking the pain reaction cycle. Refer to figure 1.18 in chapter 1 for a drawing of a neurostimulator generator and a lead. The generator is placed in a subcutaneous pocket using an open approach. The lead is tunneled to the nerve using a percutaneous approach. In addition, device values are assigned for various tissue substitutes used in the root operations of Bypass, Supplement, Replacement, and Revision. A Cesium-131 collagen implant is a radioactive "seed" encased in a collagen matrix. It is placed into the brain following resection of a brain tumor to eliminate any remaining cells.

There are three common device trade names representing devices used to supplement the dura or spinal meninges: Durafoam, DuraGen, and Durepair. They all are manufactured from bone (animal) tissue and are coded to the device value of K, Nonautologous Tissue Substitute because device value 8, Zooplastic is not available for coding in the Nervous System tables. DuraSeal is a cranial sealant and is not considered a device because it is absorbed into the body after a few weeks. Table 8.2 displays the devices used in coding procedures performed on the nervous system.

Table 8.2. Devices for the nervous system

Device Value	Devices—Central Nervous System and Cranial Nerves (0)	Device Value	Devices—Peripheral Nervous System (1)
0	Drainage Device	0	Drainage Device
2	Monitoring Device	2	Monitoring Device
3	Infusion Device	7	Autologous Tissue Substitute
4	Radioactive Element, Cesium-131 Collagen Implant	J	Synthetic Substitute
7	Autologous Tissue Substitute	K	Nonautologous Tissue Substitute
J	Synthetic Substitute	M	Neurostimulator Lead
K	Nonautologous Tissue Substitute	Y	Other Device
M	Neurostimulator Lead	Z	No Device
Y	Other Device		
Z	No Device		

Qualifiers Used in the Nervous System

Qualifier values that represent unique body parts within the nervous system are used with the root operations of Bypass and Transfer in the central nervous system and the root operation of Transfer in the peripheral nervous system. In addition to those, nervous system procedures may use the standard qualifiers of X for Diagnostic and Z for No Qualifier.

Qualifier value B in the central nervous system describes cerebral cisterns, which are cavities or enclosed spaces in the brain that are created between the arachnoid layer and the pia mater (*Mosby's* 2017, 375). There are several large cisterns in the brain that may be documented with unique names such as magna, cerebromedullary, pontine, superior, or ambient. These cisterns can be used when the root operation of Bypass is performed and are coded as the qualifier for the body part bypassed to. The body part value is the body part bypassed from in the ICD-10-PCS code. Table 8.3 displays the qualifiers used for nervous system coding.

Table 8.3. Qualifiers for the nervous system

Qualifier Value	Qualifiers—Central Nervous System and Cranial Nerves (0)	Qualifier Value	Qualifiers—Peripheral Nervous System (1)
0	Nasopharynx	1	Cervical Nerve
1	Mastoid Sinus	2	Phrenic Nerve
2	Atrium	4	Ulnar Nerve
3	Blood Vessel	5	Median Nerve
4	Pleural Cavity	6	Radial Nerve
5	Intestine	8	Thoracic Nerve
6	Peritoneal Cavity	B	Lumbar Nerve
7	Urinary Tract	C	Perineal Nerve
8	Bone Marrow	D	Femoral Nerve
9	Fallopian Tube	F	Sciatic Nerve
B	Cerebral Cisterns	G	Tibial Nerve
F	Olfactory Nerve	H	Peroneal Nerve
G	Optic Nerve	X	Diagnostic
H	Oculomotor Nerve	Z	No Qualifier
J	Trochlear Nerve		
K	Trigeminal Nerve		
L	Abducens Nerve		
M	Facial Nerve		
N	Acoustic Nerve		
P	Glossopharyngeal Nerve		
Q	Vagus Nerve		
R	Accessory Nerve		
S	Hypoglossal Nerve		
X	Diagnostic		
Z	No Qualifier		

 Code Building

Case #1:

PROCEDURE STATEMENT: Percutaneous biopsy of spinal cord at T6

ADDITIONAL INFORMATION: The patient is placed in the typical position used for spinal tap procedures. The area of the lesion is located and local anesthesia is administered. Imaging (this separately reportable procedure is covered in chapter 24 of this text) is used to confirm needle placement, and samples are cored from the spinal cord lesion for evaluation. The needle is removed and a dressing is applied.

ROOT AND INDEX ENTRIES FOR THE STATEMENT: Excision is the root operation performed in this procedure, defined as cutting out or off, without replacement, a portion of a body part. The Index entry is:

Excision

    Spinal cord

        Cervical   00BW

        Lumbar   00BY

        Thoracic   00BX

Code Characters:

Section	Body System	Root Operation	Body Part	Approach	Device	Qualifier
Medical and Surgical	Central Nervous System and Cranial Nerves	Excision	Thoracic Spinal Cord	Percutaneous	No Device	Diagnostic
0	0	B	X	3	Z	X

RATIONALE FOR THE ANSWER: The needle is used to cut a core of tissue from the lesion for biopsy purposes. The lesion is at the level of T6, or the thoracic spinal cord. The needle is placed percutaneously. No device is assigned and the qualifier value X, Diagnostic is assigned to indicate a biopsy. The correct code assignment is 00BX3ZX.

Case #2:

PROCEDURE STATEMENT: Endoscopic 3rd Ventriculostomy

ADDITIONAL INFORMATION: This bypass is necessary to drain excess cerebrospinal fluid (CSF) out of the ventricle and into the cerebral cistern, where it can be absorbed. To perform the procedure, the surgeon makes an incision in the scalp near the ear and passes a small endoscope into the 3rd cerebral ventricle. Using this endoscope, a small hole is made in the floor of the 3rd ventricle, making a new connection to a cerebral cistern and allowing the cerebrospinal fluid to flow freely out of the ventricle.

ROOT AND INDEX ENTRIES FOR THE STATEMENT: Bypass is the root operation performed in this procedure, defined as altering the route of passage of the contents of a tubular body part. The Index entry is:

Bypass

    Cerebral ventricle 0016

Code Characters:

Section	Body System	Root Operation	Body Part	Approach	Device	Qualifier
Medical and Surgical	Central Nervous System and Cranial Nerves	Bypass	Cerebral Ventricle	Percutaneous Endoscopic	No Device	Cerebral Cisterns
0	0	1	6	4	Z	B

RATIONALE FOR THE ANSWER: The root operation Bypass describes the procedure performed to allow cerebral spinal fluid to flow into the cerebral cistern where it can be reabsorbed normally. The approach for this procedure is percutaneous endoscopic and no device is used. The body part value of 6, Cerebral Ventricle describes the source of the bypass (part bypassed from) and the qualifier value B, Cerebral Cisterns, describes the body part bypassed to. The correct code assignment is 00164ZB.

Case #3:

PROCEDURE STATEMENT: Neurorrhaphy of radial nerve

ADDITIONAL INFORMATION: The left radial nerve was partially severed when the patient suffered a deep laceration to the upper arm at mid-humeral level. The surgeon repairs the radial nerve and closes the skin in layers.

ROOT AND INDEX ENTRIES FOR THE STATEMENT: Repair is the root operation performed in this procedure, defined as restoring, to the extent possible, a body part to its normal anatomic structure and function. The Index entry is:

Repair

   Nerve

      Radial   01Q6

Code Characters:

Section	Body System	Root Operation	Body Part	Approach	Device	Qualifier
Medical and Surgical	Peripheral Nervous System	Repair	Radial Nerve	Open	No Device	No Qualifier
0	1	Q	6	0	Z	Z

RATIONALE FOR THE ANSWER: Neurorrhaphy is defined as joining together two parts of a divided nerve and is coded with the root operation Repair. This was an open procedure because the surgeon visualized the surgical field directly to perform the procedure. The body part value is 6, Radial nerve and no device or qualifier is appropriate for this code. The correct code assignment is 01Q60ZZ.

Code Building Exercises

Work through each case and check your answers using the answer key in appendix B of the textbook before going on to the Check Your Understanding questions that follow.

Exercise 1:

PREOPERATIVE DIAGNOSIS: Right S1 nerve root syndrome secondary to a calcified disc right L5-S1

POSTOPERATIVE DIAGNOSIS: Same

PROCEDURE   Right L5-S1 keyhole hemilaminotomy, mesial facetectomy and foraminotomy with microscopic magnification

OPERATIVE PROCEDURE: The patient was brought to the operating room and general endotracheal anesthesia induced. A midline skin incision from L5 through the sacrum was performed. Subcutaneous tissue and fascia were dissected sharply. Subperiosteal takedown of L5 and S1 performed on the right side. Lateralizing x-ray confirmed the level and then a right L5-S1 keyhole hemilaminotomy and mesial facetectomy was performed with microscopic magnification using a high speed drill. The S1 nerve root appeared to be compressed from a combination of calcified disc and hypertrophy of the facet joint. The ligamentum flavum was incised and removed and then the S1 nerve root was decompressed along its entire length. Similar procedure was then done for the L5 root. There was some hypertrophy and ligamentum flavum compressing the L5 root as it came around the pedicle. This was all removed. The L5 root was then well decompressed from the pedicle until it exited. Bone wax applied. Small pledgets of Gelfoam were placed in the epidural space. The wound was irrigated copiously with saline until clear. Bleeding controlled with bipolar cautery. The fascia was approximated with interrupted 0 Vicryl, subcutaneous tissue with interrupted inverted 2-0 Vicryl and the skin in layers. Sterile dressings applied.

Questions:

1.1. What was the objective of this procedure?

1.2. Are the keyhole hemilaminotomy, mesial facetectomy, and foraminotomy coded separately?

1.3. What code(s) would be assigned?

Exercise 2:

DIAGNOSIS:	Left acoustic Schwannoma
PROCEDURE:	Microsurgical resection of left cerebellar pontine angle acoustic Schwannoma with Stealth stereotactic guidance, complex patch duraplasty
INDICATION:	The patient presented to us with a hearing dysfunction and was found to have a 2 cm vestibulocochlear nerve mass on MRI.

PROCEDURE: The patient was taken to the MRI scanner for normal Stealth MRI registration prep. Afterwards, the patient was taken to the OR and general anesthesia was administered. The head was registered against the Stealth computer. An incision was fashioned and the flap was elevated and held in retraction. We turned a standard craniotomy and opened the dura. We then opened the cerebellar pontine angle cistern and identified the tumor. We did central debulking and were able to mobilize the edge of the tumor to identify cranial nerve VIII as it arose from the brainstem. We continued to debulk until we had removed tumor to the extent possible. The wound was carefully irrigated with antibiotic saline multiple times. The dura was closed via patch duraplasty with Durepair dural patch and a running 4-0 nylon suture and Fibrin glue. The bone flap was replaced with multiple micro plates and screws. Soft tissue closure was carried out in standard fashion.

Questions:

2.1. Knowing the type of tumor will help you determine the body part value. What is a Schwannoma?

2.2. The tumor is found in which body part?

2.3. Would you assign a code for the duraplasty with Durepair? If so, what is the root operation?

2.4. Research Durepair to determine the type of device value to assign. What is the appropriate choice and why?

2.5. In addition to 8E090BH for the Stealth Stereotaxis (computer-assisted navigation), what code(s) would be assigned?

Check Your Understanding

Coding Knowledge Check

1. A surgeon sutures a lacerated cubital nerve branch of the right hand. How is this coded?
   a. 01840ZZ
   b. 01Q40ZZ
   c. 01JY0ZZ
   d. 01S50ZZ

2. In ICD-10-PCS, the spiral ganglion is classified as part of the _____ body part.

3. Cerebromedullary, pontine, and superior are examples of names of
   a. Ganglia
   b. Meninges
   c. Cisterns
   d. Nerves

4. The surgeon documents: Resection of tumor of meninges from the temporal lobe, sent for frozen section identification. How is this coded?
   a. 00B10ZX
   b. 00B70ZX
   c. 00C10ZZ
   d. 00T70ZZ

5. Ventriculoperitoneostomy is a bypass between the _____ ventricle and the _____ cavity and is coded as 00160J6.

Procedure Statement Coding

Assign ICD-10-PCS codes to the following procedure statements and scenarios. List the root operation selected and the code assigned.

1. Submuscular transposition of ulnar nerve, right elbow, open, for cubital tunnel syndrome

2. Release of tethered lumbar spinal cord, open approach

3. Percutaneous denervation by neurolytic agent, common fibular nerve

4. Mapping of right hemisphere of the brain, open approach to locate epilepticogenic zones

5. Percutaneous biopsy of cervical spinal cord to rule out tumor

6. Radiofrequency destruction of left trigeminal nerve, percutaneous approach to treat trigeminal neuralgia

7. Percutaneous mapping of basal ganglia

8. Remove clogged drainage tube from the existing burr hole in the parietal lobe of the brain and insert new drainage tube

_____

9. A craniectomy is performed and a parietal lobe tumor is microsurgically excised using an operating microscope. The morphology of the tissue is unknown, and the tissue is sent for pathological identification.

_____

10. Fasciotomy with median nerve release

_____

Case Studies

Assign ICD-10-PCS codes to the following case studies.

1. Operative Report

PREOPERATIVE DIAGNOSIS:	Shunt malfunction
POSTOPERATIVE DIAGNOSIS:	Shunt valve malfunction
OPERATION:	Replacement of ventriculoperitoneal shunt valve

INDICATION FOR PROCEDURE: The patient has been watched for overdrainage. He had a shunt malfunction over 5 years ago, which provided the same symptoms of overdrainage headaches. We adjusted the placement and increased the pressure, and these improved for the intervening years. He is again experiencing headaches and is here to have the shunt checked and possibly replaced. Even with a replacement, there is still a risk of overdrainage, and if that occurs, he would likely need to undergo a new procedure where we would place a new valve or use a different type of distal tubing that creates more resistance. The patient understands all of the issues and risks and elects to proceed. Signed consent is on the record prior to arrival in the operating room.

PROCEDURE: The patient was brought to the operating room. Standard operative time out was performed. The patient was identified, and site and side of surgery were confirmed. The patient was intubated via general endotracheal anesthesia without difficulty and positioned for a left-sided shunt revision. The patient's hair was trimmed with clippers. We identified his multiple prior incisions and marked the cranial incision with a small extension for the revision. Once this was done, the patient was prepped and draped in the usual sterile fashion. We began surgery by taking a Colorado tip needle and opening the cranial incision, extending it down. We identified the Rickham reservoir and the valve. The flap was held back in place with a suture, and antibiotic-impregnated sponges were placed around the periphery of the incision. Next, we disconnected the Rickham reservoir from the valve and found it to be running smoothly. The distal runoff was higher than the programmed value, and the valve was subsequently removed and replaced with a new Strata valve set at 1.5. The shunt tubing appeared patent and unobstructed. Both connection points were secured with 2-0 silk ties. The wound and reservoir were copiously irrigated with bacitracin irrigation. The wound was closed. We closed with interrupted 3-0 Vicryl and 3-0 Monocryl for primary skin closure. Skin glue was applied, as was a sterile dressing. The patient remained stable throughout the case and will be taken to the recovery room in stable condition.

2. Operative Report

PREOPERATIVE DIAGNOSIS:	Gunshot wound to the spine
POSTOPERATIVE DIAGNOSIS:	Gunshot wound to the spine
PROCEDURE PERFORMED:	Thoracic T12 laminectomy with removal of bullet fragments and repair of dural tear

HISTORY: This 45-year-old sustained a gunshot wound to the spine. The bullet was lodged directly within the canal and into the spinal cord. The patient was reported to be paraplegic. He was intubated and sedated and not really able to be examined. We discussed with the family the treatment options, including conservative management versus bullet removal. They elected to proceed with this procedure.

OPERATIVE PROCEDURE: The patient was brought into the operating theater. Following the induction of general anesthesia, the patient was turned from the supine to the prone position on the radiolucent Wilson frame. We used C-arm to localize the bullet. The patient actually had two bullets, one in the subcutaneous layer at about L2 and one in the spinal cord at T12. With localizing this, we made our skin incision directly over both of these. We incised down through the fascia and removed the more superficial one, and then we opened the thoracolumbar fascia, staying on the patient's left side, dissecting the muscle attachments off, exposing the spinous process and lamina of T12. We drilled through this, entering into the epidural space. Once we cleaned off the bone and ligamentum flavum, we got to the cerebrospinal fluid. There was a very large rent in the dura. We were able to work through this rent and we identified the bullet fragment; it was intact, and we removed it. It came out in, of course, piecemeal fashion. Once we explored looking for the bullet fragment, we could see some lacerated nerve roots as well. Obviously the patient sustained quite significant intradural injury. Following removal of this, we used several 4-0 Nurolon stitches to suture up the large dural rent. We could see there were some dural root sleeves torn as well. These were, of course, unamenable to direct closure. Then we used fibrin glue to seal this off. We closed the thoracolumbar fascia with 0 Nurolon, the dermis with inverted interrupted 2-0 Vicryl, the skin with staples. Following this procedure, all instrument, sponge, needle, and patty counts were correct.

3. Operative Report

PREOPERATIVE DIAGNOSIS:	Left-sided subdural hematoma
POSTOPERATIVE DIAGNOSIS:	Left-sided subdural hematoma
PROCEDURE PERFORMED:	Left frontal temporoparietal craniotomy and evacuation of subdural hematoma
DRAINS:	Jackson-Pratt in subgaleal space

INDICATION: This patient is a 69-year-old African-American male who has had some difficulty with mentation, some speech impairment consistent with aphasia, and some right-sided weakness. Computerized tomographic scanning of the brain revealed a large hematoma in the subdural space about the left convexity. It appeared to be chronic and subacute in appearance. At this time, due to his progressive neurological deteriorating course and the findings on computerized tomographic scanning of the brain, it was felt that consideration for removal was undertaken. The risks and indications were explained to the family because the patient was unable to consent and, after their questions were answered and the implications were discussed, consent was secured.

PROCEDURE: The patient was brought to the main operating room and, after he settled into anesthesia and his intubation tube was secured, he had his head turned to the right approximately 45 degrees and a sandbag placed under his left shoulder. His hair was removed. His scalp was prepped and draped in normal fashion for craniotomy and an incision was made no more than 1 cm anterior to the tragus of the left ear and carried in a gentle sloping fashion posteriorly and anteriorly. A myocutaneous scalp flap was reflected over towel rolls, with rubber bands and hemostats helping to effect exposure. Multiple burr holes were created and a free bone flap was elevated based on a temporalis flap. The dura was quite tense and nonpulsatile and, after we tented up about the circumference of the craniotomy site, opened the dura. Egress of subdural machine oil–colored fluid with septated membranes was identified. The membranes were resected and I coagulated back to the edge of the craniotomy, and the inner membrane was also opened in hope that the brain would re-expand. We irrigated copiously with saline solution with clear return and the subdural was both machine oil–colored in appearance, some fresh clot, and minimal amber-colored fluid loculated. At this time the dura was reapproximated after hemostasis was secured with FloSeal, bipolar coagulation, and thrombonin-soaked Gelfoam. The bone plate was placed back within the craniotomy site. A drain was left in the subgaleal space and the edge. The patient tolerated the procedure well and was transferred to the recovery room with stable vital signs.

4. Operative Report

NOTE: Do not code intraoperative imaging on this case.

DIAGNOSIS: Low back pain, failure of conservative management, chronic facet syndrome of the lumbar spine, lumbar radiculopathy, spinal stenosis

PROCEDURE PERFORMED: Neural modulation with spinal cord stimulator, permanent implant of the leads under fluoroscopic guidance

INTERIM HISTORY: Patient had undergone a trial of spinal cord stimulation. This has helped her with significant pain relief. She was able to handle this pain without much problem. Patient's only concern was that though her left-sided pain, which is more than the right side, was very well covered with the stimulator, she continued to have some persistent pain in the right lower extremity and she was wondering if we could help this. I had a detailed discussion with the patient and offered her a two-lead placement, which would cover bilaterally. Patient would like to go ahead with this. Patient understands the risks and benefits of this procedure.

PROCEDURE: After taking informed consent, with the patient in prone position and monitored anesthesia care provided by the anesthesiologist, patient's back was prepped and draped aseptically. Patient was monitored under AP view of fluoroscopy. The L1 interspinous process was identified. Local was infiltrated using 1 percent lidocaine and 0.25 percent preservative-free Marcaine, a 50/50 combination. A no. 14-gauge epidural needle was then advanced under the pedicle at the L1 level under continuous AP, then under continuous lateral fluoroscopy, to reach the epidural space, with loss of resistance technique. Once reaching the epidural space, there was no aspiration of CSF or blood, and no paresthesia at any point. An eight-contact Bionics lead was then advanced with the help of navigation. Depth was confirmed both with the lateral and AP view. At this time, I was able to thread the lead in the posterior epidural space to the level of T9. A second lead was then placed at the same level but medial to the entry of the needle on the left side, again by loss of resistance technique, to reach the epidural space under continuous fluoroscopy with a negative aspiration for CSF or blood. A second eight-contact Bionics lead was advanced to T8–T9 level. At this time, with the help of a Bionics representative, we analyzed the position of the lead. A good coverage was obtained both on the right and left sides of her back as well as in lower extremities. The patient had complete satisfaction of covering most of her pain. At this time, she did not have any paresthesia that was uncomfortable. Both the leads were then anchored and secured at the 11–2 level. At this time, general surgery took over the patient and created the pocket and tunnel (dictated separately). Patient tolerated the whole procedure very well. Patient was then moved to the recovery room where, with the help of the Bionics representative, again a good coverage was confirmed. Patient understands that if she is uncomfortable or she has to reprogram her stimulator, she has to reach me or reach the representative.

5. Operative Report

PREOPERATIVE DIAGNOSIS: Right sphenoid wing meningioma

POSTOPERATIVE DIAGNOSIS: Right sphenoid wing meningioma

PROCEDURE PERFORMED: Right frontal temporal craniotomy and zygomatic osteotomy and resection of meningioma

SPECIMENS: Meningioma

INDICATIONS FOR SURGERY: The patient is a 55-year-old gentleman who has been found during a workup to have an instrumentally large tumor spreading from the sphenoid wing laterally and growing into the brain with significant mass effect and midline shift with edema around the tumor. Tumor measures approximately 6 cm and is growing from the temporal fossa into the frontoparietal area. Informed consent is signed.

DESCRIPTION OF PROCEDURE: The patient was intubated, placed in the supine position with the head tilted to the left and was prepped and draped in a sterile fashion. Then, a large frontotemporoparietal flap was made with an incision using a #10 blade scalpel and Bovie coagulators. The incision was carried out to the temporalis muscle. The zygomatic arch was sharply cut and the muscle was retracted and then frontotemporoparietal craniotomy was performed. The middle fossa was exposed extensively and so the tumor was coagulated completely on its base. After the devascularization of the tumor, attention was directed to the dura, which was opened all around the base of the tumor, which has now gone from a skull-based tumor to a complexity tumor. The tumor was then resected with the use of ultrasonic aspirators and Bovie loops. At the end of the case, the entire tumor was resected at the base and the tumor bed was then controlled for bleeding and Flowseal was used. At this point, the dura was patched with DuraGuard bovine pericardium, and reinforced with DuraGen and Tisseal. The bone flap was put back and fixed in place with miniplates. The skull flap which was infiltrated with tumor was replaced with a titanium mesh. A JP drain was left in the subgaleal space. The muscle was closed with #2-0 Vicryl sutures. Subcutaneous tissue was closed with #3-0 Vicryl sutures and the skin was closed with staples.

6. Operative Report

PREOPERATIVE DIAGNOSIS: Nerve damage, lateral plantar nerve, and flexor digiti minimi brevis tendon, left foot

POSTOPERATIVE DIAGNOSIS: Severed superficial branch of lateral plantar nerve and flexor digiti minimi brevis tendon, left foot

CLINICAL HISTORY: This patient injured his foot using a razor-sharp garden hoe in his yard and severed the superficial branch of the lateral plantar nerve and the flexor digiti minimi brevis tendon in his left foot. The patient experienced loss of sensation on the outer side of the fifth toe and across the side of the foot, so a neurology consultation was requested, and the patient was taken directly to surgery.

PROCEDURE: Following exploration of the wound and identification of the nerve avulsion, a repair of the nerve was undertaken using a nerve graft from the sural nerve. A lateral incision was made on the lateral malleolus of the ankle. The nerve was identified and freed for grafting, and the proximal and distal sural nerve endings were anastomosed. The wound was dissected, and the damaged area of the nerve was removed. The innervation of the external digital nerve was restored by suturing the 1.5-cm graft to the proximal and digital ends of the damaged lateral plantar nerve, using the operating microscope. Tenoplasty was performed on the tendon injury, and the wound was closed in layers.

Sense Organs

The sense organs included in this chapter are the eyes, the ears, and the nose, along with the associated sinuses. The tongue, the sense organ of taste, is discussed in chapter 10, and the skin, the sense organ of touch or sensation, is discussed in chapter 14. The second character values for the Sense Organs are:

8—Eye
9—Ear, Nose, and Sinus

Functions of the Sense Organs

The eye sends visual images to the brain for interpretation as pictures. The ear sends sound waves to the brain for interpretation, and the nose sends messages regarding airborne material to the brain for interpretation as environmental fragrances. The nose and its sense of smell also play an important role in the sense of taste, along with the tongue.

Organization of the Sense Organs

ICD-10-PCS has separate body systems for the eye and for the grouping of the ear, nose, and sinuses.

Ocular (Eye) System

In ICD-10-PCS, the structures of the ocular system affecting procedural code assignment include the anterior chamber, vitreous, sclera, cornea, choroid, iris, retina, retinal vessel, lens, extraocular muscle, eyelid, conjunctiva, lacrimal gland, and lacrimal duct. The eye has three layers: the fibrous layer, the vascular layer, and the nervous layer. Each layer contains:

- **Fibrous layer**—Sclera and cornea
- **Vascular layer**—Choroid, ciliary body, and iris
- **Nervous layer**—Retina, optic nerve, and retinal blood vessels

The eye contains both an anterior cavity (containing an anterior and posterior chamber) and a posterior cavity. The anterior chamber is in front of the iris and behind the cornea. The posterior chamber is in front of the lens and behind the iris. Both the anterior and posterior chambers of the anterior cavity contain aqueous humor. The posterior or vitreous cavity contains the vitreous humor (Rizzo 2016, 264). The vitreous is also referred to as the vitreous body. It is filled with a clear, gelatinous substance and presses the retina against the wall of the eye, helping to maintain the shape of the eye (Applegate 2011, 208). Blood vessels, which supply and drain the retina, include the central retinal artery and its branches along with the central retinal vein and its branches. Figure 9.1 displays the structures of the eyeball.

Figure 9.1. Structures of the eye

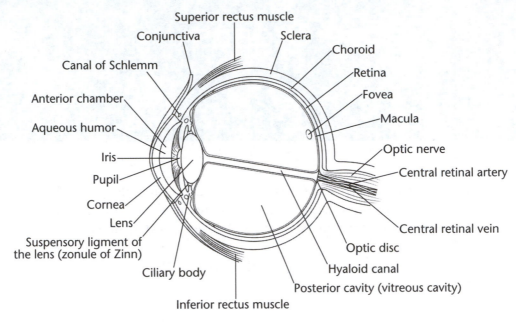

© AHIMA 2019

Anatomy Alert

ICD-10-PCS classifies all eye muscles to a single body part value of extraocular muscles and differentiates between extraocular muscles of the right and left eye.

The oculomotor muscles that move the eye are shown in figure 9.2. They are the medial rectus, lateral rectus, superior rectus, inferior rectus, inferior oblique, superior oblique, musculus orbitalis, and levator palpebrae superioris (*Mosby's* 2017, 666).

The orbital structures are shown in figure 9.3. The lacrimal (tear) gland and duct are part of the lacrimal apparatus, a tear-forming and tear-conducting system. The lacrimal gland is located above and lateral to the eye in the orbit. Other names for the lacrimal duct are lacrimal canaliculi or lacrimal canals, and they are located

Figure 9.2. Muscles of the eye

Figure 9.3. Orbital structures

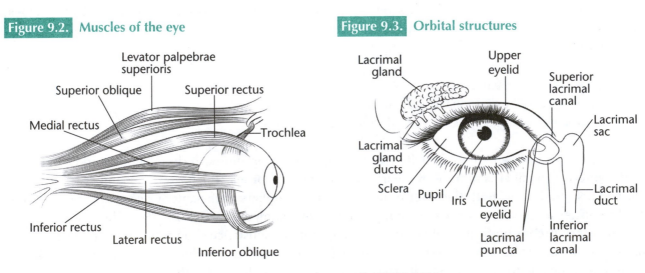

© AHIMA 2019   © AHIMA 2019

within each eyelid. The nasolacrimal duct extends from the lacrimal sac to the inferior meatus of the nose (Applegate 2011, 205).

Ear, Nose, and Sinus

In ICD-10-PCS, the structures of the ear, nose, and sinus affecting procedural code assignment include the following: external ear, auditory canal, middle ear, tympanic membrane, auditory ossicle, mastoid sinus, inner ear, eustachian tube, nasal mucosa and soft tissue, nasal turbinate, nasal septum, nasopharynx, accessory sinus, maxillary sinus, frontal sinus, ethmoid sinus, and sphenoid sinus.

Figure 9.4 shows the various parts of the ear. The external, or outer, ear is the visible area including the pinna and earlobe along with the external auditory canal, which leads to the tympanic membrane or eardrum. The external ear is also called the auricle. Components of the middle ear are the eardrum, the ossicles or ear bones, and the air cells behind the eardrum in the mastoid cavities. As illustrated, the ossicles are the hammer (malleus), anvil (incus), and stirrup (stapes). Located within the temporal bone, the semicircular canals, vestibule, and cochlea comprise the inner (internal) ear. Beneath and to the back of the ear are the mastoid air cells. These honeycombed, air-filled spaces are found in the mastoid process of the temporal bone (McKinley 2017, 187).

Figure 9.4. **Structures of the ear**

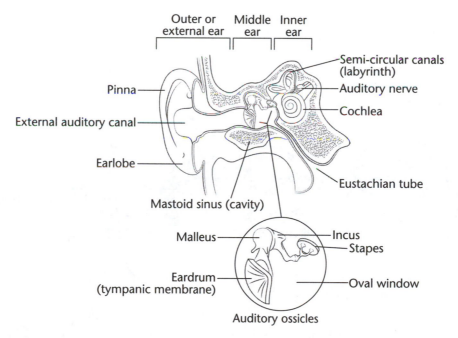

© AHIMA 2019

Figure 9.5 displays the structures of the nose. Nasal turbinates are also called nasal conchae. The remainder of the structures of the mouth and throat will be addressed in chapter 10 on the Mouth, Throat, and Respiratory System.

The four paranasal or accessory sinuses are identified in figure 9.6. "The paranasal sinuses ('the sinuses') are air-filled cavities located within the bones of the face and around the nasal cavity and eyes. Each sinus is named for the bone in which it is located" (ARS 2015). These sinuses are:

- **Ethmoid sinus**—Within the ethmoid bone between the nose and the eyes
- **Frontal sinus**—Within the frontal bone behind the forehead

- **Maxillary sinus**—Within the maxillary bone under the eyes
- **Sphenoid sinus**—Within the sphenoid bone at the center of the skull base under the pituitary gland (Applegate 2011, 329)

In addition, the mastoid sinus, or mastoid cavity, is found within the mastoid process of the temporal bone behind and beneath the ear.

Figure 9.5. **Structures of the nose**

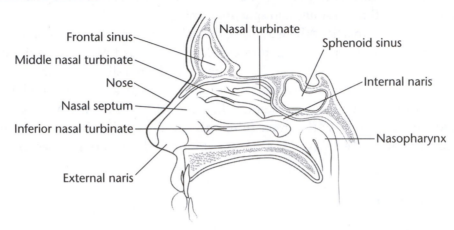

© AHIMA 2019

Figure 9.6. **Paranasal sinuses**

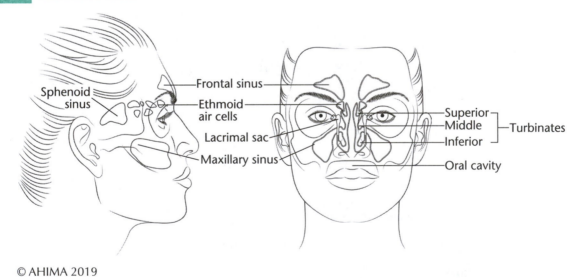

© AHIMA 2019

Common Root Operations Used in Coding Procedures Performed on the Sense Organs

The root operation of Alteration is found in the body systems related to the sense organs, because the eyes, ears, and nose are frequently altered for cosmetic purposes. Both the Eye and the Ear, Nose, and Sinuses body systems have tubular body parts included within them and, therefore, the root operations of Dilation, Occlusion, and Restriction are available here for use in assigning codes for procedures done on these systems.

The root operation Extraction is used when an ocular lens is removed without replacement by an intraocular lens implant. If a prosthetic lens is inserted at the same operative session, it is coded to the root operation

Replacement because Replacement includes the removal of the native tissue. Corneal transplant procedures are coded to the root operation Replacement because the cornea is a body part and not an organ or significant portion of an organ. The cornea is replaced by a biological or synthetic material.

Coding Tip

Corneal transplant procedures are coded to the root operation Replacement because transplant procedures in ICD-10-PCS describe organs or large sections of organs. The cornea is a body part that is replaced by biological or synthetic material.

Radial keratotomy procedures are coded to the root operation Repair because the procedure restores the body part to its normal anatomic structure and function. Scleral buckling of the retina is coded to the root operation Supplement because the buckle placed around the eyeball physically reinforces the eye and holds the retina in place.

Placement of tympanostomy or myringotomy tubes into the ears is coded to the root operation Drainage and coded with the device value of 0, Drainage Device. The body part being drained is the middle ear. The tubes are placed through the tympanic membrane to complete the drainage. Tympanoplasty is the root operation Repair, usually performed to repair a ruptured tympanic membrane. Procedures performed on the ossicles of the ear are coded based on the entire chain of ossicles. If one ossicle is removed, the root operation Excision is coded. If all of the ossicles are removed, the root operation Resection is coded.

Anatomy Alert

ICD-10-PCS classifies the ossicles (the malleus, incus, and stapes) together as one body part. Therefore, the root operation of Excision is used when one ossicle is removed, rather than the root operation of Resection.

Sinus endoscopy is coded to the actual root operation performed within the sinuses. The endoscopy is the approach to the sinus and not a procedure in itself. Diagnostic sinus endoscopy is coded to the root operation Inspection. Control of nasal hemorrhage, also called epistaxis, is coded in the Ear, Nose and Sinus body system in the 093 table. Control is coded when the nasal mucosa or soft tissue is repaired or destroyed to stop the bleeding. In addition, packing used to stop epistaxis is also coded to Control in this body system.

Be sure to research any procedure that is unfamiliar to ensure correct coding. If the documentation includes an eponym (procedure named for a person) and the intent of the procedure is unclear, query the physician for specifics.

Body Part Values for the Sense Organs

The external ear is also called the auricle. The inner ear is composed of the oval window (round window), the semicircular canal (bony labyrinth or bony vestibule), and the cochlea. Numerous synonyms are available for various parts of the eye. In the sinuses, terms such as "mastoidectomy" or "sphenoidectomy" typically refer to excision of the sinus, rather than excision of the bone in which the sinus is found. Referencing the pathology report may help to verify the exact tissue being excised in these procedures. Table 9.1 shows the body part values assigned to the sense organs. If the documentation includes specific body parts that are not included in these lists, refer to the body part key for other body part synonyms and alternative terms.

Table 9.1.   Body parts in the sense organs

Body Part Value	Body Parts—Eye (8)	Body Part Value	Body Parts—Ear, Nose, and Sinus (9)
0	Eye, Right	0	External Ear, Right
1	Eye, Left	1	External Ear, Left
2	Anterior Chamber, Right	2	External Ear, Bilateral
3	Anterior Chamber, Left	3	External Auditory Canal, Right
4	Vitreous, Right	4	External Auditory Canal, Left
5	Vitreous, Left	5	Middle Ear, Right
6	Sclera, Right	6	Middle Ear, Left
7	Sclera, Left	7	Tympanic Membrane, Right
8	Cornea, Right	8	Tympanic Membrane, Left
9	Cornea, Left	9	Auditory Ossicle, Right
A	Choroid, Right	A	Auditory Ossicle, Left
B	Choroid, Left	B	Mastoid Sinus, Right
C	Iris, Right	C	Mastoid Sinus, Left
D	Iris, Left	D	Inner Ear, Right
E	Retina, Right	E	Inner Ear, Left
F	Retina, Left	F	Eustachian Tube, Right
G	Retinal Vessel, Right	G	Eustachian Tube, Left
H	Retinal Vessel, Left	H	Ear, Right
J	Lens, Right	J	Ear, Left
K	Lens, Left	K	Nasal Mucosa and Soft Tissue
L	Extraocular Muscle, Right	L	Nasal Turbinate
M	Extraocular Muscle, Left	M	Nasal Septum
N	Upper Eyelid, Right	N	Nasopharynx
P	Upper Eyelid, Left	P	Accessory Sinus
Q	Lower Eyelid, Right	Q	Maxillary Sinus, Right
R	Lower Eyelid, Left	R	Maxillary Sinus, Left
S	Conjunctiva, Right	S	Frontal Sinus, Right
T	Conjunctiva, Left	T	Frontal Sinus, Left
V	Lacrimal Gland, Right	U	Ethmoid Sinus, Right
W	Lacrimal Gland, Left	V	Ethmoid Sinus, Left
X	Lacrimal Duct, Right	W	Sphenoid Sinus, Right
Y	Lacrimal Duct, Left	X	Sphenoid Sinus, Left
		Y	Sinus

Coding Tip

Body part values for the "accessory sinuses" and the "sinus" are available as generic terms when the specific sinus is not identified in the documentation or the exact location of the procedure is not necessary for coding purposes.

Approaches Used for the Sense Organs

The approaches that describe procedures performed on the sense organs include Open, Percutaneous, Percutaneous Endoscopic, Via Natural or Artificial Opening, Via Natural or Artificial Opening Endoscopic, and External. Note that the ethmoid and sphenoid paranasal sinuses cannot be approached via a natural or artificial opening without going through their associated bones, making their approach values Percutaneous Endoscopic when initial endoscopic sinus surgery is performed. Once the bone is removed, a subsequent endoscopic procedure can access these sinuses through the artificial opening. The maxillary and frontal sinuses can be reached through the natural nasal opening with an endoscope.

Devices Common to the Sense Organs

Device value 0, Synthetic Substitute, Intraocular Telescope in the Eye system is also called an Implantable miniature telescope, or IMT. The IMT provides central vision for age-related macular degeneration patients when implanted in one eye, while the nonimplant eye provides the peripheral vision.

Device value B, Intraluminal device, airway is available for coding the insertion of an airway device into the nasopharynx. Also known as a nasal trumpet, a nasopharyngeal airway (NPA) is inserted through one nostril to create an air passage between the nose and nasopharynx. These airways are preferred in certain patients due to injury or because of the need for a reduced gag reflex reaction (American National Red Cross 2011, 1, 4).

Three different hearing devices are assigned device values in the Ear, Nose, and Sinus system. Cochlear prostheses, both single channel and multiple channel, have device values, as does the bone conduction device (a bone-anchored hearing aid, or BAHA). In addition, these hearing devices are a combination of two devices. The receptors are inserted into the inner ear, and the external hearing device is either secured to the temporal bone or inserted into it. Refer to figure 1.17 in chapter 1 for drawing of the cochlear implant hearing device. Table 9.2 lists the devices available to coding procedures performed on the sense organs.

Table 9.2. Devices for the sense organs

Device Value	Devices—Eye (8)	Device Value	Devices—Ear, Nose, and Sinus (9)
0	Drainage Device	0	Drainage Device
0	Synthetic Substitute, Intraocular Telescope	4	Hearing Device, Bone Conduction
1	Radioactive Element	5	Hearing Device, Single Channel Cochlear Prosthesis
3	Infusion Device	6	Hearing Device, Multiple Channel Cochlear Prosthesis
5	Epiretinal Visual Prosthesis	7	Autologous Tissue Substitute
7	Autologous Tissue Substitute	B	Intraluminal Device, Airway
C	Extraluminal Device	D	Intraluminal Device
D	Intraluminal Device	J	Synthetic Substitute
J	Synthetic Substitute	K	Nonautologous Tissue Substitute
K	Nonautologous Tissue Substitute	S	Hearing Device
Y	Other Device	Y	Other Device
Z	No Device	Z	No Device

Qualifiers Used in the Sense Organs

The qualifier value for both these body systems describes the body part to which a bypass is created. The qualifier value of 3, Nasal Cavity is coded with the location lacrimal duct. The qualifier value of 4, Sclera is coded with the location anterior chamber of the eye.

The qualifier value 0, Endolymphatic in the Ear, Nose, and Sinuses system is coded with the location that the inner ear is bypassed to during a bypass procedure. The endolymphatic duct and the endolymphatic sac are the nonsensory components of the endolymph-filled, membranous labyrinth. The endolymphatic duct and sac lead from the vestibule through the vestibular aqueduct to terminate in the epidural space of the posterior cranial fossa (Lo et al. 1997, 881). These body systems may also use the standard qualifiers of X for Diagnostic and Z for No Qualifier. Table 9.3 summarizes all of the qualifiers used for coding procedures performed on these systems.

Table 9.3. Qualifiers for the sense organs

Qualifier Value	Qualifiers — Eye (8)	Qualifier Value	Qualifiers — Ear, Nose, and Sinus (9)
3	Nasal Cavity	0	Endolymphatic
4	Sclera	X	Diagnostic
X	Diagnostic	Z	No Qualifier
Z	No Qualifier		

 Code Building

Case #1:

PROCEDURE STATEMENT: Excision of left extraocular muscle for strabismus

ADDITIONAL INFORMATION: The muscle is isolated with a muscle hook. The muscle tension is increased by resection of a small piece of muscle, with reattachment of the muscle. The muscles are secured with sutures.

ROOT AND INDEX ENTRIES FOR THE STATEMENT: Excision is the root operation performed in this procedure, defined as cutting out or off, without replacement, a portion of a body part. The Index entry is:

Excision

    Muscle

        Extraocular

            Left   08BM

            Right   08BL

Code Characters:

Section	Body System	Root Operation	Body Part	Approach	Device	Qualifier
Medical and Surgical	Eye	Excision	Extraocular Muscle, Left	Open	No Device	No Qualifier
0	8	B	M	0	Z	Z

RATIONALE FOR THE ANSWER: The root operation Excision is used because a small piece of muscle is removed to tighten the muscle of the eye. An Open approach is used to access the muscle. No device value or qualifier value is appropriate for this code. The correct code assignment is 08BM0ZZ.

Case #2:

PROCEDURE STATEMENT: Incision and drainage infected cyst of right upper eyelid

ADDITIONAL INFORMATION: No drainage device is inserted. The specimen is sent for pathogen identification.

ROOT AND INDEX ENTRIES FOR THE STATEMENT: Drainage is the root operation performed in this procedure, defined as taking or letting out fluids and/or gases from a body part. The Index entry is:

Drainage

    Eyelid

        Upper

            Left   089P

            Right   089N

Code Characters:

Section	Body System	Root Operation	Body Part	Approach	Device	Qualifier
Medical and Surgical	Eye	Drainage	Upper Eyelid, Right	Open	No Device	Diagnostic
0	8	9	N	0	Z	X

RATIONALE FOR THE ANSWER: Incision and drainage is the root operation Drainage. ICD-10-PCS identifies individual body part values for upper and lower eyelids, as well and left and right eyes. The approach is open because an incision is made. No device value is appropriate for the code. The qualifier X, Diagnostic is assigned because the specimen is sent for identification. The correct code assignment is 089N0ZX.

Case #3:

PROCEDURE STATEMENT: Suturing of left external ear laceration

ADDITIONAL INFORMATION: The laceration of the ear extends through multiple layers.

ROOT AND INDEX ENTRIES FOR THE STATEMENT: Repair is the root operation performed in this procedure, defined as restoring, to the extent possible, a body part to its normal anatomic structure and function. The Index entry is:

Repair

    Ear

        External

            Bilateral   09Q2

            Left   09Q1

            Right   09Q0

Code Characters:

Section	Body System	Root Operation	Body Part	Approach	Device	Qualifier
Medical and Surgical	Ear, Nose, Sinus	Repair	External Ear, Left	Open	No Device	No Qualifier
0	9	Q	1	0	Z	Z

RATIONALE FOR THE ANSWER: The root operation for suturing of a laceration is Repair. The approach is Open because the laceration extends through multiple layers. No device value or qualifier value is appropriate for the code. The correct code assignment is 09Q10ZZ.

Code Building Exercises

Work through each case and check your answers using the answer key in appendix B of the textbook before going on to the Check Your Understanding questions that follow.

Exercise 1:

DIAGNOSIS: Retinal detachment in the right eye

PROCEDURE: Repair of retinal detachment with pars plana vitrectomy, placement of scleral buckle and retinopexy with 1000 centistoke silicone oil insertion.

OPERATIVE PROCEDURE: The eye was properly prepped and draped in the usual sterile fashion for intraocular surgery. The conjunctiva and Tenon's capsule were retracted. Scleral tunnels were created approximately 4 mm posterior to the insertion of the rectus. A 41 band was strung underneath the rectus muscles and through the scleral tunnels and was cinched down in the superotemporal quadrant with a 71 sleeve. Two trocars were placed and vitrectomy was undertaken to gain access to the retina. There were several retinal holes superiorly ×2 and then one inferiorly. Endocautery was then used to mark the retinal holes and air-fluid exchange was done, draining the fluid. The retina was tacked around the retinal tears. A 1000 centistoke silicone oil was inserted as a tamponade. This was done because the patient has a complete retinal detachment in the other eye and would not be functional under gas. A total of approximately 7 mL was used. Trocars and infusion line were removed. The eye was under normal physiological pressure. The sclerotomy, conjunctiva and Tenon's capsule were closed. Subconjunctival Vancomycin and Decadron were injected. The patient tolerated the procedure well and will be seen in clinic tomorrow. He will schedule oil removal, as appropriate, after that visit.

Questions:

1.1. How many procedures are described in this report? What are they?

_____

1.2. Why is the vitrectomy performed?

_____

1.3. What is the intent of these procedures?

_____

1.4. What code(s) would be assigned?

_____

Exercise 2:

DIAGNOSIS: Chronic maxillary sinusitis secondary to polyps

PROCEDURE PERFORMED: Bilateral endoscopic sinus surgery with removal of polyps

DESCRIPTION OF PROCEDURE: After the patient was induced under anesthesia with endotracheal tube in place, 4% cocaine was used topically intranasally and 1% Xylocaine with epinephrine was infiltrated in the usual fashion for nasal and sinus surgery. Using the zero degree endoscope, inspection revealed almost complete airway obstruction bilaterally of both nasal passageways. The left side was approached and with the aid of the microdebrider, polyps were removed from the left nasal passageway to the ostiomeatal area. The natural ostium and the maxillary sinus cavity were cleaned of obstructing polyps. Neo-Synephrine pledgets were placed while attention was turned to the opposite side where once again the microdebrider was used to remove polyps from the right nasal passageway. The natural ostium and the maxillary sinus cavity were freed of all obstructing polyps. Once again, Neo-Synephrine pledgets were placed for hemostatic purposes. At the completion all Neo-Synephrine pledgets were removed. Merocel sinus packs were placed in the ostiomeatal area with Vaseline packing impregnated with Bactroban cream placed bilaterally. The patient tolerated the procedure well. He was able to be awakened and extubated while still in the operating room and taken to the recovery room in stable condition.

Questions:

2.1. How many procedures are described in this report? What are they?

_____

2.2. What root operation(s) is assigned and why?

_____

2.3. What code(s) would be assigned?

_____

✔ **Check Your Understanding**

Coding Knowledge Check

1. The eustachian tube connects the middle ear and the _____.
   a. Inner ear
   b. Nasal turbinates
   c. Pharynx
   d. Maxillary sinus

2. Incision and drainage of a cyst of the right auricle is coded as _____.
   a. 09500ZZ
   b. 09900ZZ
   c. 099300Z
   d. 09B00ZX

3. The ethmoid sinus is located between the _____ and the _____.

4. Removal of a metallic sliver from the right sclera is coded as _____.
   a. 08C6XZZ
   b. 08CSXZZ

(Continued)

  c. 08N6XZZ

  d. 08T0XZZ

5. The intraluminal airway device inserted in the Ear, Nose, and Sinuses system creates an air passage between the _____ and the _____ .

Procedure Statement Coding

Assign ICD-10-PCS codes to the following procedure statements and scenarios. List the root operation selected and the code assigned.

1. The patient had an intraocular lens implant placed several months ago in the right eye. Today the lens has an anterior dislocation and repositioning was not possible. The lens was retrieved through the previous scleral slit. A new intraocular lens was implanted and the scleral slit was sewn and watertight. The conjunctiva was tacked closed.

  _____

2. Stapes mobilization, left ear for otosclerotic deafness, open

  _____

3. Removal of blood clot from anterior chamber of right eye, percutaneous approach

  _____

4. Repair of laceration of left conjunctiva

  _____

5. Implantation of a multiple channel cochlear implant hearing device on the left side

  _____

6. Sinus endoscopy with repair of cerebrospinal fluid leak of right ethmoid sinus wall

  _____

7. Placement of bilateral lacrimal duct plugs via the lacrimal puncta for dry eye

  _____

8. Lamellar keratoplasty, with donor corneal tissue, bilateral percutaneous

  _____

9. Placement of a synthetic shunt from the anterior chamber of the left eye to the sclera to treat persistent glaucoma

  _____

10. Septoplasty with reinforcement by siliconized Dacron mesh implant, open

  _____

Case Studies

Assign ICD-10-PCS codes to the following case studies.

1. Operative Report

PREOPERATIVE DIAGNOSIS: Cataract, left eye

POSTOPERATIVE DIAGNOSIS: Same

OPERATIVE PROCEDURE: Phacoemulsification with intraocular lens implant, left eye

PROCEDURE: On arrival in the OR, the patient's left eye was administered with Tetracine drops. Ocular akinesia was obtained with retrobulbar injection of 0.75 percent Sensorcaine and Wydase in the amount of 4 cc. Five minutes of intermittent digital pressure was applied. A superior rectus bridle suture was placed. After routine preparation and draping, a small fornix-based conjunctival flap was raised superiorly. Bleeding points were cauterized. A 7-mm step incision was made above. The anterior chamber was entered under the flap with a 5531 blade. The anterior capsule was removed under Healon with a cystotome. The nucleus was emulsified in the posterior capsule. Cortex was removed with the I & A tip. The posterior capsule was vacuumed. Healon was placed in the anterior chamber and capsular bag. The wound was extended to 7 mm. A 23.5-diopter, 3161B lens was positioned in the bag horizontally. The wound was closed with a shoelace 9-0 nylon suture. After the Healon was removed from the anterior chamber with the I & A tip, intracameral Miostat was injected. The wound was tested for water tightness. Superior rectus suture was removed. Vasocidin ointment was applied along the lid margins. An eye shield was applied. The patient tolerated the procedure well and was taken to the recovery room in good condition.

2. Operative Report

PREOPERATIVE DIAGNOSIS: Hypertropia

POSTOPERATIVE DIAGNOSIS: Same

PROCEDURE: Recess right superior rectus muscle 5.0 mm

DESCRIPTION OF PROCEDURE: The patient was taken to the operating room and given general anesthesia by LMA. The right eye was prepared and draped in a normal sterile ophthalmic fashion. A lid speculum was placed in the right eye and traction sutures placed with the eye rotated down and out. The conjunctiva was opened. The right superior rectus muscle was then isolated from a Formix open approach with care taken to make sure the entire muscle was incorporated on the hook. A double-armed 6-0 Vicryl suture was then woven through the distal muscle tendon in locking fashion and the muscle disinserted from the globe. Hemostasis was obtained with bipolar cautery. The needles were then passed through superficial sclera 5.0 mm posterior to the original insertion and the muscle tied down firmly into this position. The conjunctival wound was closed with interrupted 7-0 Vicryl sutures. Erythromycin ointment was applied to the right eye. The patient was awakened and taken to the recovery room in good condition.

3. Operative Report

PREOPERATIVE DIAGNOSIS: Retinoblastoma, stage V, right eye

POSTOPERATIVE DIAGNOSIS: Same

OPERATION: Enucleation, right eye

SURGICAL INDICATION: This is a 6-month-old healthy infant who was diagnosed two months ago with stage V retinoblastoma, right eye. The child has had two courses of chemotherapy. Because of persistent tumor, especially vitreous seeding, enucleation of the right eye was recommended. The benefits, risks, and nature of the procedure and alternative procedures were discussed in great depth with the family. The family opted for enucleation of the right eye.

SURGICAL PROCEDURE: The child was brought to the operating room after adequate preoperative medications. She was induced with facemask anesthesia, at which time an intravenous line was inserted. A cardiac monitor, blood pressure cuff, precordial stethoscope, EKG leads, and pulse oximeter were attached. The child was then intubated. Both pupils were dilated with adult Kupffer solution, and each retina was examined, including scleral depression for 360 degrees. In the right eye there was a large tumor centered in the region between the optic nerve and macula that measured six disc diameters. It showed a typical cottage cheese pattern of regression. However, overlying this tumor was extensive particulate vitreous seeding. In view of this extensive vitreous seeding, the decision was made to proceed with enucleation of the right eye. The left eye was examined. The disc, vessels, macula, and retinal periphery were normal. No tumors were noted.

The patient's face was then draped and prepared in the usual sterile fashion. A lid speculum was put into place on the right. A 360-degree peritomy was made with Westcott scissors and 0.12 Bishop-Harmon forceps. Then sequentially each of the extraocular muscles were isolated on the Stevens hook and onto a large Green's hook. A double-armed 6-0 Vicryl suture was woven through the insertion site and locked at each end respectively. The muscle was then detached from the globe and the sutures were secured to a bulldog clip. The stump of the medial rectus muscle was cross-clamped and the eye was proptosed. A fine-tipped Metzenbaum scissors was then introduced behind the orbit from the optic nerve, and then the optic nerve was cut. At this point, the globe was removed from the orbit and digital pressure was applied to the socket to obtain adequate hemostasis. Inspection of the globe revealed that it was intact. There was no extrascleral extension of tumor. A tangential portion of optic nerve was obtained measuring 7 mm at one end and 9 mm at the other end.

After adequate hemostasis was obtained, a 14-mm prosthesis was wrapped in sclera that was secured along its seam with a 4-0 Prolene suture. The scleral-wrapped prosthesis was then inserted into the muscle cone. Each of the extraocular muscles was reattached to the sclera using the preplaced sutures. Then the overlying Tenon's was closed with nine interrupted 5-0 Vicryl sutures. The conjunctiva was then closed with a running 6-0 plain suture. Topical antibiotic ointment was then placed in the conjunctival cul-de-sac, and a conformer was put into place. The eye was pressure patched with two eye pads and Tegaderm that was then secured with foam tape after the skin had been pretreated with Mastisol and the entire eye bandage was secured with an ENT head wrap. The child was then weaned from general anesthesia, extubated, and brought to the recovery room in good condition without complications.

4. Operative Report

PREOPERATIVE DIAGNOSIS: Left maxillary polyposis

POSTOPERATIVE DIAGNOSIS: Left maxillary mucous retention cyst

OPERATION: Removal of contents, left maxillary sinus

PROCEDURE: The patient was taken to the OR, where general endotracheal intubation was induced. The head was draped in the usual fashion, allowing visualization of the medial canthus. The posterior insertion of the middle turbinate and lateral wall were injected, using 1 percent lidocaine with 1:100,000 epinephrine after cocaine pledgets had been placed into the nasal cavity containing 4 percent cocaine. This allowed for vasoconstriction and hemostasis. The 30-degree scope was then used to enter the left maxillary sinus and visualize the contents of the left maxillary sinus, which were photo-documented. The contents were then removed using a combination of microdebrider, micro forceps, and a straight pickup. It appeared mainly to contain mucus with minimal polypoid soft tissue. However, specimens were sent to pathology for analysis to be sure. Photo documentation was taken at the end of the case. The procedure was then terminated, and she was taken to recovery in satisfactory condition.

5. Operative Report

PREOPERATIVE DIAGNOSIS: Pupillary ectopia after repair of corneoscleral laceration repair, OS

POSTOPERATIVE DIAGNOSIS: Same

PROCEDURE: Synechiolysis, OS

FINDINGS: Adhesions of iris to wound, OS

INDICATIONS FOR PROCEDURE: This little girl had a corneoscleral laceration OS in early May of this year that was repaired primarily. She has developed adhesions of the iris to the cornea adjacent to the corneal laceration. Synechiolysis was undertaken to treat the pupillary ectopia that resulted.

PROCEDURE: After the patient was prepped and draped in the usual sterile ophthalmic fashion, a lid speculum was inserted to the lids. Inspection revealed that the pupil was peaked temporally and that the iris was adherent to the wound temporally. A corneal incision was made superotemporally near the limbus. Healon was instilled into the anterior chamber to maintain it. A cyclodialysis spatula was inserted into the anterior chamber, and blunt dissection was used to tease the adhesions down from the cornea. Gonioscopy was used with the operating microscope to ensure that all adhesions were removed. The anterior chamber was irrigated with Balanced Salt Solution to remove the Healon. The wound was then closed with a simple, interrupted 10-0 Vicryl suture. Attention was then directed to the 10-0 nylon sutures in the cornea from the initial trauma. These were removed with an eye knife and a tying forcep.

6. Operative Report

PREOPERATIVE DIAGNOSIS: Status post repair of right lower lid and canalicular laceration

POSTOPERATIVE DIAGNOSIS: Status post repair of right lower lid and canalicular laceration

PROCEDURE:
1. Removal of right indwelling silicone tube lacrimal stent
2. Right nasolacrimal duct probing

INDICATIONS FOR SURGERY: Sufficiency of time since lacrimal repair

PROCEDURE IN DETAIL: In the operating room in the supine position after satisfactory general anesthesia had been obtained, the right nostril was packed with Afrin packing. The packing was removed. The distal end of the stent was grabbed in the nose. The proximal end of the stent was cut, and the stent was removed from the right nostril intact. A #0-Bowman probe passed smoothly through the lower punctal canalicular system down the duct into the nose. The probe was removed. TobraDex drops were placed. The patient was awakened and taken from the operating room in satisfactory condition.

The respiratory system provides the body with a supply of oxygen through breathing, also known as ventilation. Breathing moves air through the passages between the outside atmosphere and the lungs (Applegate 2011, 329). Respiration takes place at two levels, external and internal. External respiration is the exchange of gases between the lungs and the blood. Internal respiration happens when the blood transports the gases to and from the tissue cells throughout the body. The second character values for the respiratory system and mouth and throat system are:

B—Respiratory System
C—Mouth and Throat

Functions of the Respiratory System

The respiratory system manages the breathing and respiration process. In addition, the respiratory system works with the circulatory system to deliver oxygen to the cells and removes the waste products of metabolism from the cells. It also plays a role in regulating the pH of the blood (Applegate 2011, 329).

Organization of the Mouth, Throat, and Respiratory System

ICD-10-PCS classifies some portions of the traditional respiratory system as separate body systems. The nose and sinuses were introduced previously in chapter 9 on sense organs and form a portion of the upper respiratory system. The mouth and throat are discussed here and are common to the respiratory system and the digestive system.

Mouth and Throat

In ICD-10-PCS, the structures of the mouth and throat affecting procedural code assignment include the following: lip (upper and lower), palate (hard and soft), buccal mucosa, gingiva (upper and lower), tongue, parotid gland, salivary gland, parotid duct, sublingual gland, submaxillary (submandibular) gland, minor salivary gland, pharynx, uvula, tonsils, adenoids, epiglottis, larynx, vocal cord, teeth (upper and lower), and the generic "mouth and throat."

Figure 10.1 shows the structures of the mouth, also known as the oral cavity. Primary teeth erupt at approximately one year of age and are identified with letters of the alphabet. Permanent teeth start erupting at approximately age six and replace primary teeth. Permanent teeth are identified with numbers. Letters or numbers begin in the upper right of the oral cavity, running sequentially around to the upper left, then continue from the lower left to the lower right of the oral cavity. Teeth #1, #16, #17, and #32 are also referred to as wisdom teeth. Surrounding both the upper and lower teeth are the gingiva, or gums.

Figure 10.1. Oral cavity

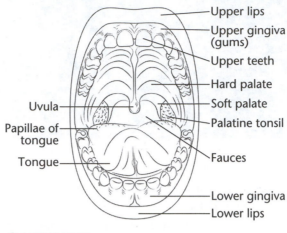

Upper lips
Upper gingiva (gums)
Upper teeth
Hard palate
Soft palate
Palatine tonsil
Uvula
Papillae of tongue
Fauces
Tongue
Lower gingiva
Lower lips

© AHIMA 2019

- **Upper primary teeth**—A through J
- **Upper permanent teeth**—1 through 16
- **Lower primary teeth**—K through T
- **Lower permanent teeth**—17 through 32 (*Stedman's* 2014)

The palate is the floor of the nasal cavity and the roof of the mouth. The front portion of the palate is the hard palate, supported by bone above it. The rear portion of the palate is the soft palate, which is not supported by bone. The posterior portion of the soft palate has an appendage called the uvula, which aids in swallowing.

The term "salivary gland" describes one of the major salivary glands, or the parotid glands, submandibular glands, and sublingual glands. The parotid glands lie on the sides of the face, immediately below and in front of the ear. The submandibular glands are in the neck, located in the space bound by the two bellies of the digastric muscle and the angle of mandible. The sublingual glands lie anterior to the submandibular gland under the tongue, beneath the mucous membrane of the floor of the mouth (NLM 2011a). The salivary glands are an accessory organ of digestion but are grouped as part of the mouth and throat system in ICD-10-PCS due to their location. Figure 10.2 displays the salivary glands. The following structures are not displayed and can be found as indicated:

- **Buccal mucosa**—Lining of the oral cavity, including mucosa of the gums, the palate, the lip, the cheek, floor of the mouth, and other structures (Rizzo 2016, 379–380).
- **Minor salivary gland**—The smaller, largely mucus-secreting, exocrine glands of the oral cavity, consisting of labial, buccal, molar, lingual, and palatine glands, and the anterior lingual gland (*Dorland's* 2012, 781).

Figure 10.3 displays the structures from the mouth to the tracheoesophageal junction, just below the voice box. The throat is divided into the nasopharynx, oropharynx, and laryngopharynx, or hypopharynx. Pharyngeal tonsils, also called adenoids, are located in the wall of the nasopharynx, but the palatine and lingual tonsils (base of the tongue) are located in the oropharynx. "The larynx is formed by nine cartilages that are connected to each other by muscles and ligaments. The three largest cartilages are the thyroid, cricoids, and epiglottis. There are two pairs of folds in the larynx. The upper pair are the vestibular folds and the lower pair are the true vocal cords. The opening between the vocal cords is the glottis" (Applegate 2011, 345). Figure 10.4 provides the detail within the voice box, including the vocal cords, the epiglottis, and the trachea.

Figure 10.2. Salivary glands

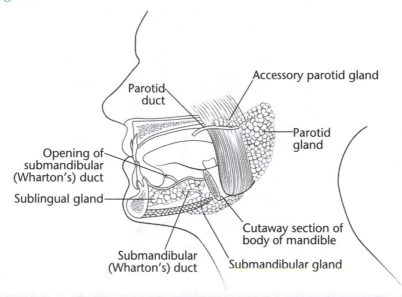

© AHIMA 2019

Figure 10.3. Mouth, pharynx, and larynx

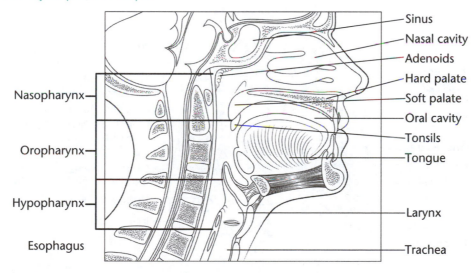

© AHIMA 2019

Coding Tip

ICD-10-PCS differentiates between the palatine and lingual tonsils. Lingual tonsils are coded to the pharynx body part, based on the body part key.

Respiratory System

In ICD-10-PCS, the structures of the respiratory system affecting procedural code assignment include: tracheo-bronchial tree, trachea, carina, bronchus (main, upper lobe, middle lobe, lower lobe, lingula), lung (lower lobe, upper lobe, middle lobe, lingual), pleura, and diaphragm. Figure 10.5 shows the organs and structures of the trachea and lungs.

Figure 10.4. Voice box

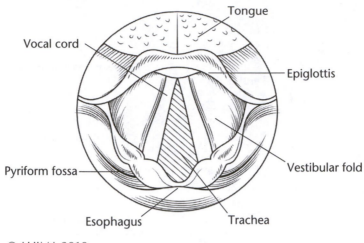

© AHIMA 2019

Figure 10.5. Trachea and lungs

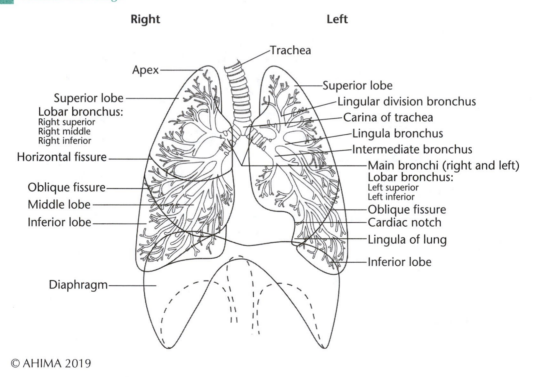

© AHIMA 2019

The tracheobronchial tree includes the trachea, bronchi, and bronchioles. A triangular ridge at the base of the trachea that separates into the openings of the right and left main bronchi is called the carina of trachea.

The superior lobe of the lung is also known as the upper lobe. The intermediate lobe is also known as the middle lobe, and the inferior lobe is also known as the lower lobe of the lung. Each lobe has a corresponding bronchus. Figure 10.6 shows the pleura, a thin serous membrane enveloping the lungs (visceral pleura), lining the thoracic cavity (parietal pleura), and the diaphragm (diaphragmatic pleura). The inner, visceral pleura is just next to the pulmonary parenchyma and the outer parietal pleura.

Figure 10.6. Pleura of the lung

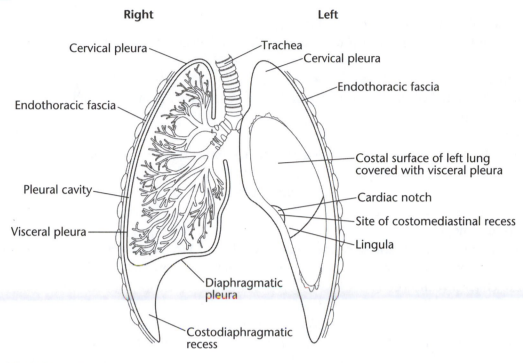

© AHIMA 2019

Anatomy Alert

The left and right lung fields are different. The left lung has upper and lower lobes with the lingula in the middle. The right lung has upper, middle, and lower lobes.

Coding Tip

Procedures performed specifically on the pleural cavity, rather than the pleura itself, are classified to the Anatomical Regions body system in ICD-10-PCS. See chapter 7 on Anatomical Regions.

Common Root Operations Used in Coding Procedures on the Mouth, Throat, and Respiratory System

Procedures frequently performed on the throat and respiratory system are laryngoscopy and bronchoscopy, along with other procedures performed through the scope. If no other procedure is performed at that time, the root operation of Inspection is performed, using a body part value of 0, Tracheobronchial Tree.

Bronchoscopy-Based Procedures

Bronchial tissue and lung tissue can both be accessed through the bronchoscope. Bronchial tissue is found inside the lumen of the bronchus and is identified with unique body parts for the bronchus of each lobe. Lung tissue is found on the outside of the bronchial wall and is accessed by taking an instrument through the wall of the bronchus. Lung tissue is also found in the alveoli, which are the air sacs that form at the end of the bronchioles. The alveolar tissue is lung tissue because it performs the work of gas exchange.

The following procedures can be performed on bronchial tissue through the bronchoscope:

- Endobronchial biopsy, also called bronchial biopsy
  - Biopsy of tissue from inside the bronchi, coded as Excision of bronchus with diagnostic qualifier
- Brush biopsy
  - Using a brush to cells from the surface of the bronchi, coded as Extraction of bronchus with the diagnostic qualifier
- Drainage
  - Removal of bronchial secretions, coded as Drainage, either diagnostic or therapeutic
- Removal of formed or inhaled foreign bodies
  - Extirpation of formed foreign bodies within the bronchi (called mucus plugs) or inhaled foreign bodies, coded as Extirpation
- Bronchial thermoplasty
  - Destruction of some of the smooth muscle of the bronchi to treat severe asthma, performed using a special radiofrequency wand on one or two bronchi per session, coded as Destruction
- Endobronchial valve insertion
  - An endobronchial valve is an implantable, self-expanding device, delivered by flexible bronchoscopy into the bronchus. The valve that looks like a miniature umbrella acts as a one-way valve to obstruct the airflow into certain areas of the lung but still allow distal air and mucus flow. The primary use is to decrease hyperinflation frequently found in emphysema (Kuehn 2018, 111–112). The endobronchial valve is pictured in figure 1.14 in chapter 1 and is coded as Insertion.
- Tracheal or bronchial dilation
  - Widening the air passage, with or without the placement of an intraluminal stent to hold open the passage, coded to Dilation.

The following procedures can be performed on lung tissue through the bronchoscope:

- Transbronchial biopsy
  - Biopsy of lung tissue through the wall of the bronchi, coded as Excision
- Bronchoalveolar Lavage (BAL)
  - Drainage procedure used to diagnose respiratory disease. As the segment of the lung tissue is lavaged (washed), the fluid is captured and sent for analysis. This is coded as Drainage of lung with the diagnostic qualifier.
- Whole lung lavage
  - Whole lung lavage is different than BAL because it is therapeutic. It irrigates the entire lung to remove pulmonary alveolar proteinosis (PAP). This is performed one lung at a time and may be performed on the second lung at a different operative session, after the first lung has recovered. This is coded as Irrigation in the 3E1 table, covered in chapter 21.

The list of codes on a bronchoscopy case can be numerous. There are eight locations that could require diagnosis or treatment, including the main right and left bronchus, the three lobes on the right, and the two lobes plus the lingula on the left. Keep track of the procedures performed in each bronchus and follow the multiple procedure guideline for code assignment. When drainage and extirpation are performed together in the same bronchus, code only the extirpation because fluid is typically used to loosen the mucus plug to allow its removal in one piece.

Thoracoscopy- or Thoracotomy-Based Procedures

Thoracoscopy or thoracotomy procedures are performed on lung structures, the pleura or the pleural cavity. Pleural cavity procedures were discussed in chapter 7. The following procedures can be performed through the chest wall:

- Excision
  - Excision can be either diagnostic or therapeutic and includes the common term "wedge resection," which is removing a small piece of a lobe in the form of a wedge.
- Resection
  - Removing an entire lobe of the lung or the entire right or left lung.
- Destruction
  - Destruction of tumors of the lung or pleura using heat or cold cautery.
- Release
  - Also called Decortication, this procedure involves removing a restrictive layer of tissue from around the lung. This layer can be called a rind or a peel and typically forms following an infection called empyema. Once this is removed, the lung is able to expand fully and again exchanges gases for the body. This is coded to Release of the specific lobe or lung from which the rind is removed.
- Lung transplantation
  - Transplanting one or both lungs from a donor.

The mouth and throat procedures of tonsillectomy and adenoidectomy are coded based on a variety of removal methods. Possible root operations are Destruction (cautery or coblation), Excision (partial removal for reduction), and Resection (scalpel or snare method to remove all of the tonsils), based on the extent of the procedure and the actual method used to perform the procedure. The tonsillectomy procedure is pictured in figure 1.7 in chapter 1 as an example of the external approach.

B3.11a. Inspection of a body part(s) performed in order to achieve the objective of a procedure is not coded separately.

Example: Fiberoptic bronchoscopy is performed for irrigation of bronchus (only the irrigation procedure is coded).

Be sure to research any procedure that is unfamiliar to assure correct coding. If the documentation includes an eponym (procedure named for a person) and the intent of the procedure is unclear, query the physician for specifics.

Body Part Values for the Mouth, Throat, and Respiratory System

Each lobe of the lung and each bronchus of the lung is defined in ICD-10-PCS by a unique body part. Therefore, if an entire lobe of the lung is removed, the root operation is Resection, rather than Excision. Depending on the root operation, it may be necessary to know which body part—the right, left, or both—was involved in the procedure to properly assign a code. Table 10.1 shows the body part values assigned to the mouth, throat, and respiratory system. If the documentation includes specific body part names that are not included in these lists, refer to the body part key for other body part synonyms and alternative terms.

Coding Tip

Surgeon documentation can provide important details about the amount of lung tissue being resected. A segmentectomy is excision of a portion of a lung lobe. A lobectomy is resection of the entire lung lobe. A pneumonectomy is resection of the entire left or right lung.

Table 10.1. Body parts in the mouth, throat, and respiratory system

Body Part Value	Body Parts—Mouth and Throat (C)	Body Part Value	Body Parts—Respiratory System (B)
0	Upper Lip	0	Tracheobronchial Tree
1	Lower Lip	1	Trachea
2	Hard Palate	2	Carina
3	Soft Palate	3	Main Bronchus, Right
4	Buccal Mucosa	4	Upper Lobe Bronchus, Right
5	Upper Gingiva	5	Middle Lobe Bronchus, Right
6	Lower Gingiva	6	Lower Lobe Bronchus, Right
7	Tongue	7	Main Bronchus, Left
8	Parotid Gland, Right	8	Upper Lobe Bronchus, Left
9	Parotid Gland, Left	9	Lingula Bronchus
A	Salivary Gland	B	Lower Lobe Bronchus, Right
B	Parotid Duct, Right	C	Upper Lung Lobe, Right
C	Parotid Duct, Left	D	Middle Lung Lobe, Right
D	Sublingual Gland, Right	F	Lower Lung Lobe, Right
F	Sublingual Gland, Left	G	Upper Lung Lobe, Left
G	Submaxillary Gland, Right	H	Lung Lingula
H	Submaxillary Gland, Left	J	Lower Lung Lobe, Left
J	Minor Salivary Gland	K	Lung, Right
M	Pharynx	L	Lung, Left
N	Uvula	M	Lungs, Bilateral
P	Tonsils	N	Pleura, Right
Q	Adenoids	P	Pleura, Left
R	Epiglottis	Q	Pleura
S	Larynx	T	Diaphragm
T	Vocal Cord, Right		
V	Vocal Cord, Left		
W	Upper Tooth		
X	Lower Tooth		
Y	Mouth And Throat		

B3.8. PCS contains specific body parts for anatomical subdivisions of a body part, such as lobes of the lungs or liver and regions of the intestine. Resection of the specific body part is coded whenever all of the body part is cut out or off, rather than coding Excision of a less specific body part.

Example: Left upper lung lobectomy is coded to Resection of upper lung lobe, left rather than Excision of lung, left.

Approaches Used in the Mouth, Throat, and Respiratory System

Many of the structures of the mouth and throat are accessed without the aid of instruments and can be visualized when the mouth is open. Therefore, the approach of X, External is commonly used when procedures are performed on the structures of the mouth and throat.

B5.3a. Procedures performed within an orifice on structures that are visible without the aid of any instrumentation are coded to the approach External.

Example: Resection of tonsils is coded to the approach External.

Devices Common to the Mouth, Throat, and Respiratory System

An endotracheal airway is a tube placed through the mouth and into the trachea to maintain an open airway in patients who are unconscious or unable to breathe on their own. This tube provides a temporary airway. This device is pictured in figure 1.4 in chapter 1 as an example of the Via Natural or Artificial Opening approach. A tracheostomy device is placed to form a more permanent airway. It is inserted either using a percutaneous approach or an open approach to create a bypass between the trachea and the skin to allow respiration directly into the trachea. The tracheostomy device is pictured in figure 1.10 in chapter 1.

Diaphragmatic pacemaker leads can be implanted laparoscopically into both sides of the diaphragm to set the respiratory rate for patients with diaphragm paralysis. The leads are attached to a pacing unit that is worn by the patient on the outside of the body. The pacemaker works by stimulating the diaphragm to expand and contract the chest wall, drawing air in and pushing it out at a regular rate. In some cases, this pacemaker can eliminate the need for mechanical ventilation by rhythmically moving the diaphragm. The root operation Insertion is used to code the placement of these pacemaker leads. Table 10.2 shows the devices that are commonly used in procedures performed on the mouth, throat, and respiratory system.

Table 10.2. Devices for the mouth, throat, and respiratory system

Device Value	Devices—Mouth and Throat (C)	Device Value	Devices—Respiratory System (B)
0	Drainage Device	0	Drainage Device
1	Radioactive Element	1	Radioactive Element
5	External Fixation Device	2	Monitoring Device
7	Autologous Tissue Substitute	3	Infusion Device
B	Intraluminal Device, Airway	7	Autologous Tissue Substitute
C	Extraluminal Device	C	Extraluminal Device
D	Intraluminal Device	D	Intraluminal Device
J	Synthetic Substitute	E	Intraluminal Device, Endotracheal Airway
K	Nonautologous Tissue Substitute	F	Tracheostomy Device
Y	Other Device	G	Intraluminal Device, Endobronchial Valve
Z	No Device	J	Synthetic Substitute
		K	Nonautologous Tissue Substitute
		M	Diaphragmatic Pacemaker Lead
		Y	Other Device
		Z	No Device

Coding Tip

Insertion of the endotracheal (ET) tube to be used for a mechanical ventilation procedure is coded in addition to the mechanical ventilation, other than when solely used during a surgical procedure (AHA 2014, 3). The insertion of the ET tube is coded as 0BH17EZ because the tube is inserted with the use of a laryngoscope, not via (through) the laryngoscope. Mechanical ventilation is coded using the root operation Performance in the Extracorporeal Assistance and Performance section of ICD-10-PCS.

Qualifiers for the Mouth, Throat, and Respiratory System

The mouth and throat body system uses qualifiers to define the number of teeth involved in the procedure, such as a single tooth, multiple teeth, or all of the teeth. Qualifiers in the respiratory system describe tissues used for replacement or for the formation of a bypass and the source of a transplanted lung. Table 10.3 lists the qualifiers used in coding procedures performed on the mouth, throat, and respiratory system.

Table 10.3. Qualifiers for the mouth, throat, and respiratory system

Qualifier Value	Qualifiers—Mouth and Throat (C)	Qualifier Value	Qualifiers—Respiratory System (B)
0	Single	0	Allogeneic
1	Multiple	1	Syngeneic
2	All	2	Zooplastic
X	Diagnostic	4	Cutaneous
Z	No Qualifier	6	Esophagus
		X	Diagnostic
		Z	No Qualifier

 Code Building

Case #1:

PROCEDURE STATEMENT: Tracheal dilation for laryngotracheal stenosis

ADDITIONAL INFORMATION: The procedure is performed with a rigid bronchoscope.

ROOT AND INDEX ENTRIES FOR THE STATEMENT: Dilation is the root operation performed in this procedure, defined as expanding an orifice or the lumen of a tubular body part. The Index entry is:

Dilation

    Trachea   0B71

Code Characters:

Section	Body System	Root Operation	Body Part	Approach	Device	Qualifier
Medical and Surgical	Respiratory System	Dilation	Trachea	Via Natural or Artificial Opening Endoscopic	No Device	No Qualifier
0	B	7	1	8	Z	Z

RATIONALE FOR THE ANSWER: The root operation Dilation is coded to describe the stretching of the trachea. This procedure is performed through a bronchoscope, or approach value 8, Via Natural or Artificial Opening, Endoscopic, because the scope is an endoscopic instrument. There is no device or qualifier for this code. The correct code assignment is 0B718ZZ.

Case #2:

PROCEDURE STATEMENT: Placement of an implant in the tooth socket of a front, upper tooth

ADDITIONAL INFORMATION: The tooth was broken off by trauma to the face. The fractured tooth root was removed, and a synthetic tooth was implanted into the tooth socket.

ROOT AND INDEX ENTRIES FOR THE STATEMENT: Replacement is the root operation performed in this procedure, defined as putting in or on biological or synthetic material that physically takes the place and/or function of all or a portion of a body part. The Index entry is:

Replacement

    Tooth

        Lower 0CRX

        Upper 0CRW

Code Characters:

Section	Body System	Root Operation	Body Part	Approach	Device	Qualifier
Medical and Surgical	Mouth and Throat	Replacement	Upper Tooth	External	Synthetic Substitute	Single
0	C	R	W	X	J	0

RATIONALE FOR THE ANSWER: The synthetic tooth is a synthetic material that takes the place of all of a body part. The root operation Replacement is used. The removal of the fractured tooth root is included in the replacement procedure and not coded separately. The approach is X, External because the tooth can be visualized without the use of an incision or instruments. The device value is J for Synthetic Substitute and the qualifier value is 0 for Single Tooth. The correct code assignment is 0CRWXJ0.

Case #3:

PROCEDURE STATEMENT: Bilateral lung transplant

ADDITIONAL INFORMATION: The transplant source is a donor organ.

ROOT AND INDEX ENTRIES FOR THE STATEMENT: Transplantation is the root operation performed in this procedure, defined as putting in or on all or a portion of a living body part taken from another individual or animal to physically take the place and/or function of all or a portion of a similar body part. The Index entry is:

Transplantation

    Lung

        Bilateral   0BYM0Z

Code Characters:

Section	Body System	Root Operation	Body Part	Approach	Device	Qualifier
Medical and Surgical	Respiratory System	Transplantation	Lungs, Bilateral	Open	No Device	Allogeneic
0	B	Y	M	0	Z	0

RATIONALE FOR THE ANSWER: The root operation Transplantation is coded for this bilateral lung transplant. The body part value is M for Lungs, bilateral. The approach is open. There is no device value and the qualifier value is 0 for Allogeneic because the organs were donated. The correct code assignment is 0BYM0Z0.

Code Building Exercises

Work through each case and check your answers using the answer key in appendix B of the textbook before going on to the Check Your Understanding questions that follow.

Exercise 1:

PREOPERATIVE DIAGNOSIS: Diaphragmatic hernia

POSTOPERATIVE DIAGNOSIS: Same

OPERATION PERFORMED: Repair of diaphragm, crural reconstruction with Composix E/X mesh patch

DESCRIPTION OF OPERATION: The patient is brought to the operating room and placed under general endotracheal anesthesia. The patient was kept supine and the abdomen prepped and draped in standard fashion. We made a periumbilical incision, passed the Veress needle, insufflated with carbon dioxide, passed the trocar and 10-mm 30-degree scope. I made another incision, passed a trocar and retractor to elevate the left lobe of the liver and made two counter incisions in the left upper quadrant and one in the right upper quadrant to gain access to the right crus of the diaphragm and the left crus of the diaphragm. These were visualized as well as the stomach going up into the mediastinum.

We grasped the stomach and folded it back into the abdomen and cut the hernia sac in the mediastinum. We were thus able to bring the stomach and gastroesophageal junction back into an intra-abdominal location without tension. We took great care to avoid injury to the vagus nerve. We then performed a crural plication and tacked the left and right crus of the diaphragm over a bougie to avoid making this too tight. We then placed a Composix mesh patch, which we had carefully sized to the repaired diaphragmatic crus and tacked this to the left diaphragm, the posterior decussation, right crus of the diaphragm. We ensured that hemostasis was adequate and removed the trocars. We used deep fascial sutures and the subcuticular stitch for the skin. We are very pleased with the construct and the patient is brought to the recovery room in stable condition.

Questions:

1.1. What does the term "plication" mean?

_____

1.2. Use the Device Key or an Internet search to determine the device value for the mesh used in this procedure. What value would you assign?

_____

1.3. What code(s) would be assigned?

_____

Exercise 2:

PREOPERATIVE DIAGNOSIS: Right recurrent pleural effusion

POSTOPERATIVE DIAGNOSIS: Right recurrent pleural effusion

PROCEDURE: Mechanical pleurodesis

PROCEDURE IN DETAIL: The patient was brought into the operating room and placed on the operating table in the supine position. The patient was intubated and anesthesia was administered through a double-lumen tube.

The patient was positioned to a lateral decubitus position with the right chest up. The right chest was prepped and draped in a sterile fashion. The lateral chest wall incision was performed. Using Bovie cautery, the operative field was dissected down to the pleural lining. The patient was noted to have large, bloody-appearing pleural effusion of the right chest. Approximately four liters of pleural fluid was drained from the right chest. The patient's hemodynamics improved as pleural effusion was evacuated.

A camera and trocar were inserted into the right chest. A single, anterior incision was made and performed under direct visualization. A Bovie scratch pad was used to perform mechanical pleurodesis. A single 28 straight chest tube was placed into the apex of the right chest and a 28 angled chest tube was placed into the posterior costophrenic angle. The chest tubes were secured into position using 0 silk suture. The camera and trocar were withdrawn. The incisions were then anesthetized with 1% lidocaine and 0.25% Marcaine. The incisions were closed using two deep layers of 0 Vicryl suture. The skin was closed using a subcuticular stitch of 4-0 Monocryl.

Questions:

2.1. How many procedures are identified in this report? What are they?

_____

2.2. What is the intent of the pleurodesis procedure?

_____

2.3. What code(s) would be assigned?

_____

✔ Check Your Understanding

Coding Knowledge Check

1. The physician documents that a wedge resection of the right upper lobe of the lung was performed. Which root operation would be used to code this procedure?
    a. Destruction
    b. Excision
    c. Resection
    d. Occlusion

2. The surgeon performs a reversal of a previous lip augmentation procedure by making an incision along the length of both lips, inside the mouth. A strip of tissue is removed from each lip to thin the lips and pull them inward, because the patient was not happy with the previous augmentation. The incisions are sutured closed. How is this coded?
    a. 0CQ1XZZ, 0CQ0XZZ
    b. 0CQ10ZZ, 0CQ00ZZ
    c. 0C01XZZ, 0C00XZZ
    d. 0CB10ZZ, 0CB00ZZ

3. The carina is located at the _____ of the _____ and separates the openings to the right and left.

4. The patient had a well-circumscribed radiopaque, spherical mass in the area of the right parotid gland that was diagnosed as sialolithiasis. This mass was removed through an open incision. How is this coded?

(Continued)

    a. 0CBB0ZX

    b. 0CB80ZZ

    c. 0CC80ZZ

    d. 0CCB0ZZ

5. Tonsils completely removed by the use of a wire snare are coded to which root operation?

    a. Alteration

    b. Excision

    c. Fragmentation

    d. Resection

Procedure Statement Coding

Assign ICD-10-PCS codes to the following procedure statements and scenarios. List the root operation selected and the code assigned.

1. Endoscopic placement of an intrabronchial valve into the left lower bronchus for persistent air leak

2. Excision of left vocal cord polyp via endoscope

3. Tracheobronchoscopy

4. Open diaphragmatic hernia repair with Prolene mesh patch

5. The patient was admitted to have a thoracoscopic lobectomy performed. The patient has a malignant neoplasm of the right middle lobe of the lung. Because of extensive pleural effusion, the physician was unable to complete the endoscopic procedure that was started. They converted to an open technique, and a successful lobectomy was performed. The patient tolerated the procedure well.

6. Removal of adenoids with electrocautery

7. Frenulotomy performed on a 4-year-old boy with ankyloglossia and speech difficulties

8. Endoscopic stenting of trachea and right main bronchus for palliative treatment of bronchial carcinoma

9. Bronchial thermoplasty of left lower lobe bronchus for severe, persistent asthma

10. Repair, cleft of hard palate, open approach

Case Studies

Assign ICD-10-PCS codes to the following case studies.

1. Operative Report

PREOPERATIVE DIAGNOSIS:	Dental caries and autism
POSTOPERATIVE DIAGNOSIS:	Dental caries and autism
PROCEDURE:	Dental restorations and primary tooth extractions
INDICATION:	Multiple dental caries lesions in a patient who is unable to cooperate for restorations in clinic.

FINDINGS:

- Generalized gingival inflammation
- Permanent dentition in normal sequence. Positive overbite. No crossbites.
- Caries lesions to restore of #2, 4, 12, 15, 30, and 31.
- Wisdom tooth crowding for extraction #1, 16, 17, and 32.

PROCEDURE: The patient was brought to the operating room and intubated. A moist throat pack was placed. Under rubber dam isolation, restorations were: #2—stainless steel crown (SSC), #4 SSC, #12 composite, #15 SSC, #30 composite, #31—ferric sulfate pulpotomy + ZOE base + SSC.

1.7 mL of 2 percent lidocaine with 1:1,000,000 epinephrine was infiltrated adjacent to the teeth indicated for extraction. #1, 16, 17 and 32 were extracted. Sockets were packed with Instat to facilitate hemostasis, which was achieved. The throat pack was removed. The patient was extubated and transferred to recovery in stable condition.

2. Operative Report

PREOPERATIVE DIAGNOSES:	Cervicofacial lymphatic malformation, tracheostomy dependence
POSTOPERATIVE DIAGNOSES:	Same
PROCEDURE:	1. Bronchoscopy
	2. Cauterization of trach site granulation tissue

FINDINGS: 1) On bronchoscopy, the glottis is normal. The subglottis has a small left sessile cyst of lymphatic malformation on the L lateral wall, non-obstructive. The trachea was without collapse or granulation at stoma site. Thick secretions in bronchi on left, greater than right. Tracheotomy: circumferential skin granulation, which was cauterized with silver nitrate. New 4.5 Tracoe trach tube was placed.

INDICATIONS: That patient is now a 5-year-old male with a history of large facial, supraglottic, and oropharyngeal cystic hygroma, causing airway obstruction. Patient had trach placed in last year and no follow up endoscopy since that time. Trach tube is 4.5 Tracoe that is changed every 2 months and suction 10×/day by parents. The family complains of bleeding with trach tube changes. No exertional dyspnea. No choking.

DESCRIPTION: After verification of informed consent, the patient was brought to the operating room and placed in the supine position. General anesthesia was induced. With laryngotracheal anesthesia, bronchoscopy was performed by advancing the telescope through the true vocal folds and evaluating the glottis, subglottis, and trachea, with findings as described. The tracheotomy site was inspected and flexible fiberoptic scope passed through trach. Trach was removed momentarily and stoma skin granulation was cauterized with silver nitrate and area neutralized with saline. Trachea irrigated with saline and suctioned. Old trach removed and replaced with new 4.5 Tracoe. Then flexible bronchoscopy performed through trach to ensure removal of irrigation and debris. The patient was then turned back to the care of Anesthesia to recover. The patient tolerated the procedure well and was transferred to the recovery room in stable condition.

ESTIMATED BLOOD LOSS: Minimal

COMPLICATIONS: None

---

3. Operative Report

PROCEDURE PERFORMED:	Bronchoscopy with transbronchial biopsies of the left lower lobe
INDICATION:	Interstitial lung disease
FINDINGS:	Normal airway anatomy

ANESTHESIA: Lidocaine 500 mg applied topically to the oropharyngeal and endobronchial mucosa. Fentanyl 100 mcg IV given in small aliquots throughout the procedure. Versed 3 mg IV total.

PROCEDURE IN DETAIL: Informed consent was obtained from the patient. The patient was brought to the endoscopy room. Anesthesia was applied. The bronchoscope was passed through the left nasal cavity into the trachea. Using fluoroscopy, transbronchial biopsies were obtained in the left lower lobe and in the inferior segment of the lingula. The trachea, carina, left and right-sided airways were all within normal limits and they were inspected to the level of the segmental bronchi. Some white to yellow secretions were noted in both dependent lower lobes. The patient tolerated the procedure well. His oxygen saturation remained above 93 percent throughout the procedure. He was hemodynamically stable throughout. He was maintained on O_2 by nasal cannula. There were no complications. Transbronchial biopsies were sent for pathology.

---

4. Operative Report

PREOPERATIVE DIAGNOSIS:	Respiratory failure
POSTOPERATIVE DIAGNOSIS:	Respiratory failure
OPERATION:	Tracheostomy

INDICATION: This is a female with respiratory failure, and multiple attempts to wean from the vent failed. The family was explained the risks and benefits of tracheostomy and consent was obtained.

PROCEDURE: The patient was brought to the operating room and placed under general anesthetic. The neck was prepped and draped. 1 percent lidocaine with epinephrine was injected into the neck. The patient was extremely obese. A 3-cm incision was made approximately two fingerbreadths above the sternal notch. A large amount of subcutaneous fat was dissected and removed with Bovie cautery. The strap muscles were identified and divided in the midline, exposing a large thyroid isthmus. Bipolar cautery was taken down to the cricoid. The thyroid isthmus was divided with bipolar cautery exposing the trachea. An incision was made between the second and third tracheal ring and an inferior based tracheal flap was created with heavy Mayos. The inferior tracheal flap was sewn to the inferior skin edge, creating a skin flap in order to mature the stoma with 3-0 Vicryl. Next, the ET tube was slowly withdrawn to just above the tracheostomy site. An 8.0 XLT Shiley trach was inserted with no difficulties. The balloon was inflated and hooked up to the anesthesia circuit, and CO_2 was confirmed. The trach was secured to the skin with 2-0 silk. Straight ties were applied. Drain sponge was applied. The patient remained stable throughout the entire case.

5. Operative Report

PREOPERATIVE DIAGNOSIS: Recurrent streptococcal tonsillar pharyngitis and left chronic otitis with effusion

POSTOPERATIVE DIAGNOSIS: Recurrent streptococcal tonsillar pharyngitis

PROCEDURES:
1. Examination of ears under anesthesia
2. Coblation tonsillectomy
3. Electrosurgical adenoidectomy

DESCRIPTION OF PROCEDURE: Following induction of general orotracheal anesthesia, the ears were inspected using binocular operating microscopes. The left ear was inspected. This ear had fluid when the child was seen in the office. There was no evidence of effusion. The right ear was also inspected and no evidence of effusion was found.

Using the Rose position, the McIvor mouth gag was placed. The palate was noted to be normal. The uvula was single. There was an easily palpable posterior nasal spine. The tonsils were 2+ in size and endophytic. The adenoids were 3+, obstructing about two-thirds of the posterior nasal choana.

The tonsils were removed in sequence using the coblation wand set at 5 on coblation and 3 on coagulation. The adenoids were then inspected using a mirror, and using surgical suction cautery set at 35, the adenoid tissue was carefully trimmed primarily from the posterior choana. There was actually adenoid tissue prolapsing into the left nasal fossa. This was carefully removed using suction cautery. The total blood loss was estimated at 30 mL. Blood and mucus were suctioned from the oral cavity. There were no postoperative complications, and the patient tolerated the procedure well, leaving the operative room in satisfactory condition.

6. Operative Report

PREOPERATIVE DIAGNOSIS: Chronic serous otitis, adenoid hypertrophy

POSTOPERATIVE DIAGNOSIS: Chronic serous otitis, adenoid hypertrophy

OPERATION: Adenoidectomy, myringotomy tube placement

DESCRIPTION OF PROCEDURE: The patient was induced under general anesthesia in the supine position via an orotracheal tube. The right tympanic membrane was visualized and sized, drained of fluid, then tubed with a ventilation tube. In a similar manner, the left tympanic membrane was visualized and sized, drained, and tubed.

A McIvor mouth gag was used to expose the pharynx. The adenoids were removed with an adenoid knife and hemostasis was obtained with suction and cautery. The patient was awakened and brought to the recovery room in good condition.

The second character values for the circulatory system are:

    2—Heart and Great Vessels
    3—Upper Arteries
    4—Lower Arteries
    5—Upper Veins
    6—Lower Veins

Functions of the Circulatory System

The heart and the great vessels circulate the blood to the lungs for oxygenation and then throughout the body. The blood also eliminates waste products from the cells. If this circulation is stopped or significantly slowed, even for a few minutes, the person's life can be compromised.

Organization of the Circulatory System

The heart, great vessels, arteries, veins, and capillaries make up the circulatory system. Arteries carry blood away from the heart. Capillaries connect arteries to veins, and the veins return blood to the heart. The circulatory system has two closed circuits, one for pulmonary circulation to and from the lungs and the other for systemic circulation, to and from the remainder of the body.

Heart and Great Vessels

The heart is a muscular organ in the middle of the mediastinum that contains four chambers. The two upper chambers are called the atriums and the two lower chambers are called the ventricles. The right atrium and ventricle receive blood from the superior and inferior vena cavae and pump this deoxygenated blood to both lungs through the pulmonary arteries. Oxygenated blood returns to the heart through the pulmonary veins and enters the left atrium and ventricle, which pump the blood throughout the body through the aorta (Applegate 2011, 264).

    The heart contains two types of valves, the atrioventricular valves and the semilunar valves, and there are two of each type. The atrioventricular valves are located where the name implies, between the atria and the ventricles. The valve between the right atrium and right ventricle has three flaps, or cusps, and is called the tricuspid valve. The valve between the left atrium and left ventricle has only two cusps and is called the bicuspid valve, or mitral valve. The semilunar valves are located at the bottom of the great vessels that carry blood from the ventricles. The valve located at the right ventricular exit to the pulmonary artery is the pulmonary semilunar valve, and the valve located at the left ventricular exit to the aorta is the aortic semilunar valve (Applegate 2011, 249–250). Figure 11.1 displays the chambers of the heart and the heart valves.

Figure 11.1. Heart

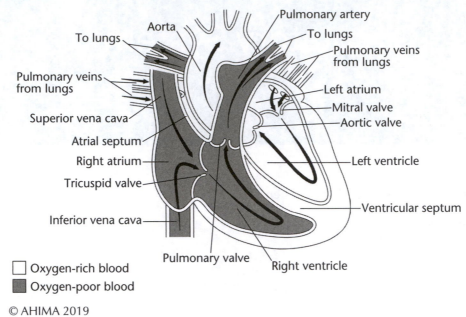

© AHIMA 2019

The great vessels of the circulatory system are the veins and arteries leaving, entering, and leaving the heart again, named the great vessels because of their relatively large diameter (Rizzo 2016, 329). They include the following:

- Aorta
  - Aortic root
  - Ascending aorta
  - Aortic arch
  - Thoracic aorta
- Vena cavae
  - Superior vena cava
  - Inferior vena cava
- Pulmonary arteries
  - Pulmonary trunk
  - Right pulmonary artery
  - Left pulmonary artery
- Pulmonary veins
  - Right superior
  - Right inferior
  - Left superior
  - Left inferior

Anatomy Alert

Body part value W, Thoracic aorta, descending in the Heart and Great Vessels body system, identifies the aorta after the arch. Body part value X, Thoracic aorta, ascending/arch includes the aortic root, the ascending aorta, and the aortic arch. Body part value 0, Abdominal aorta, is found in the Lower Arteries body system.

The coronary arteries are not part of the great vessels of the heart. They supply the heart muscle with blood, rather than supplying the rest of the body. The coronary arteries are listed below. In addition to those listed, some patients have anomalous coronary arteries called the ramus and intermediate arteries. The veins of the heart are the great, middle, and small cardiac veins.

The typical coronary arteries are the following:

- Right coronary artery
  - Right marginal
  - Right posterior descending
- Left coronary artery
  - Left anterior descending, which branches into:
    - The diagonal and septal arteries
  - Circumflex, which branches into:
    - The obtuse marginal, posterior descending and posterolateral arteries (AMA 2018, 659; McKinley 2017, 660–661)

Figure 11.2 shows the arteries of the heart.

Figure 11.2.   **Coronary arteries**

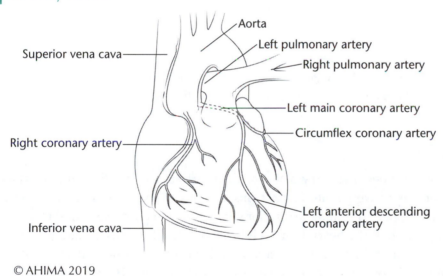

© AHIMA 2019

Coding Tip

ICD-10-PCS does not assign body part values to the names of the individual coronary arteries. The body part value for coronary arteries identifies the number of coronary arteries treated. There is one single body part value for any of the cardiac veins.

The following structures are not displayed in figures 11.1 and 11.2 and can be found as indicated:

- **Atrial septum**—Located between the two atria of the heart.
- **Chordae tendineae**—The free edge of each heart valve flap, or cusp, is anchored to the papillary muscles by the chordae tendineae.

- **Conduction mechanism**—Coordinates the contraction of the heart muscles and is made up of four structures: the sinoatrial node, the atrioventricular node, the atrioventricular bundle, and the Purkinje fibers.
- **Papillary muscle**—Two or three projections of myocardial muscle that originate in the ventricle walls and are connected to the heart valves by the chordae tendineae.
- **Pericardium**—A double-layered, loose-fitting sac around the heart. The outer layer is connective tissue. The inner layer contains the parietal pericardium on the outside and the visceral pericardium, or epicardium, closest to the heart. The pericardial space is between the inner and outer layers.
- **Ventricular septum**—Located between the two ventricles of the heart (McKinley 2017, 651–660)

Upper and Lower Arteries

The arteries are large tubes made up of elastic fibers that carry blood away from the heart to other structures. Arteries branch into smaller and smaller arteries, arterioles, and capillaries, where they exchange blood with the cells. The arteries of the body are known by many names, such as the abdominal aorta, with an alternate name of the descending aorta, and the innominate artery, with an alternate name of the brachiocephalic artery. In addition, arteries are frequently named for the areas or organs they supply with blood, such as the internal mammary artery, the temporal artery, or the thyroid artery. Figure 11.3 shows the major arteries of the body with common names.

Coding Tip

The upper arteries body system and the upper veins body system contain body parts that are found above the central dividing line of the diaphragm. The lower arteries body system and the lower veins body system contain body parts that are found below the central dividing line of the diaphragm.

Upper and Lower Veins

The veins of the body are large tubes that carry blood to the heart after it is collected from the capillaries in venules, or small veins. Venules converge into larger veins and finally converge into the superior vena cava, which returns blood from the upper body and the inferior vena cava, which returns blood from the lower body. Because veins are returning blood to the heart, there is less pressure in the veins. In addition, veins in the legs need to return blood to the heart against gravity. Therefore, veins contain venous valves, similar to very small heart valves that keep the blood flowing toward the heart rather than away. The veins of the body are known by a variety of different names and are frequently named for the area or organ that they drain of blood, such as the splenic vein, the gastric vein, or the esophageal vein. Figure 11.4 shows the major veins of the body with common names.

Figure 11.3. Major arteries of the body

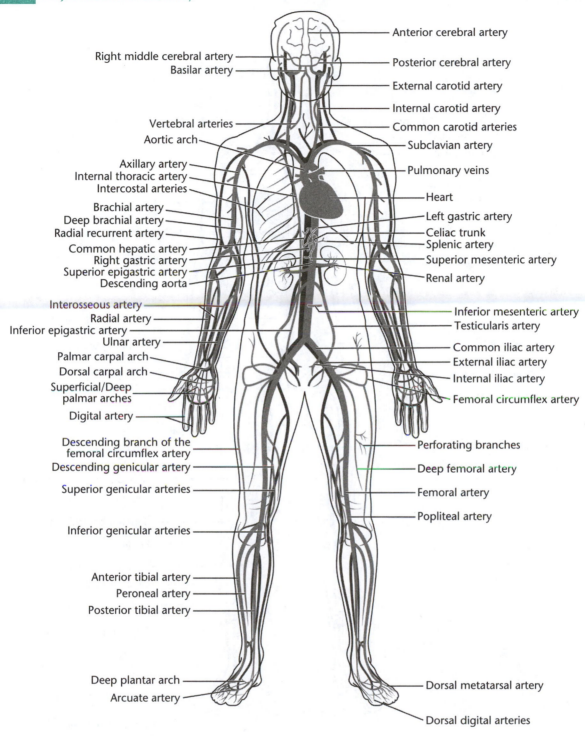

Anterior cerebral artery

Right middle cerebral artery
Basilar artery

Posterior cerebral artery

External carotid artery

Internal carotid artery

Vertebral arteries
Aortic arch

Common carotid arteries

Subclavian artery

Axillary artery
Internal thoracic artery
Intercostal arteries

Pulmonary veins

Heart

Brachial artery
Deep brachial artery
Radial recurrent artery

Left gastric artery
Celiac trunk
Splenic artery

Common hepatic artery
Right gastric artery
Superior epigastric artery
Descending aorta

Superior mesenteric artery
Renal artery

Interosseous artery
Radial artery
Inferior epigastric artery
Ulnar artery
Palmar carpal arch
Dorsal carpal arch
Superficial/Deep
palmar arches
Digital artery

Inferior mesenteric artery
Testicularis artery

Common iliac artery
External iliac artery
Internal iliac artery

Femoral circumflex artery

Descending branch of the
femoral circumflex artery
Descending genicular artery

Perforating branches

Deep femoral artery

Superior genicular arteries

Femoral artery

Popliteal artery

Inferior genicular arteries

Anterior tibial artery
Peroneal artery
Posterior tibial artery

Deep plantar arch
Arcuate artery

Dorsal metatarsal artery

Dorsal digital arteries

Figure 11.4.   Major veins of the body

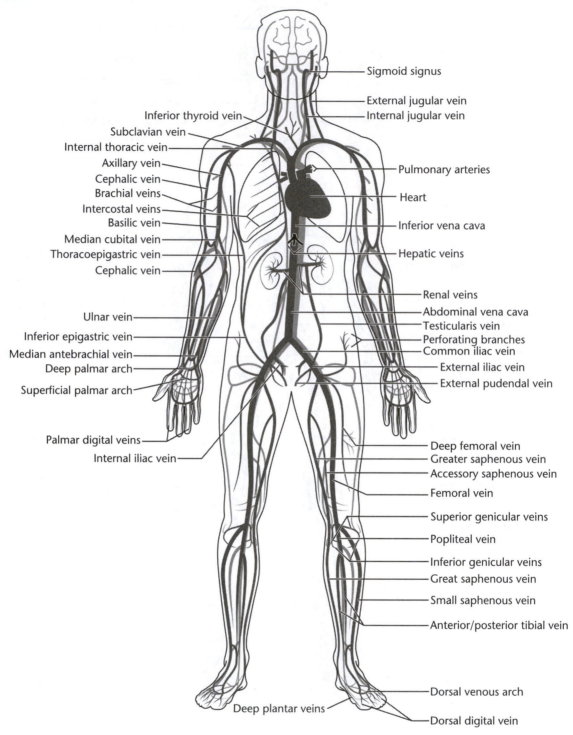

Sigmoid signus

External jugular vein
Internal jugular vein

Inferior thyroid vein

Subclavian vein
Internal thoracic vein
Axillary vein
Cephalic vein
Brachial veins
Intercostal veins
Basilic vein
Median cubital vein
Thoracoepigastric vein
Cephalic vein

Pulmonary arteries

Heart

Inferior vena cava

Hepatic veins

Renal veins
Abdominal vena cava
Testicularis vein
Perforating branches
Common iliac vein

Ulnar vein
Inferior epigastric vein
Median antebrachial vein
Deep palmar arch
Superficial palmar arch

External iliac vein
External pudendal vein

Palmar digital veins
Internal iliac vein

Deep femoral vein
Greater saphenous vein
Accessory saphenous vein

Femoral vein

Superior genicular veins

Popliteal vein

Inferior genicular veins
Great saphenous vein

Small saphenous vein

Anterior/posterior tibial vein

Dorsal venous arch

Deep plantar veins

Dorsal digital vein

© AHIMA 2019

Common Root Operations Used in Coding of Procedures on the Circulatory System

The root operations commonly assigned for circulatory system procedures involve the four root operations performed on tubular body parts, as well as those that must involve a device. Root operations for removing, draining, and repairing body parts are also assigned based on the documentation. In addition, the root operation of Map is assigned in the Heart and Great Vessels body system. The most common root operations and related procedures are discussed here in detail.

Insertion of Devices

The following is a discussion of various devices that can be inserted into the circulatory system. These are non-biological devices that monitor, assist, perform, or prevent a physiological function but do not take the place of the body part, such as pacemakers and vascular access devices.

Cardiac Rhythm–Related Devices

The most common cardiac devices inserted are those that regulate the rhythm of the heart or defibrillate the heart if it stops. The devices available in ICD-10-PCS are:

- **Pacemaker, Single Chamber**—Regulates the rhythm by the use of one lead
- **Pacemaker, Single Chamber Rate Responsive**—Regulates the rhythm by the use of one lead in response to variable activity levels such as sleeping versus walking or running
- **Pacemaker, Dual Chamber**—Regulates the rhythm by the use of two leads
- **Cardiac Resynchronization Pacemaker**—Regulates the rhythm by the use of three leads. Leads are placed in the right atrium and right ventricle, just as in a dual chamber pacemaker, but a third lead is placed in or on the left ventricle to keep the left and right side of the heart synchronized as it beats. This may be documented as a biventricular pacemaker because leads are in two ventricles.
- **Intracardiac Pacemaker**—Regulates the rhythm without the use of leads. The pacemaker is small, cylindrical, and placed via a catheter to the inside of the right ventricle. It contains the battery and electrodes within the one unit.
- **Defibrillator Generator**—Internal heart monitor that delivers an electrical shock to the heart when an abnormal rhythm is detected. This returns the rhythm to normal by the use of two leads.
- **Cardiac Resynchronization Defibrillator Generator**—Combination of the defibrillator function and the cardiac resynchronization function is one unit, by the use of three leads

Each of these units, except the intracardiac pacemaker, is approximately the size of a 50-cent piece. It is implanted in a pocket in the subcutaneous layer of the chest using an Open approach. This is coded in the 0JH table of ICD-10-PCS. If the device contains a defibrillator, code a device value that identifies a defibrillator in the title.

The leads are placed percutaneously through the veins of the chest and into the appropriate chamber(s) of the heart, called transvenous leads. The leads are coded to where the tip rests within the heart with the root operation of Insertion in the 02H table of ICD-10-PCS. The device value for the lead is matched to the type of unit the patient is having inserted, pacemaker or defibrillator.

Leads may also be placed as epicardial (directly on the heart) leads at the time of open heart surgery in preparation for later placement of the pacemaker or defibrillator unit. The approach value for epicardial leads is 0, Open. This is frequently done in infants or other patients whose veins cannot accommodate the number of leads required.

A typical transvenous dual chamber pacemaker insertion is coded as:

0JH606Z Insertion of Pacemaker, Dual Chamber into Chest Subcutaneous Tissue and Fascia, Open Approach

02H63JZ Insertion of Pacemaker Lead into Right Atrium, Percutaneous Approach

02HK3JZ Insertion of Pacemaker Lead into Right Ventricle, Percutaneous Approach

Coding Tip

Traditional pacemaker insertions require a minimum of two codes—one for the generator and one for the lead. Be sure to match the number of leads to the generator device type. A single chamber device requires one lead, a dual chamber device requires two leads, and a resynchronization device requires three leads.

Heart Assist Devices

Another type of device that is inserted is the heart assist device, which can be implantable or external. Heart assist devices have a conduit that moves blood from the left ventricle to the systemic circulation through the aorta. The device uses a pump to perform this function. Some units are biventricular with an additional conduit from the right ventricle to the pulmonary trunk. These devices either allow the heart to rest while it heals or allow patients to function while they are waiting for a heart transplant.

External heart assist devices have a controller unit that is at the patient's bedside with tubes entering and exiting the body through small holes in the abdomen. These patients are not ambulatory. Implantable heart assist devices are similar, with an internal pump in the conduit between the left ventricle and the aorta. Patients wear a controller and battery pack outside of the body, allowing them to be ambulatory while the device is in place.

External heart assist devices are coded as:

> Left ventricular: 02HA0RZ Insertion of Short-term External Heart Assist System into Heart, Open Approach
> Biventricular: 02HA0RS Insertion of Biventricular Short-term External Heart Assist System into Heart, Open Approach

Implantable heart assist devices are coded as:

> 02HA0QZ Insertion of Implantable Heart Assist System into Heart, Open Approach

Inferior Vena Cava Filter

An IVC filter is a vascular filter that is placed using a percutaneous approach into the inferior vena cava. It is meant to stop the movement of emboli from the lower extremities through the venous system and into the heart and lungs.

The filter is coded as an intraluminal device in ICD-10-PCS with code 06H03DZ. To remove the filter, the catheter deactivates the device, closing the filter, like closing an umbrella. It is then removed. The code for removal is 06PY3DZ.

Vascular Access Devices

The role of a vascular access device is to provide access for infusion of substances, drawing of blood, or both. A basic vascular access device is coded to the device value of 3, Infusion Device in ICD-10-PCS. Catheters, like leads, are coded to the location where the tip resides. All catheter insertions involve the placement of the infusion device. In addition, catheters meant for longer-term use have additional vascular access devices used in combination with the infusion device. This is a list of the various types of catheters, their uses and various parts, and coding information for ICD-10-PCS:

- **Peripheral IVs**—Not typically coded in the inpatient setting but would be coded to the hand, arm, foot, or leg vein into which they are placed.

- **Peripherally Inserted Central Catheter (PICC)**—Used for short-term access, placed percutaneously through a vein in the arm or leg, with the preferred end location of the Superior Vena Cava or Inferior Vena Cava. Coded as an infusion device, inserted to where the tip resides.

  Example: PICC to Superior Vena Cava (SVC) is 02HV33Z Insertion of Infusion Device into Superior Vena Cava, Percutaneous Approach

- **Central Venous Catheter (CVC)**—Used for short term access, placed percutaneously through a large vein in the chest, vein or groin, with the preferred end location of the Superior Vena Cava or Inferior Vena Cava. Coded as an infusion device, inserted to where the tip resides.

  Example: CVC to Superior Vena Cava (SVC) is 02HV33Z Insertion of Infusion Device into Superior Vena Cava, Percutaneous Approach

  Note: The PICC and CVC to the superior vena cava are both coded the same way. It does not matter where the catheter enters—it is coded to where the tip resides.

- **Tunneled Catheters (Broviac, Hickman, and Quinton)**—Used for longer-term access, containing two parts. The infusion device is placed just as the CVC is placed. An extender portion is tunneled through the subcutaneous tissue from the entry point in the chest or neck to a more distal location on the chest. Figure 1.15 in chapter 1 displays a tunneled vascular access device. The infusion device is coded as a CVC and the extender is coded as a vascular access device, tunneled in the subcutaneous tissue and fascia of the chest with a percutaneous approach.

  Example: Hickman catheter to the SVC is 02HV33Z and 0JH63XZ Insertion of Vascular Access Device, Tunneled into Chest Subcutaneous Tissue and Fascia, Percutaneous Approach

- **Totally Implantable Ports (Port-a-cath)**—Used for long-term access, containing two parts. The infusion device is placed just as the CVC is placed. A pocket is created for the port in the subcutaneous tissue and fascia of the chest using an open approach and the catheter is connected to the port and the skin is closed. The port is a vascular access device, totally implantable, placed with an open approach.

  Example: Port-a-Cath to the SVC is 02HV33Z and 0JH60WZ Insertion of Vascular Access Device, Totally Implantable into Chest Subcutaneous Tissue and Fascia, Open Approach

Removal

Any device placed on or within the body can be removed. For devices that are placed below the skin level, the root operation used is Removal. If a new device is required, both the removal and the placement of the new device are coded. A complete redo of a procedure is coded to the root operation performed. This happens when a device such as a pacemaker comes to the end of its battery life. The pacemaker is removed and a new pacemaker is inserted. Both procedures are coded.

Revision

If the device has become dislodged and has to be moved back into the correct position, the root operation of Revision is assigned. This happens if a cardiac lead becomes disconnected from the wall of the heart. Many times, the lead can be reattached to the wall and the device then functions normally. This is the root operation of Revision.

Heart Valve Procedures

When heart valves do not function correctly, the overall cardiac function suffers. Dilation of the heart valve can sometimes be all that is required. Dilation techniques include balloon dilation, debridement of calcification of the leaflets or commissurotomy at the base of the leaflets. All of these can be performed to allow the valve to open and close correctly.

More invasive steps may be required when the valve leaflets have become "sloppy" or have torn. Using open-heart surgery, the valve leaflet tear can be reinforced with sutures and the valve annulus, or base, can be supplemented with a mesh ring to reinforce the opening and closing function.

If the valve is badly damaged or has congenital malformation beyond repair, the valve can be replaced with a number of device options. Table 02R shows that valves can be replaced using an open, percutaneous or percutaneous endoscopic approach. Mechanical valves are coded as the device value of J, Synthetic Substitute. Valves that contain tissue leaflets are coded based on the type of tissue that makes up the leaflets. Animal tissue is common for valves, which is coded as 8, Zooplastic Tissue. It is important to note that all valves have a synthetic ring at their base. This ring is used to attach the valve in place.

Percutaneous placement of valves involves breaking the native valve open by balloon dilation and then passing a catheter-delivered valve into its place. The valve commonly has bovine pericardial leaflets attached to a synthetic ring, similar to a stent. The stent holds the new valve in place by attaching to the annulus of the native valve that was broken open. This is called transcatheter valve replacement. In either the open or percutaneous replacement, the work of removing or breaking open the native valve is not coded separately.

Coding Tip

Heart valve devices are coded based on the type of leaflets they contain. Metal leaflets are synthetic and leaflets made from animal tissue are zooplastic.

Creation

The root operation Creation is used in the circulatory system to describe the process of forming a new body part to replicate the anatomic structure or function of an absent body part. This procedure is performed when the heart has congenital anomalies such as truncus arteriosus or atrioventricular (AV) canal. In both cases, the 024 table identifies the body part as the valve being created and the qualifier as the original, deformed valve.

In truncus arteriosus, the aorta and the pulmonary trunk fail to separate during development. The combined vessel is called a truncus. This anomaly is treated by creating an aorta from the truncus and replacing the pulmonary trunk with allograft tissue or zooplastic tissue, frequently including a new pulmonary valve. The single truncal valve that was present is created into an aortic valve. If remodeling is necessary, CMS advises that the root operation of Creation be assigned. If the truncal valve is used as the aortic valve with no changes, no procedure is coded.

In the atrioventricular canal deformity, the central portion of the heart does not develop correctly. The infant is missing parts of both of the septums that separate all four chambers of the heart, often having a common atrioventricular valve rather than individual mitral and tricuspid valves. The common treatment for this deformity is to repair or supplement the ventricular septum, which separates the common valve into a mitral or tricuspid valve. If the common valve is repaired or supplemented, the appropriate root operation is assigned and the qualifier is selected to match the valve involved in the procedure. If one or both of the valves is remodeled in some other way, CMS advises that the root operation of Creation be assigned.

Aneurysms

Two common types of aneurysms develop in the walls of the arteries. A small outpocketing in an artery wall forms an aneurysm known as a sacular, berry, dome, or button aneurysm. These names describe the outpocketing that is connected to the main artery by a neck or stalk. The other type of aneurysm involves larger areas of the artery wall and is commonly called a fusiform aneurysm.

Restriction is used to treat the sacular aneurysm. Using an open approach, the neck of the aneurysm is clipped using an extraluminal device. The extraluminal device reduces the width of the artery at the aneurysm site back to its normal size. This type of extraluminal device is pictured in figure 1.12 in chapter 1. Restriction is also coded when a bioactive coil is threaded into a cerebral aneurysm. This procedure is done percutaneously with the help of guidance. This is frequently performed when the aneurysm is located in an artery inside the head. ICD-10-PCS contains only one body part value for all of the arteries in the head, which is G, Intracranial artery. The 03V table for Upper Artery Restriction contains a special device value for these coils. They are coded as device value B, Intraluminal Device, Bioactive.

Abdominal aortic aneurysms can also be treated with restrictive stents using a percutaneous approach. As the name indicates, the root operation for that procedure is Restriction rather than Supplement because the aorta is returned to its normal size and the fusiform aneurysm sac is walled off, preventing rupture. This restriction is done with an intraluminal device. If the aneurysm involves the area around the renal arteries, the intraluminal device may need to be fenestrated, or have openings, to allow blood to flow through the aortic stent and into the renal arteries. If the aneurysm extends downward and into the iliac artery or arteries, the intraluminal device may need to be branched to allow directed flow of blood into external and internal iliac arteries as they branch off of the iliac artery. Figure 1.13 in chapter 1 displays an intraluminal device used to treat an abdominal aortic aneurysm.

When the abdominal aortic aneurysm is very large or the wall is extremely weak, this aneurysm is commonly removed and replaced with a synthetic graft. The removal of the native piece of the aorta is not coded separately. The 04R table is used to code this procedure, which is typically performed using an open approach. If performed with a synthetic replacement such as Hemashield, this is coded as 04R00JZ Replacement of Abdominal Aorta with Synthetic Substitute, Open Approach.

B3.12. If the objective of an embolization procedure is to completely close a vessel, the root operation Occlusion is coded. If the objective of an embolization procedure is to narrow the lumen of a vessel, the root operation Restriction is coded.

Examples: Tumor embolization is coded to the root operation Occlusion, because the objective of the procedure is to cut off the blood supply to the vessel. Embolization of a cerebral aneurysm is coded to the root operation Restriction, because the objective of the procedure is not to close off the vessel entirely, but to narrow the lumen of the vessel at the site of the aneurysm where it is abnormally wide.

Map and Ablation of Cardiac Mechanism

The root operation Map is available for coding procedures in only two systems, the nervous system and the circulatory system. In the circulatory system, mapping is done as intraoperative cardiac mapping during open heart surgery or during a heart catheterization procedure. The Map procedure is performed to identify the exact location causing cardiac arrhythmia, such as atrial fibrillation. Once located, the location can be ablated, also referred to as scarring or destruction, to stop the flow of electrical activity.

The root operation of Map is coded separately in addition to the Destruction procedure. The body part being mapped and destroyed is the Conduction Mechanism and the approach is Percutaneous.

Heart Transplantation

Heart transplantation is performed when the heart does not function well enough to support the patient and the heart is not able to be repaired in any other way. In this procedure, the great vessels are cut and the diseased heart is removed. The new heart is sutured to the superior and inferior vena cava, the aorta and the pulmonary trunk. The removal of the native heart or heart and lungs is included in the transplant procedure, but the use of the cardiopulmonary bypass machine during the procedure is coded separately.

Cardiac (Heart) Catheterization

A cardiac, or heart, catheterization is a percutaneous procedure to diagnose cardiac disease. This is classified to the Measurement and Monitoring section of ICD-10-PCS because it is a diagnostic test. In this case, the insertion of the catheter is not coded separately. The insertion of the catheter is not the procedure itself but the access route for the physician to measure the pressure within the heart and allow the collection of blood samples for oxygen saturation. The heart cath procedure often leads directly to cardiovascular interventions such as percutaneous transluminal coronary angioplasty (PTCA) and/or thrombectomy. It may also be followed shortly by a coronary artery bypass grafting (CABG) procedure. There are three options for coding cardiac cath procedures, with only one code assigned per operative session:

- 4A023N6 Measurement of Cardiac Sampling and Pressure, Right Heart, Percutaneous Approach
  - Performed to assess the function of the right side of the heart and the pulmonary circulation
- 4A023N7 Measurement of Cardiac Sampling and Pressure, Left Heart, Percutaneous Approach
  - Performed to assess the function of the left side of the heart and the coronary and systemic circulation
- 4A023N8 Measurement of Cardiac Sampling and Pressure, Bilateral, Percutaneous Approach
  - Performed to assess both sides of the heart in a comprehensive evaluation

Imaging that can accompany a cardiac cath is fluoroscopy of the ventricles of the heart, the coronary arteries, the aorta, the pulmonary trunk, and the pulmonary arteries. The aorta, pulmonary trunk, or pulmonary artery imaging is coded in the B31 table and the heart and coronary artery imaging is found in the B21 table. Fluoroscopy in the B21 table can be of single or multiple arteries, single or multiple bypass grafts, the right or left internal mammary bypasses, or other bypass grafts, plus the right or left heart chambers. (See chapter 24 for a more detailed discussion of imaging.)

 Coding Tip

Only one cardiac catheterization code can be assigned per operative session. Assign a qualifier of Left or Right. Assign a qualifier of Bilateral if both are performed.

Percutaneous Transluminal Coronary Angioplasty (PTCA)

The root operation Dilation is used when the objective is to mechanically widen the narrowed or obstructed blood vessel, which is often performed at the time of a cardiac cath:

Once the guiding catheter is in place, a guide wire is advanced across the blockage, then a balloon catheter is advanced to the blockage site. The balloon is inflated for a few seconds to compress the blockage against the artery wall. Then the balloon is deflated. The doctor may repeat this a few times, each time pumping up the balloon a little more to widen the passage for the blood to flow through. This treatment may be repeated at each blocked site in the coronary arteries. A device called a stent may be placed within the coronary artery to keep the vessel open. (NLM 2012)

These are known as percutaneous transluminal coronary angioplasty (PTCA) procedures when performed in the coronary arteries and as percutaneous transluminal angioplasty (PTA) procedures when performed on other arteries.

 B4.4. The coronary arteries are classified as a single body part that is further specified by number of arteries treated. One procedure code specifying multiple arteries is used when the same procedure is performed, including the same device and qualifier values.

Examples: Angioplasty of two distinct arteries with placement of two stents is coded as Dilation of Coronary Artery, Two Arteries, with Two Intraluminal Devices.

Angioplasty of two distinct arteries, one with stent placed and one without, is coded separately as Dilation of Coronary Artery, One Artery with Intraluminal Device, and Dilation of Coronary Artery, One Artery with no device.

The body part value is assigned for the number of coronary arteries treated using the *same* approach, the *same* device, and the *same* qualifier. If any of those values change, then a separate code is required.

Example 1:

Two coronary arteries are treated, each with one stent (intraluminal device) using a percutaneous approach.

One coronary artery is treated with just dilation and no stent using a percutaneous approach.
This is coded as 02713EZ and 02703ZZ and *not* coded as 02723EZ. Because the last coronary artery was not treated with a device, that coronary artery must be coded separately.

Example 2:

Three coronary arteries are treated, each with one drug-eluting stent.

This is coded as 027236Z because there are three arteries for the body part and three drug-eluting stents were used and coded in the device value.

Example 3:

One coronary artery is treated with balloon angioplasty. A second coronary artery is treated with angioplasty and one bare metal stent. A third coronary artery is treated with balloon angioplasty and two drug-eluting stents.

This is coded as 02703ZZ, 02703DZ, and 027035Z because each artery is treated using a different method and, therefore, three separate codes are required.

Extirpation procedures to remove clots in the coronary arteries are often performed at the same operative session. These thrombectomy procedures are coded separately. It may help to review the names of the coronary arteries that were listed in the anatomy section earlier in this chapter.

Bypasses

Bypasses in the circulatory system can be performed using the Open approach, the Percutaneous approach and far less commonly, the Percutaneous Endoscopic approach. Coronary artery bypass grafts are performed to reroute blood to heart muscle around a coronary artery blockage. Other open bypasses can be performed in the heart or any of the upper or lower arteries or veins. Percutaneous bypasses can be performed in the Lower Arteries body system. Each of these types is described here.

Coronary Artery Bypass Grafts (CABG)

The root operation Bypass is used to code procedures where any of the tubular body parts of the circulatory system are rerouted to a different location. The root operation Bypass is coded differently with the coronary arteries. The body part value identifies the number of coronary arteries bypassed, and the qualifier specifies the vessel bypassed from (or the source of the blood flow).

Aortocoronary bypasses use a device and have the aorta as the source of the blood. A device is required to bring the blood from the aorta past the blockage and supply the coronary artery. ICD-10-PCS provides five different types of devices for open coronary artery bypass procedures including:

- 8, Zooplastic Tissue
- 9, Autologous Venous Tissue

- A, Autologous Arterial Tissue
- J, Synthetic Substitute
- K, Nonautologous Tissue Substitute

Guideline B3.9 instructs that both arterial and venous autografts harvested from a different procedure site to be used in completing the objective of a procedure should be coded separately.

B3.9. If an autograft is obtained from a different procedure site in order to complete the objective of the procedure, a separate procedure is coded.

Example: Coronary bypass with excision of saphenous vein graft, excision of saphenous vein is coded separately.

Two other coronary bypasses do not involve a device or use the aorta as the source of the blood. The left and right internal mammary arteries are close to the heart and normally supply blood to the chest wall. These arteries can be detached at the chest wall end and rerouted to send blood past an area of blockage in one or more coronary arteries. The left internal mammary artery (LIMA) is typically used on the left side of the heart and the right internal mammary artery (RIMA) is typically used on the right side of the heart. When either one of these arteries is used, there is no device identified in the 6th character because the artery was not harvested and completely disconnected. These types of grafts are called pedicle grafts because they are still connected at one end. The qualifier for the code is the artery name because the artery is the source of the blood.

Example: The LIMA is rerouted to the obtuse marginal artery as a pedicle graft. This procedure is coded as 02100Z9, Bypass Coronary Artery, One Artery from Left Internal Mammary, Open Approach.

The LIMA is often used to bypass more than one blockage. Figure 11.5 displays a coronary artery bypass graft procedure where three coronary artery sites (ramus, diagonal, and left anterior descending coronary arteries) are

Figure 11.5. Coronary artery bypass graft (CABG) procedure

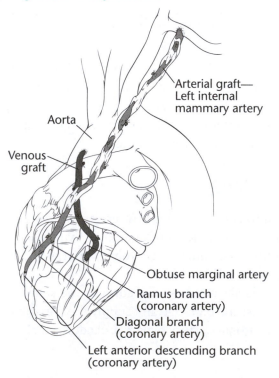

© AHIMA 2019

treated by grafting from the left internal mammary artery, and one coronary artery site is treated by grafting the saphenous venous graft to the obtuse marginal from the aorta as a free graft. If the left saphenous vein was harvested for the graft using an open approach, the codes for the procedures displayed in figure 11.5 are:

02120Z9, Bypass Coronary Artery, Three Arteries from Left Internal Mammary, Open Approach
021009W, Bypass Coronary Artery, One Artery from Aorta with Autologous Venous Tissue, Open Approach
06BQ0ZZ, Excision of Left Saphenous Vein, Open Approach

Refer to the second code building case in this chapter for a complete description of how to determine the codes for figure 11.5.

B3.6c. If multiple coronary arteries are bypassed, a separate procedure is coded for each coronary artery that uses a different device and/or qualifier.

Example: Aortocoronary artery bypass and internal mammary coronary artery bypass are coded separately.

Coding Tip

Read carefully to determine if the left and right internal mammary arteries are completely harvested from the chest wall (rare) or only detached on the distal end (common) to assure the correct device value is assigned.

Coronary artery bypass procedures performed with the use of a cardiopulmonary bypass machine require an additional code for the circulatory performance during the procedure. Refer to chapter 22 for an additional discussion of cardiopulmonary bypass procedure coding.

B3.6b. Coronary artery bypass procedures are coded differently than other bypass procedures, as described in the previous guideline. Rather than identifying the body part bypassed from, the body part identifies the number of coronary arteries bypassed to, and the qualifier specifies the vessel bypassed from.

Example: Aortocoronary artery bypass of the left anterior descending coronary artery and the obtuse marginal coronary artery is classified in the body part axis of classification as two coronary arteries, and the qualifier specifies the aorta as the body part bypassed from.

Other Open Bypasses

Bypasses of the upper and lower arteries and veins body systems are coded based on the regular rules for the root operation Bypass. Common examples of this are:

- Aorto-femoral bypass to reroute blood from the abdominal aorta to one or both femoral arteries and bypass the blocked iliac arteries. This bypass typically uses a conduit of synthetic substitute.
  If performed bilaterally, this is coded as:
  04100JK, Bypass Abdominal Aorta to Bilateral Femoral Arteries with Synthetic Substitute, Open Approach

- Femoral-popliteal bypass to reroute blood from the femoral artery to the popliteal artery and bypass a blockage in the area of the knee. This bypass can use either synthetic substitute or a greater saphenous vein autologous graft.
  If performed on the right side with a greater saphenous vein graft, this is coded as:
  041K09L, Bypass Right Femoral Artery to Popliteal Artery with Autologous Venous Tissue, Open Approach

- Axillo-femoral bypass to reroute blood from one or both axillary arteries to one or both femoral arteries and bypass the abdominal aorta. This bypass uses a conduit made of synthetic material that is tunneled from the area of the armpit along the patient's rib cage to connect at the femoral artery for patient whose abdominal aorta is tortuous or has an aneurysm.

If performed on the right side, this is coded as:

03150J6, Bypass Right Axillary Artery to Right Upper Leg Artery with Synthetic Substitute, Open Approach

Coding Tip

Bypasses are coded differently when the procedure is performed on the coronary arteries versus other non-coronary body parts. Coronary artery bypass uses the number of coronary arteries as the body part value and the source of the bypass (location blood is bypassed from) as the qualifier. Non-coronary bypasses use the body part as the starting point of the bypass and the qualifier as the destination of the bypass.

Bypass			
Non-Coronary Locations		**Coronary Arteries**	
Body Part	Qualifier	Body Part	Qualifier
From	To (Downstream Location)	Number of Coronary Arteries	From (Blood Source)

Percutaneous Bypasses

Two percutaneous bypasses can be performed in the lower extremities. These percutaneous bypasses are performed from the lower arteries to two possible destinations—a lower extremity artery or a lower extremity vein. The percutaneous bypass from a lower artery to a lower artery is called a DETOUR bypass, which uses a neighboring vein as the tunnel for the curved, synthetic conduit to reroute the blood. This curved conduit is called a TORUS stent graft. The device value assigned is J, Synthetic Substitute and the qualifier value assigned is Q, Lower Extremity Artery.

The percutaneous bypass from a lower artery to a lower vein uses a different system called the LimFlow system. The LimFlow uses a lower vein to deliver blood to the more distal leg and foot. This bypass uses a curved synthetic conduit to move blood from the artery to a vein. The one-way valves inside the vein are destroyed, allowing the vein to serve as a pathway sending oxygenated blood to the distal leg and foot. The device value assigned is J, Synthetic Substitute and the qualifier value assigned is S, Lower Extremity Vein.

Percutaneous Transluminal Angioplasty of Noncoronary Sites

Noncoronary arteries can also be dilated using the same techniques used in the coronary arteries. Extirpation of plaque or clots is also commonly performed in non-coronary vessels. At times, the plaque or clot extends from one tubular body part into another, such as the common iliac down into the internal or external iliac artery. If a procedure is performed on a continuous section of a tubular body part, code the body part value corresponding to the furthest anatomical site from the point of entry for each of the procedures performed, such as Dilation and Extirpation.

B4.1.c.   If a procedure is performed on a continuous section of a tubular body part, code the body part value corresponding to the furthest anatomical site from the point of entry.

Example: A procedure performed on a continuous section of artery from the femoral artery to the external iliac artery with the point of entry at the femoral artery is coded to the external iliac body part.

AV Fistulas and Grafts

Both an AV fistula and AV graft are made by connecting one of the patient's arteries to a vein in preparation for use in hemodialysis procedures. The fistula is a direct connection of the vessels, and a graft uses additional device material to make the connection. Both procedures are coded to the root operation Bypass. The bypass starts in the arteries and ends with the vein; therefore, the body part coded is the artery, where the bypass begins. AV fistulas are coded with a device value of Z, No Device. AV grafts are coded with a device value that describes the material used to create the graft, such as a synthetic substitute.

ICD-10-PCS deals with the coding of a thrombectomy of these structures differently. When a thrombus is removed from an AV fistula (all native tissue), the root operation of Extirpation is assigned because the thrombus is an abnormal by-product of a bodily function that needs to be removed. When a thrombus is removed from the inside an AV graft (an indwelling device), the root operation Revision is assigned because the AV graft is a malfunctioning device due to the clot. The device is connected to the artery (where the bypass started); therefore, the revision is coded to the upper or lower artery, and the device value is selected as the material being revised.

The root operation Extirpation is used to describe the process of declotting the many tubular body parts within the circulatory system, as clots are an abnormal by-product of a biological function. Embolization procedures are also performed frequently on the tubular body parts of the circulatory system. The root operation Occlusion is coded when the procedure is performed to completely close the vessel. If the intent of the procedure is to narrow the lumen of the vessel (restrict the blood flow), the root operation Restriction is assigned.

Drainage

The root operation Drainage is used to describe the removal of blood directly from a vein (venipuncture) or artery. When blood is removed through an indwelling device, such as a port or catheter, the root operation Collection is assigned in Section 8, Other Procedures.

Coding Tip

When blood is removed directly from a vein or artery, the root operation Drainage is assigned. When blood is removed through an indwelling device, such as a port or catheter, the root operation Collection is assigned in Section 8, Other Procedures.

Laser Revascularization

A specific repair procedure performed on the circulatory system is called transmyocardial laser revascularization (TMLR). A special laser is used to make very small channels into the heart muscle, making new pathways for blood to flow into the heart muscle. This is done via a small left chest incision or a midline incision when performed independently, but it can also be performed at the time of open heart surgery. TMLR is coded to the root operation of Repair, as no other root operation applies.

Be sure to research any procedure that is unfamiliar to assure correct coding. If the documentation includes an eponym (procedure named for a person) and the intent of the procedure is unclear, query the physician for specifics.

Body Part Values for the Circulatory System

Body part values are available for a variety of different arteries and veins and their associated branches. The azygos vein drains blood from the thorax and abdomen into the superior vena cava vein and is formed by the combination of the ascending lumbar veins with the right subcostal veins near the level of the 12th thoracic vertebra. The left-sided equivalent is the hemiazygos vein (vena azygos minor inferior).

The left colic vein (descending colon) leads to the inferior mesenteric vein and follows the path of the left colic artery. The middle colic vein (transverse colon) leads to the superior mesenteric vein and follows the path of the middle colic artery. The right colic (ascending colon) leads to the superior mesenteric vein and follows the path of the right colic artery. The hypogastric veins are also known as the internal iliac veins.

Generic body part values are available for body areas where arteries and veins are numerous, such as the hands and feet, the face, and the intracranial area. Individual, generic body part values are available for upper artery, upper vein, lower artery, and lower vein.

Table 11.1 lists the body parts available for coding procedures on the heart and great vessels. Table 11.2 lists the body parts available for coding procedures performed on the upper and lower arteries, and table 11.3 lists the body parts available for coding procedures performed on the upper and lower veins. If the documentation includes specific body part names that are not included in these lists, refer to the body part key for other body part synonyms and alternative terms.

Table 11.1. Body Parts in the Heart and Great Vessels

Body Part Value	Body Parts—Heart and Great Vessels (2)
0	Coronary Artery, One Artery
1	Coronary Artery, Two Arteries
2	Coronary Artery, Three Arteries
3	Coronary Artery, Four or More Arteries
4	Coronary Vein
5	Atrial Septum
6	Atrium, Right
7	Atrium, Left
8	Conductive Mechanism
9	Chordae Tendineae
A	Heart
B	Heart, Right
C	Heart, Left
D	Papillary Muscle
F	Aortic Valve
G	Mitral Valve
H	Pulmonary Valve
J	Tricuspid Valve
K	Ventricle, Right
L	Ventricle, Left
M	Ventricular Septum
N	Pericardium
P	Pulmonary Trunk
Q	Pulmonary Artery, Right
R	Pulmonary Artery, Left
S	Pulmonary Vein, Right
T	Pulmonary Vein, Left
V	Superior Vena Cava
W	Thoracic Aorta, Descending
X	Thoracic Aorta, Ascending/Arch
Y	Great Vessel

Table 11.2. **Body Parts in the Upper and Lower Arteries**

Body Part Value	Body Parts—Upper Arteries (3)	Body Part Value	Body Parts—Lower Arteries (4)
0	Internal Mammary Artery, Right	0	Abdominal Aorta
1	Internal Mammary Artery, Left	1	Celiac Artery
2	Innominate Artery	2	Gastric Artery
3	Subclavian Artery, Right	3	Hepatic Artery
4	Subclavian Artery, Left	4	Splenic Artery
5	Axillary Artery, Right	5	Superior Mesenteric Artery
6	Axillary Artery, Left	6	Colic Artery, Right
7	Brachial Artery, Right	7	Colic Artery, Left
8	Brachial Artery, Left	8	Colic Artery, Middle
9	Ulnar Artery, Right	9	Renal Artery, Right
A	Ulnar Artery, Left	A	Renal Artery, Left
B	Radial Artery, Right	B	Inferior Mesenteric Artery
C	Radial Artery, Left	C	Common Iliac Artery, Right
D	Hand Artery, Right	D	Common Iliac Artery, Left
F	Hand Artery, Left	E	Internal Iliac Artery, Right
G	Intracranial Artery	F	Internal Iliac Artery, Left
H	Common Carotid Artery, Right	H	External Iliac Artery, Right
J	Common Carotid Artery, Left	J	External Iliac Artery, Left
K	Internal Carotid Artery, Right	K	Femoral Artery, Right
L	Internal Carotid Artery, Left	L	Femoral Artery, Left
M	External Carotid Artery, Right	M	Popliteal Artery, Right
N	External Carotid Artery, Left	N	Popliteal Artery, Left
P	Vertebral Artery, Right	P	Anterior Tibial Artery, Right
Q	Vertebral Artery, Left	Q	Anterior Tibial Artery, Left
R	Face Artery	R	Posterior Tibial Artery, Right
S	Temporal Artery, Right	S	Posterior Tibial Artery, Left
T	Temporal Artery, Left	T	Peroneal Artery, Right
U	Thyroid Artery, Right	U	Peroneal Artery, Left
V	Thyroid Artery, Left	V	Foot Artery, Right
Y	Upper Artery	W	Foot Artery, Left
		Y	Lower Artery

Table 11.3 **Body parts in the Upper and Lower Veins**

Body Part Value	Body Parts—Upper Veins (5)	Body Part Value	Body Parts—Lower Veins (6)
0	Azygos Vein	0	Inferior Vena Cava
1	Hemiazygos Vein	1	Splenic Vein
3	Innominate Vein, Right	2	Gastric Vein
4	Innominate Vein, Left	3	Esophageal Vein

(Continued)   *(Continued)*

Table 11.3   Body parts in the Upper and Lower Veins (continued)

Body Part Value	Body Parts—Upper Veins (5)	Body Part Value	Body Parts—Lower Veins (6)
5	Subclavian Vein, Right	4	Hepatic Vein
6	Subclavian Vein, Left	5	Superior Mesenteric Vein
7	Axillary Vein, Right	6	Inferior Mesenteric Vein
8	Axillary Vein, Left	7	Colic Vein
9	Brachial Vein, Right	8	Portal Vein
A	Brachial Vein, Left	9	Renal Vein, Right
B	Basilic Vein, Right	B	Renal Vein, Left
C	Basilic Vein, Left	C	Common Iliac Vein, Right
D	Cephalic Vein, Right	D	Common Iliac Vein, Left
F	Cephalic Vein, Left	F	External Iliac Vein, Right
G	Hand Vein, Right	G	External Iliac Vein, Left
H	Hand Vein, Left	H	Hypogastric Vein, Right
L	Intracranial Vein	J	Hypogastric Vein, Left
M	Internal Jugular Vein, Right	M	Femoral Vein, Right
N	Internal Jugular Vein, Left	N	Femoral Vein, Left
P	External Jugular Vein, Right	P	Saphenous Vein, Right
Q	External Jugular Vein, Left	Q	Saphenous Vein, Left
R	Vertebral Vein, Right	T	Foot Vein, Right
S	Vertebral Vein, Left	V	Foot Vein, Left
T	Face Vein, Right	Y	Lower Vein
V	Face Vein, Left		
Y	Upper Vein		

Approaches Used for the Circulatory System

Coding of procedures performed on the circulatory system uses six of the seven approaches. Open, Percutaneous, and Percutaneous Endoscopic approaches are commonly assigned. The approaches of Via Natural or Artificial Opening and Via Natural or Artificial Opening Endoscopic are only available in the 06L table for occlusion of esophageal vein erosions performed through the gastrointestinal tract. The External approach is available for coding with the root operations Fragmentation, Removal, Revision, and Inspection in these systems.

Devices Common to the Circulatory System

The unique devices used in procedures performed on the circulatory system are the pressure sensor monitoring device, the short-term external heart assist system, the implantable heart assist system, the drug-eluting intraluminal device, and the bioactive intraluminal device. The implantable pressure sensor is a specialized monitoring device that is placed within the heart or great vessels to perform continuous pulmonary artery pressure (PAP) measurements through the use of wireless technology (Mobile Health News 2010).

The external heart assist system is an older-style device that involves inserting a graft to the right ventricle and the pulmonary artery or the left ventricle and the aorta with an external motor or pump to assist with the blood flow. The implantable heart assist systems are newer-style devices that are completely implantable with the same heart graft or grafts and the implantable pump placed below the diaphragm.

The drug-eluting intraluminal device, usually termed a stent, is the same as a typical intraluminal device but is covered with a special coating that releases a drug at the site of the stent placement to prevent clot production. An example of a bioactive intraluminal device is the bioactive coils that contain biodegradable polymers to encourage occlusion or thrombus formation in aneurysms and arteriovenous malformations. Tables 11.4 through 11.6 list the devices available for coding procedures performed on the circulatory system.

Coding Tip

A Swan-Ganz catheter is coded to the device value 0, Monitoring Device, Pressure Sensor because it monitors pulmonary artery output and pressure. The implantable pulmonary artery pressure sensor is a specialized pressure monitoring device and is coded to the device value 0, Monitoring device, pressure sensor.

Table 11.4. Devices for the Heart and Great Vessels

Device Value	Devices—Heart and Great Vessels (2)
0	Monitoring Device, Pressure Sensor
2	Monitoring Device
3	Infusion Device
4	Intraluminal Device, Drug-eluting
5	Intraluminal Device, Drug-eluting, Two
6	Intraluminal Device, Drug-eluting, Three
7	Intraluminal Device, Drug-eluting, Four or More
7	Autologous Tissue Substitute
8	Zooplastic Tissue
9	Autologous Venous Tissue
A	Autologous Arterial Tissue
C	Extraluminal Device
D	Intraluminal Device
E	Intraluminal Device, Two
E	Intraluminal Device, Branched or Fenestrated, One or Two Arteries
F	Intraluminal Device, Three
F	Intraluminal Device, Branched or Fenestrated, Three or More Arteries
G	Intraluminal Device, Four or More
J	Synthetic Substitute
J	Cardiac Lead, Pacemaker
K	Cardiac Lead, Defibrillator
K	Nonautologous Tissue Substitute
M	Cardiac Lead
N	Intracardiac Pacemaker
Q	Implantable Heart Assist System
R	Short-Term External Heart Assist System
T	Intraluminal Device, Radioactive
Y	Other Device
Z	No Device

Table 11.5.   Devices for the Upper and Lower Arteries

Device Value	Devices—Upper Arteries (3)	Device Value	Devices—Lower Arteries (4)
0	Drainage Device	0	Drainage Device
2	Monitoring Device	1	Radioactive Element
3	Infusion Device	2	Monitoring Device
4	Intraluminal Device, Drug-eluting	3	Infusion Device
5	Intraluminal Device, Drug-eluting, Two	4	Intraluminal Device, Drug-eluting
6	Intraluminal Device, Drug-eluting, Three	5	Intraluminal Device, Drug-eluting, Two
7	Intraluminal Device, Drug-eluting, Four or More	6	Intraluminal Device, Drug-eluting, Three
7	Autologous Tissue Substitute	7	Intraluminal Device, Drug-eluting, Four or More
9	Autologous Venous Tissue	7	Autologous Tissue Substitute
A	Autologous Arterial Tissue	9	Autologous Venous Tissue
B	Intraluminal Device, Bioactive	A	Autologous Arterial Tissue
C	Extraluminal Device	C	Extraluminal Device
D	Intraluminal Device	D	Intraluminal Device
E	Intraluminal Device, Two	E	Intraluminal Device, Two
F	Intraluminal Device, Three	E	Intraluminal Device, Branched or Fenestrated, One or Two Arteries
G	Intraluminal Device, Four or More	F	Intraluminal Device, Three
J	Synthetic Substitute	F	Intraluminal Device, Branched or Fenestrated, One or Two Arteries
K	Nonautologous Tissue Substitute	G	Intraluminal Device, Four or More
M	Stimulator Lead	J	Synthetic Substitute
Y	Other Device	K	Nonautologous Tissue Substitute
Z	No Device	Y	Other Device
		Z	No Device

Table 11.6.   Devices for the Upper and Lower Veins

Device Value	Devices—Upper and Lower Veins (5 and 6)
0	Drainage Device
2	Monitoring Device
3	Infusion Device
7	Autologous Tissue Substitute
9	Autologous Venous Tissue
A	Autologous Arterial Tissue
C	Extraluminal Device
D	Intraluminal Device
J	Synthetic Substitute
K	Nonautologous Tissue Substitute
M	Neurostimulator Lead
Y	Other Device
Z	No Device

Qualifiers Used in the Circulatory System

The qualifier values for bypass procedures of the coronary arteries are assigned using a different method than the qualifier values assigned with bypass procedures performed on other body parts. When procedures are performed on coronary arteries, the qualifier describes the vessel bypassed from, meaning the origin of the bypass.

The body part value describes the number of coronary arteries bypassed to. The qualifiers for the remainder of the body parts within the circulatory system describe the body part bypassed to.

For example, a single vessel coronary bypass graft of the left anterior descending artery using the left mammary artery with an open approach is coded as 02100Z9. The body part value of 0 refers to one coronary artery, and the qualifier value of 9 describes the origin of the bypass as the left internal mammary artery. Note that when the internal mammary artery is used to perform the bypass, no device value is assigned because the internal mammary artery is not disconnected from the blood supply (not a free graft).

In contrast, an open left femoral-popliteal artery bypass using a cadaver vein graft is coded as 041L0KL. The body part value of L refers to the source of the bypass as the left femoral artery, and the qualifier value of L describes the body part bypassed to, the popliteal artery.

A separate procedure is coded for each coronary artery that is treated with a different device or a different qualifier. Therefore, multiple codes may be required to correctly code a coronary artery bypass graft procedure of several vessels.

Drug-coated balloons deliver a time-released medication into the dilated vessel wall that helps prevent restenosis of the vessel. The use of the drug-coated balloon is captured in the qualifier of dilation code because the balloon is not a device that is left in place at the end of the procedure. Qualifier value 1, Drug-Coated Balloon is available for assignment with specific body parts in the 037, 047, and 057 tables for dilation of appropriate arteries and veins. In addition, circulatory system procedures may use the standard qualifiers of X for Diagnostic and Z for No Qualifier.

The qualifier value 7, Stent Retriever, is assigned when extirpation is performed on the extracranial arteries (all of the carotid arteries and the vertebral arteries) and all intracranial arteries using a stent retriever catheter to capture and remove the clot. Tables 11.7 through 11.9 list the qualifier values available for coding procedures performed on the circulatory system.

Coding Tip

The word "stent" in the name of the stent retriever catheter refers to the wire framework used to capture the clot, not to a stent that remains after the procedure is complete. No device is left in place following the extirpation procedure.

Table 11.7. Qualifiers for the Heart and Great Vessels

Qualifier Value	Qualifiers—Heart and Great Vessels (2)
0	Allogeneic
1	Syngeneic
2	Zooplastic
2	Common Atrioventricular Valve
3	Coronary Artery
4	Coronary Vein
5	Coronary Circulation
6	Bifurcation

(Continued)

Table 11.7. Qualifiers for the Heart and Great Vessels (continued)

Qualifier Value	Qualifiers—Heart and Great Vessels (2)
7	Atrium, Left
8	Internal Mammary, Right
9	Internal Mammary, Left
A	Innominate Artery
B	Subclavian
C	Thoracic Artery
D	Carotid
E	Atrioventricular Valve, Left
F	Abdominal Artery
G	Axillary Artery
G	Atrioventricular Valve, Right
H	Brachial Artery
H	Transapical
J	Intraoperative
J	Temporary
J	Truncal Valve
K	Left Atrial Appendage
P	Pulmonary Trunk
Q	Pulmonary Artery, Right
R	Pulmonary Artery, Left
S	Biventricular
S	Pulmonary Vein, Right
T	Ductus Arteriosus
T	Pulmonary Vein, Left
U	Pulmonary Vein, Confluence
V	Lower Extremity Artery
W	Aorta
X	Diagnostic
Z	No Qualifier

Table 11.8. Qualifiers for the Upper and Lower Arteries

Qualifier Value	Qualifiers—Upper Arteries (3)	Qualifier Value	Qualifiers—Lower Arteries (4)
0	Upper Arm Artery, Right	0	Abdominal Aorta
1	Upper Arm Artery, Left	1	Celiac Artery
1	Drug-Coated Balloon	1	Drug-Coated Balloon
2	Upper Arm Artery, Bilateral	2	Mesenteric Artery
3	Lower Arm Artery, Right	3	Renal Artery, Right
4	Lower Arm Artery, Left	4	Renal Artery, Left

(Continued)   *(Continued)*

Table 11.8. Qualifiers for the Upper and Lower Arteries (continued)

Qualifier Value	Qualifiers—Upper Arteries (3)	Qualifier Value	Qualifiers—Lower Arteries (4)
5	Lower Arm Artery, Bilateral	5	Renal Artery, Bilateral
6	Upper Leg Artery, Right	6	Common Iliac Artery, Right
6	Bifurcation	6	Bifurcation
7	Upper Leg Artery, Left	7	Common Iliac Artery, Left
7	Stent Retriever	8	Common Iliac Artery, Bilateral
8	Upper Leg Artery, Bilateral	9	Internal Iliac Artery, Right
9	Lower Leg Artery, Right	B	Internal Iliac Artery, Left
B	Lower Leg Artery, Left	C	Internal Iliac Artery, Bilateral
C	Lower Artery, Bilateral	D	External Iliac Artery, Right
D	Upper Arm Vein	F	External Iliac Artery, Left
F	Lower Arm Vein	G	External Iliac Artery, Bilateral
G	Intracranial Artery	H	Femoral Artery, Right
J	Extracranial Artery, Right	J	Temporary
K	Extracranial Artery, Left	J	Femoral Artery, Left
M	Pulmonary Artery, Right	K	Femoral Artery, Bilateral
N	Pulmonary Artery, Left	L	Popliteal Artery
V	Superior Vena Cava	M	Peroneal Artery
X	Diagnostic	N	Posterior Tibial Artery
Z	No Qualifier	P	Foot Artery
		Q	Lower Extremity Artery
		R	Lower Artery
		S	Lower Extremity Vein
		T	Uterine Artery, Right
		T	Abdominal artery
		U	Uterine Artery, Left
		X	Diagnostic
		Y	Upper Artery
		Z	No Qualifier

Table 11.9. Qualifiers for the Upper and Lower Veins

Qualifier Value	Qualifiers—Upper Veins (5)	Qualifier Value	Qualifiers—Lower Veins (6)
1	Drug-Coated Balloon	4	Hepatic Vein
X	Diagnostic	5	Superior Mesenteric Vein
Y	Upper Vein	6	Inferior Mesenteric Vein
Z	No Qualifier	9	Renal Vein, Right
		B	Renal Vein, Left
		C	Hemorrhoidal Plexus
		P	Pulmonary Trunk

(Continued)

Table 11.9. Qualifiers for the Upper and Lower Veins (continued)

Qualifier Value	Qualifiers—Lower Veins (6)
Q	Pulmonary Artery, Right
R	Pulmonary Artery, Left
T	Via Umbilical Vein
X	Diagnostic
Y	Lower Vein
Z	No Qualifier

 Code Building

Case #1:

PROCEDURE STATEMENT: Treatment of aneurysm of a cerebral artery by bioactive coil restriction

ADDITIONAL INFORMATION: A biodegradable intraluminal polymer coil is placed within the aneurysm of the cerebral artery to restrict blood flow into the aneurysm to enhance thrombus formation within the aneurysm. The coil is placed percutaneously with artery access through the neck.

ROOT AND INDEX ENTRIES FOR THE STATEMENT: Restriction is the root operation performed in this procedure, defined as partially closing an orifice or the lumen of a tubular body part. The Index entry is:

Restriction

    Artery

        Intracranial   03VG

Code Characters:

Section	Body System	Root Operation	Body Part	Approach	Device	Qualifier
Medical and Surgical	Upper Arteries	Restriction	Intracranial Artery	Percutaneous	Intraluminal Device, Bioactive	No Qualifier
0	3	V	G	3	B	Z

RATIONALE FOR THE ANSWER: The aneurysm is a widening of the artery through a weak arterial wall. The root operation Restriction is used to code this procedure because the widened area is restricted by the bioactive coil device. A cerebral artery is an intracranial artery in ICD-10-PCS. The approach value is 3, Percutaneous because the coil is threaded into the aneurysm through arterial access in the neck. The bioactive coil is device value B, Intraluminal device, bioactive. No qualifier is appropriate for this code. The correct code assignment is 03VG3BZ.

Case #2:

PROCEDURE STATEMENT: A coronary artery bypass graft procedure where three coronary arteries are treated by grafting from the left internal mammary artery (LIMA) and one coronary artery is treated by grafting the saphenous venous graft to the obtuse marginal from the aorta.

ADDITIONAL INFORMATION: This procedure is pictured in figure 11.5 of this chapter. The arteries treated by the LIMA are the left anterior descending artery, the diagonal artery, and the ramus artery. The artery treated by the saphenous venous graft is the obtuse marginal artery. The left saphenous vein was harvested using an Open approach.

ROOT AND INDEX ENTRIES FOR THE STATEMENT: Bypass is the root operation performed in this procedure, defined as altering the route of passage of the contents of a tubular body part. The Index entry for a bypass procedure is:

Bypass

    Artery

        Coronary

               Four or More arteries   0213

               One artery   0210

               Three arteries   0212

               Two arteries   0211

Code Characters for the Left Internal Mammary Bypass:

Section	Body System	Root Operation	Body Part	Approach	Device	Qualifier
Medical and Surgical	Heart and Great Vessels	Bypass	Coronary Artery, Three Arteries	Open	No Device	Internal Mammary, Left
0	2	1	2	0	Z	9

Code Characters for the Saphenous Venous Bypass:

Section	Body System	Root Operation	Body Part	Approach	Device	Qualifier
Medical and Surgical	Heart and Great Vessels	Bypass	Coronary Artery, One Artery	Open	Autologous Venous Tissue	Aorta
0	2	1	0	0	9	W

ROOT AND INDEX ENTRIES FOR THE STATEMENT: Excision is the root operation performed in this procedure, defined as cutting out or off, without replacement, a portion of a body part. The Index entry for excision procedure is:

Excision

    Vein

        Saphenous

        Left   06BQ

        Right   06BP

Code Characters for the Harvesting of the Saphenous Venous Graft:

Section	Body System	Root Operation	Body Part	Approach	Device	Qualifier
Medical and Surgical	Lower Veins	Excision	Saphenous Vein, Left	Open	No Device	No Qualifier
0	6	B	Q	0	Z	Z

RATIONALE FOR THE ANSWER: Two codes are required for the bypass procedures because different devices and qualifiers need to be assigned to the different bypass procedures performed. The body part value for the number of coronary arteries treated by each individual method using a different device or qualifier is assigned for each unique combination. The three coronary arteries treated with the bypass from the left internal mammary artery is coded with the device character of Z, No Device because the internal mammary artery is not a free graft. The qualifier for this code is 9, Internal Mammary, Left, because this is the source of the bypass. The one coronary artery treated with the free graft from the saphenous vein is coded with the device character of 9, Autologous Venous Tissue and a qualifier value of W, Aorta, because the aorta is the source of the bypass. The greater saphenous vein is a free graft and is therefore coded as a venous device in ICD-10-PCS. In addition, the harvesting of the saphenous vein is coded as the root operation Excision. The body part value Q is assigned for the left greater saphenous vein. No device or qualifier values are appropriate for this code. The correct code assignment is 02120Z9, 021009W, and 06BQ0ZZ.

Code Building Exercises

Work through each case and check your answers using the answer key in appendix B of the textbook before going on to the Check Your Understanding questions that follow.

Exercise 1:

DIAGNOSIS:	Juxtarenal aortic aneurysm
OPERATION PERFORMED:	Open aortic aneurysm repair with an 18 mm Dacron straight graft.
INDICATIONS:	An 85-year-old female with a history of known aortic aneurysm who presents for surgical repair.

DESCRIPTION OF PROCEDURE: The patient was brought to the operating theater and placed in supine position where general endotracheal tube anesthesia was achieved. Abdomen was then prepped and draped in usual sterile fashion. Midline incision was made. Soft tissue was incised and dissected sharply and the intraperitoneal space was entered sharply. The small bowel was eviscerated. Ligament of Treitz was taken down.

The aneurysm was examined and the proximal neck of the aneurysm was dissected out. An aortic clamp was positioned here. The 6000 units of heparin were given IV. After 3 minutes of circulating time, the aorta was cross clamped and then arteriotomy was made above the aneurysm sac in the proximal aorta. An 18 mm straight graft was brought up and anastomosed to the proximal aorta with a running 3-0 Prolene. An incision was made in the distal aorta below the aneurysm and the aneurysm was completely resected and sent to Pathology. The graft was cut to length and anastomosed to the aorta. This was performed with a running 3-0 Prolene. The anastomosis was forward bled, back bled, filled with heparin and saline, and suctioned. Air was evacuated and last sutures were tightened. The aortic clamp was taken down gently and the suture lines were each inspected and were satisfactory. The bowel was reorganized within the cavity. The abdomen was then closed with a running looped PDS followed by skin staples at the skin level. Sterile dressing was applied.

Questions:

1.1. Is this Repair, Supplement, or Replacement of the aorta? Why?

_____

1.2. In which body system is this portion of the aorta found?

_____

1.3. What code(s) would you assign?

Exercise 2:

DIAGNOSIS: Right-sided middle cerebral artery aneurysm

OPERATION PERFORMED: Right frontotemporal anterior skull base craniotomy and clipping of the aneurysm under operative microscope

PROCEDURE: The patient was brought to the operating room. After administration of adequate general endotracheal anesthesia, the head was secured in a three-point fixation mechanism. The scalp was prepared in a sterile fashion. The incision was made and superficial hemostasis was achieved. Multiple burr holes were made and a craniotomy bone flap was turned. After adequate exposure of the base of the skull, we opened the dura. We were able to carefully dissect away, under high power of microscope, all of the arachnoid adhesions and reached the aneurysm. The neck appeared to be quite wide. The vessel was clearly isolated and eventually a 10 mm curved clip was applied to the neck of the aneurysm. A portion of the aneurysm remained unprotected at the proximal end of the clip and required a second small clip to obliterate that part as well. Complete hemostasis was achieved. The skull was placed back and secured in place with multiple titanium plates and screws. The incision was closed in anatomical layers using 2-0 Vicryl for reapproximation of the muscle and fascia as well as galea.

Questions:

2.1. If a clip is placed on the outside of an aneurysm, what root operation is assigned?

2.2. What body system is used to code this procedure?

2.3. What body part value is assigned for the middle cerebral artery?

2.4. What code(s) would be assigned?

Exercise 3:

DIAGNOSIS: Left lower extremity claudication with high grade left popliteal artery stenosis

PROCEDURE: Atherectomy and drug-coated balloon angioplasty of left popliteal stenosis

INDICATIONS: This 56-year-old gentleman has had over 6 months of reported LLE claudication which was managed conservatively but progressed to be disabling.

DETAILS: Following conscious sedation and sterile prepping, the right common femoral artery was accessed with a micropuncture set. The needle was exchanged for a 4-French sheath and the C2 glide catheter was used to select the left common iliac artery and then the left superficial femoral artery. A 7-French sheath was advanced and angiography was performed, showing approximately 95% stenosis of the mid left popliteal artery.

The patient was heparinized with 5,000 units and an emboshield distal protection device was advanced and positioned in the distal popliteal artery. The atherectomy device was then used to traverse the lesion at 80,000 revolutions per minute. Three runs were made, which resulted in approximately 50% to 60% of residual stenosis. A 4 mm × 80 mm IN.PACT Admiral drug-coated balloon was then used to perform angioplasty up to 4 atmospheres. Protection device was removed and completion angiogram demonstrated a less than 10% residual. The long sheath was removed and pressure hemostasis was achieved.

Questions:

3.1. How many procedures are identified in this report? What are they?

_____

3.2. What is the difference between a drug-eluting stent and a drug-coated balloon? Which one is used in this case?

_____

3.3. What code(s) would be assigned?

_____

 Check Your Understanding

Coding Knowledge Check

1. A valvuloplasty of the tricuspid valve, completed with a ring prosthesis, is coded to which root operation?
   a. Bypass
   b. Dilation
   c. Restriction
   d. Supplement

2. Repositioning a previously placed cardiac pacemaker lead, percutaneous approach, is coded with which body part value?
   a. 5
   b. A
   c. M
   d. Y

3. The abdominal aorta is included in the_____body system in ICD-10-PCS.

4. Within the coronary arteries, the qualifier used in a code for the root operation Bypass indicates

   _____.

   a. Origin of the bypass
   b. The body part bypassed to
   c. The type of tissue used to form the bypass
   d. Nothing, the qualifier value of Z is assigned

5. Four coronary arteries are treated with angioplasty and one bare metal stent in each artery. What device value is assigned for this case? _____

Procedure Statement Coding

Assign ICD-10-PCS codes to the following procedure statements and scenarios. List the root operation selected and the code assigned.

1. Open excision of right internal mammary artery to be used as graft material

2. Percutaneous exchange of transvenous right atrial and ventricular leads of a pacemaker, which was initially placed three years ago; battery remains intact. No EP studies performed at this time.

3. Left temporal artery biopsy, open approach, to rule out temporal arteritis due to headaches and abnormal lab values

4. Open-heart surgery for repair of atrial septal defect with mesh

5. Declot the Circle of Willis at the skull base with a stent retriever

6. Open placement of a synthetic arteriovenous graft from the left brachial artery to the cephalic vein above the elbow in preparation for hemodialysis

7. Double aorto-coronary artery bypass, open approach (left internal mammary artery to left anterior descending; left saphenous vein to diagonal, open harvesting). (Do not code use of cardiopulmonary bypass equipment.)

8. Suture closure of patent ductus arteriosus, open

9. Open excision of left atrial appendage

10. Percutaneous transmyocardial laser revascularization of left ventricle

Case Studies

NOTE: For additional case study coding on coronary artery bypass grafting (CABG), see chapter 22, Extracorporeal Assistance and Performance, as many CABG procedures are performed with the use of cardiopulmonary bypass.

After study of the material in chapter 22, case study practice is provided for coding of all the necessary procedures performed during a CABG procedure.

For additional case study coding on cardiac catheterization procedures, see chapter 24 on Imaging, as cardiac catheterizations are performed using imaging. After study of the material in chapter 24, case study practice is provided for coding of all the necessary procedures performed through the cardiac catheter.

Assign ICD-10-PCS codes to the following case studies.

1. Operative Report

PREOPERATIVE DIAGNOSIS: Occluded right external iliac artery

POSTOPERATIVE DIAGNOSIS: Same

INDICATIONS FOR OPERATION: This is a 59-year-old white man who has undergone attempted right iliac balloon angioplasty approximately 2 weeks prior to this admission. We were unable to open the right external iliac artery, and at this point in time, the patient presents for an elective femoral bypass graft.

OPERATION: The patient was taken to the operating room and placed in the supine position. Once adequate epidural anesthesia had been obtained, the patient's lower abdomen and bilateral lower extremities were prepared and draped in the usual fashion. Incisions were made in both groins simultaneously, and each common femoral and superficial femoral artery was approached using blunt dissection to the subcutaneous tissue. The common femoral artery, superficial femoral artery, and smaller arteries were then identified and isolated with ligaloops. On the left side, the common femoral artery and superficial femoral artery were palpated and noted to have an arteriosclerotic plaque posteriorly, but a soft anterior area of the artery proximal. This point was chosen for the anastomotic site. The patient was then heparinized, and after waiting an appropriate amount of time, a 1.5-cm arteriotomy was then made. The prosthetic graft was then chosen to be a ringed Gore-Tex 8 suture. A tunnel was then created from the right groin to the left through the tissue and over to the right groin. The right common femoral artery was then examined and noted to have plaque posteriorly, but was soft anteriorly. Approximately 1- to 1.5-cm arteriotomy was then made and the graft was already brought through the groin, was then sized and the anastomosis was begun. A running 6-0 Prolene suture was used. As the anastomosis was completed, the left leg was opened, and the graft was flushed to remove any clots. As distal control was released on the right superficial femoral artery, back bleeding was noted to be poor; therefore, a thrombectomy was performed using a 4-mm Fogarty catheter. Again, back bleeding revealed good patency of the artery. The anastomosis was then completed. All ligaloops were then removed, and there was noted to be good flow through both the graft and the right lower extremity with good Doppler pulses. The groin incisions were then closed in two layers and the skin was closed with interrupted nylon suture. Dressings were placed and the patient was removed from the operating room in stable condition.

2. Operative Report

NOTE: Do not code the operative aortogram or angiography included with this case.

PREOPERATIVE DIAGNOSIS: A 9 cm infrarenal abdominal aortic aneurysm

POSTOPERATIVE DIAGNOSIS: A 9 cm infrarenal abdominal aortic aneurysm

PROCEDURE: Endovascular repair of abdominal aortic aneurysm with Gore excluder graft

HISTORY: This is an 87-year-old male who presented to the ER with back pain. He was diagnosed with a large AAA that was asymptomatic in incidental finding. He was transferred to ABC Hospital for treatment. CT scan revealed a neck that was less than 15 mm, but greater than 1 cm with approximately a 50-degree angulation of the neck. Because of the patient's age, it was felt that endovascular repair would be the best situation for this patient. After informed consent was obtained from the patient's family, they agreed and wished to proceed.

     In the operating room, transverse groin incisions were made in the common femoral and profunda femoral. Superficial femoral arteries were dissected off. Control was obtained. Subsequently on the right, an entry needle was used to access the femoral artery. A guidewire was introduced and a 5-French sheath introduced. Subsequently, a Percor catheter was introduced into the aorta and an aortogram was performed. This revealed patent bilateral renal arteries. Mesenteric artery was patent. The neck of the aneurysm was visible approximately a centimeter and a half below the left renal artery. The large aneurysmal sac was visible as well as bilateral iliac arteries, which were patent. Subsequently, an Amplatz wire was inserted and the 5-French sheath was exchanged for an 18-French sheath. On the left side, the common femoral artery was accessed with an entry needle. A guidewire was introduced and a 5-French sheath introduced. An Amplatz wire was introduced and 5-French sheath was then exchanged for a 12-French sheath. Subsequently to the right, a 26 × 14 × 14 Gore excluder main body trunk was inserted. This was measured from a previous CT scan. After angiographic localization of the left renal artery, the graft was deployed with excellent apposition to the wall, even though there was some tortuosity. The graft was then fully deployed. In order to anchor the graft on the right, the ipsilateral limb was inserted after localization of the hypogastric arteries. An 18 × 10 ipsilateral Gore excluder then was inserted and deployed with appropriate overlap. Subsequently, the left gate was cannulated. Confirmation of cannulation was obtained by spinning a pigtail catheter within the neck of the aneurysm. On the left, after angiographic localization of the hypogastric arteries, an 18 × 14 contralateral limb was inserted and deployed with appropriate overlap. Subsequently, balloon was inserted and the proximal distal attachment sites were ballooned as well as the floor divided. A completion angiogram revealed excellent flow through the excluder graft with no type 1 endo leak. There were multiple arteries visible; however, the aneurysm sac did not fill. The sheath was then withdrawn. The bilateral common femoral arteries were repaired with 5-0 Prolene sutures. There were good Doppler signals distal to the repair with triphasic flow. The groin wounds were irrigated and closed in two layers with 3-0 Vicryl and 4-0 Monocryl subcuticular for the skin. All instrument counts and sponge counts were correct as per the nursing staff. The patient was extubated and transferred to recovery in stable condition.

3. Operative Report

PREOPERATIVE DIAGNOSIS:	Severe three-vessel coronary artery disease
POSTOPERATIVE DIAGNOSIS:	Severe three-vessel coronary artery disease
OPERATION:	Coronary artery bypass grafting ×3, off pump

PROCEDURE DESCRIPTION: The patient was prepped and draped in appropriate manner, having undergone general endotracheal anesthetic. After appropriate time-out and IV antibiotics therapy, a skin incision was made in the standard fashion. I opened the chest and isolated and took down the left internal mammary artery with clips and Bovie cauterization. Papaverine was placed on and in the mammary artery. Endoscopic vein harvest was performed to remove the left saphenous vein. Ties, 4-0, and clips were placed in the vein branches.

Attention was then turned to the artery anastomosis. The left internal mammary was anastomosed to the left circumflex artery and then sequentially to the left anterior descending artery using 7-0 Prolene suture. The reverse saphenous vein graft was then anastomosed to the proximal right coronary artery using an 8-0 Prolene suture. The aorta was side-clamped and the aortotomy and anastomosis were quickly performed. The aorta was unclamped and hemostasis was verified. The mediastinum was irrigated with warm bacitracin solution and a chest tube was placed. Hemostasis was achieved throughout in standard fashion. The pericardium was closed loosely and the sternum was closed with single stranded wires. Running #1, 2-0 and a 4-0 subcuticular stitch were used. Steri-strips and dressing were applied and the patient was transferred to the cardiovascular intensive care unit in stable condition.

4. Operative Report

NOTE: Do not code intraoperative fluoroscopic guidance with this procedure.

PROCEDURE: Placement of a dual chamber pacemaker

INDICATIONS: Patient with symptomatic sick sinus syndrome, bradycardia, alternating with symptomatic palpitations and tachycardia

PROCEDURE DESCRIPTION: After informed consent, the patient is brought to the lab. The procedure was done under conscious sedation, fluoroscopic guidance. One percent Lidocaine was used to anesthetize the skin under the left clavicle and a subcutaneous pocket was made for the pacemaker generator and leads. The left subclavian vein was cannulated twice using a micro puncture set, which was up-sized to regular 035 wire, the position of which was confirmed under fluoro. A 7-French sheath and a 7-French right ventricular lead was used and placed in the right ventricular apex originally and then more proximally in the inferior wall. The numbers were suboptimal, including the R-wave sensing. I then moved the lead to the right ventricular mid to upper septum. The numbers were better. There was no diaphragmatic stimulation, and the lead was sutured down. This was an active fixation lead.

The right atrial lead was then placed using a 7-French sheath under fluoroscopic guidance. The numbers looked good. There was no diaphragmatic stimulation, and the lead was sutured down. The leads were then attached to the generator, which was sutured down in the pocket. Wound irrigated with antibiotic and inspected for hemostasis and closed in layers. Patient tolerated the procedure well without any complication.

5. Operative Report

PREOPERATIVE DIAGNOSIS: Coronary artery disease, left anterior descending coronary artery

POSTOPERATIVE DIAGNOSIS: Coronary artery disease, left anterior descending coronary artery

PROCEDURE PERFORMED: Direct stenting of the proximal-mid left anterior descending coronary artery using 2.7 × 33 mm CYPHER drug-eluting stent, Angio-Seal closure of the left femoral arteriotomy site

PROCEDURE: After a discussion of the risks, benefits, and alternatives to the therapy, informed consent was obtained. The patient was brought to the procedure room and prepped and draped in the sterile fashion. The right femoral artery was accessed and an XXB 3.56 French guide catheter was used. BMW wire was used. Immediately after the origin of the large diagonal branch, there was about 80 percent eccentric LAD disease. Mid and distal LAD otherwise appear to be unremarkable. The CYPHER stent was deployed up to 10 atmospheres, covering the entire moderately diseased proximal segment as well as proximate significant disease, and post dilator with 3.0 × 15 mm POWERSAIL balloon up to 15 atmospheres. Intracoronary nitroglycerin was given. This resulted in a fully deployed stent TIMI 3 flow. No evidence for dissection, thrombosis, or distal embolization. Diagonal branch remained fully patent as well. Guide catheter and the wires were removed. Left femoral arterial sheath was removed. 6 French Angio-Seal deployed. Hemostasis was obtained. No immediate complications were noted. The patient tolerated the procedure well.

6. Operative Report

NOTE: Exclude from coding the use of cardiopulmonary bypass equipment on this case.

PREOPERATIVE DIAGNOSIS: Critical aortic valvular stenosis

POSTOPERATIVE DIAGNOSIS: Critical aortic valvular stenosis

OPERATION: Aortic valve replacement with a 21 mm St. Jude Medical Biocor bioprosthetic porcine valve

PROCEDURE DETAILS: Under general anesthesia, with the chest, abdomen, groin, and lower extremities prepped and draped in a sterile fashion, a median sternotomy incision was made. The sternum was split along the midline using a sternal saw. The Cooley retractor was inserted, and the pericardium was opened. Pericardial stay sutures were placed. The aorta and the right atrium were cannulated in the usual manner. The patient was placed on cardiopulmonary bypass and was cooled to 28 degrees Centigrade. Once on bypass, the aortic crossclamp was applied, and the initial dose of cold oxygenated crystalloid cardioplegia was given via the aortic root, and cold topical saline slush solution was applied, and the initial dose of cold topical saline slush solution was applied to the pericardial well. When the heart was cold and quiet, the right superior pulmonary vein was exposed and opened, and a right angle vent catheter was inserted into this opening. The aorta was opened just above the coronary ostium aortic annulus, and the aortic valve was exposed through this transverse aortotomy. The valve leaflets were heavily calcified and were rigidly mobile. It appeared that the basic structure of the native valve was that of a bicuspid configuration. The leaflets of the valve were excised and the annulus was decalcified using pituitary rongeur forceps. The valve annulus was sized to a 21-mm St. Jude Biocor bioprosthetic porcine valve sizer, and a 21-mm valve was selected. This valve was sewn in place using interrupted 2-0 Tycron pledgeted sutures. Once all of the sutures had been placed, the 21-mm valve seated well in the area of the right coronary, allowing the right coronary to be easily visualized as the sutures were tied. Once all of the sutures had been tied and the sutures cut adjacent to the knots, the aortotomy was closed using a running 4-0 Prolene cardiovascular suture. Once the aortotomy was secured, the vent in the right superior pulmonary vein was removed, and this opening was secured with a 3-0 Tycron pursestring stitch.

The left side of the heart was deaired as the vent was removed, and it was further deaired through the aortic root with a Bengash needle as the aortic crossclamp was removed. Further deairing was also carried out with a 14 gauge Angiocath through the LV apex. The patient was weaned from cardiopulmonary bypass without difficulty. When adequate rewarming had taken place, all cannulation sites were inspected for hemostasis. When safely off bypass, mediastinum was drained with a 36 Argyle tube brought out through a separate stab incision inferiorly. The mediastinum was further inspected for hemostasis. When dry, the sternum was closed using interrupted stainless steel wires to approximate the sterna plates. The fascia was closed with a running 0 Vicryl. The subcutaneous tissue was closed with running 2-0 Vicryl, and the skin was closed with a subcuticular 3-0 Vicryl stitch. Sterile dressings were applied. The patient was then taken to the intensive care unit with stable vital signs.

Chapter 12

Gastrointestinal and Hepatobiliary Systems

This chapter will complete the discussion of the gastrointestinal system and describe procedures performed on the esophagus, stomach, intestines, anus, and rectum. Also included is a discussion of the hepatobiliary system because of its close connection with the gastrointestinal system. The mouth and throat were introduced in chapter 10 with the respiratory system, as they are common to both systems. The second character values for the gastrointestinal system are:

D—Gastrointestinal System
F—Hepatobiliary System and Pancreas

Functions of the Gastrointestinal System

The gastrointestinal system performs six major functions:

- Ingestion of food through the mouth
- Mechanical digestion by chewing food with the teeth and churning and mixing food in the stomach
- Chemical digestion by the addition of saliva by the salivary glands and chemicals by the stomach and liver
- Mixing and propelling movements of swallowing by the pharynx and esophagus and peristalsis from the stomach through the large intestines
- Absorption of nutrients and water by the small intestines and water by the large intestines
- Elimination of indigestible waste products as defecation by the anus (Applegate 2011, 353)

Organization of the Gastrointestinal System

The gastrointestinal system is made up of the mouth, palate, tongue, teeth, salivary glands, pharynx, esophagus, stomach, liver, gallbladder, pancreas, small intestines (duodenum, jejunum, and ileum), large intestines (ileocecal junction, cecum, appendix, ascending colon, transverse colon, descending colon, and sigmoid colon), rectum, and anus. In ICD-10-PCS, these organs are found in three separate systems of the mouth and throat (covered in chapter 10), the gastrointestinal system, and the hepatobiliary system, each with its own set of ICD-10-PCS tables. Figure 12.1 displays the major structures of the gastrointestinal tract from the esophagus to the anus. Also included in the figure is the spleen, to provide orientation to its location in the abdomen in relationship to the stomach and the intestines.

Digestive System

In ICD-10-PCS, the structures of the digestive system affecting procedural code assignment include the following portions of this system: upper intestinal tract, esophagus (upper, middle, lower), esophagogastric junction, stomach, pylorus, small intestine, duodenum, jejunum, ileum, ileocecal valve, lower intestinal tract, large intestine,

Figure 12.1. Gastrointestinal tract

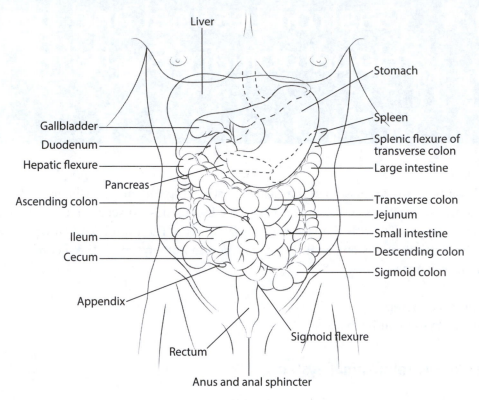

© AHIMA 2019

cecum, appendix, ascending colon, transverse colon, descending colon, sigmoid colon, rectum, anus, anal sphincter, omentum (greater and lesser), mesentery, and peritoneum.

The stomach is the large digestive organ in the thorax where the process of food digestion takes place. The stomach is divided into areas called the cardia, fundus, body, antrum, and pylorus (Rizzo 2016, 385). Figure 12.2 shows the divisions of the stomach. The pylorus is the only division of the stomach that is identified by an individual body part value in ICD-10-PCS.

The digestive tract is a long, tubular structure that is found within the abdominal and peritoneal cavities. The small intestine is a long and narrow tube that loops back and forth within the lower abdomen and is surrounded

Figure 12.2. Stomach

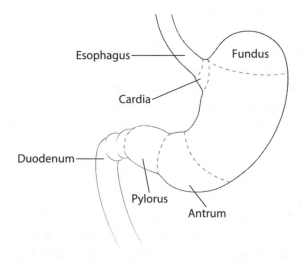

© AHIMA 2019

by the large intestine. These structures stay in place because of the supportive structures of the omentum and the mesentery. The omentum and the mesentery also contain blood vessels and nerves that supply the intestines. The mesentery is a fan-shaped projection of the parietal peritoneum that is found from the lumbar region to the posterior abdominal wall. The greater omentum is a continuation of the serosa of the greater curvature of the stomach and the first part of the duodenum into the transverse colon. The lesser omentum attaches from the liver to the lesser curvature of the stomach and the first part of the duodenum (*Mosby's* 2017, 1025). Figure 12.3 shows a cross-section of the abdomen and pelvis. The mesentery and the omentum can be seen providing support to the tubular structures and helping to maintain the proper position of each part of the digestive system.

Figure 12.3.   Mesentery and omentum

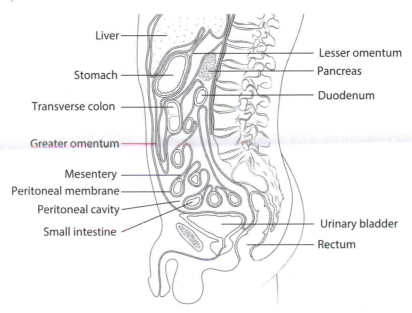

© AHIMA 2019

Additional gastrointestinal structures identified with body part values in ICD-10-PCS that are not displayed in the figures in this chapter are defined here:

- **Esophagogastric junction**—The area covering the terminal portion of esophagus and the beginning of stomach at the cardiac orifice
- **Ileocecal valve**—The valve at the junction of the cecum with the colon that guards the opening where the ileum enters the large intestine
- **Anal sphincter**—The terminal segment of the large intestine, beginning from the ampulla of the rectum and ending at the anus
- **Peritoneum**—A membrane of squamous epithelial cells, the mesothelial cells, covered by apical microvilli that allow rapid absorption of fluid and particles in the peritoneal cavity. The peritoneum is divided into parietal and visceral components. The parietal peritoneum covers the inside of the abdominal wall. The visceral peritoneum covers the intraperitoneal organs. The double-layered peritoneum forms the mesentery that suspends these organs from the abdominal wall (Rizzo 2016, 97).

Anatomy Alert

The peritoneum is a double-layered covering of the intraperitoneal organs that forms the mesentery that suspends the organs from the abdominal wall.

Hepatobiliary System

In ICD-10-PCS, the structures of the hepatobiliary system and pancreas affecting procedural code assignment include the following: liver (right and left lobe), gallbladder, hepatic ducts, cystic duct, common bile duct, hepatobiliary duct, ampulla of Vater, pancreatic duct, accessory pancreatic duct, and pancreas.

Hepatobiliary refers to the liver and bile ducts. Bile ducts are channels that collect and transport the bile secretion from the bile canaliculi, the smallest branch of the biliary tract in the liver, through the bile ductules, through the bile ducts out of the liver, and to the gallbladder for storage (Applegate 2011, 365). An accessory pancreatic duct is an additional duct that may be found in some patients. Figure 12.4 illustrates the relationship between the liver, the gallbladder, the pancreas, the hepatobiliary ducts, and the duodenum.

Figure 12.4. Liver, gallbladder, pancreas, and ducts

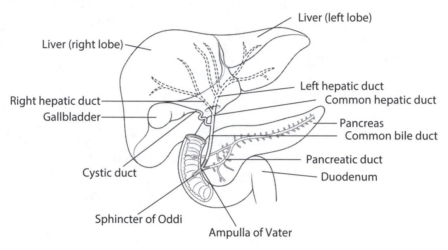

© AHIMA 2019

Common Root Operations Used in Coding of Procedures on the Gastrointestinal System

The gastrointestinal system is comprises tubular body parts. Therefore, these sections of ICD-10-PCS include the root operations of Dilation, Occlusion, and Restriction. Organs in the gastrointestinal tract are transplanted from donors and, therefore, the root operation of Transplantation is included here.

Guideline B3.2c discusses when to code multiple procedures and specifically instructs the coding professional to assign multiple codes when distinct objectives are performed on the same body part. Therefore, if a lesion is destroyed, excised, or resected from a tubular body part, codes are assigned for the removal method. Multiple lesions or polyps removed within the same body part are only coded once per body part. For example, two lesions of the stomach are only coded as one excision with a body part value of 6, Stomach.

When a section of the gastrointestinal system is removed, either by excision or resection, the anastomosis necessary to reconnect the remaining portions of the tubular body part in their correct order is not coded separately, based on Guideline B3.1b. The root operation Bypass is only coded when the route of passage of a tubular body part is altered, meaning that the gastrointestinal system is rerouted to an abnormal route. For example, the Roux-en-Y bariatric procedure creates a bypass between the stomach and the jejunum, causing a rerouting of the contents of the tubular body part. However, not all bariatric procedures are coded with the root operation Bypass. Adjustable gastric banding is coded to the root operation Restriction because the band restricts the size of the stomach. Sleeve gastrectomy procedures actually reduce the size of the stomach by excising the greater curvature and therefore are coded with the root operation Excision. A special qualifier is available to describe this Excision as vertical.

Other common bypass procedures in the gastrointestinal system are the colostomy or the ileostomy procedure where a portion of the intestine is rerouted to the outside of the body. These are traditional bypasses and are therefore coded with the body part value as the origin of the bypass (colon or ileum) and the qualifier coded as the destination of the bypass, qualifier value 4, Cutaneous.

Take-down of a colostomy or ileostomy (patient no longer requires the ostomy) requires two codes because every bypass procedure has two ends. Ostomy take-downs involve repair of the large or small intestine that was previously exteriorized and the open repair of the abdominal wall where the through-and-through connection to the outside is no longer needed.

B3.1b. Components of a procedure specified in the root operation definition and explanation are not coded separately. Procedural steps necessary to reach the operative site and close the operative site, including anastomosis of a tubular body part, are also not coded separately.

Examples: Resection of a joint as part of a joint replacement procedure is included in the root operation definition of Replacement and is not coded separately. Laparotomy performed to reach the site of an open liver biopsy is not coded separately. In a resection of sigmoid colon with anastomosis of descending colon to rectum, the anastomosis is not coded separately.

B3.2c. During the same operative episode, multiple procedures are coded if multiple root operations with distinct objectives are performed on the same body part.

Example: Destruction of sigmoid lesion and bypass of sigmoid colon are coded separately.

Coding Tip

Adjunct information about the anastomotic technique used to complete a colectomy procedure (such as side-to-end or end-to-end) is not specified in ICD-10-PCS. The specific root operation of Destruction, Excision, or Resection is assigned. Bypass is not coded separately if the remaining portions of the gastrointestinal system are reconnected in their proper order.

Assigning root operations to the various myotomy procedures in the gastrointestinal system should be completed by determining the intent of the procedure. The pyloromyotomy procedure is an example of the root operation Dilation because the intent of the procedure is to dilate the pylorus. In a pyloromyotomy, "the surgeon makes an incision in the wall of the pylorus. The lining bulges through the incision, opening a channel from the stomach to the small intestine" (Mayo Clinic 2018a). This assignment is also true for other muscular structures of the gastrointestinal system such as the esophagogastric junction and the anal sphincter. Cutting the muscle to expand the tube is the root operation Dilation. Dilation can also be performed using a balloon, as in treatment of a Schatzki ring, a ring of tightened mucosa in the distal esophagus.

The esophagus may also require Restriction instead of Dilation. The fundoplication procedure can be performed to restrict the esophagogastric junction. Plication means wrapping and a fundoplication is specific to the fundus of the stomach. A Nissen fundoplication is the wrapping of the fundus of the stomach around the esophagogastric junction and the stitching of the stomach onto itself to restrict the junction and help prevent gastroesophageal reflux.

Coding Tip

The root operation Dilation is coded when the objective of the procedure is to enlarge the diameter of a tubular body part or orifice. Dilation includes both intraluminal or extraluminal methods of enlarging the diameter. A device placed to maintain the new diameter is an integral part of the Dilation procedure and is coded to sixth-character device value in the Dilation procedure code. Dilation can also be accomplished by cutting the wall of a tubular body part to achieve the dilation.

Reduction of a volvulus, intussusception, or malrotation of the gastrointestinal system is the root operation of Reposition and is coded to the body part where the abnormality is located. Fixation procedures such as rectopexy, proctopexy, or gastropexy are also coded to the root operation of Reposition because the intent of the procedure is to place the body part into the correct or other suitable location. The fixation itself is the method used to maintain the body part in that position. Enterolysis, or mobilization of intestinal adhesions, is coded to the root operation of Release and the body part value is assigned based on the body part being freed if this is the intent of the procedure. If lysis of adhesions is performed to gain access to a body part, it is part of the approach, such as the open or percutaneous endoscopic approach.

B3.13.   In the root operation Release, the body part value coded is the body part being freed and not the tissue being manipulated or cut to free the body part.

Example: Lysis of intestinal adhesions is coded to the specific intestine body part value.

B3.11c.   When both an Inspection procedure and another procedure are performed on the same body part during the same episode, if the Inspection procedure is performed using a different approach than the other procedure, the Inspection procedure is coded separately.

Example: Endoscopic Inspection of the duodenum is coded separately when open Excision of the duodenum is performed during the same procedural episode.

Ulcer repair is frequently done with an omental patch called a Graham patch. When the surgeon uses an omental patch to repair a peptic ulcer, the patch is not typically disconnected from the omentum. It is pulled up to cover the perforated ulcer and stitched in place. In ICD-10-PCS, when the patch material is not completely disconnected from the source, it does not qualify as a device. The repair using the local tissue that is stitched in place is the root operation of Repair. Because the tissue was not harvested and made into a device for the procedure, it cannot be coded to the root operation of Supplement. When a body part is restored without the use of a device, it is Repair. When a body part is restored with the use of a device, it is Supplement.

Be sure to research any procedure that is unfamiliar to ensure correct coding. If the documentation includes an eponym (procedure named for a person) and the intent of the procedure is unclear, query the physician for specifics.

Body Parts for the Gastrointestinal and Hepatobiliary Systems

The Upper Intestinal Tract, body part value 0, includes organs above the diaphragm plus the stomach and duodenum below the diaphragm. The Lower Intestinal Tract, body part value D, includes organs below the diaphragm starting with the jejunum. These two body part values have limited use for procedures involving the root operations of Change, Removal, Inspection, and Revision. The esophagus is divided into the three parts of upper, middle, and lower in the tables for some root operations. The upper esophagus is also called the cervical esophagus. The middle esophagus is also called the thoracic esophagus. The lower esophagus is also called abdominal esophagus.

B4.8.   In the Gastrointestinal body system, the general body part values Upper Intestinal Tract and Lower Intestinal Tract are provided as an option for the root operations Change, Inspection, Removal, and Revision. Upper Intestinal Tract includes the portion of the gastrointestinal tract from the esophagus down to and including the duodenum, and Lower Intestinal Tract includes the portion of the gastrointestinal tract from the jejunum down to and including the rectum and anus.

Example: In the root operation Change table, change of a device in the jejunum is coded using the body part Lower Intestinal Tract.

The large intestine is the site of many types of procedures. Surgeons use terms such as right hemicolectomy, left hemicolectomy, and colectomy. Body part value F, Large Intestine, Right is a combination body part including a small portion of the terminal ileum, the ileocecal valve, appendix, cecum, ascending colon, and the transverse colon to the right of the midline (Mayo Clinic 2018b). Body part value G, Large Intestine, Left is a combination body part including the transverse colon to the left of midline, descending and the sigmoid colon. Body part value E, Large Intestine contains all of the parts of the large intestine (Mayo Clinic 2018c).

Table 12.1 lists the body part values associated with the gastrointestinal and hepatobiliary systems. If the documentation includes specific body part names that are not included in these lists, refer to the body part key for other body part synonyms and alternative terms.

Coding Tip

The body part values of 0 for Upper intestinal tract and D for Lower intestinal tract have limited use for procedures involving the root operations of Change, Removal, Inspection, and Revision. Upper and lower intestinal tract are not synonymous with small and large intestines. Upper intestinal tract ends at the duodenum and lower intestinal tract start at the jejunum.

Table 12.1.   Body parts in the Gastrointestinal and Hepatobiliary systems

Body Part Value	Body Parts—Gastrointestinal System (D)	Body Part Value	Body Parts—Hepatobiliary System and Pancreas (F)
0	Upper Intestinal Tract	0	Liver
1	Esophagus, Upper	1	Liver, Right Lobe
2	Esophagus, Middle	2	Liver, Left Lobe
3	Esophagus, Lower	4	Gallbladder
4	Esophageal Junction	5	Hepatic Duct, Right
5	Esophagus	6	Hepatic Duct, Left
6	Stomach	7	Hepatic Duct, Common
7	Stomach, Pylorus	8	Cystic Duct
8	Small Intestine	9	Common Bile Duct
9	Duodenum	B	Hepatobiliary Duct
A	Jejunum	C	Ampulla Of Vater
B	Ileum	D	Pancreatic Duct
C	Ileocecal Valve	F	Pancreatic Duct, Accessory
D	Lower Intestinal Tract	G	Pancreas
E	Large Intestine		
F	Large Intestine, Right		
G	Large Intestine, Left		
H	Cecum		
J	Appendix		
K	Ascending Colon		
L	Transverse Colon		
M	Descending Colon		
N	Sigmoid Colon		
P	Rectum		
Q	Anus		
R	Anal Sphincter		
U	Omentum		
V	Mesentery		
W	Peritoneum		

Anatomy Alert

The pylorus is the only portion of the stomach that is identified with an individual body part value in ICD-10-PCS.

Approaches Used for the Gastrointestinal and Hepatobiliary Systems

The gastrointestinal system contains two natural body openings; therefore, the approaches of Via Natural or Artificial Opening and Via Natural or Artificial Opening, Endoscopic are extremely common in procedures performed on this system. Open procedures performed with the assistance of instruments in a percutaneous endoscopic approach are coded to Open based on Guideline B5. At the completion of the procedure, the laparoscopic instruments and trocars are still in the abdomen. The completion of the procedure takes place through a separate open incision. In this procedure, the approach value would be 0, Open. In a laparoscopic converted to open procedure, the trocars are removed when the conversion decision takes place. In this procedure, two codes are assigned, as indicated in Guideline B.3.2d. One code is assigned for the Inspection with a percutaneous endoscopic approach and another code is assigned for the definitive procedure with an Open approach. To visualize the difference between a percutaneous endoscopic and open cholecystectomy, refer to figure 1.2 in chapter 1.

B5.2. Procedures performed using the Open approach with percutaneous endoscopic assistance are coded to the approach Open.

Example: Laparoscopic-assisted sigmoidectomy is coded to the approach Open.

The gastrointestinal system also contains approach value F, Via Natural or Artificial Opening with Percutaneous Endoscopic Assistance for use in coding the Excision or Resection of a portion of the large intestine through the anal opening with the assistance of a laparoscope. The procedure is called a rectal pull-through, and the laparoscopes and instruments are used to disconnect the structures that hold the intestines in place, such as the mesentery or arteries and veins. Once the intestines are loosened from their attachments, they are pulled out through the rectum and anus until a point past the level of disease. The intestine is then disconnected at the level of the rectum or proximal anus and removed. The healthy intestine is then anastomosed to the remaining rectum or anus to complete the procedure. This process can be visualized as the technique used to pull a sleeve lining out through the wrist hole in the sleeve, with the lining then cut and resewn to the remaining sleeve lining. Figure 1.6 in chapter 1 shows this approach when assigned for a laparoscopic-assisted vaginal hysterectomy, which uses a very similar technique.

Devices Common to the Gastrointestinal System

When a patient cannot eat through the oral route, feeding tube insertion is required and is coded to the location where the tip of the tube comes to rest with the Insertion root operation. Feeding tubes are typically inserted into either the stomach or the jejunum, but the 0DH table allows for placement in multiple places in the gastrointestinal system. A gastrostomy (G-tube) is the common feeding tube placement. The physician may refer to this as a "percutaneous endoscopic gastrostomy" or PEG tube because the insertion of the G-tube is done with the assistance of the scope. However, in ICD-10-PCS, the approach value is 3, Percutaneous, because the tube is not delivered into the stomach through the endoscope. The endoscope helps determine the best placement for the tube. This is coded as 0DH63UZ.

A jejunostomy tube is a feeding tube placed through the skin directly into the jejunum when the stomach cannot be used for digestion. This tube may be placed with the assistance of a laparoscope, but the tube is not delivered through the skin with the scope. This is coded as 0DHA3UZ.

A combination gastrostomy and jejunostomy feeding tube, called a PEG/J or a G-J tube, is another option available for patients. These tubes are placed in the stomach like a regular PEG tube but have a special internal channel that holds the jejunostomy tube within the lumen of the PEG tube. The PEG is placed first, and the J-tube is threaded through the special PEG. The J-port is used for feeding and the G-port is used for venting, trial feeding, or medications. The PEG/J tube insertion is coded to 0DH63UZ and 0DHA7UZ because the J-tube is inserted through the opening previously made by the G-tube. The advantage of the G-J tube is only one opening is created into the abdomen.

Esophageal airways, also called gastric tube airways or obturator airways, are inserted through the mouth and placed into the esophagus. The inflatable bulb that rests in the esophagus blocks air entry into the gastro-intestinal tract and forces air into the trachea from the pump and mask. These are coded to the device value, B, Intraluminal device, airway.

Muscle damage or laxity, pelvic floor dysfunction, or previous surgical interventions can all cause fecal incontinence. To help restore bowel control, an artificial anal sphincter can be inserted. Figure 12.5 is a drawing of the artificial sphincter device, placed to restore bowel continence. The device has an internal pump that is used to move fluid from the balloon reservoir into the artificial sphincter cuff to maintain continence. When released, the fluid returns to the reservoir to allow the bowels to empty. The sphincter cuff is placed around the anus and the pump and reservoir are placed in the subcutaneous layer of the perineum.

Figure 12.5.   Artificial sphincter device

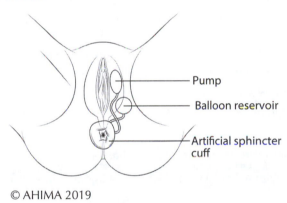

Pump

Balloon reservoir

Artificial sphincter cuff

© AHIMA 2019

When the nerves to the anal sphincter are damaged, a stimulator lead can be inserted to trigger muscle contraction and relaxation with a stimulator generator placed into the back or abdomen. A gastric stimulator acts like a pacemaker for the stomach. It is a two-part device with the stimulator generator implanted into a subcutaneous pocket of the abdomen near the stomach using an open approach and two stimulator leads tunneled percutaneously to the surface of the stomach. Table 12.2 lists the device values associated with the gastrointestinal system.

Table 12.2.   Devices for the Gastrointestinal and Hepatobiliary systems

Device Value	Devices—Gastrointestinal System (D)	Device Value	Devices—Hepatobiliary System (F)
0	Drainage Device	0	Drainage Device
1	Radioactive Element	1	Radioactive Element
2	Monitoring Device	2	Monitoring Device
3	Infusion Device	3	Infusion Device
7	Autologous Tissue Substitute	7	Autologous Tissue Substitute
B	Intraluminal Device, Airway	C	Extraluminal Device

(Continued)   *(Continued)*

Table 12.2. Devices for the Gastrointestinal and Hepatobiliary systems (continued)

Device Value	Devices—Gastrointestinal System (D)	Device Value	Devices—Hepatobiliary System (F)
C	Extraluminal Device	D	Intraluminal Device
D	Intraluminal Device	J	Synthetic Substitute
J	Synthetic Substitute	K	Nonautologous Tissue Substitute
K	Nonautologous Tissue Substitute	Y	Other Device
L	Artificial Sphincter	Z	No Device
M	Stimulator Lead		
U	Feeding Device		
Y	Other Device		
Z	No Device		

Qualifiers Used in the Gastrointestinal and Hepatobiliary Systems

The qualifiers used in the gastrointestinal system are used with the root operations of Bypass, Transfer, and Transplantation. The qualifiers in the hepatobiliary system and pancreas body system are used with the root operations of Bypass, Destruction and Transplantation. The qualifier of Irreversible Electroporation (IRE) is used to describe a destruction technique of using micro-electrical pulses to destroy the cell wall. The pulses make the cell wall porous, which causes cell death. Both systems use the standard qualifiers of X for Diagnostic or Z, No Qualifier. Table 12.3 lists the qualifiers in use in these body systems.

B3.6a. Bypass procedures are coded by identifying the body part bypassed "from" and the body part bypassed "to." The fourth character body part specifies the body part bypassed from, and the qualifier specifies the body part bypassed to.

Example: Bypass from stomach to jejunum; stomach is the body part and jejunum is the qualifier.

Table 12.3. Qualifiers for the Gastrointestinal and Hepatobiliary systems

Qualifier Value	Qualifiers—Gastrointestinal System (D)	Qualifier Value	Qualifiers—Hepatobiliary System (F)
0	Allogeneic	0	Allogeneic
1	Syngeneic	1	Syngeneic
2	Zooplastic	2	Zooplastic
3	Vertical	3	Duodenum
4	Cutaneous	4	Stomach
5	Esophagus	5	Hepatic Duct, Right
6	Stomach	6	Hepatic Duct, Left
9	Duodenum	7	Hepatic Duct, Caudate
A	Jejunum	8	Cystic Duct
B	Ileum	9	Common Bile Duct
H	Cecum	B	Small Intestine
K	Ascending Colon	C	Large Intestine
L	Transverse Colon	F	Irreversible Electroporation

(Continued)   *(Continued)*

Table 12.3. Qualifiers for the Gastrointestinal and Hepatobiliary systems (continued)

Qualifier Value	Qualifiers—Gastrointestinal System (D)	Qualifier Value	Qualifiers—Hepatobiliary System (F)
M	Descending Colon	X	Diagnostic
N	Sigmoid Colon	Z	No Qualifier
P	Rectum		
Q	Anus		
X	Diagnostic		
Z	No Qualifier		

 Code Building

Case #1:

PROCEDURE STATEMENT: Cauterization of a peptic erosion

ADDITIONAL INFORMATION: The erosion is cauterized using a gastroscope to promote healing.

ROOT AND INDEX ENTRIES FOR THE STATEMENT: Destruction is the root operation performed in this procedure, defined as physical eradication of all or a portion of a body part by the direct use of energy, force, or a destructive agent. The Index entry is:

Destruction

   Stomach   0D56

Code Characters:

Section	Body System	Root Operation	Body Part	Approach	Device	Qualifier
Medical and Surgical	Gastrointestinal System	Destruction	Stomach	Via Natural of Artificial Opening, Endoscopic	No Device	No Qualifier
0	D	5	6	8	Z	Z

RATIONALE FOR THE ANSWER: Cauterization is the root operation Destruction. A peptic erosion is found in the stomach. Body part value 6, Stomach is assigned. The approach value 8, Via Natural or Artificial Opening, Endoscopic describes the use of the gastroscope to perform the procedure. No device value or qualifier value are appropriate for this code. If the ulcer was the source of acute bleeding, the root operation of Control would have been assigned. For this case, the correct code assignment is 0D568ZZ.

Case #2:

PROCEDURE STATEMENT: Pancreas transplant

ADDITIONAL INFORMATION: The procedure is performed using an open approach, and the native pancreas is not removed. The organ is from an unrelated, matched donor.

ROOT AND INDEX ENTRIES FOR THE STATEMENT: Transplantation is the root operation performed in this procedure, defined as putting in or on all or a portion of a living body part taken from another individual or animal to physically take the place and/or function of all or a portion of a similar body part. The Index entry is:

Transplantation

  Pancreas   0FYG0Z

Code Characters:

Section	Body System	Root Operation	Body Part	Approach	Device	Qualifier
Medical and Surgical	Hepatobiliary System and Pancreas	Transplantation	Pancreas	Open	No Device	Allogeneic
0	F	Y	G	0	Z	0

RATIONALE FOR THE ANSWER: The index provides 6 of the 7 characters as 0FYG0Z. The qualifier of 0, Allogeneic is assigned because the organ was from a matched donor. The correct code assignment is 0FYG0Z0.

Case #3:

PROCEDURE STATEMENT: Adhesiolysis

ADDITIONAL INFORMATION: There are adhesions of the lower esophagus to the diaphragm causing painful respiration and swallowing. The percutaneous endoscopic approach is used.

ROOT AND INDEX ENTRIES FOR THE STATEMENT: Release is the root operation performed in this procedure, defined as freeing a body part from an abnormal physical constraint causing symptoms. The Index entry is:

Release

Esophagus   0DN5

        Lower   0DN3

        Middle   0DN2

        Upper   0DN1

Code Characters:

Section	Body System	Root Operation	Body Part	Approach	Device	Qualifier
Medical and Surgical	Gastrointestinal System	Release	Esophagus, Lower	Percutaneous Endoscopic	No Device	No Qualifier
0	D	N	3	4	Z	Z

RATIONALE FOR THE ANSWER: The root operation Release is used to code lysis of adhesions because the adhesions are an abnormal physical constraint. The body part value 3, Esophagus, lower is coded because that is the body part being released. The percutaneous endoscopic approach value is 4. No device value or qualifier value is appropriate for this code. The correct code assignment is 0DN34ZZ.

Code Building Exercises

Work through each case and check your answers using the answer key in appendix B of the textbook before going on to the Check Your Understanding questions that follow.

Exercise 1:

PREOPERATIVE DIAGNOSIS: Gastroesophageal reflux disease with unsatisfactory medical management

POSTOPERATIVE DIAGNOSIS: Same

OPERATION PERFORMED: Nissen Fundoplication

DESCRIPTION OF OPERATION: The patient is brought to the operating room and placed under general endotracheal anesthesia. The patient was prepped and draped in standard fashion. We made a periumbilical incision, passed the Veress needle, insufflated with carbon dioxide passed the trocars. I made two counter incisions in the left upper quadrant and one in the right upper quadrant.

We grasped the stomach with the grasper, folded it posteriorly and made a circumferential 360-degree wrap around the gastroesophageal junction, tacking it from the left fundus to the esophagus to the right fundus. We used three sutures like this and then we used two EndoStitches to tack the stomach to the left diaphragm and then to the right diaphragm to minimize the chance of gastric torsion or herniation.

This fundoplication was performed over the bougie and we were very satisfied with the result. We ensured that hemostasis was adequate and removed the trocars. We used deep fascial sutures and the subcuticular stitch for the skin. The patient was taken to PACU in good condition.

Questions:

1.1. What is the intent of this procedure?

_____

1.2. Which root operation is assigned?

_____

1.3. What code(s) should be assigned?

_____

Exercise 2:

PRE-OPERATIVE DX: Pneumoperitoneum

POST-OPERATIVE DX: Perforated Gastric Ulcer with enteric peritonitis

PROCEDURE:
1. Diagnostic Laparoscopy
2. Laparoscopic Oversew of Gastric Ulcer with Graham Patch

INDICATIONS: Pt is a 62-year-old female who presented with 5 hours of severe, acute epigastric pain. Abdominal films revealed possible free air under the diaphragm.

PROCEDURE: The patient was taken to the OR in the supine position. She was then placed under general anesthesia and intubated. Entry into the abdomen was obtained with a 2.0 cm incision just inferior to the umbilicus. Scopes were inserted.

Upon inspection of the stomach, there was purulent fluid in the right upper quadrant around the liver and stomach. The suction irrigator was used to suction out the purulent fluid. There was an obvious ulcer on the anterior stomach in the pre-pyloric position. The edges of the ulcer were then cleaned and the ulcer was then oversewn with three 3-0 Vicryl sutures in figure of eight fashion. The needles were left on the figure of eight sutures and omentum was pulled over the ulcer to buttress it. The Vicryl sutures were placed through the omentum and tied over the ulcer to create a Graham Patch. A temporary wound drain was brought out through the RUQ port. Ports were removed and sites closed with a 0 Vicryl using an endoclose technique.

Questions:

2.1. Research the Graham Patch to determine how the procedure is performed. Is the Graham Patch a device in ICD-10-PCS and why or why not?

_____

2.2. What root operation would you assign for the oversewing of the gastric ulcer? Why?

_____

2.3. What code(s) would be assigned?

_____

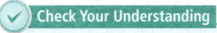
Check Your Understanding

Coding Knowledge Check

1. A colonoscopy without an additional procedure is coded as which root operation?
   a. Excision
   b. Inspection
   c. Introduction
   d. Map

2. Reduction of a volvulus is coded to the root operation _____.

3. Laparoscopic removal of an infected suture from the mesentery is coded as
   a. 0DBV0ZX
   b. 0DBV4ZZ
   c. 0DCV3ZZ
   d. 0DCV4ZZ

4. Insertion of an artificial anal sphincter is coded as _____.
   a. 0DHQ0LZ
   b. 0DHQ3LZ
   c. 0DHE0LZ
   d. 0DHR4LZ

5. The cystic duct connects the _____ and the _____.

Procedure Statement Coding

Assign ICD-10-PCS codes to the following procedure statements and scenarios. List the root operation selected and the code assigned.

1. Drainage of infected gallbladder with placement of drainage device, done laparoscopically

_____

2. Open right hemicolectomy

_____

3. Creation of a colostomy at the descending colon level, open approach

4. An open Kasai procedure was performed to treat biliary atresia. The jejunum was connected to the common hepatic duct at the base of the liver.

5. Open pyloromyotomy for stenosis

6. Rectal pull-through procedure was performed for resection of all of the sigmoid colon and excision of some of the descending colon with the assistance of a laparoscope.

7. Placement of a GI tube endoscopically into the jejunum for parenteral nutrition through the nose

8. Laparoscopic appendectomy

9. Extracorporeal shock wave lithotripsy of common bile duct stone

10. Open suturing of a liver laceration

Case Studies

Assign ICD-10-PCS codes to the following case studies.

1. Operative Report

PREOPERATIVE DIAGNOSIS: Pyloric stenosis

POSTOPERATIVE DIAGNOSIS: Pyloric stenosis

OPERATION: Laparoscopic pyloromyotomy

INDICATIONS: This baby has been having emesis since birth and it has been projectile at times. The mother has done an exceptional job of keeping the baby hydrated with stable weight by breastfeeding almost around the clock. Upper GI and ultrasound have both confirmed the presence of pyloric stenosis. Therefore, we are exploring to confirm the diagnosis and to perform a pyloromyotomy.

PROCEDURE: The patient was prepped and draped in the usual sterile fashion. A small incision was made in the infraumbilical location and a Kocher used to grasp the fascia. A Veress needle was then introduced into the abdomen and the abdomen insufflated to 10 cm of pressure after confirmation with a saline test. We then brought in a 3-mm trocar to this location and secured it in place with a nylon suture. The camera was then brought in and did confirm the diagnosis. Stab incisions were made in the left upper quadrant and right upper quadrant for placement of the arthrotomy knife in the left and a grasper in the right.

We held the duodenum and then used the arthrotomy knife to create a pyloromyotomy. It was very difficult to spread this pyloromyotomy once we had adequate incision made. The tissue was not quite the same as a normal pylorus but, clearly, this baby had pyloric stenosis. We had it adequately spread using a pyloric spreader through the left upper quadrant incision. We performed the test to confirm that half of the ring was independent and then we also had the anesthesiologist insufflate with air to be sure a perforation did not exist. When both of these tests were satisfactory, we then removed all of our devices and allowed the abdomen to desufflate. The incision over the umbilicus was then closed with a 4-0 Vicryl followed by Dermabond at each site. The patient was awoken in the operating room and taken to recovery in satisfactory condition.

2. Operative Report

PREOPERATIVE DIAGNOSIS: Carcinoma of the sigmoid colon

POSTOPERATIVE DIAGNOSIS: Carcinoma of the sigmoid colon

OPERATION: Sigmoid colon resection

INDICATION: This is a 71-year-old white female who has history of lung cancer who had some change in bowel habits, had a colonoscopy, and was found to have a sigmoid colon cancer at 30 cm. The patient had partial resection of a polypoid lesion that revealed an infiltrating carcinoma in a villous adenoma. The lesion was not completely resected, and surgical resection is recommended at this time.

OPERATION: The patient was brought to the operating room, prepped, and draped in the usual fashion. A lower midline incision was used. On exploring, the abdomen, liver, gallbladder, pancreas, stomach, and small bowel were normal. The patient's uterus, ovaries, and fallopian tubes were normal also. The patient had a firm lesion in the distal sigmoid colon just above the peritoneal reflection. The sigmoid colon was mobilized, the left ureter was identified, and the sigmoid colon was then resected, dividing the colon at the junction between the sigmoid colon and the rectum with a roticulating stapler, taking the mesentery of the sigmoid colon, dividing it proximally at approximately 7–10 cm proximal to the lesion. In doing this, the patient had a large amount of redundant sigmoid colon and we were able to do a side-to-side anastomosis between the upper rectum and the proximal sigmoid colon. This was done with a GI stapler and the roticulating stapler, as well. Once this was completed, the wound was irrigated and good hemostasis was obtained, the incision was closed with #1 Vicryl for the fascia, and staples were used for the skin. The patient tolerated the procedure well.

3. Operative Report

PREOPERATIVE DIAGNOSES: 1. Respiratory failure

                                     2. Intracranial hemorrhage

POSTOPERATIVE DIAGNOSES: 1. Respiratory failure

                                     2. Intracranial hemorrhage

PROCEDURE PERFORMED: 1. Tracheostomy tube

                                     2. Percutaneous endoscopic gastrostomy placement

DESCRIPTION OF PROCEDURE: The patient was a head injury with a bleed, unable to be successfully weaned from the vent. The risks and benefits of PEG and tracheostomy were explained to the patient's family. Consent was obtained. The patient was brought to the operating room and laid in the supine position on the operating room table. General endotracheal anesthesia was administered by the anesthesia department. The area around the neck was first draped and prepped in the usual sterile fashion. Using #15 scalpel a vertical incision was made above the sternal notch. Dissection was carried down through subcutaneous tissue, splitting the strap muscles and easily identifying the trach. Two stay sutures of Vicryl suture material were placed on each side of the trach. The trach was pulled farther into the field, and then a cut was made between the first and second tracheal rings. The endotracheal tube was removed and a #8 cuffed Shiley tracheostomy tube was placed without difficulty into the trachea. Once this was completed the trach was secured in all quadrants. The skin incision was further closed using nylon suture and good end-tidal CO_2 was noted. The trach was in good position. The patient was saturating at 100 percent. Once the trach was secured with trach ties, our attention was then turned to the patient's abdomen. An endoscope was passed into the patient's stomach. The stomach was easily transilluminated through the abdominal wall. A percutaneous stick was made into the stomach through the abdominal wall. A wire was then placed into the stomach and grasped and pulled out through the patient's mouth. The feeding tube was then secured and then pulled back in through the scope and pulled into the patient's stomach, where it was secured in place. We then confirmed that the PEG tube was in appropriate position in the stomach. The tube was then secured in place to the patient's skin with silk suture. Clean sterile dressings were applied. The patient was transferred back to the intensive care unit in critical but stable condition.

4. Operative Report

PREOPERATIVE DIAGNOSIS:	Obstruction of the rectum in patient with known colon cancer
POSTOPERATIVE DIAGNOSIS:	Obstruction of the rectum due to compression from tumor
OPERATION PERFORMED:	Diverting transverse loop colostomy

INDICATION FOR PROCEDURE: The patient is a 45-year-old white female who underwent a sigmoid colectomy approximately 18 months ago for colon cancer and then underwent adjuvant therapy. She presents today with crampy abdominal pain and underwent CT of the abdomen which demonstrated peritoneal implants as well as tumor in her pelvis and large tumor growth near her rectum.

PROCEDURE: After informed consent was obtained, the patient was taken to the OR and place in the supine position. After successful induction of general endotracheal anesthesia, the patient's abdomen was prepped and draped in the sterile fashion. A #10 blade was used to make a small transverse incision overlying a mark in the left upper quadrant which had been marked preoperatively. Dissection was taken down through the subcutaneous tissue to the level of the fascia which was divided sharply in the lateral aspect of the rectus abdominis muscle and also divided with the electrocautery. The peritoneum was entered and extended the length of the incision. The transverse colon was readily identified and this was grasped and mobilized into the wound. The omentum was dissected off of the colon and a mesenteric defect created and a stomal rod passed underneath the colon, thus supporting the loop up into the wound. The electrocautery was then used to make a transverse opening in the colon and then the ostomy was matured using interrupted 3-0 Vicryl sutures in a standard fashion. A suction was then placed down each limb of the loop colostomy to allow for decompression. A colostomy appliance was then applied. The patient tolerated the procedure well and was awakened and extubated without difficulty. She was taken to the PACU in stable condition.

5. Operative Report

PREOPERATIVE DIAGNOSIS:	Acute dysphagia
POSTOPERATIVE DIAGNOSIS:	Foreign body in esophagus, removed
PROCEDURE:	EGD

INDICATION FOR PROCEDURE: The patient presents with acute dysphagia following ingestion of egg roll and chicken last night. He has a background history of hesitancy of swallowing and a remote history some 30 years ago of some sort of balloon dilation.

PROCEDURE: With the patient in the left lateral decubitus position, the Olympus Video Endoscope was atraumatically inserted by mouth and advanced into the esophagus. In the distal esophagus, a foreign body was identified. This appeared to be meat. The endoscope was advanced to the area and the foreign body gently pushed into the stomach without difficulty. Inspection of the stomach revealed florid erosions in the gastric antrum. A biopsy was taken in the stomach for Helicobacter status. The duodenum appeared normal. The endoscope was then withdrawn. Inspection of the lower esophagus revealed some inflammatory change. It was difficult to know whether this was simply a contact trauma secondary to the meat infection or whether he has mild esophagitis. The patient tolerated the procedure well and was sent to recovery in good condition.

6. Operative Report

PROCEDURE NAME:	Sphincterotomy and stone extraction
INDICATION FOR PROCEDURE:	Paroxysmal right upper quadrant pain associated with disturbed liver function that is post-cholecystectomy

PROCEDURE DESCRIPTION: The Olympus Video side-viewing duodenoscope was atraumatically introduced into esophagus and advanced with slide-by technique into the stomach. The gastric mucosa was normal. The pyloric channel was normal and easily intubated. The first and second parts of the duodenum were visualized. The ampulla appeared normal. Initial cannulation with a precurved catheter revealed a normal pancreatic duct. A single injection was made into the pancreas. Repositioning was accomplished with the assistance of a straight 0.035 guidewire and free cannulation of the common duct was obtained, revealing a large multifaceted free floating stone within the common bile duct. The intrahepatic biliary system appeared normal. The extrahepatic biliary system appeared dilated. An exchange was made with a 20-mm sphincterotome and a sphincterotomy was performed with perfect hemostasis. The duct was then swept with a 15-mm stone extraction balloon and the stone was pulled into the duodenal lumen and removed. The duct was "swept" 2 more times with negative results. The procedure was terminated with the patient in satisfactory condition and she was returned to the recovery area for observation.

ASSESSMENT: Choledocholithiasis associated with recurring obstruction and biliary colic in a post-cholecystectomy patient.

Chapter 13

Endocrine and Lymphatic Systems

This chapter will cover the subjects of the endocrine and lymphatic systems for coding in ICD-10-PCS. These systems are both fairly small but serve unique and important functions in the body. The endocrine system releases hormones that direct functions of the body, and the lymphatic system drains fluid from the tissues and helps to protect the body from disease. The endocrine system is covered first, followed by the lymphatic system. The 2nd character values for these systems are:

G—Endocrine System
7—Lymphatic and Hemic Systems

Functions of the Endocrine System

The endocrine system consists of a series of small glands that secrete hormones into the blood. Even though these glands are small, they are very powerful in their effects on the remainder of the body. The endocrine glands regulate body activities by producing hormones that influence those cells that have receptor sites for that hormone (Applegate 2011, 225).

Organization of the Endocrine System

The endocrine glands consist of the pituitary, the pineal body, the thyroid and parathyroids, the adrenals, the Islets of Langerhans found in the pancreas, and the gonads found in the testes and ovaries (Rizzo 2016, 285). Some hormone-secreting organs considered to be part of the endocrine system are found in other sections of ICD-10-PCS. These include the hypothalamus located with the central nervous system, the pancreas with the hepatobiliary system, the ovary with the female reproductive system, and the testes with the male reproductive system. Figure 13.1 shows the location of the structures associated with the endocrine system.

Additional body parts not displayed in figure 13.1, their synonyms, and their locations are:

- **Carotid body (glomus caroticum, intercarotid body, nodulus caroticus)**—"A small structure containing neural tissue at the bifurcation of the carotid arteries. It monitors the pressure and oxygen content of the blood and therefore assists in regulating blood pressure and respiratory rate." (*Mosby's* 2017, 300)
- **Para-aortic body (corpus glomera aortica, aortic body, organs of Zuckerkandl)**—"One of several small structures on the arch of the aorta that contain neural tissue sensitive to the chemical composition of arterial blood." (*Mosby's* 2017, 121)
- **Coccygeal glomus (corpus coccygeum, arteriococcygeal gland or body)**—"A small group of arterioles connecting directly to veins and having a rich nerve supply." (*Mosby's* 2017, 770)
- **Glomus jugulare**—"An ovoid body found in the adventitia of the upper part of the superior bulb of the internal jugular vein" (*Dorland's* 2012, 235)
- **Paraganglion extremity**—Paraganglia structure found along the iliac and femoral vessels, particularly around the iliac bifurcation

Figure 13.1. Endocrine system

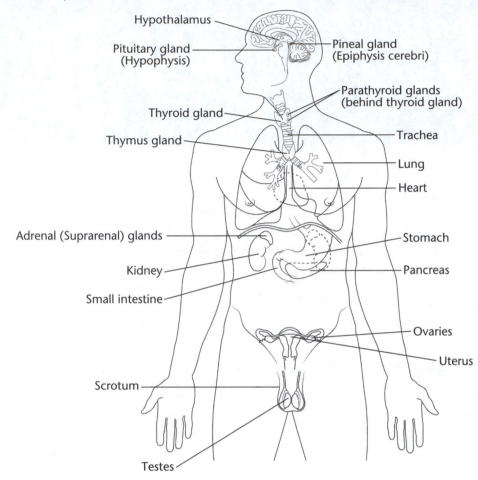

© AHIMA 2019

Common Root Operations Used in Coding Procedures on the Endocrine System

The endocrine system contains small, isolated organs that do not have ducts. Therefore, there are no root operations that describe procedures on tubular body parts. In addition, endocrine glands are not transplanted, and therefore Transplantation is not an available root operation. The most common root operations performed on endocrine structures are Excision (both diagnostic and therapeutic) and Resection. Be sure to research any procedure that is unfamiliar to assure correct coding. If the documentation includes an eponym (procedure named for a person) and the intent of the procedure is unclear, query the physician for specifics.

Body Part Values for the Endocrine System

In ICD-10-PCS, the structures of the endocrine system affecting procedural code assignment include the following portions of this system: pituitary gland, pineal body, adrenal gland, carotid body, para-aortic body, coccygeal glomus, glomus jugulare, aortic body, paraganglion extremity, thyroid gland, superior parathyroid gland, inferior parathyroid gland, and the generic term "endocrine gland." Additional organs, such as the ovaries and testes, are classified in other body systems. Table 13.1 lists the body parts within the endocrine system in ICD-10-PCS. If the documentation includes specific body part names that are not included in this list, refer to the body part key for other body part synonyms and alternative terms.

Table 13.1. **Body parts in the Endocrine system**

Body Part Value	Body Parts—Endocrine System (G)
0	Pituitary Gland
1	Pineal Body
2	Adrenal Gland, Left
3	Adrenal Gland, Right
4	Adrenal Glands, Bilateral
5	Adrenal Gland
6	Carotid Body, Left
7	Carotid Body, Right
8	Carotid Bodies, Bilateral
9	Para-aortic Body
B	Coccygeal Glomus
C	Glomus Jugulare
D	Aortic Body
F	Paraganglion Extremity
G	Thyroid Gland, Lobe, Left
H	Thyroid Gland, Lobe, Right
J	Thyroid Gland Isthmus
K	Thyroid Gland
L	Superior Parathyroid Gland, Right
M	Superior Parathyroid Gland, Left
N	Inferior Parathyroid Gland, Right
P	Inferior Parathyroid Gland, Left
Q	Parathyroid Glands, Multiple
R	Parathyroid Gland
S	Endocrine Gland

Anatomy Alert

The carotid body is not part of the carotid artery. It is a small epithelioid structure located just above the bifurcation of the common carotid artery on each side.

Approaches Used in the Endocrine System

The endocrine glands are completely enclosed within the body and are not accessible except through the skin. Therefore, the approaches of Open, Percutaneous, and Percutaneous endoscopic are available for coding in the endocrine system. The External approach is used when changing, removing, or revising a device within the endocrine system.

Devices Common to the Endocrine System

The endocrine system has a limited number of devices that can be placed during a procedure. Drainage, monitoring, and infusion devices are classified with device values. The standard device values of Y, Other Device, and Z, No Device are also available. Table 13.2 shows the device values available for coding procedures performed on the endocrine system.

Table 13.2. Devices for the Endocrine system	
Device Value	**Devices—Endocrine System (G)**
0	Drainage Device
2	Monitoring Device
3	Infusion Device
Y	Other Device
Z	No Device

Qualifiers for the Endocrine System

There are no unique qualifier values assigned for the endocrine system. Table 13.3 shows that only the standard qualifiers of X, Diagnostic and Z, No Qualifier are available for use in coding procedures performed on the endocrine system.

Table 13.3. Qualifiers for the Endocrine system	
Qualifier Value	**Qualifiers—Endocrine System (G)**
X	Diagnostic
Z	No Qualifier

Functions of the Lymphatic System

The lymphatic system returns excess interstitial fluid to the blood, absorbs fat and fat-soluble vitamins from the digestive tract, and provides defense against invading microorganisms and disease. Lymph is similar in consistency to blood plasma (Applegate 2011, 323).

Organization of the Lymphatic System

The lymphatic system is made up of lymph vessels, lymph nodes, the tonsils, the spleen, and the thymus. ICD-10-PCS classifies the tonsils in the mouth and throat body system. The remainder of the system is discussed here, in addition to the bone marrow.

The lymph vessels return lymph to the venous system and take fluids away from the cells. The lymph nodes are small, oval structures about 2 cm in size that filter the lymph. The greatest concentration of lymph nodes is found in the cervical, axillary, and inguinal areas. The thoracic duct is the largest lymph vessel in the body. It starts at the cisterna chyli in the lower abdomen that drains the lymph from the extremities. The thoracic duct empties into the left subclavian vein.

The thymus is found in mid-chest, anterior to the ascending aorta and posterior to the sternum. It matures and releases T lymphocyte cells that fight infection. Refer to figure 12.1 in the gastrointestinal system chapter for the position of the spleen, just below the stomach. The spleen is structured like a very large lymph node, and it filters blood in a similar way. It removes damaged erythrocytes from circulation and stores excess blood for later use. Figure 13.2 displays the lymphatic organs, nodes, and ducts.

Figure 13.2.   Lymph nodes and ducts

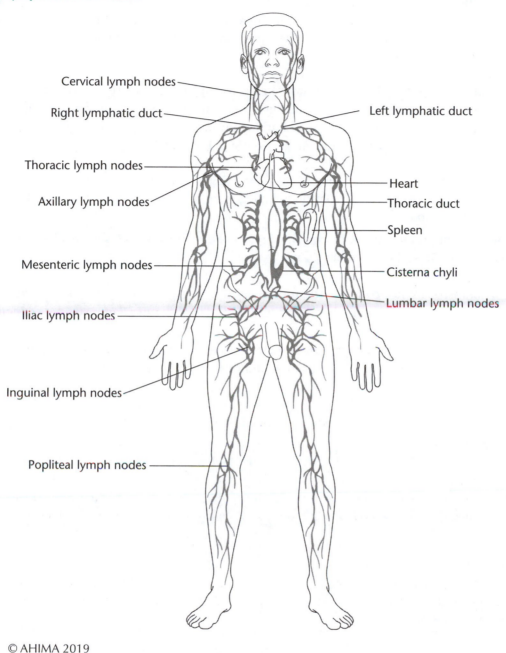

Cervical lymph nodes

Right lymphatic duct

Left lymphatic duct

Thoracic lymph nodes

Axillary lymph nodes

Heart

Thoracic duct

Spleen

Mesenteric lymph nodes

Cisterna chyli

Lumbar lymph nodes

Iliac lymph nodes

Inguinal lymph nodes

Popliteal lymph nodes

© AHIMA 2019

Bone marrow is the spongy tissue inside some of the large bones. It contains immature cells, called stem cells. These stem cells can develop into the red blood cells that carry oxygen through the body, the white blood cells that fight infections, and the platelets that help with blood clotting (NLM 2011b).

Common Root Operations Used in Coding Procedures on the Lymphatic System

The lymphatic system contains tubular body parts, and therefore the root operations of Dilation, Occlusion, and Restriction are available for use in coding procedures performed on the lymphatic system. The body part value for each lymphatic location is the entire lymph node chain, also called a level. Therefore, if an entire lymph node chain (level) is cut out, the appropriate root operation is Resection. When a lymph node(s) is cut out, the root operation is Excision.

Coding Tip

When an entire lymph node chain is cut out, the appropriate root operation is Resection. When a lymph node(s) is cut out, the root operation is Excision. Physicians may refer to a lymph node chain as a lymph node level. Level and chain are synonymous.

The thymus and the spleen are organs that can be transplanted, and therefore the root operation of Transplantation is available for use, defined as putting in a mature and functioning living body part taken from another individual or animal. However, putting in autologous or nonautologous bone marrow, pancreatic islet cells, or stem cells is coded to the Administration section of ICD-10-PCS.

B3.16. Putting in a mature and functioning living body part taken from another individual or animal is coded to the root operation Transplantation. Putting in autologous or nonautologous cells is coded to the Administration section.

Example: Putting in autologous or nonautologous bone marrow, pancreatic islet cells, or stem cells is coded to the Administration section.

Bone marrow biopsies are not coded to the root operation Excision. They are coded to the root operation Extraction because bone marrow is pulled or stripped out. The qualifier of Diagnostic is assigned, as this procedure is a biopsy.

Be sure to research any procedure that is unfamiliar to assure correct coding. If the documentation includes an eponym (procedure named for a person) and the intent of the procedure is unclear, query the physician for specifics.

B3.4a. Biopsy procedures are coded using the root operations Excision, Extraction, or Drainage and the qualifier Diagnostic.

Examples: Fine needle aspiration biopsy of fluid in the lung is coded to the root operation Drainage with the qualifier Diagnostic.

Biopsy of bone marrow is coded to the root operation Extraction with the qualifier Diagnostic. Lymph node sampling for biopsy is coded to the root operation Excision with the qualifier Diagnostic.

Coding Tip

Bone marrow biopsies are not coded to the root operation Excision. They are coded to Extraction, with the qualifier of Diagnostic. Bone marrow transplant procedures are coded in Section 3, Administration to the root operation Transfusion.

Body Part Values for the Lymphatic System

The lymphatic system in ICD-10-PCS contains the lymphatic ducts and nodes throughout the body, the thoracic duct, the cisterna chyli, the thymus, the spleen, and the bone marrow. The body parts for bone marrow are defined as sternum, iliac, and vertebral, as these are the primary places where bone marrow is extracted.

If the body part name includes the word lymphatic, the body part value refers to the lymph nodes of that particular region or area of the body. The lymph nodes contained within the chest and the abdominal cavities provide challenges in coding. The lymph nodes are classified by the body part region they drain, but this is not easy to determine without help understanding the anatomy.

The most helpful information about the lymph nodes found within ICD-10-PCS is the feature called Definitions, found in the CMS ICD-10-PCS file following the index. Table 13.4 is an excerpt from the Definitions related to body parts that are related to the lymphatics of these cavities.

If any of these lymph nodes are named, the body part key will be of assistance. The definitions are the body part key in reverse, but neither one names all of the nodes. Especially problematic are nodes identified in the documentation as "peri-renal" or "peri-adrenal." Both the kidneys and the adrenal glands are found in the retroperitoneal space and are, therefore, aortic nodes. The retroperitoneal space contains the adrenal glands, kidneys, ureters, aorta, inferior vena cava, esophagus, duodenum, ascending and descending colon, and rectum.

This system contains the generic terms of "lymphatic" and "bone marrow" for coding when the exact location is not necessary for coding, such as with the root operations Insertion, Inspection, Removal, or Revision. Table 13.5 shows the body parts associated with the lymphatic system. If the documentation includes specific body part names that are not included in this list, refer to the body part key for other body part synonyms and alternative terms.

Table 13.4. Definitions of Lymphatic body part values within body cavities

Body Part Value	Body Part Name	Lymph Nodes Included
7	Lymphatic, Thorax	Intercostal Lymph Node
		Mediastinal Lymph Node
		Parasternal Lymph Node
		Paratracheal Lymph Node
		Tracheobronchial Lymph Node
B	Lymphatic, Mesenteric	Inferior Mesenteric Lymph Node
		Pararectal Lymph Node
		Superior Mesenteric Lymph Node
C	Lymphatic, Pelvis	Common Iliac (Subaortic) Lymph Node
		Gluteal Lymph Node
		Iliac Lymph Node
		Inferior Epigastric Lymph Node
		Obturator Lymph Node
		Sacral Lymph Node
		Subaortic (Common Iliac) Lymph Node
		Suprainguinal Lymph Node
D	Lymphatic, Aortic	Celiac Lymph Node
		Gastric Lymph Node
		Hepatic Lymph Node
		Lumbar Lymph Node
		Pancreaticosplenic Lymph Node
		Para-aortic Lymph Node
		Retroperitoneal Lymph Node

Table 13.5. Body parts in the Lymphatic system

Body Part Value	Body Parts—Lymphatic System (7)
0	Lymphatic, Head
1	Lymphatic, Right Neck
2	Lymphatic, Left Neck
3	Lymphatic, Right Upper Extremity
4	Lymphatic, Left Upper Extremity
5	Lymphatic, Right Axillary
6	Lymphatic, Left Axillary
7	Lymphatic, Thorax
8	Lymphatic, Internal Mammary, Right
9	Lymphatic, Internal Mammary, Left
B	Lymphatic, Mesenteric
C	Lymphatic, Pelvis
D	Lymphatic, Aortic
F	Lymphatic, Right Lower Extremity
G	Lymphatic, Left Lower Extremity
H	Lymphatic, Right Inguinal
J	Lymphatic, Left Inguinal
K	Thoracic Duct
L	Cisterna Chyli
M	Thymus
N	Lymphatic
P	Spleen
Q	Bone Marrow, Sternum
R	Bone Marrow, Iliac
S	Bone Marrow, Vertebral
T	Bone Marrow

Approaches Used in the Lymphatic System

The approaches of Percutaneous and Percutaneous Endoscopic are available to code procedures in this section. The External approach is used when changing, removing, or revising a device within the lymphatic system.

Devices Common to the Lymphatic System

Extraluminal and intraluminal devices are used within the tubular body parts of the lymphatic system. In addition, various tissues types are used in the root operations Removal, Supplement, and Revision. Drainage and infusion devices are frequently inserted into the lymphatic system. Table 13.6 lists the available devices for coding procedures performed on the lymphatic system.

Table 13.6. Devices for the Lymphatic system

Device Value	Devices—Lymphatic System (7)
0	Drainage Device
3	Infusion Device
7	Autologous Tissue Substitute
C	Extraluminal Device
D	Intraluminal Device
J	Synthetic Substitute
K	Nonautologous Tissue Substitute
Y	Other Device
Z	No Device

Qualifiers for the Lymphatic System

Qualifiers for the lymphatic system describe the source of transplanted tissue. The standard X, Diagnostic and Z, No Qualifier are also included. Table 13.7 lists the qualifiers available for coding procedures performed on the lymphatic system.

Table 13.7. Qualifiers for the Lymphatic system

Qualifier Value	Qualifiers—Lymphatic System (7)
0	Allogeneic
1	Syngeneic
2	Zooplastic
X	Diagnostic
Z	No Qualifier

 Code Building

Case #1:

PROCEDURE STATEMENT: Ablation of adenoma of the left inferior parathyroid gland

ADDITIONAL INFORMATION: Percutaneous radiofrequency ablation (RFA) of an inferior parathyroid adenoma is performed in a patient with clinically untreatable hypercalcemia.

ROOT AND INDEX ENTRIES FOR THE STATEMENT: Destruction is the root operation performed in this procedure, defined as physical eradication of all or a portion of a body part by the direct use of energy, force, or a destructive agent. The Index entry is:

Destruction

    Parathyroid Gland 0G5R

        Inferior

                Left   0G5P

                Right   0G5N

Code Characters:

Section	Body System	Root Operation	Body Part	Approach	Device	Qualifier
Medical and Surgical	Endocrine System	Destruction	Inferior Parathyroid Gland, Left	Percutaneous	No Device	No Qualifier
0	G	5	P	3	Z	Z

RATIONALE FOR THE ANSWER: Ablation is the radiofrequency destruction of all or part of a body part. This procedure was performed percutaneously. The parathyroid glands are classified as part of the endocrine system in ICD-10-PCS. No device value or qualifier value is appropriate for this code. The correct code assignment is 0G5P3ZZ.

Case #2:

PROCEDURE STATEMENT: Suture of thoracic duct

ADDITIONAL INFORMATION: Thoracoscopic suture repair of iatrogenic chylothorax following thoracic duct injury during mediastinal surgery

ROOT AND INDEX ENTRIES FOR THE STATEMENT: Repair is the root operation performed in this procedure, defined as restoring, to the extent possible, a body part to its normal anatomic structure and function. The Index entry is:

Repair

    Lymphatic

        Thoracic Duct 07QK

Code Characters:

Section	Body System	Root Operation	Body Part	Approach	Device	Qualifier
Medical and Surgical	Lymphatic and Hemic Systems	Repair	Thoracic Duct	Percutaneous Endoscopic	No Device	No Qualifier
0	7	Q	K	4	Z	Z

RATIONALE FOR THE ANSWER: The root operation Repair is coded because injury to the thoracic duct caused a defect. The intent of the root operation Repair is to return a body part to its normal anatomic structure and function. The thoracoscopic approach is approach value 4, Percutaneous endoscopic. No device value or qualifier value is appropriate for this code. The correct code assignment is 07QK4ZZ.

Case #3:

PROCEDURE STATEMENT: Thymus gland transplant into infant

ADDITIONAL INFORMATION: Thymus transplant is performed to treat congenital absence of the thymus gland in DiGeorge syndrome. The thymus is transplanted using an open approach and is provided by organ donation.

ROOT AND INDEX ENTRIES FOR THE STATEMENT: Transplantation is the root operation performed in this procedure, defined as putting in or on all or a portion of a living body part taken from another individual or animal to physically take the place and/or function of all or a portion of a similar body part. The Index entry is:

Transplantation

    Thymus   07YM0Z

Code Characters:

Section	Body System	Root Operation	Body Part	Approach	Device	Qualifier
Medical and Surgical	Lymphatic and Hemic Systems	Transplantation	Thymus	Open	No Device	Allogeneic
0	7	Y	M	0	Z	0

RATIONALE FOR THE ANSWER: The root operation Transplantation is coded because the thymus is a living organ from a donor. The procedure is performed with an Open approach. No device value is appropriate for this code. The qualifier value of 0, Allogeneic is assigned because the source of the thymus is an organ donation from another human being. The correct code assignment is 07YM0Z0.

Code Building Exercises

Work through each case and check your answers using the answer key in appendix B of the textbook before going on to the Check Your Understanding questions that follow.

Exercise 1:

PREOPERATIVE DIAGNOSIS: Right upper lobe lung mass

POSTOPERATIVE DIAGNOSIS: Right upper lobe lung mass

PROCEDURE: Right thoracoscopic upper lobe apical segmentectomy and lymph node biopsy of level 7 lymph nodes

DESCRIPTION OF OPERATION: The patient was brought to the operating room and all lines were placed and anesthesia administered. We then put the patient in the right-side-up position with all pressure points being padded. I placed a 5 mm trocar. I had good visualization of the lung. There was a lesion noted on the apical portion of the upper lobe that correlated with our CT scan.

    To that end, we placed all our other ports appropriately. We followed the arterial and venous distributions of the RUL and performed an apical segmentectomy. I sent this to pathology for frozen section. We then proceeded with our lymph node biopsies, sampling the level 7 lymph nodes and also sent those for frozen. The pathologist called into the room stating the lung lesion, scar tissue, and lymph nodes were negative.

    We irrigated and also sprayed Progel, as an air leak sealing adjunct, as well as FloSeal into the dissection bed posteriorly. A chest tube, which was placed under direct vision, was secured and placed through the

50 mm port site. The trocars were removed. All sponge and lap counts, instrument counts were correct. The wounds were closed in three layers in a standard fashion with Dermabond to the skin.

Questions:

1.1. Is a segmentectomy the removal of some or all of the right upper lobe of the lung?

_____

1.2. What root operation is assigned for the segmentectomy?

_____

1.3. Research the level 7 lymph nodes and determine where the level is located. There are several good pictures on the Internet that will help identify the location. What body part value is assigned?

_____

1.4. What code(s) would be assigned?

_____

Exercise 2:

Case Scenario: A patient with known rectal cancer underwent a core needle biopsy of the spleen to characterize a solid splenic lesion. The procedure was performed in the interventional radiology suite and ultrasound guidance was used to perform the procedure.

Questions:

2.1. Which group of root operations would be used to select the root operation for this procedure and why?

_____

2.2. Which root operation is assigned for this procedure and why?

_____

2.3. What approach value would be assigned for a core needle biopsy performed with ultrasound guidance?

_____

2.4. What code(s) should you assign? (Do not code the ultrasound guidance used in this case.)

_____

✔ Check Your Understanding

Coding Knowledge Check

1. The parasternal lymph nodes are classified to Lymphatic, _____.

2. The thyroid isthmus is transected into two pieces. Which root operation value is assigned for this procedure?
   a. 8, Division
   b. B, Excision
   c. D, Extraction
   d. T, Resection

(Continued)

3. Percutaneous endoscopic adhesiolysis of the spleen is coded as _____.
   a. 07BP0ZX
   b. 07NP4ZZ
   c. 07SP0ZZ
   d. 07TP4ZZ

4. Removal of a calcification of a lymph node is coded to the root operation of _____.
   a. Excision
   b. Extirpation
   c. Extraction
   d. Resection

5. The para-aortic body is also known as the corpus _____ aortica.

Procedure Statement Coding

Assign ICD-10-PCS codes to the following procedure statements and scenarios. List the root operation selected and the code assigned.

1. The entire left thyroid lobe is excised using an open approach.

   _____

2. Excision of right carotid body tumor, open approach

   _____

3. Drainage of cyst of left lobe of thyroid and placement of drain, open approach

   _____

4. Parathyroid biopsy, open

   _____

5. Craniectomy with infratentorial excision of pineal tumor

   _____

6. Open total thymectomy

   _____

7. Open excision of the entire right axillary lymph node chain

   _____

8. Right thyroid isthmus lumpectomy, open approach

   _____

9. Autotransplantation of right inferior parathyroid gland, open approach

   _____

10. Percutaneous right adrenal biopsy

    _____

Case Studies

Assign ICD-10-PCS codes to the following case studies.

1. Operative Report

PREOPERATIVE DIAGNOSIS:	Uninodular non-toxic goiter, left
POSTOPERATIVE DIAGNOSIS:	Follicular adenoma
OPERATION:	Left thyroid lobectomy
FINDINGS:	Massive left thyroid lobe with intra-lobe nodule. Frozen section diagnosis showed no evidence of well-differentiated thyroid carcinoma.

DESCRIPTION OF PROCEDURE: After an adequate general endotracheal anesthetic, the neck was prepped and draped in the usual manner. A previous low collar incision had been marked in the holding area. The incision was made and subplatysmal flaps were elevated. The diastasis of the strap musculature was identified and the straps were gently elevated off the massively enlarged left thyroid lobe. Superior pedicle was meticulously skeletonized. Each vessel was clamped, cut, and either cauterized or tied. The gland was delivered medially, gently dissecting the soft tissue off the capsule of the thyroid. The superior parathyroid was easily identified and its vasculature preserved. The recurrent nerve was easily identified shortly after this as coursing toward the cricothyroid membrane. A biopsy was taken and examined. The abovementioned findings were noted. The gland was delivered farther up onto the ventral surface of the trachea. The connections were clamped, cut, and tied. A running 3-0 chromic stitch was placed across the junction of the right thyroid and the isthmus. A small Jackson-Pratt drain was placed. The wound was closed in layers. The patient was awakened and taken to recovery in good condition. There were no complications.

2. Operative Report

PREOPERATIVE DIAGNOSIS:	Conn's syndrome with abnormal aldosterone secretion from the left adrenal gland
POSTOPERATIVE DIAGNOSIS:	Conn's syndrome with abnormal aldosterone secretion from the left adrenal gland
OPERATION PERFORMED:	Laparoscopic left adrenalectomy
SPECIMENS:	Left adrenal gland

INDICATIONS FOR PROCEDURE: This 46-year-old woman has hypertension and hypokalemia. Workup revealed hyperaldosteronism that, after adrenal vein sampling, appeared to localize specifically to the left adrenal gland with markedly elevated levels of aldosterone. After the risks and benefits of the procedure and possible complications were explained, the patient elected to undergo laparoscopic left adrenalectomy.

DESCRIPTION OF PROCEDURE: Under general anesthesia, initial access to the abdomen was obtained using a direct cut-down technique below the left ribs. Insertion of a blunt cannula was undertaken, and the abdomen was insufflated under direct visualization. Under direct visualization, we placed a medial 5.0-mm trocar and two 5.0-mm trocars more lateral to our initial access site.

We proceeded to mobilize the left colon from the left sidewall using harmonic shears and we adequately mobilized the colon out of the way and rolled the inferior pole of the spleen medially and superiorly, rolling the spleen off its left lateral attachments. We then opened up Gerota's fascia gently, where we identified the adrenal gland in place, which appeared to be somewhat long and flat in appearance.

Meticulous dissection was carried out inferiorly and medially, where we identified a solitary left adrenal vein, which we triply clipped and divided. We then dissected the adrenal gland off its bed using L-hook cautery with excellent hemostasis. We then placed the gland into an impermeable entrapment sac and removed it through the initial access site, passing it off the field. There was no evidence of bleeding. We then proceeded to close our initial access trocar site with 0 Vicryl suture on a suture-passer using a figure-of-eight technique. We replaced the left colon back into the left upper abdomen. We removed our instruments under direct visualization, desufflating the abdomen completely. There was no bleeding from the trocar sites. The skin was closed with 4-0 monocryl subcuticular stitch. Steri-Strips were applied. Sterile dressing was applied.

3. Operative Report

PREOPERATIVE DIAGNOSIS: Hodgkins, nodular sclerosis

POSTOPERATIVE DIAGNOSIS: Same

PROCEDURE: Bone marrow aspiration

Procedure performed in OR under anesthesia. Patient identified and consent obtained.

Bone marrow studies performed today as patient is having a mediport placed by general surgery during same operative session, dictated separately. 11-gauge Jamshidi biopsy needle used. Bone marrow biopsy sample obtained from right posterior iliac crest and sent to pathology. Tolerated procedure without complications and was handed to surgery team for placement of port.

4. Operative Report

PREOPERATIVE DIAGNOSIS: Hypertrophic pyloric stenosis

POSTOPERATIVE DIAGNOSES: Hypertrophic pyloric stenosis; thrombosed accessory spleen

OPERATION: 1. Laparoscopic pyloromyotomy

        2. Excision of thrombosed accessory spleen

INDICATIONS FOR SURGERY: Patient is a 4-week-old boy with a 1-week history of progressively projectile vomiting. Patient was brought to the emergency department, where he underwent ultrasound evaluation. Ultrasound findings revealed a pyloric channel of 15 mm in length with a wall thickness of 3.8 mm, consistent with hypertrophic pyloric stenosis.

FINDINGS: Moderately hypertrophied pylorus. No evidence of mucosal perforation. There was a 1 cm × 2 cm dark purple mass on the omentum, consistent with a thrombosed accessory spleen. This was excised without difficulty and sent for pathologic evaluation.

PROCEDURE: After adequate endotracheal anesthesia had been administered, his stomach was decompressed and his bladder was emptied, and his abdomen was prepared and draped in the usual sterile fashion. After infiltration with a local anesthetic, the base of the umbilicus was everted and a vertical 5-mm incision was made. A Veress needle was introduced and pneumoperitoneum was established to 8 mm Hg pressure at 1 L/minute flow. Laparascope was introduced and stab incisions were made in the right upper quadrant and left upper quadrant. Examination revealed a 1 cm × 2 cm dark purplish mass attached to the omentum near the spleen. This was separate from the spleen. He had a normal appearing lobulated spleen in the left upper quadrant. This mass was consistent with a thrombosed accessory spleen. This was dissected free using electrocautery and placed in an endocatch bag. It was removed through the umbilical trocar and sent for pathologic review. The pylorus was stabilized. The Arthro blade was extruded approximately 2 mm and used to incise the pylorus. The blade was then retracted and the blunt tip was used to initiate the pyloromyotomy.

This then was replaced with a pyloric spreader, which was used to complete the pyloromyotomy. The mucosa was seen bulging without evidence of mucosal perforation. Forty cc of air was inflated into the stomach by the anesthesiologist. This revealed no evidence of a mucosal perforation. The stomach was then decompressed.

Reexamination of the intraperitoneal cavity revealed good hemostasis. All instruments and trocars were removed and the pneumoperitoneum was deflated. The fascia of the right upper quadrant trocar site and the umbilical trocar site were closed with 2-0 Vicryl in figure-of-eight stitch fashion. The umbilical skin incision was closed with 5-0 plain gut in interrupted stitch fashion. The other upper quadrant incisions were closed with Monocryl in subcuticular running stitch fashion. All incisions were cleaned and infiltrated with a local anesthetic. The umbilical trocar site was dressed with sterile gauze and Tegaderm. The other incisions were dressed with Steri-Strips.

5. Operative Report

PREOPERATIVE DIAGNOSIS:	1. Idiopathic thrombocytopenia purpura
	2. Arteriovenous malformations with bleeding in small bowel
	3. Anemia related to above
POSTOPERATIVE DIAGNOSIS:	1. Idiopathic thrombocytopenia purpura
	2. Arteriovenous malformations with bleeding in small bowel
	3. Anemia related to above
OPERATION:	Laparoscopic splenectomy

INDICATIONS: The patient is a 74-year-old man with arteriovenous malformations and idiopathic thrombocytopenia purpura with chronic gastrointestinal bleeding. He has had several blood transfusions and platelet count resides in the 60s recently. The procedure, benefits, risks, and alternatives of splenectomy in this situation have been detailed. He wished to proceed.

PROCEDURE: After obtaining adequate general endotracheal anesthesia, the abdomen was prepped with Hibiclens and draped in the usual sterile fashion. The patient was in semi-right decubitus position with appropriate orientation and padding. He had been given his vaccines preoperatively.

The abdomen was accessed through a left subcostal endopath technique and a 12-mm trocars was placed there. A 12-mm trocars was placed more medially and a 5-mm trocars was placed in the flank. The ligamentous attachments to the spleen were divided hemostatically with a harmonic scalpel. Medial and lateral mobilization gave very nice access to the hilum. Three loads of a 45-mm white load stapler were applied with excellent hemostasis and there was absolutely no problem at all from bleeding. The spleen was placed into a bag intact and then removed from one of the 12-mm port sites without any problem. The surgical field was evaluated and had complete hemostasis. A couple of clips were placed on the staple line at the point where the vessels were identified. The ports were removed. There was no bleeding from within or without. The 12-mm port site fascia sites were closed with interrupted 0 Vicryl suture under direct vision. The skin was irrigated and closed with subcuticular Vicryl suture. Steri-strips and sterile dressings were applied. The patient was awakened and extubated in the operating room and taken to the recovery room in good condition. He tolerated the procedure well and had no hemodynamic or pulmonary problems throughout the procedure.

6. Operative Report

PREOPERATIVE DIAGNOSIS: Primary hyperparathyroidism.

POSTOPERATIVE DIAGNOSIS: Primary hyperparathyroidism.

NAME OF PROCEDURE: Left superior parathyroidectomy.

INTRAOPERATIVE FINDINGS: Normal-appearing thyroid gland with left superior parathyroid gland enlarged and excised. Intact PTH level decreased from 101.9 at the beginning of the procedure to 7.9 fifteen minutes after excision of the left superior parathyroid gland. Left inferior parathyroid gland unable to be identified.

INDICATIONS: The patient is a 35-year-old female with a history of renal stones. She was subsequently diagnosed with primary hyperparathyroidism. A sestamibi scan was suspicious for a left inferior parathyroid adenoma. After discussion of the risks, benefits, and alternatives, the patient was consented to undergo the above procedure.

DESCRIPTION OF PROCEDURE: Under general anesthesia and endotracheal intubation, a shoulder roll was placed to provide neck extension. A time out was conducted, confirming the identity of the patient as well as the procedure to be performed. A small amount of 1% lidocaine with 1:100,000 epinephrine was locally injected into the planned left parasagittal cervical incision. The neck was then prepped and draped in the usual fashion.

A 2.5 cm incision was created at the previous site marking in a pre-existing skin crease. Dissection continued through the dermis, subcutaneous tissues, and platysmal muscle. The strap muscles were divided along the midline raphe, and the left strap muscles were lateralized to encounter the left thyroid lobe. Blunt dissection was performed down the inferior aspect of the gland, near the inferior thyroid artery and tracheoesophageal groove. The recurrent laryngeal nerve was identified in this area, and its integrity was confirmed with nerve stimulation. Blunt dissection was then performed along the inferior and posterior aspects of the thyroid lobe as well as the central neck compartment.

The incision was then enlarged 1 cm both medially and laterally. Continued dissection around the thyroid gland was performed, with division of the middle thyroid vein. The suspected superior parathyroid gland was subsequently identified and noted to be enlarged. It was resected and sent for frozen section analysis, which confirmed the presence of parathyroid tissue. Then 15 minutes status post excision, a venous blood draw was performed. This confirmed an intact parathyroid level decreased from 101.9 to 7.9. This concluded the procedure. The wound was thoroughly irrigated with normal saline, and hemostasis was ensured. Incision was closed in layers with deep 3-0 Vicryl sutures within the strap muscles and 4-0 Vicryl sutures within the platysma and deep dermis. A 5-0 Monocryl subcutaneous suture was used to reapproximate the skin edges. Benzoin ointment and Steri-Strips were applied. The patient was returned to anesthesia, awakened, extubated, and taken to the PACU in stable condition.

SPECIMENS SENT: Left superior parathyroid totally resected and sent for frozen section pathology, with confirmation of parathyroid tissue, unable to determine cellularity.

Integumentary System

The 2nd character values for the integumentary system are:

H—Skin and Breast
J—Subcutaneous Tissue and Fascia

Functions of the Integumentary System

The integumentary system is the flexible yet rugged covering of the body that regulates the body temperature and protects it from harmful ultraviolet rays and other harmful external irritants. It also detects environmental changes in temperature and pressure. Skin can repair itself from minor damage, but larger structural interruptions must be surgically repaired (Rizzo 2016, 113).

Organization of the Integumentary System

ICD-10-PCS divides the integumentary system into two main parts, the skin and breast (including the nails and hair) and the subcutaneous tissue and fascia.

Skin and Breast

The skin is made up of epidermis and dermis. The epidermal layer does not contain blood vessels. The epidermis receives its nutrients from the cells that are growing underneath, called the basement membrane. The epidermis is pushed up by the growing basement membrane, and the surface cells slowly die from lack of nutrients and are sloughed off (Applegate 2011, 89). The dermal layer is thicker and below the epidermis, containing both collagenous and elastic fibers to make it strong and flexible. The dermis contains small blood vessels and nerves, as well as hair follicles. The term "partial thickness of the skin" refers to the epidermis only. The term "full thickness of the skin" refers to both the epidermis and the dermis.

The subcutaneous tissue is found below the dermis and is made up of connective tissue. It is also referred to as subcutaneous fat, or the hypodermis (McKinley et al. 2017, 128). Below the subcutaneous tissue is the fascia, a connective tissue covering that connects the subcutaneous tissue to the muscle. Figure 14.1 displays the layers of the skin, the subcutaneous tissue, and fascia. These are all found above the muscle layer, which will be covered in chapter 15. The breast, also called the mammary gland, is the organ of milk production in the female. They are present in both males and females but normally only develop in the female. Each breast contains ducts that collect milk and deliver it to the nipple, the central raised area surrounded by the areola. Figure 14.2 shows a cross-section of the breast in relationship to the underlying muscle layers.

Figure 14.1. **Layers of Integumentary system**

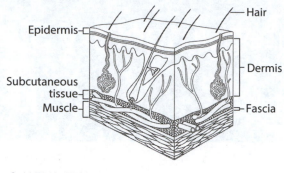

© AHIMA 2019

Figure 14.2. **Breast**

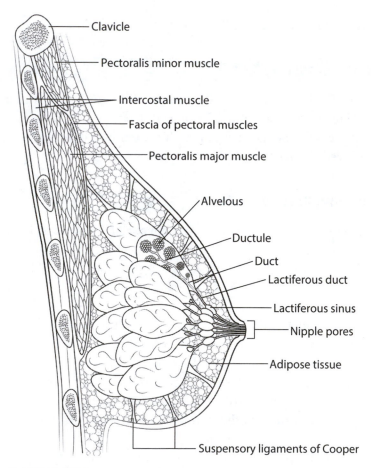

© AHIMA 2019

Anatomy Alert

ICD-10-PCS makes a clear distinction between skin and subcutaneous tissue. Skin includes both the epidermis and the dermis. The subcutaneous tissue is the layer below the dermis. Physicians may document the word "skin" and mean skin and the subcutaneous tissue layers. Subcutaneous tissue can also be called "fat" or "soft tissue." Be careful to determine the body system being identified.

The nails are thin plates of very hard dead tissue at the end of each finger and toe. The nail body is the visible portion of the nail, while the nail root is at the proximal end of the nail and covered by skin and cuticle. The nail matrix is also at the proximal end of the nail and is the location of nail growth. Figure 14.3 shows the frontal view and a cross-section view of the fingernail and associated structures.

Figure 14.3. The nail

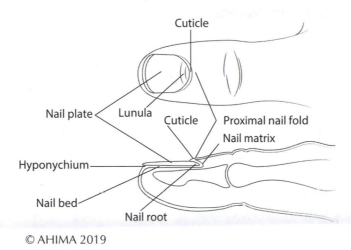

© AHIMA 2019

Coding Tip

ICD-10-PCS does not differentiate among the parts of the nail. The nail bed and nail plate are both coded to the body part values of Q, Fingernail or R, Toenail. The cuticle and the proximal nail fold are coded to the skin of the hand or foot, as appropriate.

Subcutaneous Tissue and Fascia

The subcutaneous layer is below the dermal layer and above the fascia. This layer is technically not a part of the skin. It consists mainly of adipose tissue and loose connective tissue fibers that are continuous with those of the dermis, leaving no clear dividing line. The adipose tissue forms a cushion for the underlying structures of the body and is also referred to as the soft tissue of the body (Applegate 2011, 91). When a surgeon performs undermining, the connections between the skin and the subcutaneous tissue are broken using a scalpel, allowing the epidermis and dermis to stretch for wound closure. The fascia is a connective tissue that surrounds muscles, groups of muscles, blood vessels, and nerves, binding those structures together. These structures are pictured in figure 14.1.

Common Root Operations Used in Coding Procedures Performed on the Integumentary System

Liposuction is performed on the subcutaneous tissue layer. When liposuction is performed for medical reasons, such as obtaining the patient's own fat tissue to use as an autologous tissue substitute, the root operation Extraction is coded. When the liposuction is performed for cosmetic purposes, the root operation Alteration is coded.

The root operations Reattachment and Reposition can be used to code procedures performed on the skin but cannot be used to code procedures performed on the subcutaneous tissue and fascia. Similar procedures on the subcutaneous tissue and fascia are coded to the root operation of Repair.

Tissue rearrangement through the use of flaps is the root operation of Transfer because the flap is still connected to the vascular and nervous supply. In contrast, a free skin graft is disconnected from all connections to the body; therefore, a free skin graft is a device and the placement of the graft is coded to the root operation of Replacement using a device value of 7, Autologous Tissue Substitute. The harvesting of the skin graft is coded separately as Excision, based on Guideline B3.9. The Excision or Resection of the diseased or damaged skin being replaced is not coded separately based on the definitions of both Excision and Resection.

Mastectomy and Reconstruction Procedures

Various types of mastectomy procedures can be performed based on the extent of the disease. They are:

- **Lumpectomy**—Removes small piece of breast tissue and can be performed for diagnostic or therapeutic purposes. Lymph node sampling may be done at the same session and is coded separately.
- **Partial mastectomy**—More extensive than lumpectomy but not the removal of the entire breast.
- **Simple or total mastectomy**—Removes the entire breast but no nodes or muscles.
- **Modified radical mastectomy**—Removes the entire breast and the axillary lymph nodes but no muscle tissue is removed.
- **Radical mastectomy**—Removes the entire breast, the axillary, infraclavicular and supraclavicular lymph node chains, and chest wall muscle from below the breast.

When a mastectomy procedure is performed and not followed at the same operative session with a Replacement procedure, the mastectomy is coded. Tissue expanders are not a device used to replace the breast.

A tissue expander is a device that is placed into the remaining breast after excision or into the new breast mound after replacement if the tissue is not generous enough to accommodate a permanent replacement implant. The tissue expander has an injection port that allows additional fluid to be added at regular intervals until the desired size is obtained. At that point, the tissue expander is removed and a permanent saline or silicone implant is placed into the breast to complete the Replacement procedure. Refer to figure 1.9 in chapter 1 to see the placement of the tissue expander and how the tissue expander is filled.

Replacements

When a mastectomy procedure is performed and is followed at the same operative session with a Replacement procedure, the mastectomy is not coded because Replacement procedures always include the removal of the native body part.

Breast replacements use a manufactured device, donated tissue, or patient's own tissue that has been completely disconnected. The patient's own tissue that has been disconnected is called a free graft or free flap. Free flaps are multiple layers of tissue that have been excised to become a graft. The Replacement procedure is used when a graft takes the place of a body part. Microanastomosis of arteries and veins is frequently documented as the surgeon reconnects the grafted tissue because the vascular connections must be reestablished.

The DIEP free flap is a subcutaneous-based flap with the associated skin, raised from the abdomen. It includes the deep inferior epigastric perforator artery and vein, for which it is named. These vessels are connected to the vessels of the chest wall that bring blood to and take blood from the flap. This is qualifier 7 in the 0HR table for Replacement. When Replacements are coded, remember to code what is being replaced.

Reconstruction with a Transfer

Muscle transfers are also used to create a breast reconstruction. Muscle transfers are commonly called flaps or pedicle flaps. Abdominal muscles are frequently transferred to the breast through a tissue tunnel to create a new breast mound. In a transverse rectus abdominis myocutaneous (or TRAM) flap, the base of the flap is muscle. The associated subcutaneous tissue and skin are also transferred with the muscle.

The TRAM pedicle flap is transferred from the abdomen area through a tunnel up the middle of the chest, between the subcutaneous tissue and fascia of the chest. For coding, we select the transferred body part as abdominal muscle, left or right. The qualifier for this code is 6, Transverse Rectus Abdominis Myocutaneous Flap. When transfers are coded, remember to code what is moving. Any Excision or Resection of a diseased body part should also be coded because Transfer does not include these other procedures.

Another very common flap reconstruction is done using the latissimus dorsi myocutaneous flap. Like the TRAM, this flap is muscle-based. ICD-10-PCS classifies the latissimus dorsi muscle as a trunk muscle, and it is coded as the body part being transferred. Use the qualifier of 5, Latissimus Dorsi Myocutaneous Flap for this transfer.

Breast Implants

Breast implants can be used as either a reconstruction (Replacement) device or as an Alteration device. They are coded as the device value J, Synthetic Substitute for either procedure.

When a biopsy is performed and the same body part is excised, resected, or destroyed at the same procedure site, both the biopsy and the definitive procedure are coded.

Coding Tip

Body parts that are still connected on at least one side are not considered devices in ICD-10-PCS. This type of harvesting is typically done in preparation for a transfer procedure. If the body part is completely disconnected from the body and is used in another procedure, it is considered a device and coded with the device value of 7, Autologous Tissue Substitute. This complete harvesting to create a tissue device is coded separately based on Coding Guideline B3.9.

B3.4b. If a diagnostic Excision, Extraction, or Drainage procedure (biopsy) is followed by a more definitive procedure, such as Destruction, Excision, or Resection at the same procedure site, both the biopsy and the more definitive treatment are coded.

Example: Biopsy of the breast followed by partial mastectomy at the same procedure site; both the biopsy and the partial mastectomy procedure are coded.

The root operation Division is used to describe the endoscopic repair of a contracted plantar fascia, often documented as a plantar fasciotomy. The root operation Insertion is coded when the intent of the procedure is to insert a device into a body part and the insertion is not a part of another root operation. The subcutaneous tissue is a common place for devices to reside. Neurostimulator generators, pacemaker generators, and defibrillator generators are all inserted into subcutaneous pockets in different areas of the body.

A totally subcutaneous implantable cardioverter-defibrillator and the leads for the unit are all placed in the subcutaneous tissue layer. This device does not have leads that are transvenous or epicardial. These leads defibrillate the heart but without being inside the chest cavity. A long lead runs through the subcutaneous layer of the chest. It senses and corrects irregular rhythm or lack of rhythm. The device value for the cardioverter-defibrillator is 8, Defibrillator Generator and the device value for the lead is P, Cardiac Rhythm Related Device (AHA 2012, 104–106).

Be sure to research any procedure that is unfamiliar to ensure correct coding. If the documentation includes an eponym (procedure named for a person) and the intent of the procedure is unclear, query the physician for specifics.

Body Part Values for the Integumentary System

Two important guidelines pertain to coding in the integumentary system. Guideline B4.6 describes the appropriate body parts associated with the joints of the body when procedures are performed on the skin, subcutaneous tissue, or fascia overlying one of these joints. Shoulder is coded to the upper arm body part, while the elbow and wrist are both coded to the lower arm body part. The hip is coded to the upper leg body part. The knee is coded to the lower leg body part, and the ankle is coded to the foot body part.

B4.6. If a procedure is performed on the skin, subcutaneous tissue, or fascia overlying a joint, the procedure is coded to the following body part:

- Shoulder is coded to Upper arm
- Elbow is coded to Lower arm
- Wrist is coded to Lower arm
- Hip is coded to Upper leg
- Knee is coded to Lower leg
- Ankle is coded to Foot

Guideline B3.5 answers the question of how to code procedures that are performed on overlapping layers of the skin, subcutaneous tissue, fascia, muscle, and bone. This guideline tells the coder to assign the body part value specifying the deepest layer.

B3.5. If the root operations Excision, Repair, or Inspection are performed on overlapping layers of the musculoskeletal system, the body part specifying the deepest layer is coded.

Example: Excisional debridement that includes skin and subcutaneous tissue and muscle is coded to the muscle body part.

Table 14.1 lists the body part values available for coding procedures performed on the integumentary system. If the documentation includes specific body part names that are not included in these lists, refer to the body part key for other body part synonyms and alternative terms.

Table 14.1. Body parts in the Integumentary system

Body Part Value	Body Parts—Skin and Breast (H)	Body Part Value	Body Parts—Subcutaneous Tissue and Fascia (J)
0	Skin, Scalp	0	Subcutaneous Tissue and Fascia, Scalp
1	Skin, Face	1	Subcutaneous Tissue and Fascia, Face
2	Skin, Right Ear	4	Subcutaneous Tissue and Fascia, Right Neck
3	Skin, Left Ear	5	Subcutaneous Tissue and Fascia, Left Neck
4	Skin, Neck	6	Subcutaneous Tissue and Fascia, Chest
5	Skin, Chest	7	Subcutaneous Tissue and Fascia, Back
6	Skin, Back	8	Subcutaneous Tissue and Fascia, Abdomen
7	Skin, Abdomen	9	Subcutaneous Tissue and Fascia, Buttock
8	Skin, Buttock	B	Subcutaneous Tissue and Fascia, Perineum
9	Skin, Perineum	C	Subcutaneous Tissue and Fascia, Pelvic Region
A	Skin, Inguinal	D	Subcutaneous Tissue and Fascia, Right Upper Arm
B	Skin, Right Upper Arm	F	Subcutaneous Tissue and Fascia, Left Upper Arm

(Continued)   *(Continued)*

Table 14.1. Body parts in the Integumentary system (continued)

Body Part Value	Body Parts—Skin and Breast (H)	Body Part Value	Body Parts—Subcutaneous Tissue and Fascia (J)
C	Skin, Left Upper Arm	G	Subcutaneous Tissue and Fascia, Right Lower Arm
D	Skin, Right Lower Arm	H	Subcutaneous Tissue and Fascia, Left Lower Arm
E	Skin, Left Lower Arm	J	Subcutaneous Tissue and Fascia, Right Hand
F	Skin, Right Hand	K	Subcutaneous Tissue and Fascia, Left Hand
G	Skin, Left Hand	L	Subcutaneous Tissue and Fascia, Right Upper Leg
H	Skin, Right Upper Leg	M	Subcutaneous Tissue and Fascia, Left Upper Leg
J	Skin, Left Upper Leg	N	Subcutaneous Tissue and Fascia, Right Lower Leg
K	Skin, Right Lower Leg	P	Subcutaneous Tissue and Fascia, Left Lower Leg
L	Skin, Left Lower Leg	Q	Subcutaneous Tissue and Fascia, Right Foot
M	Skin, Right Foot	R	Subcutaneous Tissue and Fascia, Left Foot
N	Skin, Left Foot	S	Subcutaneous Tissue and Fascia, Head and Neck
P	Skin	T	Subcutaneous Tissue and Fascia, Trunk
Q	Finger Nail	V	Subcutaneous Tissue and Fascia, Upper Extremity
R	Toe Nail	W	Subcutaneous Tissue and Fascia, Lower Extremity
S	Hair		
T	Breast, Right		
U	Breast, Left		
V	Breast, Bilateral		
W	Nipple, Right		
X	Nipple, Left		
Y	Supernumerary Breast		

Approaches Used for the Integumentary System

The approaches of Open, Percutaneous, and External are all used for coding procedures performed on the integumentary system. In addition, the approaches of Via Natural or Artificial Opening and Via Natural or Artificial Opening, Endoscopic are also available when coding procedures performed on the breast and nipple, through the natural opening of the nipple pores into the mammary ducts.

It is important to remember the approach definitions when coding integumentary procedures. The definition of an external procedure says that the procedure is performed on the outside of the body and does not go through the skin. Therefore, procedures performed on the skin can be coded with the External approach. The definition of an open procedure says that instruments go through the skin. Therefore, procedures performed on the subcutaneous tissue and fascia are not performed with an External approach. Those procedures typically utilize another approach such as Open or Percutaneous. Procedures performed manually from the outside of the body may be performed and coded with an External approach, such as Inspection or Release.

Devices Common to the Integumentary System

Replacement procedures can use tissue-cultured epidermal autograft. This type of graft is from the patient's own skin that was previously harvested and grown in a laboratory to a larger size to be used as a skin replacement approximately 14 days later. This type of tissue is coded with the device value of 7, Autologous Tissue Substitute because the origin is the patient's own skin.

Device values for the Subcutaneous Tissue and Fascia body system include several types of implantable devices that are commonly placed in subcutaneous pockets, such as contraceptive devices (capsules), stimulator generators, tissue expanders, cardiac rhythm–related devices (pacemakers), infusion pumps, and vascular access devices (tunneled and totally implantable ports). Specific device values are available for coding the insertion of devices. Cardiovascular devices were discussed in chapter 11. More generic device values are available for coding the removal or revision of devices.

Coding Tip

Totally implantable ports used to gain access to a central vein are coded with the device value of W, Vascular Access Device, Totally Implantable. These vascular access devices are inserted into a subcutaneous pocket using an open approach. The associated infusion device is coded separately to the location where the tip rests. Tunneled vascular access devices are coded to X, Vascular Access Device, Tunneled. The associated infusion device is coded separately to the location where the tip rests. See chapter 11 for a complete discussion.

Neurostimulators are inserted to provide deep brain stimulation for Parkinson's disease or essential tremor or for chronic pain management. The stimulator generator is placed in a subcutaneous pocket (using an open approach) and the lead (or leads) is placed at the body part where the stimulation is required (using either a percutaneous or open approach, depending upon the body part). Neurostimulators are coded just like pacemakers. A single array stimulator has one port where one lead can be connected. A multiple array stimulator has two or more ports where two or more leads can be connected (Kuehn 2015). Table 14.2 lists the device values used to code procedures performed on the integumentary system.

Table 14.2.   Devices for the Integumentary system

Device Value	Devices—Skin and Breast (H)	Device Value	Devices—Subcutaneous Tissue and Fascia (J)
0	Drainage Device	0	Drainage Device
1	Radioactive Element	0	Monitoring Device, Hemodynamic
7	Autologous Tissue Substitute	1	Radioactive Element
J	Synthetic Substitute	2	Monitoring Device
K	Nonautologous Tissue Substitute	3	Infusion Device
N	Tissue Expander	4	Pacemaker, Single Chamber
Y	Other Device	5	Pacemaker, Single Chamber Rate Responsive
Z	No Device	6	Pacemaker, Dual Chamber
		7	Autologous Tissue Substitute
		7	Cardiac Resynchronization Pacemaker Pulse Generator
		8	Defibrillator Generator
		9	Cardiac Resynchronization Defibrillator Pulse Generator
		A	Contractility Modulation Device
		B	Stimulator Generator, Single Array
		C	Stimulator Generator, Single Array Rechargeable
		D	Stimulator Generator, Multiple Array
		E	Stimulator Generator, Multiple Array Rechargeable
		H	Contraceptive Device
		J	Synthetic Substitute
		K	Nonautologous Tissue Substitute

(Continued)

Table 14.2. Devices for the Integumentary system (continued)

Device Value	Devices—Subcutaneous Tissue and Fascia (J)
M	Stimulator Generator
N	Tissue Expander
P	Cardiac Rhythm–Related Device
V	Infusion Device, Pump
W	Vascular Access Device, Totally Implantable
X	Vascular Access Device, Tunneled
Y	Other Device
Z	No Device

Qualifiers Used in the Integumentary System

Qualifier values are available to describe the types of flaps used in the root operation Replacement. In the Skin and Breast body system, qualifiers are available to describe both full-thickness and partial-thickness procedures performed on the skin and breast. The qualifier value for tissue-cultured epidermal autograft is value 4, Partial Thickness because only the epidermis is tissue cultured for use as a tissue replacement for the patient. Free skin grafts of both epidermal and dermal layers are coded with qualifier value 3, Full Thickness, because the epidermal and dermal layers together make up the full thickness of the skin. Grafts containing only dermis are considered partial thickness grafts, qualifier value 4, because they are less than the full thickness of skin. There is also a qualifier to designate that multiple lesions were destroyed during the same operative session, rather than coding individual codes for each lesion destroyed.

In the Subcutaneous Tissue and Fascia body system, qualifiers are used to specify when more than one tissue layer was used in the Transfer procedure. Table 14.3 lists the qualifiers available for use in coding procedures performed on the integumentary system.

Coding Tip

When tissue flaps are coded with the root operation of Transfer, the body system value describes the deepest tissue layer in the flap. The qualifier is used to describe when more than one tissue layer is transferred.

Table 14.3. Qualifiers for the Integumentary system

Qualifier Value	Qualifiers—Skin and Breast (H)
3	Full Thickness
4	Partial Thickness
5	Latissimus Dorsi Myocutaneous Flap
6	Transverse Rectus Abdominus Myocutaneous Flap
7	Deep Inferior Epigastric Artery Perforator Flap
8	Superficial Inferior Epigastric Artery Flap
9	Gluteal Artery Perforator Flap
D	Multiple
X	Diagnostic
Z	No Qualifier

Qualifier Value	Qualifiers—Subcutaneous Tissue and Fascia (J)
B	Skin and Subcutaneous Tissue
C	Skin, Subcutaneous Tissue and Fascia
X	Diagnostic
Z	No Qualifier

Code Building

Case #1:

PROCEDURE STATEMENT: Removal of implanted infusion port from patient's chest

ADDITIONAL INFORMATION: The implantable port is removed from the patient's subcutaneous layer following incision.

ROOT AND INDEX ENTRIES FOR THE STATEMENT: Removal is the root operation performed in this procedure, defined as taking out or off a device from a body part. The Index entry is:

Removal of device from

    Subcutaneous tissue and fascia

      Trunk   0JPT

Code Characters:

Section	Body System	Root Operation	Body Part	Approach	Device	Qualifier
Medical and Surgical	Subcutaneous Tissue and Fascia	Removal	Subcutaneous Tissue and Fascia, Trunk	Open	Vascular Access Device, Totally Implantable	No Qualifier
0	J	P	T	0	W	Z

RATIONALE FOR THE ANSWER: The root operation Removal is coded when devices are taken out or off from a body part. The implantable port is a vascular access device that was implanted in the subcutaneous layer of the patient's chest. Removal of implantable devices requires an incision and therefore the approach value of 0, Open is assigned. The device value is W, Vascular Access Device, Totally Implantable. The correct code assignment is 0JPT0WZ.

Case #2:

PROCEDURE STATEMENT: Destruction of three skin lesions on back

ADDITIONAL INFORMATION: Three full-thickness lesions are removed from the patient's right upper back using cryocautery.

ROOT AND INDEX ENTRIES FOR THE STATEMENT: Destruction is the root operation performed in this procedure, defined as physical eradication of all or a portion of a body part by the direct use of energy, force, or a destructive agent. The Index entry is:

Destruction

    Skin

      Back   0H56XZ

Code Characters:

Section	Body System	Root Operation	Body Part	Approach	Device	Qualifier
Medical and Surgical	Skin and Breast	Destruction	Skin, Back	External	No Device	Multiple
0	H	5	6	X	Z	D

RATIONALE FOR THE ANSWER: The root operation Destruction is used to code the removal of the lesions using cryocautery because the lesions are completely eradicated. The body part value of 6, Skin, back is used. The exact location of right and upper back is not classifiable in ICD-10-PCS. Destruction of a skin lesion uses the External approach. Three lesions destroyed and, therefore, the qualifier of D, Multiple is assigned. The correct code assignment is 0H56XZD.

Case #3:

PROCEDURE STATEMENT: Incision and drainage of an axillary abscess of the soft tissue

ADDITIONAL INFORMATION: The patient has a non-healing abscess of the soft tissue of the right axilla. The abscess is drained through an incision. No device remains at the end of the procedure.

ROOT AND INDEX ENTRIES FOR THE STATEMENT: Drainage is the root operation performed in this procedure, defined as taking or letting out fluids and/or gases from a body part. The Index entry is:

Drainage

    Subcutaneous tissue and fascia

        Upper arm

            Left   0J9F

            Right   0J9D

Code Characters:

Section	Body System	Root Operation	Body Part	Approach	Device	Qualifier
Medical and Surgical	Subcutaneous Tissue and Fascia	Drainage	Subcutaneous Tissue and Fascia, Right Upper Arm	Open	No Device	No Qualifier
0	J	9	D	0	Z	Z

RATIONALE FOR THE ANSWER: The root operation Drainage is used to code an incision and drainage procedure. Guideline B4.6 instructs the coder that the shoulder is part of the upper arm, and, therefore, the axilla is part of the upper arm body part. This is coded in the Subcutaneous Tissue and Fascia body system because the "soft tissue" layer is identified. The body part of axilla, found in the Anatomical Regions, Upper Extremities body system is only used when a specific body layer is not mentioned in the documentation. Incision and drainage procedures use an Open approach. No device value or qualifier value are appropriate for this code. The correct code assignment is 0J9D0ZZ.

Code Building Exercises

Work through each case and check your answers using the answer key in Appendix B of the textbook before going on to the Check Your Understanding questions that follow.

Exercise 1:

PREOPERATIVE DIAGNOSIS:	Abdominal wall abscess
POSTOPERATIVE DIAGNOSIS:	Incisional abscess
PROCEDURE:	Incision and drainage (I&D) of abdominal abscess, excisional debridement of nonviable skin, subcutaneous tissue and fascia

INDICATIONS: Patient is a pleasant 60-year-old gentleman who initially had a sigmoid colectomy for diverticular abscess. Came in approximately 24 hours ago with pain across his lower abdomen and an oozing incision site. CT scan demonstrated presence of an abscess beneath the incision.

FINDINGS: The patient was found to have an abscess that went down to the level of the fascia. The anterior layer of the fascia was fibrinous and some portions necrotic. This was excisionally debrided using the Bovie cautery and scalpel.

TECHNIQUE: Patient was identified, then taken into the operating room where, after induction of anesthesia, his abdomen was prepped with Betadine solution and draped in a sterile fashion. The wound opening where it was draining was explored using a curette. The extent of the wound marked with a marking pen and using the Bovie cautery, the abscess was opened and evacuated. I then noted that there was a significant amount of necrosis below this. Bovie cautery and scalpel were used to remove the necrotic fascia. The wound was irrigated and after achievement of excellent hemostasis, the wound was packed with antibiotic-soaked gauze. A dressing was applied. Patient tolerated the procedure well, and he was taken to recovery room in stable condition.

Questions:

1.1. Is there a guideline that helps determine the body system involved in this procedure? If so, which one?

_____

1.2. In which body system is this procedure coded?

_____

1.3. What code(s) would be assigned?

_____

Exercise 2:

PREOPERATIVE DIAGNOSIS:	Full thickness open wound, right foot, 70 sq cm
POSTOPERATIVE DIAGNOSIS:	Full thickness open wound, right foot, 70 sq cm
OPERATION:	Debridement of recipient site of right foot skin wound and split-thickness autograft from right thigh to right foot

INDICATIONS: This young man developed a deep venous thrombosis resulting in an ischemic injury to his right foot resulting in tissue necrosis. He is now ready for skin grafting.

PROCEDURE: The patient was placed on the operating table in the supine position under general anesthesia with orotracheal intubation. The foot and thigh were prepped with Betadine and draped in a sterile fashion. The right lateral foot wound had healthy granulation tissue for the majority, but there was some soft eschar remaining. Approximately 15 sq cm of skin were debrided using a #15 blade in a tangential excision until healthy, bleeding tissue was encountered. This resulted in a 7 × 10 cm wound. A split-thickness graft at 12/1000 of an inch was harvested from the right thigh using a Padgett dermatome. The skin graft was meshed 1:1 and placed unexpanded over the distal aspect of the wound. This would allow maximal take of the graft. The graft was sutured in placed using 5-0 gut sutures continuously. The wound was dressed with Adaptic, followed by cotton gauze soaked in mineral oil and a dry dressing. The patient was extubated and left the OR in stable condition.

Questions:

2.1. Based on ICD-10-PCS definitions and guidelines, how many procedures will be coded for this documentation and why?

_____

2.2. Which definition and/or guideline supports your decision?

_____

2.3. What are the procedures to be coded?

_____

 Check Your Understanding

Coding Knowledge Check

1. A laceration of the skin and subcutaneous tissue of the right wrist is repaired. Which body part value is assigned?
   a. B, Skin of right lower arm
   b. G, Subcutaneous tissue and fascia, right lower arm
   c. F, Skin of right hand
   d. J, Subcutaneous tissue and fascia, right hand

2. When a qualifier value of 6 is assigned for a breast procedure, the procedure is called a _____ flap.

3. The patient was bitten in the head by a dog, creating a flap laceration of a 4 cm × 3 cm piece of scalp, including the subcutaneous layer. Which root operation is used to code the restoration completed by the surgeon?
   a. Alteration
   b. Reattachment
   c. Repair
   d. Transfer

4. The surgeon performs a biopsy of the breast, which is confirmed as adenocarcinoma by frozen section. The surgeon performs a mastectomy at the same operative session. How many procedures are coded?

   _____

5. Using a surgical scissors, the podiatrist cuts away the ingrown toenail of a patient with diabetes to reduce the patient's pain while walking. Which root operation(s) is(are) coded for this procedure?
   a. Alteration
   b. Excision

(*Continued*)

c. Extraction
d. Extirpation

Procedure Statement Coding

Assign ICD-10-PCS codes to the following procedure statements and scenarios. List the root operation selected and the code assigned.

1. Cryocautery of five skin lesions of the inguinal region

   _____

2. Skin lesion removal, left inguinal area

   _____

3. Repair of laceration of subcutaneous tissue and fascia of the left foot with layered closure

   _____

4. Needle drainage of left breast cyst for evaluation

   _____

5. Evacuation of subungual hematoma, fingernail

   _____

6. Bilateral breast augmentation with silicone implants, open approach

   _____

7. The patient presents for repair of a 3rd-degree burn of the right forearm caused when a chemical splashed on his arm at work. The burn measures 2 cm × 3 cm and the burn eschar is excised before the skin and subcutaneous tissue advancement flap is created. The advanced flap measures 3 cm × 4 cm.

   _____

8. Placement of a rechargeable multiple array stimulator generator into the fat layer of the patient's back, open approach

   _____

9. Incision of scar contracture of the skin of the right elbow

   _____

10. Incision of pilonidal cyst

   _____

Case Studies

Assign ICD-10-PCS codes to the following case studies.

1. Operative Report

PREOPERATIVE DIAGNOSIS:	Full-thickness burn injuries to bilateral buttocks, left thigh, and right thigh
POSTOPERATIVE DIAGNOSIS:	Full-thickness burn injuries to bilateral buttocks, left thigh, and right thigh
PROCEDURE PERFORMED:	Application of cultured epidermal graft to full-thickness burn injuries previously excised, to bilateral buttocks and bilateral thighs

INDICATIONS FOR PROCEDURE: The patient is a 4-year-old male who previously had undergone wound preparation with excision and removal of an old allograft and granulation tissue from bilateral buttocks and bilateral thighs. This was done in preparation for application of cultured epidermal graft today.

DESCRIPTION OF THE PROCEDURE: The patient was brought to the operating room and placed in the supine position on the OR table. General anesthesia and endotracheal intubation were accomplished without difficulty. The patient was then turned to the prone position, where the previously placed operative dressings were removed. After this was done, bleeding was controlled with the electrocautery unit and warm laparotomy pads. After the wounds had been prepared and hemostasis obtained, cultured skin applications were done on the above area. They were secured with staples in all corners of the areas and then dressed with fine mesh gauze dressing, followed by wet burn dressing, irrigation catheters, and Spandex to secure the dressings to the wound. After this was done, the patient was turned to the supine position without difficulty or incident, and he was transferred to the recovery room in good condition.

2. Operative Report

PREOPERATIVE DIAGNOSIS: Ductal carcinoma in situ of right breast

POSTOPERATIVE DIAGNOSIS: Ductal carcinoma in situ of right breast

PROCEDURE: Right needle-localized lumpectomy

INDICATIONS: The patient is a 68-year-old woman who was noted to have abnormal calcifications at roughly the 6 o'clock position of the areola. These were biopsied and found to be ductal carcinoma in situ. She has requested to proceed with the needle-localized lumpectomy. The risks of bleeding, infection, poor wound healing, and unappealing cosmetics were discussed. The possibility that we could find invasive carcinoma was also discussed. The need for postoperative radiation therapy was also discussed. She was well aware of the possibility of positive margins which would lead to further surgery or mastectomy. The localization needle was placed in the inferior aspect of the right breast at the Breast Diagnostic Center by radiology just prior to this procedure and is dictated separately.

PROCEDURE: The patient was moved to the surgical suite, where general anesthesia was again verified. A curvilinear incision was made on the inferior aspect of the areola. This was taken down to the subcutaneous tissue. Flaps were raised in each direction for approximately 2 cm and taken down to the chest wall. A long stitch was placed medially, a short stitch superiorly. The specimen was then removed. The cavity was then thoroughly irrigated. 0.25 percent Marcaine was used for local anesthesia. The subcutaneous tissue was then approximated using 3-0 Monocryl. The skin was approximated using 4-0 Monocryl in a running subcuticular fashion. A sterile dressing was then applied. The patient tolerated the procedure well and was taken to the recovery room.

3. Operative Report

DIAGNOSIS: Complex congenital heart disease with ongoing need for vascular access

NAME OF PROCEDURE: Placement of a Broviac catheter (4.2-French Broviac via left saphenous vein).

INDICATIONS: I was asked to place a Broviac catheter in this 8-day-old baby with complex heart disease who has had an initial repair with delayed sternal closure. A lower vein Broviac is requested due to lack of available space or vessels in chest.

DESCRIPTION OF PROCEDURE: With the patient in the supine position under general anesthesia, the lower abdomen, inguinal region and genitalia, and anterior left thigh were all prepped with Betadine and draped in a sterile fashion. We made a small transverse incision just below the inguinal crease and noted meticulous hemostasis as we dissected down onto the saphenous vein. The saphenous was isolated with 5-0 silk ties. We fashioned a subcutaneous tunnel from further down on the left thigh a few centimeters above the knee up to groin incision and brought a 4.2-French pediatric Broviac catheter through the tunnel, placing the cuff just inside the insertion site. The insertion site was snugged around the catheter with a 4-0 nylon that was also used to affix the catheter to the leg and an additional nylon used to further affix the catheter to the leg. An appropriate length of catheter was cut. A small venotomy was made in the saphenous and the catheter was threaded proximally. Fluoroscopy identified the tip lie in the inferior vena. I used a 6-0 Prolene suture to secure the catheter in place. The catheter seemed to function very well in terms of infusion and withdrawal, and the femoral vein itself was not compromised in terms of its overall diameter. A 0.25% plain Marcaine block was administered. We noted hemostasis and then closed the groin wound with interrupted 5-0 Vicryl subcuticular sutures. The wound was dressed with a Tegaderm. A Biopatch disc was applied at the catheter skin insertion site. The catheter was curled under a Tegaderm. The entire system was then heparinized with 1.5 mL of standard heparin saline flush.

4. Operative Report

PREOPERATIVE DIAGNOSIS: Pacemaker malfunction

POSTOPERATIVE DIAGNOSIS: Same

OPERATION PERFORMED: Replacement of pacemaker generator and electrode

PROCEDURE: The patient was positioned on the fluoroscopy table and the right chest was prepared and draped. Local anesthesia was obtained with 1 percent lidocaine with epinephrine. The pocket was reopened and the generator removed. Analysis of the lead showed intermittent R waves obtained. At this point, it was elected to proceed with insertion of a new lead and generator. A Medtronic lead, model #4024-52, serial number KJH124391W, was placed into the apex of the right ventricle. The lead was sutured in place using 2-0 silk and connected to a Medtronic generator. This was a DVI single chamber pacer programmed at a rate of 70. Inspection was made to be certain that hemostasis was adequate. The old lead was capped and abandoned. The wound was closed using 3-0 Vicryl for subcutaneous tissue and 3-0 nylon for skin. Dry dressings were applied, and the patient was returned to the recovery room in satisfactory condition.

5. Operative Report

PREOPERATIVE DIAGNOSIS: Advanced ovarian cancer

POSTOPERATIVE DIAGNOSIS: Advanced ovarian cancer

PROCEDURE PERFORMED: Insertion of venous access port

HISTORY: The patient is a 59-year-old female who underwent a hysterectomy last week as well as omental and abdominal washing sampling for advanced ovarian cancer. The patient now is to start on chemotherapy and actually has received a dose already, but Oncology has requested placement of a port. The procedure for this, risks, options, and expected post-op course were discussed with the patient, and she agreed to surgery.

WHAT WAS DONE: With the patient first in supine position, the left chest, shoulder, and neck area were prepped and draped in the usual fashion. On the first stick the subclavian vein was identified, blood flowed and aspirated easily into the syringe, and a flexible guidewire was passed into the right atrium under fluoroscopy. 1 percent Xylocaine with epinephrine was then instilled over the anterior chest wall, and a subcutaneous pocket was made. I then made a tunnel from the pocket up to this site of the wire that exited the subclavian area. Through this tunnel I would pass the catheter. At this point, the vein dilator and introducer sheath were then placed over the wire, the wire and the dilator were removed, and the catheter was threaded through the sheath as it was peeled away, and under fluoroscopic control we put the tip into the superior vena cava. At this point at the chest wall site I cut the catheter to the appropriate length, hooked it up to the port, and anchored the port to the anterior chest wall with silk sutures. I then tested the port three or four times, and each time it easily infused heparinized saline and each time it easily aspirated blood. I then percutaneously placed an angled Huber needle hooked up to a butterfly through-and-through the skin and subcutaneous tissue through the area so that I accessed the port. I then tested this three or four times. Each time it easily instilled heparinized saline and easily aspirated blood, and then I flushed it with heparinized saline and capped it. At this point, I checked once more with fluoroscopy to make sure the catheter tip was in good position, and it appeared to be in the superior vena cava. At this point, the incisions were closed in layers with chromic to the subcutaneous tissue and a running PDS subcuticular stitch to close the skin followed by Benzoin, Steri-Strips, gauze dressings, and Tegaderm. The patient tolerated the procedure well and left the operating room for the recovery room.

6. Operative Report

PREOPERATIVE DIAGNOSIS:
1. Stage IV right trochanteric pressure sore
2. Partial quadriplegia
3. Osteomyelitis right trochanter

POSTOPERATIVE DIAGNOSIS:
1. Stage IV right trochanteric pressure sore
2. Partial quadriplegia
3. Osteomyelitis right trochanter

PROCEDURE(S) PERFORMED:
1. Excision of stage IV right trochanteric pressure sore (with ostectomy)
2. Right tensor fascia lata (TFL) fasciocutaneous flap closure of stage IV right trochanteric pressure sore

SPECIMEN: Excised soft tissue and bone right trochanter

HISTORY: A 30-year-old male who, five years ago, sustained a head injury and was left with partial quadriplegia. He had a longstanding history of a non-healing wound to the right trochanter. He now returns after IV antibiotics and local wound care. The plan today is to excise the bone and close the wound with a well-vascularized flap. The patient understands the risks of the procedure to include but not limited to infection, hematoma, delayed wound healing, a partial or total loss of the flap, need for further surgery, and ongoing infection in the bone, and all of his questions were answered.

DETAILS OF PROCEDURE: The patient was brought to the operating room and placed supine on the operating room table. An endotracheal tube could not be placed due to the patient's anteriorly placed trachea and neck fusion. He was placed with his right side up. He was prepped and draped in a sterile fashion.

The wound was painted with methylene blue, including some undermined edges. The wound edges were freshened up with a #10 blade. All of the methylene blue-stained tissue was excised. This took us down to some remainder of the greater trochanter, which was cleaned and osteotome was used to resect the visible portion.

A tensor fascia lata flap was designed to close this large wound. It was incised, taken down through the subcutaneous tissue to the fascia. The fascia was incised and from an inferior to superior direction, dissection was carried out to free the flap from the surrounding tissue. The pedicle was identified medially and preserved. The flap was rotated into place. All the wounds had been irrigated with antibiotic irrigation through the Pulsava jet irrigator. Hemostasis was achieved with cautery. Closed suction drains were placed, and the flap was inset and the donor site closed using interrupted 0 Vicryl, 2-0 Vicryl, and 3-0 nylon suture. There was a 3-cm portion where the donor site met the flap medially which could not be closed without stressing the flap, and therefore, this was left open. This area was packed with saline-soaked gauzes. The remainder was covered with Xerofrom dressing, dry sterile dressings, and Tegaderm. The patient was transferred directly into a Clinitron bed, and was taken to the recovery room in stable conditions.

Chapter

15

Muscular System: Muscles, Tendons, Bursae, and Ligaments

This chapter begins the discussion of the musculoskeletal system with the musculature, the ICD-10-PCS sections on muscles, tendons, bursae, and ligaments. The 2nd character values for the muscular system are:

K—Muscles
L—Tendons
M—Bursae and Ligaments

Functions of the Muscular System

The four functions of the muscular system are to:

- **Produce movement**—Muscle contractions create the movement of the body
- **Maintain the posture of the body**—Sitting or standing cannot be accomplished without muscle contraction
- **Provide joint stability**—Tendons extend over joints to protect them
- **Produce the heat necessary to maintain body temperature**—Muscle metabolism creates nearly 85 percent of the heat produced in the body (Applegate 2011, 164)

The muscular system holds the bones and joints together. Bones and joints cannot move without the help of muscles, tendons, and ligaments. The bursa help these structures move more effectively. All voluntary movement happens by contraction of skeletal muscle, and in addition to this role in movement, the muscles help determine the outer shape of the body.

Organization of the Muscular System

The ICD-10-PCS code structure for procedures performed on the musculoskeletal system includes sections on muscles, tendons, bursae, and ligaments; head and facial bones; upper bones; lower bones; upper joints; and lower joints. This chapter and chapter 16 describe the specific root operations, body parts, approaches, devices, and qualifiers commonly used on procedures performed on these structures.

Muscles

Muscles are bundles of individual muscle fibers that are wrapped by a connective tissue covering. Each individual muscle bundle is covered by epimysium. Fascia surrounds the epimysium and separates each muscle. Fascia is categorized in ICD-10-PCS in the same section as subcutaneous tissues, covered in chapter 14. These outer coverings support and protect the cells and aid in their contraction (Applegate 2011, 141). The origin of a muscle is the fixed or more stable end of the muscle. The insertion of the muscle is the more movable attachment of the muscle. The anterior muscular system is displayed in figure 15.1, and the posterior muscular system is displayed in figure 15.2.

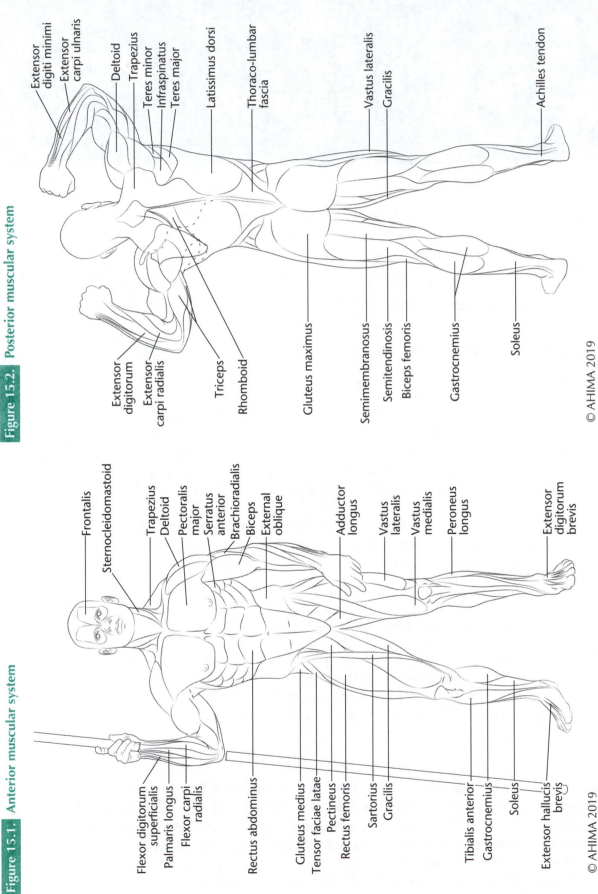

Figure 15.2.   Posterior muscular system

Extensor digiti minimi
Extensor carpi ulnaris
Deltoid
Trapezius
Teres minor
Infraspinatus
Teres major
Latissimus dorsi
Thoraco-lumbar fascia
Vastus lateralis
Gracilis
Achilles tendon

Extensor digitorum
Extensor carpi radialis
Triceps
Rhomboid
Gluteus maximus
Semimembranosus
Semitendinosis
Biceps femoris
Gastrocnemius
Soleus

© AHIMA 2019

Figure 15.1.   Anterior muscular system

Frontalis
Sternocleidomastoid
Trapezius
Deltoid
Pectoralis major
Serratus anterior
Brachioradialis
Biceps
External oblique
Adductor longus
Vastus lateralis
Vastus medialis
Peroneus longus
Extensor digitorum brevis

Flexor digitorum superficialis
Palmaris longus
Flexor carpi radialis
Rectus abdominus
Gluteus medius
Tensor faciae latae
Pectineus
Rectus femoris
Sartorius
Gracilis
Tibialis anterior
Gastrocnemius
Soleus
Extensor hallucis brevis

© AHIMA 2019

Tendons

"A tendon is a ropelike extension of the connective tissue coverings of a muscle that attaches a muscle to a bone" (Applegate 2011, 164). An aponeurosis is a broader, flatter, sheet-like tendon that connects a muscle to a bone. The hands and the feet are a complex combination of muscles, tendons, and ligaments. The tendons are almost always named for the muscle that they attach to bone. The notable exception is the Achilles tendon, found at the back of the lower leg connecting the gastrocnemius muscles to the calcaneus bone on the bottom of the foot (Rizzo 2016, 209). The tendons of the hand are displayed in figure 15.3, and the tendons of the foot are displayed in figure 15.4.

Bursae and Ligaments

A bursa is a flat, fluid-filled sac found between a bone and a tendon or muscle that forms a cushion to help the tendon or muscle slide smoothly over the bone. Figure 15.5 shows the subacromial bursa, which forms a cushion between the deltoid tendon and the supraspinatus tendon. Figure 15.6 shows the bursae of the knee, cushioning the many tendons and ligaments that form the knee joint capsule.

Ligaments are shiny, flexible bands of fibrous tissue connecting together articular parts of bones. Figure 15.7 details the ligaments of the knee.

Figure 15.3 **Extensor tendons of the hand**

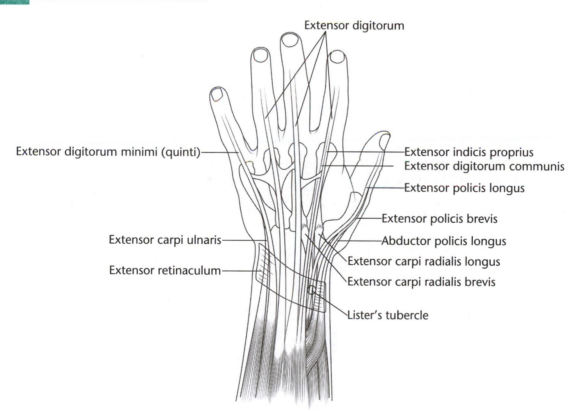

© AHIMA 2019

Figure 15.4. Tendons of the foot

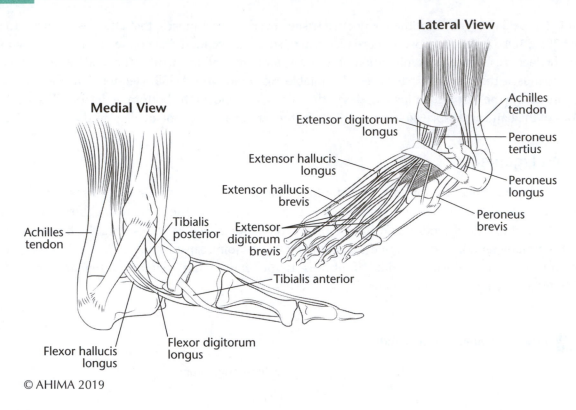

Lateral View

Medial View

Extensor digitorum
longus

Achilles
tendon

Peroneus
tertius

Extensor hallucis
longus

Peroneus
longus

Extensor hallucis
brevis

Tibialis
posterior

Peroneus
brevis

Achilles
tendon

Extensor
digitorum
brevis

Tibialis anterior

Flexor hallucis
longus

Flexor digitorum
longus

© AHIMA 2019

Figure 15.5. Subacromial bursa

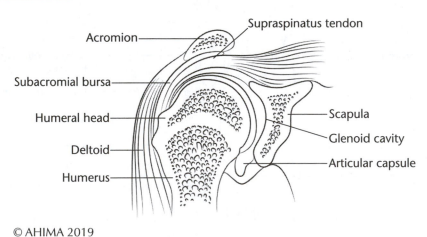

Acromion

Supraspinatus tendon

Subacromial bursa

Humeral head

Scapula

Deltoid

Glenoid cavity

Humerus

Articular capsule

© AHIMA 2019

Figure 15.6. Knee bursae

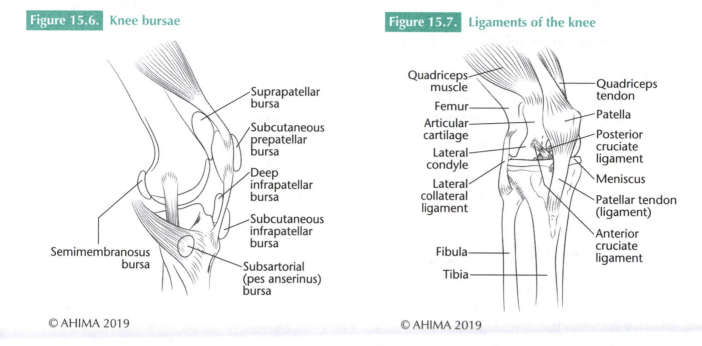

Suprapatellar bursa

Subcutaneous prepatellar bursa

Deep infrapatellar bursa

Subcutaneous infrapatellar bursa

Semimembranosus bursa

Subsartorial (pes anserinus) bursa

© AHIMA 2019

Figure 15.7. Ligaments of the knee

Quadriceps muscle

Femur

Articular cartilage

Lateral condyle

Lateral collateral ligament

Fibula

Tibia

Quadriceps tendon

Patella

Posterior cruciate ligament

Meniscus

Patellar tendon (ligament)

Anterior cruciate ligament

© AHIMA 2019

Common Root Operations Used in Coding of Procedures on the Muscular System

Some of the more common procedures performed on tendons are tenolysis, tenotomy, and tenodesis.

- Tenolysis is the freeing of a tendon from adhesions and is coded to the root operation of Release.
- A tenotomy is cutting of the tendon and is coded to the root operation of Division.
- Tenodesis is surgical anchoring of a tendon to a bone with sutures and may be coded as the root operation Reposition if the tendon is moved, such as in a biceps tenodesis where the biceps tendon is moved to the humerus. Tenodesis may also be coded to the root operation of Reattachment if the tendon has ruptured from the bone (completely separated, avulsed) and must be sutured to the bone in the same location. If the tendon is lacerated through the tendon itself, the root operation of Repair is assigned when the tendon is sutured to itself.

Decompression fasciotomy procedures are performed to release trapped muscles, such as those found in compartment syndrome. These procedures are coded with the root operation Release and the body part value is the muscle being released. Surgical debridement of damaged muscle may also be required in the same procedure, coded to the root operation Excision.

Coding Tip

The root operation Division is coded when the sole objective of the procedure is to cut into, transect, or otherwise separate all or a portion of a body part. When the objective is to cut or separate the area around a body part or the attachments to a body part that are causing abnormal constraint, then the root operation Release is coded instead.

Bursitis can be treated with drainage or removal, based on the extent of the inflammation. Removal of an entire bursa would be coded to the root operation Resection.

When an injury occurs to multiple layers, such as the skin, subcutaneous tissue, and muscles, the repair is coded to the deepest layer repaired, based on guideline B3.5. Repair of the outer layers is included in the procedure, as the closure of any open procedure is included in the definitive procedure performed. The same concept applies for Excision and the newer Extraction tables in the muscles, tendons and bones body systems. Extraction is used to code nonexcisional debridement of these structures.

B3.5. If the root operations Excision, Repair, or Inspection are performed on overlapping layers of the musculoskeletal system, the body part specifying the deepest layer is coded.

Example: Excisional debridement that includes skin and subcutaneous tissue and muscle is coded to the muscle body part.

Be sure to research any procedure that is unfamiliar to assure correct coding. If the documentation includes an eponym (procedure named for a person) and the intent of the procedure is unclear, query the physician for specifics.

Body Parts for the Muscular System

Body part values in the muscular system can include multiple individual structures rather than naming each structure with a value. For example, the muscle body part value of R, Upper Leg Muscle, Left includes 14 individual muscles of the upper leg. The same is true for tendons. Tendon body part values are determined by their associated muscle name. Therefore, documentation should be assessed carefully to determine if the procedure is being performed on a muscle or a tendon, as either could be named using a similar name. For example, the lower leg contains both the flexor digitorum longus muscle and the flexor digitorum longus tendon.

If a specific tendon, ligament, or bursa supporting a joint is the focus of a procedure at a joint, the procedure should be coded to that body part. If the procedure is performed on joint structures themselves, the procedure is coded to the joint body system, covered in chapter 16. Muscles of the finger are considered part of the hand muscle body part and those of the toes are considered part of the foot muscle body part. The same is true for tendons and ligaments of the fingers and toes.

In addition, laterality is important in the muscular system. Depending on the root operation, it is necessary to know which body part, the right or the left, was involved in the surgery in order to assign a code. If the same root operation is performed on multiple body parts, and those body parts are separate and distinct body parts classified to a single ICD-10-PCS body part value, multiple procedures are coded. The muscles and tendons are good examples of where this is possible. Table 15.1 shows the body part values assigned to the muscular system. If the documentation includes specific body part names that are not included in these lists, refer to the body part key for other body part synonyms and alternative terms.

Table 15.1. Body part values

Body Part Value	Body Parts— Muscles (K)	Body Part Value	Body Parts— Tendons (L)	Body Part Value	Body Parts—Bursae and Ligaments (M)
0	Head Muscle	0	Head and Neck Tendon	0	Head and Neck Bursa and Ligament
1	Facial Muscle	1	Shoulder Tendon, Right	1	Shoulder Bursa and Ligament, Right
2	Neck Muscle, Right	2	Shoulder Tendon, Left	2	Shoulder Bursa and Ligament, Left
3	Neck Muscle, Left	3	Upper Arm Tendon, Right		
4	Tongue, Palate, Pharynx Muscle	4	Upper Arm Tendon, Left	3	Elbow Bursa and Ligament, Right
		5	Lower Arm and Wrist Tendon, Right		
5	Shoulder Muscle, Right			4	Elbow Bursa and Ligament, Left
6	Shoulder Muscle, Left	6	Lower Arm and Wrist Tendon, Left	5	Wrist Bursa and Ligament, Right
7	Upper Arm Muscle, Right	7	Hand Tendon, Right		

(Continued)

(Continued)

(Continued)

Table 15.1.   Body part values (continued)

Body Part Value	Body Parts—Muscles (K)	Body Part Value	Body Parts—Tendons (L)	Body Part Value	Body Parts—Bursae and Ligaments (M)
8	Upper Arm Muscle, Left	8	Hand Tendon, Left	6	Wrist Bursa and Ligament, Left
9	Lower Arm and Wrist Muscle, Right	9	Trunk Tendon, Right	7	Hand Bursa and Ligament, Right
B	Lower Arm and Wrist Muscle, Left	B	Trunk Tendon, Left	8	Hand Bursa and Ligament, Left
C	Hand Muscle, Right	C	Thorax Tendon, Right	9	Upper Extremity Bursa and Ligament, Right
D	Hand Muscle, Left	D	Thorax Tendon, Left	B	Upper Extremity Bursa and Ligament, Left
F	Trunk Muscle, Right	F	Abdomen Tendon, Right	C	Upper Spine Bursa and Ligament
G	Trunk Muscle, Left	G	Abdomen Tendon, Left	D	Lower Spine Bursa and Ligament
H	Thorax Muscle, Right	H	Perineum Tendon	F	Sternum Bursa and Ligament
J	Thorax Muscle, Left	J	Hip Tendon, Right	G	Rib(s) Bursa and Ligament
K	Abdomen Muscle, Right	K	Hip Tendon, Left	H	Abdomen Bursa and Ligament, Right
L	Abdomen Muscle, Left	L	Upper Leg Tendon, Right	J	Abdomen Bursa and Ligament, Left
M	Perineum Muscle	M	Upper Leg Tendon, Left	K	Perineum Bursa and Ligament
N	Hip Muscle, Right	N	Lower Leg Tendon, Right	L	Hip Bursa and Ligament, Right
P	Hip Muscle, Left	P	Lower Leg Tendon, Left	M	Hip Bursa and Ligament, Left
Q	Upper Leg Muscle, Right	Q	Knee Tendon, Right	N	Knee Bursa and Ligament, Right
R	Upper Leg Muscle, Left	R	Knee Tendon, Left	P	Knee Bursa and Ligament, Left
S	Lower Leg Muscle, Right	S	Ankle Tendon, Right	Q	Ankle Bursa and Ligament, Right
T	Lower Leg Muscle, Left	T	Ankle Tendon, Left	R	Ankle Bursa and Ligament, Left
V	Foot Muscle, Right	V	Foot Tendon, Right	S	Foot Bursa and Ligament, Right
W	Foot Muscle, Left	W	Foot Tendon, Left	T	Foot Bursa and Ligament, Left
X	Upper Muscle	X	Upper Tendon	V	Lower Extremity Bursa and Ligament, Right
Y	Lower Muscle	Y	Lower Tendon	W	Lower Extremity Bursa and Ligament, Left
				X	Upper Bursa and Ligament
				Y	Lower Bursa and Ligament

Approaches Used for the Muscular System

There are no natural orifices and typically no artificial orifices within the muscular system. Therefore, the approaches available for use in coding procedures performed on this system are Open, Percutaneous, Percutaneous endoscopic, and External.

Devices Common to the Muscular System

Device values for the muscular system are limited. The muscles, tendons, and bursae and ligaments all contain the same device values with the addition of Device value M, Stimulator lead to the muscular system. Muscles contract based on electrical signals sent from the brain through the nerves and into the muscles. Stimulator leads are inserted within the muscles to cause muscle contractions and prevent muscle atrophy after extensive trauma. Table 15.2 lists the Device values available for use in the muscular system.

Table 15.2. Devices for the muscles, tendons, bursae, and ligaments

Device Value	Devices—Muscles (K)	Device Value	Devices—Tendons (L)	Device Value	Devices—Bursae and Ligaments (M)
0	Drainage Device	0	Drainage Device	0	Drainage Device
7	Autologous Tissue Substitute	7	Autologous Tissue Substitute	7	Autologous Tissue Substitute
J	Synthetic Substitute	J	Synthetic Substitute	J	Synthetic Substitute
K	Nonautologous Tissue Substitute	K	Nonautologous Tissue Substitute	K	Nonautologous Tissue Substitute
M	Stimulator Lead	Y	Other Device	Y	Other Device
Y	Other Device	Z	No Device	Z	No Device
Z	No Device				

Qualifiers Used in the Muscular System

Qualifier values represent the body layers transferred in addition to the muscle included in the procedure, when the root operation of Transfer is being performed. In the Transfer procedure, myocutaneous flaps are differentiated from muscle flaps by the qualifier. If only the muscle is transferred, the qualifier value of Z, No Qualifier is assigned. This means that the muscle was moved locally to take over the function of another weaker or absent muscle. This is different than a myocutaneous flap transfer in which the muscle and all of the tissue above it are transferred locally. In this case, the qualifier value of 2, Skin and Subcutaneous Tissue is assigned because the entire flap of tissue is transferred. If a specific flap name is identified as a qualifier option, the specific qualifier is assigned. This is typically done to reconstruct an area for major tissue loss. Muscular system procedures may also use the standard qualifiers of X for Diagnostic and Z for No Qualifier. Table 15.3 lists the qualifier values available for use with the Muscular system.

Table 15.3. Qualifiers for the muscles, tendons, bursae, and ligaments

Qualifier Value	Qualifiers—Muscles (K)	Qualifier Value	Qualifiers—Tendons (L)	Qualifier Value	Qualifiers—Bursae and Ligaments (M)
0	Skin	X	Diagnostic	X	Diagnostic
1	Subcutaneous Tissue	Z	No Qualifier	Z	No Qualifier
2	Skin and Subcutaneous Tissue				
5	Latissimus Dorsi Myocutaneous Flap				
6	Transverse Rectus Myocutaneous Flap				
7	Deep Inferior Epigastric Artery Perforator Flap				
8	Superficial Inferior Epigastric Artery Flap				
9	Gluteal Artery Perforator Flap				
X	Diagnostic				
Z	No Qualifier				

Code Building

Case #1:

PROCEDURE STATEMENT: Cutting of the sternocleidomastoid tendon

ADDITIONAL INFORMATION: This open procedure was performed to release torticollis on the right side of the neck. The tendon that connects the sternocleidomastoid muscle to the sterno-clavicular joint is tight and is cut to release the muscle.

ROOT AND INDEX ENTRIES FOR THE STATEMENT: Release is the root operation performed in this procedure, defined as cutting into a body part without draining fluids and/or gases from the body part in order to separate or transect the body part. The body part being released is coded. The Index entry is:

Sternocleidomastoid muscle

    use Neck muscle, Right

    use Neck muscle, Left

and

Release

    Muscle

    Neck

        Left   0KN3

        Right 0KN2

Code Characters:

Section	Body System	Root Operation	Body Part	Approach	Device	Qualifier
Medical and Surgical	Muscles	Release	Neck Muscle, Right	Open	No Device	No Qualifier
0	K	N	2	0	Z	Z

RATIONALE FOR THE ANSWER: The body part key tells the coder that the sternocleidomastoid muscle is a muscle of the neck. The root operation Release is coded because the intent of the procedure was to release the muscle by cutting the tendon to relieve the torticollis, caused by a contracture of the tendon. The approach is open and no device value or qualifier value is appropriate for the code. The correct code assignment is 0KN20ZZ.

Case #2:

PROCEDURE STATEMENT: Removal of embedded foreign body in the subcutaneous infrapatellar bursa

ADDITIONAL INFORMATION: The patient fell forward onto the right knee and lodged a rough piece of gravel inside the bursa. The foreign body is removed via an incision.

ROOT AND INDEX ENTRIES FOR THE STATEMENT: Extirpation is the root operation performed in this procedure, defined as taking or cutting out solid matter from a body part. The Index entry is:

Extirpation

    Bursa and Ligament

Knee

Left   0MCP

Right   0MCN

Code Characters:

Section	Body System	Root Operation	Body Part	Approach	Device	Qualifier
Medical and Surgical	Bursae and Ligaments	Extirpation	Knee Bursa and Ligament, Right	Open	No Device	No Qualifier
0	M	C	N	0	Z	Z

RATIONALE FOR THE ANSWER: The infrapatellar bursa is a bursa of the knee. The root operation Extirpation is coded for the removal of the foreign body from the bursa. The approach is open through an incision. No device value or qualifier value is appropriate for this code. The correct code assignment is 0MCN0ZZ.

Case #3:

PROCEDURE STATEMENT: Masseter muscle transfer

ADDITIONAL INFORMATION: The procedure is performed to correct an angulation of the corner of the mouth and allow closure of the lips. No other layers were transferred and the procedure is performed through an incision in the mouth.

ROOT AND INDEX ENTRIES FOR THE STATEMENT: Transfer is the root operation performed in this procedure, defined as moving, without taking out, all or a portion of a body part to another location to take over the function of all or a portion of a body part. The Index entry is:

Masseter muscle

   use Head muscle

   and

   Transfer

   Muscle

      Head   0KX0

Code Characters:

Section	Body System	Root Operation	Body Part	Approach	Device	Qualifier
Medical and Surgical	Muscles	Transfer	Head Muscle	Open	No Device	No Qualifier
0	K	X	0	0	Z	Z

RATIONALE FOR THE ANSWER: The root operation Transfer is used because the muscle is not disconnected from the vascular and nervous supply. The body part key directs the coder to use the body part value 0, Head Muscle for the masseter muscle. The approach was open because the procedure was performed through an incision in the mouth. No device value or qualifier value is appropriate for this code. The correct code assignment is 0KX00ZZ.

Code Building Exercises

Work through each case and check your answers using the answer key in appendix B of the textbook before going on to the Check Your Understanding questions that follow.

Exercise 1:

DIAGNOSIS: Torn anterior cruciate ligament of the right knee

PROCEDURE: Reconstruction of the anterior cruciate ligament using patellar tendon graft

INDICATIONS: This is a 31-year-old male who sustained an ACL injury to his right knee during a surfing accident.

DESCRIPTION: The patient was placed under general anesthesia. The right knee was prepped and draped with the limb free. Tourniquet was applied to the thigh. Arthroscopic ports were placed and we found that the anterior cruciate ligament was torn away from the wall lateral femoral condyle. It was quite lax as well. Using a shaver, the ligament was trimmed and all the soft tissue was removed from around and up into the notch.

The arthroscopy was terminated. The tourniquet was elevated. An incision was made from the mid patella to the tibial tubercle, with dissection carried down to the patellar tendon. The middle third of the patellar tendon, approximately 10 to 11 mm, was harvested with bone plugs from tibia and patella. The patellar and tibial portions were marked and a small saw was used to cut the bone plugs from each end. The patellar defect was smoothed and tendon defect was approximated and closed.

The guide for the tibial tunnel was then put in place just in front of the posterior tibial tendon. A 10-mm channel was reamed with a bulldog reamer. The bone posterior to this was reamed for the plug plus 5 mm. The passer was put through the guide, and the guide was removed. The tendon graft was passed up into the channel and seemed to fit well. A biodegradable plug screw was set in place in the femur. This was approximately 9 × 25 mm. The position and tightness were excellent, and drawer test at this point was trace, as was the Lachman. There was no impingement of the graft with extension, and no change in the length. The 9 × 25 mm tibial plug screw was put into place. This, again, was quite tight, and the Lachman test was just a trace positive. The joint moved well and was irrigated with arthroscopic fluid. The wound was irrigated and the subcutaneous tissues were closed with 2-0 Vicryl. The skin was closed with 4-0 nylon, as was each of the ports. Dressing was applied as well as a Bledsoe brace.

Questions:

1.1. What is the intent of this procedure?

1.2. Are the bone plugs coded separately for this procedure? Why or why not?

1.3. Is the arthroscopy coded separately for this procedure? Why or why not?

1.4. Are there any other procedures to code?

1.5. What code(s) should be assigned?

Exercise 2:

DIAGNOSIS: Avulsed right patellar tendon at inferior pole of patella

PROCEDURE: Patellar tendon repair

INDICATION: The patient overflexed the right knee during a fall on the ice in which she collapsed with full weight onto the right knee. The tendon ruptured from the patella, requiring repair in the OR today.

DESCRIPTION: General anesthesia was administered, and the patient was prepped and draped, with tourniquet applied at the mid femur. The patient was positioned supine with a bump under the hip. A longitudinal incision was made from the inferior pole of the patella to the tibial tubercle and dissected down to the level of the tendon. The patellar space was irrigated and cleared of clots. The patellar bone sleeve is identified and is reduced without difficulty. A guide hole was drilled through the tendon and patellar bone sleeve. A partially threaded cannulated screw over a washer was introduced as a lag screw. Another lag screw was placed through the tibial tubercle at the base of the patellar tendon as an anchor for the patellotibial cerclage wire. A guide hole was drilled in the superior pole of the patella, parallel to the avulsion. The cerclage wire was looped under the anchor screw, turned in a figure-of-eight, tunneled through the superior pole of the patella, and cinched. The lag screw was tightened until the patellar bone sleeve was completely reduced and the tendon was in appropriate alignment. The wound was irrigated with antibiotic solution, and the wound was closed in layers. The knee was immobilized in extension in knee immobilizer. Passive ROM ordered through PT for post-op day #1.

Questions:

2.1. Research the repair of an avulsed patellar tendon. This may also be called a patellar sleeve fracture because the tendon pulls away a small piece of bone as it ruptures from the bone. What root operation describes the process of repairing this tendon avulsion?

   _____

2.2. Where does the body part key classify the patellar tendon?

   _____

2.3. What code(s) should be assigned?

   _____

 Check Your Understanding

Coding Knowledge Check

1. A finger muscle is coded to which body part value?
    a. Upper Muscle
    b. Lower Muscle
    c. Lower Arm and Wrist Muscle
    d. Hand Muscle

2. The insertion of a _____ into a lower muscle is coded as 0KHY0MZ.

3. A biceps tenodesis to the humerus is coded to which root operation?
    a. Reattachment
    b. Reposition

    c. Replacement

    d. Supplement

4. True or false? A tendon is often named for the bone of its insertion. _____

5. A _____ is between a bone and a tendon and forms a cushion to help the tendon slide.

Procedure Statement Coding

Assign ICD-10-PCS codes to the following procedure statements and scenarios. List the root operation selected and the code assigned.

1. Incision and drainage of infected right shoulder bursa

    _____

2. Following a previous MOHS surgery with deep excision of a tumor, an open myocutaneous flap was transferred on the right forearm.

    _____

3. Open repair of ruptured right deltoid muscle

    _____

4. Open palmaris longus tendon transfer of the right hand

    _____

5. Incision of the tendon sheath of the constricted extensor digitorum brevis in the right foot, percutaneous approach

    _____

6. Put back the avulsed left Achilles tendon, open approach

    _____

7. Percutaneous biopsy of right gastrocnemius muscle

    _____

8. Percutaneous removal of foreign body from the right abductor hallucis muscle

    _____

9. Open excision of lesion from right Achilles tendon

    _____

10. Pulling fluid from the left infrapatellar bursa, percutaneous approach

    _____

Case Studies

Assign ICD-10-PCS codes to the following case studies:

1. Operative Report

PREOPERATIVE DIAGNOSIS: 1. Circular saw injury with complex laceration of left index finger with laceration of extensor tendon and joint capsule

                                     2. Laceration collateral ligament, radial side

POSTOPERATIVE DIAGNOSIS:
1. Circular saw injury with complex laceration of left index finger with laceration of extensor tendon and joint capsule
2. Laceration collateral ligament, radial side

OPERATION PERFORMED:
1. Debridement and repair extensor tendon and joint capsule
2. Repair radial collateral ligament and wound closure

This is a 42-year-old white male who accidentally injured his left index finger on a circular saw while working at home in his garage. The patient sustained a jagged laceration over the dorsal radial aspect of the index finger at the proximal interphalangeal joint. The wound was deep, involving the joint capsule, extensor tendon, and collateral ligament. The sensation to the tip of the finger was intact, especially all of the radial side. The wound measured about 3 cm in length.

PROCEDURE: Local anesthetic digital block administered as 0.5 percent Marcaine. After anesthesia had been obtained, the hand was prepped and draped in the usual manner. Tourniquet then was placed at the base of the fingers. The wound was then debrided. After satisfactory debridement, the joint capsule and extensor tendon then were repaired with 5-0 PDS suture material. The radial collateral ligament also was repaired with the same suture material. The skin then was carefully approximated with 5-0 nylon. After completion, a dressing was applied. The tourniquet was released and there was good perfusion throughout the fingers. An aluminum splint was placed.

---

2. Operative Report

PREOPERATIVE DIAGNOSIS: Trigger finger, right index finger

POSTOPERATIVE DIAGNOSIS: Trigger finger, right index finger

OPERATION: Tenovaginotomy for triggering, right index finger

PROCEDURE DESCRIPTION: Under satisfactory sedation and monitoring by anesthesia, the right hand and arm were widely prepped and draped with Betadine in the standard fashion. A mid metacarpal digital block was carried out for anesthesia with 1 percent plain Xylocaine. The entire procedure was carried out under 4.5-power loupe magnification.

A transverse incision was made adjacent to the distal palmar crease at the proximal flexor sheath. Dissection was carried straight down to the A1 pulley, which was incised and partially excised for an adequate tenovaginotomy. The patient then had full active flexion and extension of the index finger. Hemostasis was secured.

The skin was closed with a running horizontal mattress suture of 5-0 Prolene. A Xeroform gauze, carefully molded and conforming hand dressing was applied. On release of the tourniquet, there was good circulation throughout the hand.

The patient tolerated the procedure well and was taken to the recovery room in stable and satisfactory condition.

---

3. Operative Report

PREOPERATIVE DIAGNOSIS: Carpometacarpal arthritis left thumb

POSTOPERATIVE DIAGNOSIS: Carpometacarpal arthritis left thumb

PROCEDURE: Left trapezial excision, tendon transfer

INDICATIONS: The patient is a 52-year-old gentleman with symptomatic carpometacarpal joint arthritis. He has failed conservative treatment and now is admitted for trapezial excision.

OPERATION: The patient was brought to the operating room, placed on the operating table in the supine position. General anesthesia was administered via LMA and the left arm was prepped and draped in the customary sterile fashion. An upper arm tourniquet was applied. The arm was exsanguinated and the tourniquet was placed at 250 torr. A C-shaped incision was made over the basilar joint and was brought down through the subcutaneous tissue. The branch of radial nerves were identified and protected. The dorsal capsule was then opened. The trapezium was identified. This was confirmed with the use of mini-C-arm, and then a trapezial excision was made as far as possible into the trapezium. Removed the entire trapezium in piecemeal fashion with a rongeur and knife. The flexor carpi radialis was protected. Its sheath was then opened and then an incision was made in the forearm. The flexor carpi radialis tendon was split with a #28 gauge wire and at this time an osteotomy was placed in the dorsal surface of the metacarpal with a rotating burr. A second one was placed over the base of the metacarpal and a K-wire was driven retrograde through the base of the metacarpal up to the skin. At this time the flexor carpi radialis tendon was brought through the osteotomy at the base of the metacarpal through the dorsal incision. It was sewn to itself. The position was then checked with the C-arm again and the K-wire was driven in order to hold the space in place at the center. The remainder of the flexor carpi radialis tendon was wound around the K-wire to keep it in place. The ends of the flexor carpi radialis were then sewn to itself and the dorsal capsule was repaired with interrupted ligatures of 3-0 Ethibond suture. Next, the tourniquet was let down. Hemostasis was obtained. The wounds were then closed with a layered closure of 4-0 Monocryl suture with a deep layer and then a subcutaneous layer. Steri-Strips were then applied and a thumb spica cast. The patient tolerated the procedure well and was discharged to the recovery room in good condition.

4. Operative Report

PREOPERATIVE DIAGNOSIS: Complex laceration of the dorsal aspect of the left index finger with laceration of extensor tendon and the PIP joint

POSTOPERATIVE DIAGNOSIS: Complex laceration of the dorsal aspect of the left index finger with laceration of extensor tendon and the PIP joint

OPERATION PERFORMED: Repair of extensor tendon, wound closure and splint

INDICATIONS: This is a 20-year-old male who accidentally injured his left index finger with a knife. The patient sustained a laceration of the dorsal aspect of his left index finger at the proximal interphalangeal joint. The wound measures about 1.5 cm in length. The wound was deep and lacerated the central slit of the extensor tendon over 80 percent. The tendon needed to be repaired; otherwise it would cause a deformity.

PROCEDURE: 0.5 percent Marcaine was used as local anesthetic, and after anesthesia had been obtained, the hand was then prepped and draped in the usual manner. A tourniquet was then placed at the base of the finger. The wound then was explored. The extensor tendon was repaired with 5-0 PDS suture material. After completion, the skin was then closed with 5-0 nylon. The tourniquet was released. There was good perfusion throughout the finger. The dressing was applied. An aluminum splint was placed. The patient tolerated the procedure well.

5. Operative Report

NOTE: Do not code any intraoperative imaging documented in this report.

PREOPERATIVE DIAGNOSIS: Right thumb crush injury

POSTOPERATIVE DIAGNOSIS: Right thumb crush injury

PROCEDURES:
1. Open fracture of head of proximal thumb
2. Extensor pollicis longus tendon restoration

PROCEDURE DETAILS: The patient was taken to the operating room. Given preoperatively 1g of Ancef and 80 mg of tobramycin IV in the emergency room. Axillary block was previously administered, as well as a standard metacarpal block, by myself. Standard prep and drape was done. The extremity was exsanguinated and tourniquet was inflated to 250 mm Hg. The entire procedure was performed with 3.5 loupe magnification. The complex, radially based laceration was opened, vigorously irrigated with normal saline and bacitracin. Neurovascular bundle identified, visualized, and noted to be intact, though contused. Laceration was extended dorsally to facilitate exposure. Because of the complexity of the fracture, the entire fracture was opened. Fracture site was irrigated and debrided. Fracture site was curetted. Multiple loose bone fragments were removed. The proximal fracture was stabilized with 0.35 crossed K-wires, resulting in excellent bony fixation. The fracture was then anatomically reduced and transfixed with transverse 0.35 K-wires to the distal phalanx. This was confirmed clinically and then with intra-operative AP and lateral C-arm. Fracture was clinically stable and anatomically reduced.

The area was irrigated with normal saline with bacitracin again. All potential bleeders were electrocauterized. The distal interphalangeal joint was stabilized in 0 degrees of extension with a 0.45 K-wire that was originally driven retrograde followed by antegrade with excellent purchase. Extensor pollicis longus was formally repaired with interrupted 4-0 MERSILENE followed by 6-0 nylon epitenon repair. Strong anatomic repair was achieved. The area was again irrigated. Skin was closed with interrupted 4-0 and 5-0 nylon with no skin loss. At this point, the hand was cleansed with hydrogen peroxide. Proximal metacarpal and median nerve block was performed with 0.5 percent Marcaine. The hand was then further dressed with Neosporin, Adaptic, 4 × 4, 1-inch TubeGauz. A complex static volar splint was then applied, which was forearm-based and covering the thumb. Tourniquet was released. Patient tolerated the procedure well and was transferred to the recovery room in stable condition. Estimated blood loss was none.

6. Operative Report

PREOPERATIVE DIAGNOSIS: Left quadriceps tendon rupture

POSTOPERATIVE DIAGNOSIS: Left quadriceps tendon rupture

PROCEDURE: Repair of left quadriceps tendon rupture

PROCEDURE: The patient was brought to the operating room, and after the instillation of a satisfactory spinal anesthesia, the left lower extremity was appropriately prepared and draped in the usual sterile fashion. A midline incision was made and centered over the patella and carried down to the quadriceps mechanism. Medial and lateral dissection was carried out to expose the retinaculum, which was torn approximately 2 cm laterally and medially. There was a direct avulsion of the quadriceps tendon off the patella with a small fleck of osteophytic bone. The quadriceps tendon was freshened. Also, the bony surface of the patella was debrided of soft tissue, and hematoma, and fibrous tissue. Once this was repaired, three holes: center, mid lateral, and mid medial were marked. Following this, a #5 Ethibond and #2 fiber-wire were placed in the quadriceps mechanism both medially and laterally, beginning in the midportion with a Krackow suture. Following this, three drill holes were made longitudinally from superior to inferior through the patella, and a suture passer was used to retrieve the ends of the suture. When these were secured, the quad tendon was brought down into the patellar bed. Following this, #2 Ethibond retinacular sutures were added from the superolateral and superomedial junction of the patella laterally and medially. These were then tightened. As they were tightened, the sutures in the patella were securely tightened as well. The retinacular sutures were then tightened. Supplemental 2-0 Vicryl anteriorly into the quad tendon and patellar soft tissue and retinaculum was then accomplished. This knee could be flexed to about 30 degrees before there was significant tension on this quadriceps tendon. Therefore, we will be holding him in extension. Following this, a thorough Water Pik irrigation was accomplished. The subcutaneous was closed with interrupted 2-0 Vicryl and the skin closed with skin clips. A sterile dressing and a knee immobilizer were placed. The patient was taken to the recovery room in satisfactory condition.

Chapter 16

Skeletal System: Bones and Joints

This chapter completes the discussion of the musculoskeletal system and concentrates on procedures performed on the bones and joints. The 2nd character values for the body systems included in this chapter are:

N—Head and Facial Bones
P—Upper Bones
Q—Lower Bones
R—Upper Joints
S—Lower Joints

Functions of the Bones and Joints

Bones support the soft organs of the body and protect other soft internal body parts. Bones also store minerals, especially calcium, and form new blood cells in red bone marrow. The joints of the body allow movement, in combination with the muscles, tendons, bursae, and ligaments that were covered in chapter 15.

Organization of the Bones and Joints

ICD-10-PCS organizes the skeletal system into groupings of the bones of the head and face, upper and lower bones, and upper and lower joints. The body is a combination of short bones, flat bones, long bones, and irregular bones.

Anatomy Alert

The Medical and Surgical section of ICD-10-PCS does not classify bones in the traditional anatomical divisions of axial and appendicular skeleton. Bones and joints are classified as head and facial bones, upper and lower bones, and upper and lower joints.

Bones

Short bones are smaller bones that are approximately equal in all dimensions. These bones are mainly found in the ankles and wrists. Flat bones are thin and contoured to fit the body space. Cranial bones are an example of flat bones. Irregular bones have varying shapes and are found in numerous parts of the body, such as the face and the vertebra. Long bones are longer than they are wide, having a long shaft with enlarged ends. Long bones make up the extremities, with the shaft of a long bone also called the diaphysis. This structure is hollow with an internal space called the medullary cavity. The ends of the long bones are called the epiphysis. The surfaces of the epiphysis are covered with smooth, articular cartilage that facilitates movement within the joints.

Other areas of the bone are covered by connective tissue called periosteum, which contains nerves, lymph vessels, and blood vessels (Rizzo 2016, 139).

Common terms used to describe areas of the bone surfaces are:

- **Condyle**—A round prominence at the end of a bone, forming part of a joint (distal femur)
- **Crest**—A ridge on the bone's surface (iliac crest)
- **Epicondyle**—A smaller prominence at the end of a bone or a small bump above a condyle (medial epicondyle of humerus)
- **Facet**—A smooth, flat articular surface (vertebrae)
- **Fissure**—A natural cleft in a bone (auricular fissure of the temporal bone)
- **Foramen**—A natural opening in a bone, used as a passage for other structures (foramen magnum of occipital bone)
- **Fossa**—A broad, shallow depression (temporomandibular joint fossa)
- **Fovea**—A small, cuplike depression on the end of a bone (submandibular fovea)
- **Head**—Enlarged, round end of a bone (humeral head)
- **Meatus**—A tunneled passageway in a bone (nasal meatus)
- **Process**—A projection of a bone (mastoid process or spinous process of vertebrae)
- **Sinus**—A hollow space in a bone (maxillary sinus)
- **Spine**—A slender projection from a bone (scapular spine)
- **Trochanter**—A large, blunt, irregular projection from a bone (greater and lesser trochanter of the femur)
- **Tubercle**—A small, rounded knob on a bone (pubic tubercle)
- **Tuberosity**—A rounded knob on a bone, larger than a tubercle (ischial tuberosity) (Applegate 2011, 106)

Recognizing the names of these bone markings in the documentation can assist the coder in determining the appropriate body part value to assign to a procedure. For example, the humerus has a head at the proximal end and epicondyles at the distal end. The femur has a head, neck, and trochanter at the proximal end and condyles at the distal end.

Figure 16.1 displays the bones of the head and neck. Figure 16.2 displays the bones of the skull and face. The orbit is bordered by the frontal bone, the zygomatic bone, the maxilla, and the lacrimal bone. The palatine bone is between the maxilla and the pterygoid process of the sphenoid bone and is located behind the nasal cavity.

Anatomy Alert

The orbit is formed by the combination of the frontal bone, the zygomatic bone, the maxilla, and the lacrimal bone.

Vertebrae are irregular-shaped bones that form the spinal column, the protective bony covering over the spinal cord. Figure 8.5 in chapter 8 depicts the vertebral column and the associated peripheral nerves. The vertebral column is made up of cervical, thoracic, and lumbar vertebrae. Also sometimes included in the discussion of the vertebral column are the sacrum and coccyx, the flat bones that follow the lumbar vertebrae at the bottom of the column.

There are specific naming conventions for vertebral bones. An individual vertebral bone is described in an operative report using the name of a single vertebra, such as C5 or L2. If procedures are performed on two individual vertebrae, the vertebrae are described by naming each individually, separated by a comma, such as T8, T9. A vertebral joint is the intersection of two vertebrae. This joint is described in an operative report using the names of the two vertebrae on either side, separated by a dash, such as C4–C5 or L1–L2.

Figure 16.1. Head and neck bones

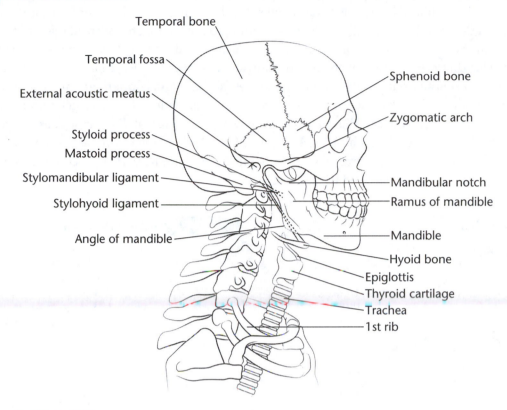

Temporal bone
Temporal fossa
External acoustic meatus
Sphenoid bone
Zygomatic arch
Styloid process
Mastoid process
Stylomandibular ligament
Stylohyoid ligament
Mandibular notch
Ramus of mandible
Angle of mandible
Mandible
Hyoid bone
Epiglottis
Thyroid cartilage
Trachea
1st rib

© AHIMA 2019

Figure 16.2. Skull and facial bones

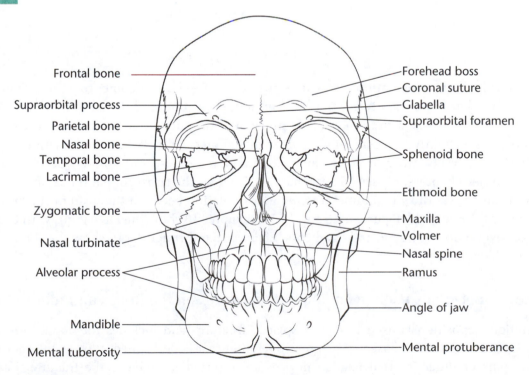

Frontal bone
Forehead boss
Coronal suture
Supraorbital process
Glabella
Parietal bone
Supraorbital foramen
Nasal bone
Temporal bone
Sphenoid bone
Lacrimal bone
Zygomatic bone
Ethmoid bone
Maxilla
Nasal turbinate
Volmer
Nasal spine
Alveolar process
Ramus
Angle of jaw
Mandible
Mental tuberosity
Mental protuberance

© AHIMA 2019

C1 (the atlas) is the first vertebra. Together, C1 and C2 (the axis) form a pivot joint that allows the head to rotate from side to side, while also moving up and down. C3 through L5 are all shaped in a similar manner, with a body (corpus) on the anterior side and processes extending to the lateral and posterior sides. These processes interlock and form the movable joints of the spine. They also provide the surfaces necessary for the insertion of the back muscles that create the movement. An individual vertebra is also called a vertebral segment. The space between two vertebral bodies is called the intervertebral space and contains an intervertebral disc. These discs are made of an outer fibrocartilage ring that surrounds the nucleus pulposus, a gelatinous substance. The disc acts as a shock absorber between the vertebrae as they move. Vertebral discs are documented in the same manner as intervertebral joints, such as L3–L4. Figure 16.3 shows a single lumbar vertebra and figure 16.4 shows the view of a lumbar intervertebral joint from the posterior view. ICD-10-PCS contains body part values for the major bones of the body, pictured in figure 16.5.

| Figure 16.3. Vertebra | Figure 16.4. Posterior view of lumbar vertebral joint |

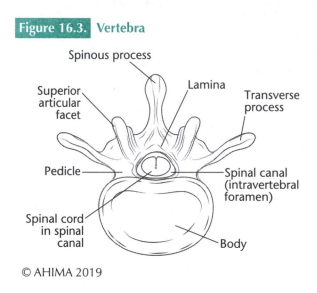

© AHIMA 2019

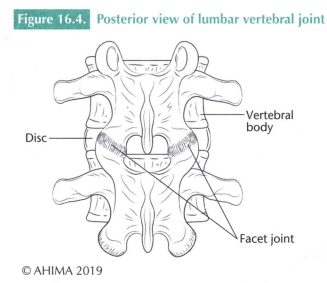

© AHIMA 2019

Joints

The joint, also called an articulation, is where two or more bones come together. Synarthroses, amphiarthroses, and diarthroses are terms that further define the joint and the amount of movement in a particular joint. A synarthrosis is an immovable joint, such as the sutures between the bones of the head. An amphiarthrosis is a slightly movable joint, such as the connection between the ribs and the sternum, and a diarthrosis is a freely movable joint, such as shoulders, knees, and elbows. Several joints have been pictured in other chapters. Figure 15.5 in chapter 15 shows the subacromial bursa and a part of the shoulder joint. It illustrates the glenohumeral joint, an articulation between the head of the humerus and the glenoid cavity of the scapula. Figures 15.6 and 15.7 in chapter 15 show the knee joint, with the complex combination of several bones, bursa, and ligaments. Figures 16.6 through 16.10 show the shoulder, elbow, wrist, hip, and ankle joints.

Common Root Operations Used in Coding of Procedures on the Bones and Joints

The root operation Reposition is used to code displaced fractures and includes the application of a cast. Nondisplaced fractures are coded based on the root operation that is performed, such as the root operation Insertion when pins or other internal fixation devices are inserted to stabilize the fracture. Casting of a nondisplaced fracture is coded to the root operation Immobilization in section 2, Placement, but cast application is rarely, if ever, coded in the inpatient setting. Placing a dislocated or subluxed joint back into the correct

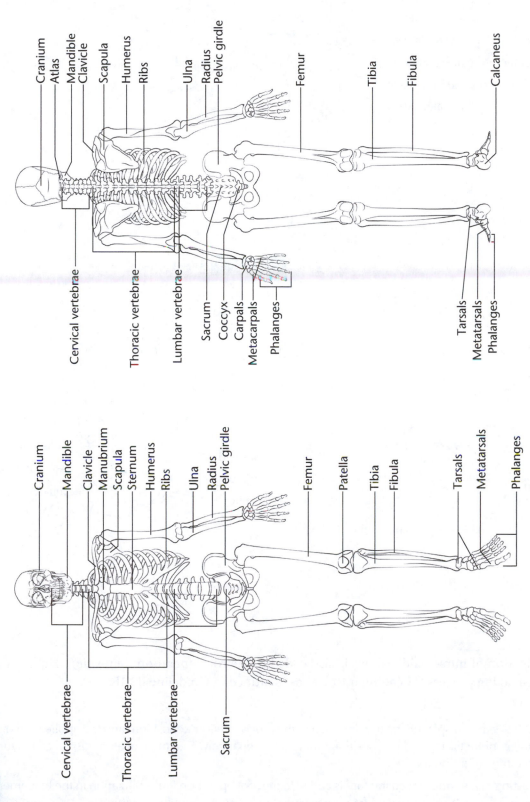

Figure 16.5. Bones of the body

© AHIMA 2019

Cranium
Atlas
Mandible
Clavicle
Scapula
Humerus
Ribs
Ulna
Radius
Pelvic girdle
Femur
Tibia
Fibula
Calcaneus

Cervical vertebrae
Thoracic vertebrae
Lumbar vertebrae
Sacrum
Coccyx
Carpals
Metacarpals
Phalanges
Tarsals
Metatarsals
Phalanges

Cranium
Mandible
Clavicle
Manubrium
Scapula
Sternum
Humerus
Ribs
Ulna
Radius
Pelvic girdle
Femur
Patella
Tibia
Fibula
Tarsals
Metatarsals
Phalanges

Cervical vertebrae
Thoracic vertebrae
Lumbar vertebrae
Sacrum

Figure 16.6.   Shoulder joint

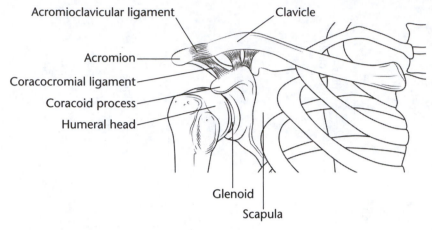

© AHIMA 2019

Figure 16.7.   Elbow joint

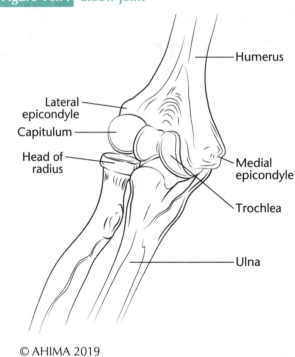

© AHIMA 2019

Figure 16.8.   Wrist joint

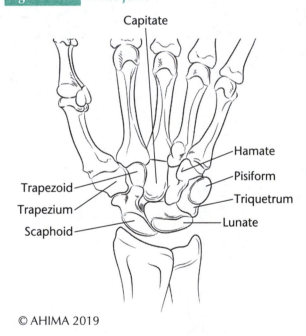

© AHIMA 2019

position, such as reduction of nursemaid's elbow, is also coded to the root operation Reposition. Figure 16.11 displays the decision-making process for coding fractures as identified in Guideline B3.15.

B3.15.   Reduction of a displaced fracture is coded to the root operation Reposition, and the application of a cast or splint in conjunction with the Reposition is not coded separately. Treatment of a nondisplaced fracture is coded to the procedure performed.

Example: Casting of a nondisplaced fracture is coded to the root operation Immobilization in the Placement section. Putting a pin in a nondisplaced fracture is coded to the root operation Insertion.

Figure 16.9. Hip joint

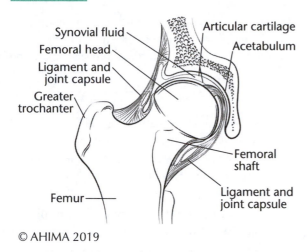

© AHIMA 2019

Figure 16.10. Ankle joint

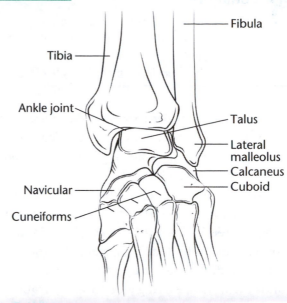

© AHIMA 2019

Figure 16.11. Fracture coding

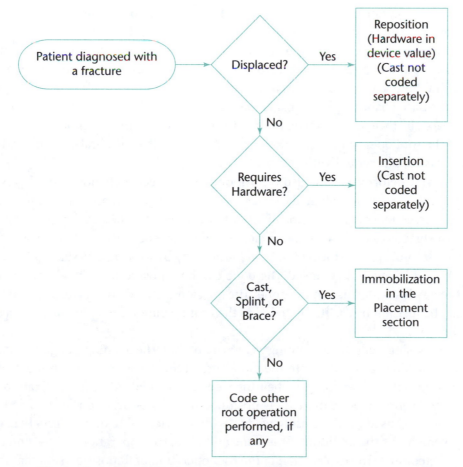

©Kuehn Consulting, LLC. Used with permission.

Coding Tip

If the fracture is repositioned using an external approach, but the hardware is placed using a different approach, code the Reposition root operation with the approach used to place the device. Debridement at the site of an open fracture is included in the Reposition procedure. The surgeon must clean up the fracture site before the bone can be repositioned and the site closed.

Internal fixation devices are placed anywhere within or along the bone. Device value 6, Internal Fixation Device, Intramedullary, is only available for use in coding procedures performed on the upper and lower extremities, the location of the long bones of the body. Intramedullary devices are specialized internal fixation devices that are placed within the intramedullary space of a long bone to stabilize the bone.

External fixation devices are found in a variety of different styles. A monoplanar or uniplane device is a specific type of external fixation device that holds the fracture in one plane or one direction. A typical monoplanar device is pictured in figure 1.11 in chapter 1 in the discussion of devices. A limb-lengthening device is similar to a monoplanar device that has expandable rods along the limb. The rods are expanded in small increments to encourage longitudinal bone growth. A ring device is also called a multiplane external fixation device because it surrounds the limb like a ring and provides fixation in two or more planes (AMA 2018, 120–121).

Prophylactic nailing and cementing are performed to reinforce fragile bones that have a potential for fracture. Either of these procedures is coded to the root operation Supplement, because both the nail and the cement are physically reinforcing the bone.

Vertebroplasty is performed when the vertebral body is fractured with the bone fragments that have not migrated and there is not significant loss of height in the vertebral body. The fractured vertebral body is a nondisplaced fracture, which is stabilized with the introduction of acrylic bone cement to maintain vertebral height, prevent further injury, and to relieve pain. This is coded with the root operation Supplement because the bone cement was used to supplement the vertebral body. Kyphoplasty is performed when the fracture is displaced. The vertebral body has loss of height and needs to be repositioned. The fracture is first repositioned by the use of a catheter-based balloon placed inside the vertebra and inflated to bring the vertebra back to its full height. The space created by the balloon is then filled with acrylic bone cement to hold the fracture in place. This requires two codes. The root operation Reposition is coded because the vertebral body has suffered a displaced fracture and the bone is supplemented with cement.

Bones and joints with deformities are also repositioned to correct their position. This is common in the lower extremities when bones are not aligned to bear weight properly, such as in the femur, tibia, or the bones of the feet. Surgical correction of these deformities often involves the osteotomy procedure. Based on the correction needed, the osteotomy may be either a closing wedge osteotomy or an opening wedge osteotomy.

A closing wedge osteotomy is performed to realign the body by making a V-shaped incision that cuts out a wedge of bone. Once the wedge is removed, the bone can be repositioned into alignment to properly bear weight by closing the newly created gap in the bone. The incision into the bone is held in place with an internal fixation device while the incision heals. This is coded to the root operation of Reposition with a device value of 4, Internal Fixation Device.

The opposite of the closing wedge is an opening wedge osteotomy. The opening wedge osteotomy is performed to realign the body by making an incision into the bone and forcing the bone to open into a V-shape opening. A bone graft is placed into the space created when the wedge is opened. An internal fixation device holds the bone graft in place and keeps the bone in the new position. This procedure requires two codes. The first code is the same Reposition code used on the closing wedge, with a device value of 4, Internal Fixation Device. The second code is Supplement for the addition of the bone graft. The root operation of Division is not coded with either type of wedge osteotomy. The explanation of the root operation of Reposition says that the body part may or may not be cut out or off to be moved to the new location, indicating that the cutting of the bone is an operative step for this procedure. Guideline B3.1b says that components of the procedure are not coded separately.

B3.1b. Components of a procedure specified in the root operation definition and explanation are not coded separately. Procedural steps necessary to reach the operative site and close the operative site, including anastomosis of a tubular body part, are also not coded separately.

Example: Resection of a joint as part of a joint replacement procedure is included in the root operation definition of Replacement and is not coded separately. Laparotomy performed to reach the site of an open liver biopsy is not coded separately. In a resection of the sigmoid colon with anastomosis of descending colon to rectum, the anastomosis is not coded separately.

Replacement of Bones and Joints

Joint replacement surgery is assigned to the root operation of Replacement. The common hip and knee replacement procedures are coded in the 0SR table for Lower Joints. There are options for total joint replacement, called arthroplasty, as well as hemiarthroplasty, or replacement of half of the joint. The hip is made up of two parts, the femur side and the acetabular side. The prosthesis used for the replacement is made up of four parts, two parts for each half:

Femoral Half:	1. Femoral stem placed inside the intramedullary canal of the femur
	2. Femoral head, attached to the femoral stem (bearing surface)
Acetabular Half:	1. Acetabular cup, also called a shell, screwed into the acetabular socket of the pelvic bone
	2. Acetabular liner, placed into the cup (bearing surface)

The device values for these prostheses are designed to describe the material that comprises the bearing surface. The stem and the cup are always made of metal and do not affect the coding. The following device values are available to describe the bearing surfaces for the total hip replacement procedure:

- **1, Synthetic substitute, Metal**—Both surfaces are metal
- **2, Synthetic substitute, Metal on Polyethylene**—Head is metal and liner is polyethylene
- **3, Synthetic substitute, Ceramic**—Both surfaces are ceramic
- **4, Synthetic substitute, Ceramic on Polyethylene**—Head is ceramic and liner is polyethylene
- **6, Synthetic substitute, Oxidized Zirconium on Polyethylene**—Head is a special oxidized zirconium surface and liner is polyethylene
- **J, Synthetic substitute**—Bearing surfaces made of other materials or unknown

When a hemiarthroplasty is performed, the device values are appropriate for the half being replaced. Polyethylene is only available for the acetabular liner surface.

The knee prosthesis is identified with only two options: synthetic substitute and synthetic substitute, oxidized zirconium on polyethylene. The knee prosthesis has two halves with an optional piece to replace part of the patella:

Femoral Half:	Femoral replacement for the condylar cartilage surface (typically metal)
Tibial Half:	1. Tibial plateau with stem into the intramedullary canal of tibia (typically metal)
	2. Meniscal replacement cups (typically polyethylene), sometimes called a liner
Patellar Portion:	Optional piece replacing the back portion of the patella with polyethylene (surface not coded)

There are special device values available for the unicondylar knee replacement of either the medial or lateral compartment when only one compartment of the knee is replaced. Unicondylar means that only one side of the knee is replaced (one femoral condyle along with one meniscus). The patellofemoral compartment can also be replaced separately. All hip and knee synthetic prosthesis replacements require a qualifier that identifies whether cement was or was not used to secure the prosthesis.

Replacement of the shoulder joint is coded in the 0RR table for Upper Joints. Shoulder prostheses are designed like the hip prosthesis with a humeral half (stem into the humerus with an attached head) and a glenoid half (cup screwed into the scapula with an attached liner). The device value is J, Synthetic Substitute. Hemiarthroplasties of the shoulder are indicated with a qualifier describing humeral surface or glenoid surface. A special device value is available for the reverse ball and socket prosthesis that places the ball on the glenoid side and the socket on the humeral side. This prosthesis is used when the traditional, heavier prosthesis cannot be supported on the humeral side or when the shoulder joint is too damaged to accept the traditional type. Guideline B3.1b clarifies that the resection of the joint to be replaced is included in the root operation Replacement.

Infected prostheses may need to be removed until the infection in the joint heals and a second replacement can take place. In the first step of the process, the entire prosthesis is removed, called explantation, and a static (meaning nonmovable) spacer is left in its place during the healing process. In the second step of the process, the static spacer is removed and the joint is replaced again. The following is an example of the steps for an infected right hip prosthesis, including a new ceramic, cemented prosthesis:

Step 1: Remove right hip prosthesis, 0SP90JZ

Insert static spacer into right hip, 0SH908Z

Step 2: Remove static spacer from right hip, 0SP908Z

Replace right hip joint with all ceramic prosthesis using cement, 0SR9039

When the prosthesis is recalled or is worn, the process is straightforward. The prosthesis is removed and the hip is replaced again. The following is an example for the right hip with a worn prosthesis and the same new ceramic, cemented hip prosthesis:

Remove right hip prosthesis, 0SP90JZ

Replace right hip joint with all ceramic prosthesis using cement, 0SR9039

Note that the removal code is the difference between a first-time replacement and one that is a repeat procedure. In addition to the static spacer that provides little or no movement of the joint, an articulating spacer is also available for coding. As the name implies, the articulating spacer allows both movement and the ability to bear weight and walk. The articulating spacers are coded to the root operation of Replacement because they can be used as a permanent replacement in some cases, such as in the elderly, who may not be able to undergo the additional procedure required by a static spacer.

Revision of a joint prosthesis is coded with one code because the prosthesis is not completely removed. Remember that the joint has two halves. In the example of the hip joint, if the acetabular liner becomes cracked, but the acetabular cup remains intact in the pelvic bone, only one part of that half needs attention. Removing and inserting a new liner is the root operation of Revision because that entire half is not removed. This is similar to the classic example of a plate and screw device used to treat a fracture. If one of the screws becomes loose and is removed and a new one inserted, the root operation is Revision because the entire device is not removed. The same is true of the femoral head. If the head is damaged but the stem is secure inside the femur, the exchange of the head is coded to Revision.

Resurfacing of a joint surface is also a Replacement procedure. The definition of Replacement states that biological or synthetic material physically takes the place and/or function of all or a portion of a body part. Resurfacing involves removing the worn surfaces from the joint. Once a portion of the body part is removed and replaced with a device, the root operation of Replacement is assigned, based on the complete definition of Replacement.

Replacement of bone can also be performed. This is done to replace bone damaged by disease or severe injury and is not as common as replacement of joints. If the procedure involves the removal of damaged or diseased bone and bone is put in its place, the root operation of Replacement is assigned and the excision of the native bone is not coded separately.

Repair of Joints

Capsulorrhaphy is coded as Repair, upper or lower joints because the capsule, synovium, and labrum are joint structures. Other repair procedures involve anchoring a partially torn labrum in either the shoulder or hip or suturing a torn meniscus in the knee. Guideline B4.5 clarifies that tendons, ligaments, bursae, and fascia supporting a joint are coded to their respective body systems, not the joint itself.

Coding Tip

The capsule, synovium, and labrum of joints are classified to their associated joints in ICD-10-PCS.

Be sure to research any procedure that is unfamiliar to ensure correct coding. If the documentation includes an eponym (procedure named for a person) and the intent of the procedure is unclear, query the physician for specifics.

Body Parts for Bones and Joints

The adult human body has 206 bones and over 250 joints. ICD-10-PCS does not assign body part values to all of the bones and joints in the body. To allow proper coding of all these body parts, Guideline B4.1a clarifies that if a procedure is performed on a portion of a body part that is not identified with a body part value, the body part value corresponding to the whole body part should be coded. The generic body part value Y for upper or lower bone or upper or lower joint can also be assigned when a procedure is performed on a specific bone or joint that does not have an individual body part value identified.

B4.1a. If a procedure is performed on a portion of a body part that does not have a separate body part value, code the body part value corresponding to the whole body part.

Example: A procedure performed on the alveolar process of the mandible is coded to the mandible body part.

Guideline B4.3 also clarifies that bilateral body part values are available for some body parts. If a bilateral body part value is not available, the procedure should be coded individually for each side of the body, assigning the correct body part values for right and left. Table 16.1 lists the body part values for the bones of the body. If the documentation includes specific body part names that are not included in these lists, refer to the body part key for other body part synonyms and alternative terms. Table 16.2 lists the body part values for the joints of the body.

B4.3. Bilateral body part values are available for a limited number of body parts. If the identical procedure is performed on contralateral body parts, and a bilateral body part value exists for that body part, a single procedure is coded using the bilateral body part value. If no bilateral body part value exists, each procedure is coded separately using the appropriate body part value.

Example: The identical procedure performed on both fallopian tubes is coded once using the body part value Fallopian Tube, Bilateral. The identical procedure performed on both knee joints is coded twice using the body part values Knee Joint, Right and Knee Joint, Left.

Anatomy Alert

Upper bones and upper joints in ICD-10-PCS are defined as bones and joints above the level of the first lumbar vertebra plus the upper extremities. Lower bones and lower joints in ICD-10-PCS are defined as bones and joints of the first lumbar vertebra and below, plus the lower extremities.

Table 16.1.   Body part values for the bones

Body Part Value	Body Parts—Head and Face Bones (N)	Body Part Value	Body Parts—Upper Bones (P)	Body Part Value	Body Parts—Lower Bones (Q)
0	Skull	0	Sternum	0	Lumbar Vertebra
1	Frontal Bone	1	Ribs, 1 to 2	1	Sacrum
3	Parietal Bone, Right	2	Ribs, 3 or More	2	Pelvic Bone, Right
4	Parietal Bone, Left	3	Cervical Vertebra	3	Pelvic Bone, Left
5	Temporal Bone, Right	4	Thoracic Vertebra	4	Acetabulum, Right
6	Temporal Bone, Left	5	Scapula, Right	5	Acetabulum, Left
7	Occipital Bone	6	Scapula, Left	6	Upper Femur, Right
B	Nasal Bone	7	Glenoid Cavity, Right	7	Upper Femur, Left
C	Sphenoid Bone	8	Glenoid Cavity, Left	8	Femoral Shaft, Right
F	Ethmoid Bone, Right	9	Clavicle, Right	9	Femoral Shaft, Left
G	Ethmoid Bone, Left	B	Clavicle, Left	B	Lower Femur, Right
H	Lacrimal Bone, Right	C	Humeral Head, Right	C	Lower Femur, Left
J	Lacrimal Bone, Left	D	Humeral Head, Left	D	Patella, Right
K	Palatine Bone, Right	F	Humeral Shaft, Right	F	Patella, Left
L	Palatine Bone, Left	G	Humeral Shaft, Left	G	Tibia, Right
M	Zygomatic Bone, Right	H	Radius, Right	H	Tibia, Left
N	Zygomatic Bone, Left	J	Radius, Left	J	Fibula, Right
P	Orbit, Right	K	Ulna, Right	K	Fibula, Left
Q	Orbit, Left	L	Ulna, Left	L	Tarsal, Right
R	Maxilla	M	Carpal, Right	M	Tarsal, Left
T	Mandible, Right	N	Carpal, Left	N	Metatarsal, Right
V	Mandible, Left	P	Metacarpal, Right	P	Metatarsal, Left
W	Facial Bone	Q	Metacarpal, Left	Q	Toe Phalanx, Right
X	Hyoid Bone	R	Thumb Phalanx, Right	R	Toe Phalanx, Left
		S	Thumb Phalanx, Left	S	Coccyx
		T	Finger Phalanx, Right	Y	Lower Bone
		V	Finger Phalanx, Left		
		Y	Upper Bone		

Table 16.2. Body part values for the joints

Body Part Value	Body Parts—Upper Joints (R)	Body Part Value	Body Parts—Lower Joints (S)
0	Occipital-cervical Joint	0	Lumbar Vertebral Joint
1	Cervical Vertebral Joint	1	Lumbar Vertebral Joints, 2 or More
2	Cervical Vertebral Joints, 2 or More	2	Lumbar Vertebral Disc
3	Cervical Vertebral Disc	3	Lumbosacral Joint
4	Cervicothoracic Vertebral Joint	4	Lumbosacral Disc
5	Cervicothoracic Vertebral Disc	5	Sacrococcygeal Joint
6	Thoracic Vertebral Joint	6	Coccygeal Joint
7	Thoracic Vertebral Joints, 2 to 7	7	Sacroiliac Joint, Right
8	Thoracic Vertebral Joints, 8 or More	8	Sacroiliac Joint, Left
9	Thoracic Vertebral Disc	9	Hip Joint, Right
A	Thoracolumbar Vertebral Joint	A	Hip Joint, Acetabular Surface, Right
B	Thoracolumbar Vertebral Disc	B	Hip Joint, Left
C	Temporomandibular Joint, Right	C	Knee Joint, Right
D	Temporomandibular Joint, Left	D	Knee Joint, Left
E	Sternoclavicular Joint, Right	E	Hip Joint, Acetabular Surface, Left
F	Sternoclavicular Joint, Left	F	Ankle Joint, Right
G	Acromioclavicular Joint, Right	G	Ankle Joint, Left
H	Acromioclavicular Joint, Left	H	Tarsal Joint, Right
J	Shoulder Joint, Right	J	Tarsal Joint, Left
K	Shoulder Joint, Left	K	Tarsometatarsal Joint, Right
L	Elbow Joint, Right	L	Tarsometatarsal Joint, Left
M	Elbow Joint, Left	M	Metatarsal-Phalangeal Joint, Right
N	Wrist Joint, Right	N	Metatarsal-Phalangeal Joint, Left
P	Wrist Joint, Left	P	Toe Phalangeal Joint, Right
Q	Carpal Joint, Right	Q	Toe Phalangeal Joint, Left
R	Carpal Joint, Left	R	Hip Joint, Femoral Surface, Right
S	Carpometacarpal Joint, Right	S	Hip Joint, Femoral Surface, Left
T	Carpometacarpal Joint, Left	T	Knee Joint, Femoral Surface, Right
U	Metacarpophalangeal Joint, Right	U	Knee Joint, Femoral Surface, Left
V	Metacarpophalangeal Joint, Left	V	Knee Joint, Tibial Surface, Right
W	Finger Phalangeal Joint, Right	W	Knee Joint, Tibial Surface, Left
X	Finger Phalangeal Joint, Left	Y	Lower Joint
Y	Upper Joint		

Approaches Used for the Bones and Joints

The approaches of Open, Percutaneous, Percutaneous Endoscopic, and External are used to code procedures performed on the bones and joints. The term arthrotomy means that a joint capsule was incised, indicating that an open procedure was performed. Closed reductions of fractures are performed without opening the skin and are coded to the approach value External. When a displaced fracture is repositioned using an external approach (closed reduction) and an internal fixation device is placed using the Percutaneous approach, such as a K wire, the procedure is coded to the Percutaneous approach.

B5.3b. Procedures performed indirectly by the application of external force through the intervening body layers are coded to the approach External.

Example: Closed reduction of fracture is coded to the approach External.

Devices Common to the Bones and Joints

Many of the device values in the bones and joints body systems deal with fractures and joint replacements. An internal fixation device not associated with fractures is a rigid plate. This plate is a device used to close the sternum following open chest surgery rather than the more traditional closure using wires. The rigid plate fixation device provides easier access if emergency re-entry is required into the chest cavity. Device value N, Neurostimulator Generator, is only available for use in coding procedures performed on the skull.

Many of the remaining device values deal with the root operation of Fusion, which is joining together portions of an articular body part rendering the articular body part immobile. Articular body parts are the joints of the body, found in the 0R, Upper Joints and 0S, Lower Joints body systems with lumbar vertebra 1 as the dividing line. The process of fusion takes place when bone is in contact with other bone or a bone graft. Over time, these two bones heal together into a fusion, just as if it had been a fracture of a single bone. The process of fusion takes months or years. Coding of the fusion process of the spine is detailed here. Coding fusion of nonspinal joints is less complicated.

Coding of Spinal Fusion

Spinal fusion coding involves making complex decisions involving body part values, device values, and qualifiers. Therefore, spinal fusion coding and related subjects are discussed here as a complete topic, along with case examples, before completing the discussion on qualifiers used in other bone and joint procedures.

Selecting the Body Part Value for Spinal Fusion

The naming scheme for vertebral bones and joints is detailed in the anatomy section of this chapter. As you code a spinal fusion, be sure that all the joint combinations are accounted for. The coding tip that follows reviews how to identify joints, including the joints that connect the different regions of the spine.

Coding Tip

Identify the number of spinal joints involved in the fusion to assure that the correct body parts are assigned. As an example, the surgeon fuses the interbody joints of T10 through L2. The details would look like this:

Joint	Body System and Body Part Values
T10-T12	0R, Upper Joints, 7, Thoracic Vertebral Joints, 2 to 7
T12-L1	0R, Upper Joints, A, Thoracolumbar Vertebral Joint
L1-L2	0S, Lower Joints, 0, Lumbar Vertebral Joint

Three codes are required to fully identify the fusion of all four joints.

B3.10a. The body part coded for a spinal vertebral joint(s) rendered immobile by a spinal fusion procedure is classified by the level of the spine (e.g., thoracic). There are distinct body part values for a single vertebral joint and for multiple vertebral joints at each spinal level.

Example: Body part values specify Lumbar Vertebral Joint, Lumbar Vertebral Joints, 2 or more, and Lumbosacral Vertebral Joint.

Selecting the Device Value for Spinal Fusion

Guideline B3.10c describes how to assign the device value for spinal fusion. Figure 16.12 provides the decision process used to determine the device value. It shows that if an interbody fusion device (also called a cage) is used, alone or with bone, device value A, Interbody Fusion Device is the only device value assigned. If there is no interbody fusion device used, then bone must have been used to create the fusion. If autologous bone is the only bone used, assign device value 7, Autologous Tissue Substitute. If nonautologous bone is the only bone used, assign device value K, Nonautologous Tissue Substitute. If a mixture of both types of bone are used, assign only device value 7, Autologous Tissue Substitute. Autologous bone harvested from a different procedure site to complete the Fusion process is coded to Excision, based on Guideline B3.9.

Figure 16.12. Fusion device coding

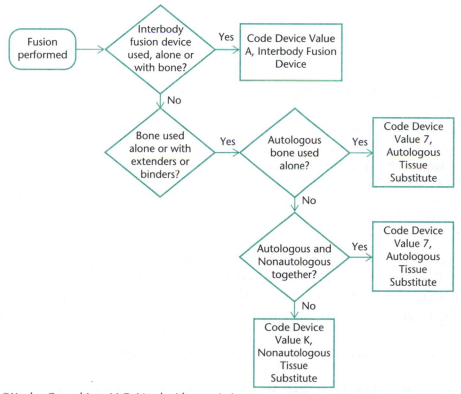

©Kuehn Consulting, LLC. Used with permission.

B3.10c. Combinations of devices and materials are often used on a vertebral joint to render the joint immobile. When combinations of devices are used on the same vertebral joint, the device value coded for the procedure is as follows:

- If an interbody fusion device is used to render the joint immobile (alone or containing other material, such as bone graft), the procedure is coded with the device value Interbody Fusion Device.

- If bone graft is the *only* device used to render the joint immobile, the procedure is coded with the device value Nonautologous Tissue Substitute or Autologous Tissue Substitute.
- If a mixture of autologous and nonautologous bone graft (with or without biological or synthetic extenders or binders) is used to render the joint immobile, code the procedure with the device value Autologous Tissue Substitute.

Example: Fusion of a vertebral joint using a cage style interbody fusion device containing morsellized bone graft is coded to the device Interbody Fusion Device. Fusion of a vertebral joint using a bone dowel interbody fusion device made of cadaver bone and packed with a mixture of local morsellized bone and demineralized bone matrix is coded to the device Interbody Fusion Device. Fusion of a vertebral joint using both autologous bone graft and bone bank graft is coded to the device Autologous Tissue Substitute.

Devices placed at the time of a fusion procedure that stabilize the spine are not coded separately in ICD-10-PCS, based on advice in Coding Clinic, 2nd Quarter 2014. An interspinous process device is not a fusion device. It is implanted during a surgical procedure to decompress and stabilize the posterior spine but without fusing the spine. The device is placed using a minimally invasive technique to hold the two spinous processes apart, keeping the pressure off the spinal cord and nerve roots. An interspinous process device is also called an interspinous spacer or an interspinous distraction device.

Selecting the Qualifier Value for Spinal Fusion

The qualifiers available for coding procedures performed on the spine define the specific anatomical approach used for spinal fusion surgery. The spinal approach qualifiers are:

- **0, Anterior Approach, Anterior Column**—Access through the front of the body to perform a procedure on the body of the vertebra or the disc
- **1, Posterior Approach, Posterior Column**—Access through the back of the body to perform a procedure on the vertebral foramen, spinous processes, facets and/or lamina
- **J, Posterior Approach, Anterior Column**—Access through the back of the body to perform a procedure on the body of the vertebra or the disc

Anterior Column Fusion

An interbody fusion is always performed on the anterior column, because the fusion takes place between the vertebral bodies on the front of the spine. The anterior column can be approached from either the anterior (front) or the posterior (back). The abbreviation for lumbar interbody fusion is LIF. One or more letters is added before this abbreviation to identify how the anterior column was accessed, such as ALIF, or anterior lumbar interbody fusion.

The following are abbreviations for anterior lumbar fusion procedures and their descriptions:

- **ALIF (anterior lumbar interbody fusion)**—The approach is from the anterior.
- **AxiaLIF (axial lumbar interbody fusion)**—The approach from the posterior, from under the sacrum. This approach is percutaneous to approach the L5-S1 with a completely internal procedure performed with imaging guidance.
- **DLIF (direct lateral lumbar interbody fusion)**—The approach is anterior but from the lateral, or side of the patient, limiting the incision size.
- **PLIF (posterior lumbar interbody fusion)**—The approach is from the posterior.

- **TLIF (transforaminal lumbar interbody fusion)**—The approach is from the posterior but to one side of the spine, through the neuroforamen.
- **XLIF (extreme lateral interbody fusion)**—The approach is from the anterior but far to the side through a small incision or by using a series of tube dilators to create a space just large enough to see through.

Table 16.3 displays the qualifier values for each of the approaches to the anterior column.

Table 16.3.   Qualifier values for anterior fusion

Anterior Approach, Anterior Column (0)	Posterior Approach, Anterior Column (J)
ALIF	AxiaLIF
DLIF	PLIF
XLIF	TLIF

Figure 16.13 contains an operative report for an anterior cervical fusion procedure that utilizes an interbody fusion device, called a cage, filled with an allograft material. In this case, the interbody fusion device is coded in the device value, and the allograft material is not coded separately. This procedure is coded as 0RG10A0.

Coding Tip

Interbody fusion devices can only be placed in the anterior column because they are placed between the vertebral bodies, which are on the anterior side of the spine.

Figure 16.13.   Anterior cervical interbody fusion

Procedure performed: C6–C7 anterior interbody arthrodesis and C6–C7 insertion of interbody allograft.

Operative technique: The skin was prepped and draped in the standard surgical fashion and the area was marked using standard landmarks of the midline and cricoid cartilage. After infiltration of 0.5% Marcaine with epinephrine, a longitudinal neck incision was performed opposite the C6–C7 level using a #10 scalpel blade. Incision was deepened and hemostasis was obtained. The longus colli muscle was undermined and self-retaining retractors were placed. Caspar distraction pins were placed at the C6 and C7 vertebral bodies. Discectomy was carried out utilizing pituitary rongeurs, Kerrison rongeurs and curettes to widen and remove the anterior disc complex. Abrasion of the endplates was completed and the posterior disc complex was removed down to the level of the posterior longitudinal ligament. Both nerve roots and the spinal cord remained free.

The clean disc space was sized appropriately with trial interbody cage of 15.5 mm × 6 mm to achieve arthrodesis. Endplates were abraded again. The permanent interbody cage was chosen, filled with Trinity allograft and inserted into the disc space. It fit well and was snug. Pins were removed. Fluoroscopic guidance confirmed good placement of the cage. The wound was irrigated with antibiotic solution and hemostasis was achieved. All layers were closed with absorbable sutures. Counts were correct. The patient tolerated the procedure well.

> Device value A, Interbody fusion device is selected

> Allograft material is not coded separately because it's used with an Interbody fusion device at the same level.

Posterior Column Fusion

The posterior column fusion is performed through a posterior approach, or qualifier value 1, Posterior approach, posterior column. This procedure does not have a formal abbreviation, but some surgeons abbreviate it as PLF (posterior lumbar fusion) when performed on the lumbar spine. This fusion is performed by clearing any tissue causing constriction of the spinal cord or nerve roots, such as by a laminectomy or foraminotomy to remove excess bone. Pedicle-based rods and screws are placed to maintain the correct alignment and distance of the vertebral joints and stabilize the spine. To form the fusion, this bone is placed along the spinous process or as a bridge between the transverse processes of the spine. If the patient's own bone is insufficient, bone bank bone will be added. It is important to understand that the pedicle-based stabilization does not fuse the spine. The bone heals together to form the fusion. Without the bone, the spine will not fuse. The pedicle-based stabilization is not coded separately. It is integral to the fusion process.

Figure 16.14 contains an operative report for a posterior cervical fusion procedure that utilizes both autograft and allograft material. In this case, the autograft is coded in the device value and the allograft material is not coded separately, based on the guideline. This operative report has two codes, 0RG2071 for the cervical fusion and 0RG4071 for the cervicothoracic fusion.

Figure 16.14. **Posterior cervical fusion**

Both autograft and allograft are used. The autograft is coded in the device value and the allograft is not coded, based on the guideline.

Procedure performed: Posterior cervical fusion and instrumentation, C5 to T1

Operative technique: The patient is undergoing correction of her scoliosis and stabilization of the posterior spine. She was given intravenous antibiotics and placed in a Mayfield head holder. She was rolled onto the operating table in a prone position. She was able to be placed in a nearly perfectly straight alignment with positioning. A sterile field was then prepped and the skin was infiltrated. An incision was made from C4 to T2. Subperiosteal dissection ensued. Lateral mass screws were placed from C5 to T1. Vertebral bone was excised to allow rod contouring and reduction of the curvature. Bone grafts were placed which consisted of morcellized autograft from the removed spinous processes and additional allograft. Spinal stabilization rod was placed and tightened to the screws. The vertebrae were irrigated and the tissues were closed in sequential layers.

360-Degree Fusion

An anterior and posterior fusion together create a 360-degree fusion. Two codes are required for this fusion because the qualifiers are different. This is most common in the lumbar spine. A 360-degree lumbar fusion done with a PLIF, accompanied by a posterior lumbar fusion at L3–L5 is coded:

0SG10AJ   Fusion of 2 or more Lumbar Vertebral Joints with Interbody Fusion Device, Posterior Approach, Anterior Column, Open Approach
0SG1071   Fusion of 2 or more Lumbar Vertebral Joints with Autologous Tissue Substitute, Posterior Approach, Posterior Column, Open Approach

Anterior fusion with pedicle-based stabilization rods and screws on the posterior, but without bone to create the posterior fusion is not a 360-degree fusion. This fusion is an anterior column fusion only because bone is required for a fusion of the posterior column.

Coding Tip

A posterior lumbar interbody fusion (PLIF) is a fusion of the anterior column using a posterior approach and is coded to qualifier value J. This is different than a posterior lumbar fusion, which is a fusion of the posterior column using a posterior approach and coded to qualifier value 1. These two procedures can be done independently or during the same operative session. If performed together at the same joint level, code both procedures separately.

Laminectomy

A laminectomy is performed as the approach to the spinal canal or as a Release procedure because the lamina is pressing on the spinal cord or nerve roots. Review figure 16.3 to see that the lamina surrounds the spinal cord or nerve roots and overgrowth can constrict the nervous system structures. If the Release procedure is part of a Fusion procedure, the Release is not coded. It is an operative step that is necessary to perform a pain-free Fusion for the patient.

Discectomy

The discectomy is treated the same as the laminectomy. The discectomy is performed to provide room for the interbody fusion device that will take its place during Fusion and is therefore an operative step, the removal of a native body part before replacement. Guideline B3.1b says resection of a joint as part of the joint replacement procedure is included in the root operation and is not coded separately. The intervertebral disc is the joint, similar to a hip labrum or knee meniscus, and the removal of this native body part is included in the Fusion procedure. If Fusion is not performed, then the discectomy is performed because the disc is constricting the spinal cord or nerve root and the procedure is a Release procedure. If the discectomy is part of a Fusion procedure, the discectomy is not coded, nor is the Release procedure coded.

Re-fusion

Re-fusion, or the process of repeating a fusion at the same level, is coded to the root operation of Fusion in ICD-10-PCS because repeat procedures are coded to the root operation performed. Fusing a joint a second time is commonly done for pseudarthrosis, or false joint. This term is used when a fusion procedure is performed but the joint fails to heal together as a solid fusion. In this case, previous hardware is removed and the fusion is repeated.

Table 16.4 lists the devices available for coding procedures performed on the bones of the body. Table 16.5 lists the device values available for coding procedures performed on the upper and lower joints of the body.

Table 16.4. Device values for procedures performed on bones

Device Value	Devices—Head and Face Bones (N)	Device Value	Devices—Upper and Lower Bones (P and Q)
0	Drainage Device	0	Drainage Device
4	Internal Fixation Device	0	Internal Fixation Device, Rigid Plate
5	External Fixation Device	4	Internal Fixation Device
7	Autologous Tissue Substitute	5	External Fixation Device
J	Synthetic Substitute	6	Internal Fixation Device, Intramedullary
K	Nonautologous Tissue Substitute	7	Autologous Tissue Substitute
M	Bone Growth Stimulator	8	External Fixation Device, Limb Lengthening
N	Neurostimulator Generator	B	External Fixation Device, Monoplanar
S	Hearing Device	C	External Fixation Device, Ring
Y	Other Device	D	External Fixation Device, Hybrid
Z	No Device	J	Synthetic Substitute
		K	Nonautologous Tissue Substitute
		M	Bone Growth Stimulator
		Y	Other Device
		Z	No Device

Table 16.5. Devices for the Upper and Lower Joints

Device Value	Devices—Upper Joints (R)	Device Value	Devices—Lower Joints (S)
0	Drainage Device	0	Drainage Device
0	Synthetic Substitute, Reverse Ball and Socket	0	Synthetic Substitute, Polyethylene
3	Infusion Device	1	Synthetic Substitute, Metal
4	Internal Fixation Device	2	Synthetic Substitute, Metal on Polyethylene
5	External Fixation Device	3	Synthetic Substitute, Ceramic
7	Autologous Tissue Substitute	3	Infusion Device
8	Spacer	4	Synthetic Substitute, Ceramic on Polyethylene
A	Interbody Fusion Device	4	Internal Fixation Device
B	Spinal Stabilization Device, Interspinous Process	5	External Fixation Device
C	Spinal Stabilization Device, Pedicle-Based	6	Synthetic Substitute, Oxidized Zirconium on Polyethylene
D	Spinal Stabilization Device, Facet Replacement	7	Autologous Tissue Substitute
J	Synthetic Substitute	8	Spacer
K	Nonautologous Tissue Substitute	9	Liner
Y	Other Device	A	Interbody Fusion Device
Z	No Device	B	Resurfacing Device
		B	Spinal Stabilization Device, Interspinous Process
		C	Spinal Stabilization Device, Pedicle-Based
		D	Spinal Stabilization Device, Facet Replacement
		E	Articulating Spacer
		J	Synthetic Substitute
		K	Nonautologous Tissue Substitute
		L	Synthetic Substitute, Unicondylar Medial
		M	Synthetic Substitute, Unicondylar Lateral
		N	Synthetic Substitute, Patellofemoral
		Y	Other Device
		Z	No Device

Qualifiers Used for the Bones and Joints

The qualifiers available for coding procedures performed on the joints can further define devices that were coded in the 6th character, such as devices that are cemented or uncemented during insertion. Skeletal system procedures may also use the standard qualifiers of X for Diagnostic and Z for No Qualifier.

The qualifiers for the bones and joints are listed in tables 16.6 and 16.7.

Table 16.6. Qualifiers for the Head and Face Bones, Upper Bones, and Lower Bones

Qualifier Value	Qualifiers—Head and Face Bones (N)	Qualifier Value	Qualifiers—Upper Bones (P)	Qualifier Value	Qualifiers—Lower Bones (Q)
X	Diagnostic	X	Diagnostic	2	Sesamoid Bone(s) 1st Toe
Z	No Qualifier	Z	No Qualifier	X	Diagnostic
				Z	No Qualifier

Table 16.7. Qualifiers for the Upper and Lower Joints

Qualifier Value	Qualifiers—Upper Joints (R)	Qualifier Value	Qualifiers—Lower Joints (S)
0	Anterior Approach, Anterior Column	0	Anterior Approach, Anterior Column
1	Posterior Approach, Posterior Column	1	Posterior Approach, Posterior Column
6	Humeral Surface	9	Cemented
7	Glenoid Surface	A	Uncemented
J	Posterior Approach, Anterior Column	C	Patellar Surface
X	Diagnostic	J	Posterior Approach, Anterior Column
Z	No Qualifier	X	Diagnostic
		Z	No Qualifier

 Code Building

Case #1:

PROCEDURE STATEMENT: Foreign body in the fourth metatarsal-phalangeal joint, right foot

ADDITIONAL INFORMATION: X-rays in the office showed a 1.5-cm needle just plantar to the fourth MPJ on the fourth toe. During the procedure, attention was directed to the plantar aspect of the foot, MPJ, and toe where an approximately 2-cm incision was made linearly and was deepened using sharp and blunt dissection. Retraction was used to expose the plantar aspect of the foot and MPJ. Upon probing with the hemostat, a metallic object was identified, removed, and sent to pathology.

ROOT AND INDEX ENTRIES FOR THE STATEMENT: Extirpation is the root operation performed in this procedure, defined as taking or cutting out solid matter from a body part. The Index entry is:

Extirpation

    Joint

        Metatarsal-phalangeal

           Right   0SCM

Code Characters:

Section	Body System	Root Operation	Body Part	Approach	Device	Qualifier
Medical and Surgical	Lower Joints	Extirpation	Metatarsal-phalangeal Joint, Right	Open	No Device	No Qualifier
0	S	C	M	0	Z	Z

RATIONALE FOR THE ANSWER: The foreign body is removed from the metatarsal-phalangeal joint using an open approach. No device remains in place at the conclusion of the procedure and no qualifier is appropriate. The correct code assignment is 0SCM0ZZ.

Case #2:

PROCEDURE STATEMENT: Open reduction fractures of nasal bones

ADDITIONAL INFORMATION: A modified left Killian incision with perichondral and periosteal elevation of the left side was performed. The overlapping fragments of nasal bone formed an irregular hump-like heightening of nasal dorsum, which now was reshaped using osteotomes and rasp. Rechecking airway showed that this left an appropriate airway bilaterally with the vertical midline septum and good proportions and relations of lateral nasal walls. Nasal contours also were quite considerably improved. An external plastic splint was applied over Steri-Strips in the usual manner.

ROOT AND INDEX ENTRIES FOR THE STATEMENT: Reposition is the root operation performed in this procedure, defined as moving to its normal location or other suitable location all or a portion of a body part. The Index entry is:

Reposition

    Bone

        Nasal   0NSB

Code Characters:

Section	Body System	Root Operation	Body Part	Approach	Device	Qualifier
Medical and Surgical	Head and Facial Bones	Reposition	Nasal Bone	Open	No Device	No Qualifier
0	N	S	B	0	Z	Z

RATIONALE FOR THE ANSWER: The displaced nasal fracture is repositioned to its normal location using an open approach. No device remains in place at the conclusion of the procedure and no qualifier is appropriate. The correct code assignment is 0NSB0ZZ.

Case #3:

PROCEDURE STATEMENT: Posterior fusion of L5–S1

ADDITIONAL INFORMATION: L5–S1 is fused with allograft bone using a posterior approach to the posterior spine.

ROOT AND INDEX ENTRIES FOR THE STATEMENT: Fusion is the root operation performed in this procedure, defined as joining together portions of an articular body part, rendering the articular body part immobile. The Index entry is:

Fusion

    Lumbosacral   0SG3

Code Characters:

Section	Body System	Root Operation	Body Part	Approach	Device	Qualifier
Medical and Surgical	Lower Joints	Fusion	Lumbosacral Joint	Open	Nonautologous Tissue Substitute	Posterior Approach, Posterior Column
0	S	G	3	0	K	1

RATIONALE FOR THE ANSWER: One lumbosacral vertebral joint between L5 and S1 is fused using allograft bone via an open posterior approach to the posterior spine. The correct code assignment is 0SG30K1.

Code Building Exercises

Work through each case and check your answers using the answer key in appendix B of the textbook before going on to the Check Your Understanding questions that follow.

Exercise 1:

DIAGNOSIS: Infected right total hip replacement

PROCEDURE: Removal of infected right total hip replacement and insertion of articulating spacer and antibiotic cement

OPERATIVE FINDINGS: There was blood-tinged cloudy fluid in the subfascial space. Both the femoral component and acetabular components were loose with bone loss present. There was also granulation-type tissue behind the acetabular component.

DESCRIPTION OF PROCEDURE: The patient was placed under anesthesia and was prepped and draped in sterile fashion about the right hip and the right lower extremity. The previous scar was re-opened using a posterolateral approach to the hip. Multiple biopsies were taken. The femoral component was grossly loose and it was removed easily by reverse impaction. The acetabulum was carefully exposed and additional biopsies were taken. The Zimmer explant device was then used to carefully remove the acetabular component. The membrane behind the acetabular component was then sent as a specimen. The acetabular cavity was curetted. The femoral canal was curetted.

A PROSTALAC articulating spacer device had been prepared prior to the initial skin incision. The femoral component was cemented using one pack of cement with four vials of Nebcin and four vials of Vancomycin powder. Acetabulum spacer component was then cemented into place with another batch of the same cement. After the cement hardened, a reduction with trial components was performed. Excellent stability was noted. The PROSTALAC spacer head was snapped into place. The wound was copiously irrigated. The joint was closed with PDS suture in interrupted fashion. Subcutaneous tissue was closed with PDS suture. Skin was closed with staples.

Questions:

1.1. What is the objective of this procedure?

1.2. What type of spacer is used?

1.3. What root operation is assigned for placing the PROSTALAC spacer?

1.4. Which body part is selected for the biopsies that were taken?

1.5. What code(s) should be assigned?

Exercise 2:

DIAGNOSIS: Status post prior lumbar laminectomies and spinal fusions at multiple levels from T12 to L4 with severe stenosis L4–L5 and severe degenerative disks, L4–S1 with bilateral radiculopathy

OPERATIONS PERFORMED:
1. Decompressive lumbar laminectomy, facetectomy and foraminotomy of L4–5, L5–S1
2. Lumbar discectomy, L4–L5 and L5–S1, replaced with interbody device
3. Posterior spinal instrumentation, L4–S1
4. Posterolateral spinal fusion, L4–S1
5. Use of autograft and allograft

COMPLICATIONS: Dural tear, repaired

INDICATIONS: This 62-year-old female had a prior successful surgical fusion for degenerative scoliosis. The patient did well until recently when she began complaining of increasing back pain and buttock pain. She again failed conservative treatment for several months.

DESCRIPTION OF OPERATION: The patient was brought to the operating table. General anesthesia was administered and the patient was placed in a prone position on Jackson table. The back was prepped and draped in sterile fashion. A midline skin incision was made below the previous incision site to expose the spinous process of L4, L5, and S1, and the L4–L5 transverse processes bilaterally were visualized. The hardware was also cleared of the soft tissues in its distal part. At this point, the decompressive laminectomy was carried out by removing the lamina and performing facetectomy and foraminotomies. Upon attempting to do this, we did encounter a dural tear, which was repaired satisfactorily with 4-0 nylon with Gelfoam overlay.

The discectomy was carried out with curettes and disk shavers at L4–L5 and L5–S1, with the dura and the S1 nerve roots retracted. Morselized bone graft obtained from the removal of the spinous processes, laminae, and facets was placed into Staxx expandable cage at L4–L5 and expanded to 9 mm. The same process was repeated at L5–S1 with the Staxx expanded to 8 mm. We proceeded with a posterior spinal instrumentation and we placed 7.0 screws. The posterolateral spinal fusion was done by abutting the fusion mass from the prior surgery, which was found to be satisfactory. Autograft bone graft was placed in and augmented with allograft, followed by placement of the screws and a rod through the rod connectors. Final x-rays were taken and found to be very satisfactory. Closure was then performed with 0 Vicryl in interrupted fashion. 2-0 Vicryl was used for subcutaneous tissue. Skin was closed with 3-0 Monocryl subcuticularly.

Questions:

2.1. What was the objective of this procedure?

2.2. The surgeon performed the procedure on the anterior column first and then on the posterior column. What qualifiers will be assigned for the codes for the procedures?

2.3. The procedures were performed on both lumbar joints and lumbosacral joints. Which body part values will be assigned for the codes for the procedures?

2.4. Which guideline helps determine the device value assigned for these procedures?

2.5. Are the decompressive laminotomies, facetectomies, and foraminotomies coded separately?

2.6. Which body part does the body part key advise you to use for the dural repair?

2.7. What code(s) should be assigned?

Exercise 3:

DIAGNOSIS: Right shoulder massive rotator cuff tear and subacromial impingement

OPERATIONS: Right shoulder arthroscopic rotator cuff repair and subacromial decompression

INDICATIONS: The patient is a pleasant 66-year-old male who has persistent shoulder pain, visualized on MRI as a massive rotator cuff tear.

DETAILS: The patient was taken to the OR and, after adequate general anesthesia, he was placed in well-padded lateral decubitus position with the right upper extremity up. The arm was put to traction and bony landmarks noted. The skin and acromion were injected with 0.5% bupivacaine. A posterolateral portal was created and the camera introduced into the joint. The massive tear was immediately seen. The biceps tendon looked intact. The glenoid was also intact. The camera was then moved to the subacromial compartment. Overlying the rotator cuff was a large subacromial spur, consistent with subacromial impingement. Given this, a subacromial decompression was undertaken. The shaver was used to debride the soft tissue and periosteum on the underside, and an 8-mm subacromial spur was excised beginning anteriorly and laterally and progressing to the posterior and medial edge to make a type 1 acromion.

Upon completion of this decompression, the camera was then reintroduced into the posterior portal, and a side-to-side repair of the anterior and posterior leaves of the rotator cuff was undertaken. Using Orthocord and a suture shuttle, sutures were passed through the tendon and used to convert the L-shaped tear into a much smaller crescent-shaped tear. A suture anchor was used to fix the apex of the crescent to the humeral head. Additional suture anchors were placed at the corners. The humeral head was completely covered with this repair. Hemostasis was obtained and the compartment was copiously irrigated and drained and the portals were removed.

Questions:

3.1. The body part key does not provide an entry for rotator cuff. Research what structures make up the rotator cuff of the shoulder and identify how it should be classified in ICD-10-PCS. What body part would you select?

3.2. In addition to the procedure performed on the rotator cuff, what other procedure is performed? Which root operation would be assigned?

3.3. What code(s) should be assigned?

Check Your Understanding

Coding Knowledge Check

1. A procedure code in the Upper and Lower Bones body systems identifying the insertion of a bone growth stimulator would have which 6th character? _____

2. The acetabulum is located in the _____.
   a. Shoulder joint
   b. Hip joint
   c. Lower leg
   d. Skull

3. A percutaneous lumbar vertebroplasty is coded to which root operation?
   a. Release
   b. Repair
   c. Replacement
   d. Supplement

4. An intramedullary device is a(n) _____ fixation device.

5. The operative report indicates that a procedure was performed on T1. Based on the naming convention for the vertebrae of the spine, the coder can determine this procedure must be a(n) _____.
   a. Alteration
   b. Corpectomy
   c. Discectomy
   d. Fusion

Procedure Statement Coding

Assign ICD-10-PCS codes to the following procedure statements and scenarios. List the root operation selected and the code assigned.

1. Open "repair" of a displaced right pisiform fracture

   _____

2. Insertion of a Smith and Nephew Genesis II metal on polyethylene prosthesis, cemented into the left knee joint

   _____

3. Left reverse shoulder replacement, metal on polyethylene

   _____

4. Percutaneous placement of intramedullary nail into a nondisplaced fracture of right femoral shaft

   _____

5. Arthroscopic partial meniscectomy of left knee

   _____

6. Posterior lumbar interbody fusion (L4-L5), posterolateral fusion of posterior spine with an allograft (L4-L5)

7. Percutaneous removal of external fixation device from left humeral shaft

8. Closed reduction of fractured left mandible

9. Incision and drainage of abscess of right finger interphalangeal joint for postoperative infection, placement of drainage device

10. Open replacement of the metal femoral head of a left hip prosthesis. The remainder of the prosthesis was not replaced.

Case Studies
Assign ICD-10-PCS codes to the following case studies.

1. Operative Report

PREOPERATIVE DIAGNOSIS: Right femoral neck fracture

POSTOPERATIVE DIAGNOSIS: Right femoral neck fracture

OPERATION: Right hip hemiarthroplasty with #9 stem, #47 head, +0 neck

INDICATIONS FOR SURGERY: The patient is an 80-year-old female with history of a fall, sustaining a right femoral neck fracture. We discussed treatment options and recommended proceeding with a right hemiarthroplasty. All questions were answered. Consent was signed.

DESCRIPTION OF PROCEDURE: The patient was brought to the operating room and given a spinal anesthesia. She was placed in the left lateral decubitus position. The right hip was sterilely prepped and draped in a routine fashion.

Anterolateral approach of the hip was made and carried down through skin, subcutaneous tissue, IT band, and gluteus maximus. Anterior portion of the gluteus medius and minimus was elevated from the greater trochanter. The capsule was identified and opened in an H-fashion. The femoral head was removed without difficulty and sized to a size 47 metal implant.

Attention was then drawn to the femur, which was machined to fit a 9 press-fit stem. At this time, the 9 stem was placed, put through a trial range of motion and found to be stable with the leg in full extension, with maximal external rotation, flexing the hip and the knee to 90 degrees of maximal internal external rotation, and leg length appeared close and symmetrical. At this time the trial components were removed. The hip was thoroughly irrigated and the real stem was cemented with +0 neck and 47 head. Once again, it was reduced and found to be very stable in all motions tested.

The wound was then thoroughly irrigated. No. 1 Vicryl was used to close the capsule. The wound was irrigated. No. 1 Vicryl was used to close the gluteus medius and minimus. The wound was irrigated. No. 1 Vicryl was used to close the IT band and gluteus maximus. The wound was irrigated, 2-0 Vicryl for subcutaneous tissue and staples for skin. Neosporin, Adaptic 4 × 4 gauze, and foam tape were then applied.

2. Operative Report

PREOPERATIVE DIAGNOSIS: Displaced left patella fracture

POSTOPERATIVE DIAGNOSIS: Displaced left patella fracture

PROCEDURE PERFORMED: Open reduction and internal fixation of left patella using cannulated screws and 18-gauge wire

INDICATIONS: This 42-year-old female with type 1 diabetes mellitus became unsteady on her feet, fell, and had a displaced patellar fracture with bleeding into the quadriceps. All questions were answered and the consent was signed.

PROCEDURE: Regional block anesthesia was administered as patient could not be cleared for general anesthesia at this time. A cuff was placed in the upper portion of the left thigh. The leg was then prepped and draped in sterile fashion. Compressive wrap was applied distally. The leg was exsanguinated. Tourniquet was inflated.

Incision was made sharply through skin and subcutaneous tissue. Dissection was carried down to the patella fracture. A large hematoma was encountered, thoroughly evacuated and irrigated. The fracture included a fairly transverse fragment. A bone scrub was used to clean soft tissue debris from the cancellous surfaces. When a clean fracture site was achieved, the reduction forceps was used to hold the patella in a reduced position anteriorly. X-ray imaging also confirmed the reduction. Guide pin was placed and the knee was flexed slightly from superior to inferior. A 4.5 Synthes stainless steel screw system was utilized. Position was confirmed by lateral radiograph, by palpation and visualization. The second screw was then placed on the lateral aspect of the patella and again confirmed with x-ray imaging, palpation and visualization. Good purchase was achieved by both screws. A tension band wiring was then performed by threading the wire through both screws and then back upon itself. Soft tissues were then repaired laterally using interrupted Fiberwire suture and closed over the top of the hardware to prevent irritation. Subcutaneous was closed over that with Vicryl suture and the skin was closed with nylon.

3. Operative Report

PREOPERATIVE DIAGNOSIS: Infected right tibial plateau wound

POSTOPERATIVE DIAGNOSIS: Infected right tibial plateau wound

PROCEDURE: I&D right tibial incision

INDICATIONS FOR PROCEDURE: The patient is status post trauma. He sustained multiple injuries to include a right tibial plateau fracture that was fixed three weeks ago. He now has a purulence exuding from the middle aspect of his incision. After discussing the risk, benefits, and alternatives with the patient and family, it was determined that operative intervention with incision and drainage with cultures would be appropriate.

PROCEDURE: After obtaining informed consent from the patient, identifying the patient and the operative site, the patient was taken to the operating suite. Anesthesia was administered. A non-sterile bumper was placed under the patient's right hip. No tourniquet was used. The patient's right lower extremity was then prepped and draped in the usual sterile fashion. An incision was made into the knee joint following his previous incision in a curvilinear fashion, progressing over the lateral joint line. This was carried sharply through the skin. At this time, superficial cultures were taken of the gross purulence that was present. Blunt dissection was carried down to the level of the deep fascia. The deep fascia did appear to be intact and the purulence did not appear to tract to it. This deep fascia was then opened sharply. This carried us down to the level of the plate. Deep culture was taken from this area as well. The wound was then copiously irrigated with normal saline. All screws were checked for tightness and were found to be one half turn from totally tight, which was rectified at this time. The remainder of the five liter bag of irrigation was irrigated through in a pulsatile fashion. At this time, a deep drain was placed. A medium Hemovac was placed. The deep fascia was closed with 0 PDS and superficial fascia with 2-0 PDS. The skin was closed with 2-0 nylon, all in an interrupted fashion. The patient was washed and dried and placed in a sterile postoperative dressing and a nonsterile ACE wrap. All sponge, needle, and instrument counts were verified to be correct prior to the completion of the procedure. The patient was allowed to waken and was taken to PACU in a stable condition.

4. Operative Report

NOTE: Exclude from coding any intraoperative imaging on this case.

PREOPERATIVE DIAGNOSIS: Right distal radius and ulna fractures

POSTOPERATIVE DIAGNOSIS: Right distal radius and ulna fractures

OPERATION: Closed reduction and percutaneous pinning of right distal radius fracture and closed reduction of right distal ulna fracture

OPERATIVE INDICATIONS: The patient is an 11-year-old male who has right distal radius and ulna fractures. He presents for surgical treatment. I previously attempted a closed reduction in the fluoroscopy suite next to the emergency room, and his fracture was difficult to reduce without more significant sedation. He thus presents to the operating room for closed reduction and possible pinning and possible open procedure. The risks, benefits, and potential complications were explained to the parents. They understood these things and wished to proceed with surgery.

TECHNIQUE: The patient was taken to the operating room and placed supine on the OR table with all of his extremities adequately padded. The splint was removed from the right upper extremity and a closed reduction was performed after the patient was under anesthesia. Both fractures were found to reduce. Fluoroscopy was used to view the fracture in multiplanar fluoroscopy. Given the fracture pattern, I thought it would be appropriate to pin the radius to increase stability. Two K wires were then placed under direct fluoroscopic guidance across the fracture site in the radius. The growth plate was avoided. The fracture and pins were again visualized in multiplanar fluoroscopy, and the fractures and the pins were noted to be in good position. The pins were bent and cut. Final films were obtained. Sterile dressings followed by sugar tong type of splint were then applied.

5. Operative Report

NOTE: Exclude from coding any intraoperative monitoring and intraoperative imaging on this case.

OPERATION:
1. Anterior cervical decompression C5–C6
2. Arthrodesis C5–C6

INDICATIONS FOR PROCEDURE: The patient is a 27-year-old right-handed patient seen for neurosurgical evaluation because of pain in his neck and both shoulders. He reports heavy exercise on a trampoline in high school and developed a kink in his neck, which has gradually increased in severity. In addition, he was in an auto accident last year, which increased his symptoms. He had physical therapy for 3 to 4 weeks and pain medications at a pain center, and also went to a chiropractor. He has tried anti-inflammatory medications, three or four different times of physical therapy courses, and three epidural steroids, and felt worse afterwards. Pain in the back of his neck radiating to both shoulders, weakness of both arms, numbness of his neck and the left shoulder, coughing and sneezing does not increase his pain, bowel and bladder function well. The risks and reasons for surgery were described to him. His questions were answered to his satisfaction, and he desired that the operative procedure be provided, and I agreed to do so for him.

PROCEDURE: After pre-medications, the patient was brought to the operating theatre and endotracheal anesthesia was introduced. He was positioned supine with a roll beneath his shoulders. His head was slightly turned toward the left. An incision was made in one of the Langer's skin lines, horizontally in the neck. Blunt and sharp dissection allowed us to reach the anterior surface of the vertebral column. Intraoperative x-ray verified the presence of a needle placed into the disc space at the C5–C6 level. Self-retaining retractors were then positioned. The longus coli muscle was mobilized. A portion of the disc material was removed after the posterior longitudinal ligament was opened. Soft disc material was present in this region protruding against the dura and pressing on the nerve root, which was now fully exposed once the ligament was opened. The protruding disc was excised. A careful search with the use of the operating microscope for any fragments of disc was accomplished. The DSSEP (dermatomal somatosensory-evoked potential) came down to good range back into normal. An interbody fusion device was chosen to fit the opening and filled with allograft bone. EVI screws and plate of 18 mm was placed firmly into position. Final AP and lateral x-ray was obtained. The wound was closed with Vicryl with Dermabond on the skin. A collar will be provided. The patient appeared to tolerate the procedure well and will be cared for postoperatively.

6. Operative Report

PREOPERATIVE DIAGNOSIS: Chronic lateral epicondylitis, right elbow

POSTOPERATIVE DIAGNOSIS: Chronic lateral epicondylitis, right elbow

OPERATION:
1. Right elbow arthrotomy with exploration and lateral epicondylectomy
2. Fasciotomy with common extensor origin release

PROCEDURE: Following the induction of satisfactory general anesthesia, the patient's right elbow was prepped and draped sterilely. The arm was wrapped with an Ace bandage, and the pneumatic tourniquet was inflated to 250 mm Hg. A 3-cm incision was made beginning at the lateral epicondyle and extending distally over the common extensor tendon origin. The common extensor was divided in line with the skin incision and reflected from the lateral epicondyle of the elbow. All edematous granulation tissue was removed from the common extensor origin, and the elbow joint was entered. There were no articular cartilage defects or loose bodies. Sufficient lateral epicondyle of the elbow was then removed with rongeurs to create a flat cancellous bony surface. Following this, the wound was thoroughly irrigated with saline and infiltrated with local anesthesia. The deep fascia was approximated side-to-side without tension with 2-0 Vicryl suture. Subcutaneous tissue was closed with 3-0 Vicryl, followed by 4-0 Vicryl in the intradermal tissue. Steri-Strips and sterile dressings were applied. The patient was placed in a sling.

The patient was transferred to her bed and taken to the recovery room in stable condition. There were no operative complications, and the patient tolerated the procedure well. The pneumatic tourniquet was deflated at the end of the procedure.

Urinary System

The urinary system performs the function of cleansing the blood and removing waste products from the body in the form of urine. The 2nd character value for the Urinary System is T.

Functions of the Urinary System

The six functions of the urinary system are to rid the body of waste materials, regulate the fluid volume of the body, maintain electrolyte concentrations in body fluids, control blood pH levels, secrete erythropoietin, and secrete rennin (Applegate 2011, 413).

Organization of the Urinary System

The urinary system contains two major organs called kidneys, which cleanse the blood and form urine. The urine travels from the kidneys through the ureters to the bladder, an organ that stores urine until a sufficient volume has been accumulated. When the nerves of the bladder send a signal that the bladder is full, urine is expelled from the bladder through the urethra to the outside of the body. The body parts associated with the urinary system are the kidneys, the ureters, the bladder, and the urethra. The adrenal glands of the endocrine system are found on the top of the kidneys. Figure 17.1 displays the components of the urinary system.

Anatomy Alert

The body has two ureters and one urethra. Read documentation carefully for the terms uretero and urethro to determine the body part being referenced.

The process of forming urine incorporates the other functions performed by the kidney, such as regulating fluid volume and maintaining electrolyte balance. The kidney is made up of triangular divisions called the renal pyramids, found within the renal medulla, or medullary tissue. At the outer edge of each kidney is the renal cortex. The cortex contains the glomerular capsules, each containing a glomerulus. Inside the glomerulus, the blood is filtered and the waste products and fluid are removed as urine is formed. The inside of the kidney is called the renal medulla. The collecting ducts drain the urine that is formed in the glomeruli and accumulate it in the renal pelvis, the larger collection area at the proximal end of each ureter. The ureters are long, fibrous tubes that connect each kidney to the bladder. Figure 17.2 shows the frontal cross-section of the kidney with the filtering and collection systems.

As the urine is collected, it travels down each ureter to the bladder, where urine is temporarily stored. The bladder is a muscular reservoir that is located in females just adjacent to the uterus posterosuperiorly and to the vagina posteroinferiorly. In males, it is adjacent to the rectum posterosuperiorly and is superior to the prostate gland (McKinley et al. 2017, 824). The ureters enter the bladder in the trigone, the muscular area that acts as a funnel to direct urine into the urethra through the bladder neck. The bladder neck is at the apex

Figure 17.1. Urinary system

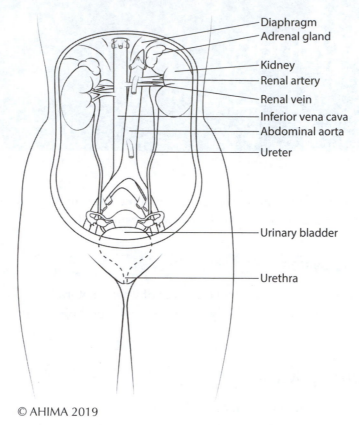

- Diaphragm
- Adrenal gland
- Kidney
- Renal artery
- Renal vein
- Inferior vena cava
- Abdominal aorta
- Ureter
- Urinary bladder
- Urethra

© AHIMA 2019

Figure 17.2. Cross-section of the kidney

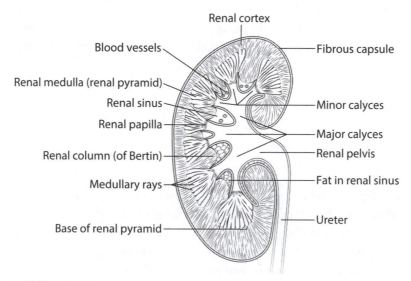

- Renal cortex
- Blood vessels
- Renal medulla (renal pyramid)
- Renal sinus
- Renal papilla
- Renal column (of Bertin)
- Medullary rays
- Base of renal pyramid
- Fibrous capsule
- Minor calyces
- Major calyces
- Renal pelvis
- Fat in renal sinus
- Ureter

© AHIMA 2019

of the trigone, along with the internal urethral sphincter. The external urethral sphincter is at the distal end of the urethra, near the external opening. The kidneys, their associated adrenal glands, and both ureters are located in the retroperitoneal space, behind the peritoneal cavity. The bladder and urethra are located in the pelvic cavity. Figure 17.3 shows a cross-section of the bladder, showing the location of the ureteral openings, the trigone, and the bladder neck.

Figure 17.3.   **Cross-section of the bladder**

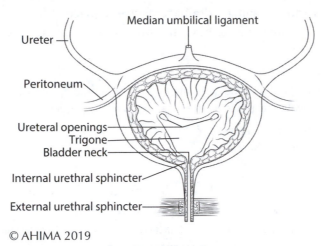

Median umbilical ligament

Ureter

Peritoneum

Ureteral openings
Trigone
Bladder neck

Internal urethral sphincter

External urethral sphincter

© AHIMA 2019

Common Root Operations Used in Coding Procedures on the Urinary System

All of the root operations that can be performed on tubular body parts can be performed on the body parts of the urinary system. Dilation of a body part in the urinary system is performed by passing sounds (metal instruments of various shapes) or filiforms (guidewires used to pass larger instruments over an obstruction) through the tubular body parts, followed by scopes or other instruments. Dilation can also be performed by cutting the wall of the tubular body part, such as incising the bladder neck or the urethral opening. When stents are inserted into the ureters, the intent of the procedure is to dilate and the stent holds open the ureter. The root operation Dilation is assigned and the device value is D, Intraluminal Device. Just as with coronary stents, there is no other root operation that can be assigned to deploy a stent in the ureter.

When the bladder, a ureter, or the urethra is no longer functional or must be removed, a bypass procedure is often performed. A vesicostomy creates a new opening between the bladder and the skin. A ureterostomy creates a new opening between the ureter and the skin. When the bladder needs to be removed, the ureters can be bypassed to a piece of the ileum in a ureteroileal conduit procedure or sigmoid bladder procedure. The portion of the colon is used to simulate a urinary bladder, and an artificial opening is created in the skin. All of these procedures are coded with the root operation Bypass.

Another common bypass procedure used to treat vesicoureteral reflux is called a cross-trigonal reimplantation of the ureter. This can be performed on one or both ureters. In this procedure, the ureter enters the back musculature of the bladder high in the dome. The ureter is then tunneled on a diagonal from one side of the bladder to the other, with the opening placed in an upward orientation. This re-routing helps stop the reflux of urine upward into the kidney and reduces infection.

Following a temporary diversion (bypass) of urine to allow healing, an undiversion procedure may be performed to restore the normal path of urine. The root operation Repair is used to code this reversal of the diversion procedure.

When the musculature around the bladder relaxes, a bladder suspension procedure is performed. The root operation Reposition is coded to describe this suspension procedure. When the bladder or the urethra is suspended by the use of mesh or other synthetic material, the root operation assigned is Supplement because the mesh physically reinforces the body part. The root operation of Reposition does not allow the use of a device for this procedure. Supplement is the not elsewhere classified (NEC) procedure when the body part is restored with a device.

Procedures performed on devices that have been placed in the urinary system are coded to the root operation performed, such as Change or Removal. Irrigation of previously placed indwelling tube is coded to the root operation Irrigation of indwelling device in the Administration section, covered in chapter 21 of this text.

Placement of a urinary catheter is coded to the root operation Drainage because the intent of the procedure is to drain the bladder, with or without leaving a drainage device in place at the end of the procedure. The root operation Insertion is not used, as the code tables do not provide a device value for a drainage device to be left at the conclusion of the procedure.

B6.1c. Procedures performed on a device only and not on a body part are specified in the root operations Change, Irrigation, Removal, and Revision and are coded to the procedure performed.

Example: Irrigation of percutaneous nephrostomy tube is coded to the root operation Irrigation of indwelling device in the Administration section.

The root operation Transplantation is used to code renal transplants from any source with the qualifier identifying the source. If the native kidney is removed to make room for the transplant, the resection is not coded separately. If a renal transplant is rejected, the later removal of the transplanted kidney is coded to the root operation Resection and the appropriate kidney, right or left.

The root operation Fragmentation is coded when a urinary calculus is broken up, such as with extracorporeal shockwave lithotripsy. If the fragments of the calculus will not pass through the urinary system on their own and must be removed, the root operation Extirpation is coded instead of the Fragmentation procedure. The fragmentation process is considered an operative step for the Extirpation procedure.

Hypospadias is a congenital anomaly of the placement of the urethral opening. Rather than in the tip of the penis, the urethral opening can be:

- **Glanular**—To the underside of the penis in the glans penis
- **Distal**—In the shaft of the penis toward the end
- **Proximal**—In the shaft of the penis toward the scrotum
- **Penoscrotal**—At the base of the penis, near the junction of the penis and the scrotum

When the hypospadias location is glanular, the urethra can be repositioned to the tip of the penis. In all other locations, there is not enough urethra present to allow repositioning. In this case, the absent urethra needs to be replaced with graft material or reconstructed using transferred prepuce (foreskin) that is still attached. Common harvesting locations for free grafts are the foreskin, buccal mucosa and bladder tissue.

Be sure to research any procedure that is unfamiliar to assure correct coding. If the documentation includes an eponym (and the intent of the procedure is unclear), query the physician for specifics.

Body Part Values for the Urinary System

The kidney pelvis and the bladder neck have individual body part values within ICD-10-PCS. Bilateral body part values are available for the kidneys and for the ureters. The male prostate, while frequently accessed through the urinary system and the cause of many urinary problems, is not a part of the urinary system in ICD-10-PCS. The prostate is a body part within the male reproductive system, covered in chapter 18 of this text.

Coding Tip

Bilateral body part values are available for the kidneys and the ureters. If procedures are performed on the renal pelvis of both the right and left kidneys, two procedures are coded with individual body part values for right and left, as no bilateral kidney pelvis body part value is identified.

B3.11b. If multiple tubular body parts are inspected, the most distal body part (the body part farthest from the starting point of the inspection) is coded. If multiple non-tubular body parts in a region are inspected, the body part that specifies the entire area inspected is coded.

Example: Cystoureteroscopy with inspection of bladder and ureters is coded to the ureter body part value. Exploratory laparotomy with general inspection of abdominal contents is coded to the peritoneal cavity body part value.

When Inspection is performed, follow Guideline B3.11b to select the body part. If multiple parts are inspected, code the most distal part. In the urinary system, this means the farthest body part from the starting point of the Inspection. If the entire urinary tract is inspected using an endoscope, including the kidney, assign code 0TJ58ZZ. The cystoscopy procedure is pictured in figure 1.5 of chapter 1.

Guideline B4.1b directs the coder to code the body part identified as the site of the procedure when the location is described in the documentation as "peri" to an anatomical structure. Periureteric adhesions would be located around the ureter. A procedure to release these adhesions would be assigned to the body part value for the affected ureter. Table 17.1 lists the body part values available for coding procedures performed on the urinary system. If the documentation includes specific body part names that are not included in these lists, refer to the body part key for other body part synonyms and alternative terms.

Table 17.1. Body parts in the Urinary system

Body Part Value	Body Parts—Urinary System (T)
0	Kidney, Right
1	Kidney, Left
2	Kidneys, Bilateral
3	Kidney, Pelvis, Right
4	Kidney, Pelvis, Left
5	Kidney
6	Ureter, Right
7	Ureter, Left
8	Ureters, Bilateral
9	Ureter
B	Bladder
C	Bladder Neck
D	Urethra

Approaches Used in the Urinary System

Different parts of the urinary anatomy are approached in the traditional open fashion or through the natural or artificial opening of the urethra. When the kidney is approached through the skin and through the wall of the kidney with only instruments and using guidance, the procedure is called a percutaneous nephrotomy. If the approach is through the skin, around the base of the kidney and directly into the renal pelvis, the procedure is called a percutaneous pyelotomy. In the pyelotomy procedure, the body of the kidney is not entered. Both of these procedures use the ICD-10-PCS Percutaneous approach. If an endoscope is introduced through this route, it is the Percutaneous Endoscopic approach.

B5.4. Procedures performed percutaneously via a device placed for the procedure are coded to the approach Percutaneous.

Example: Fragmentation of kidney stone performed via percutaneous nephrostomy is coded to the approach Percutaneous.

Devices Common to the Urinary System

Neurostimulator leads may be inserted into the bladder or urethra to treat overactive bladder or urinary retention. The neurostimulator generator is inserted into a subcutaneous pocket in the upper buttock following the same concepts used in cardiac pacemaker insertion.

Artificial sphincters are also implanted to assist with urinary control. The urethral sphincter is a muscle that allows the body to hold in urine. An inflatable artificial sphincter is an implanted device that keeps urine from leaking when the urinary sphincter no longer works well. The artificial sphincter has three parts: a cuff around the urethra, a balloon that is implanted in the abdomen, and a pump that is placed in the male scrotum or female abdomen. The pump inflates the cuff. To urinate, the cuff of the artificial sphincter can be relaxed so urine can flow out. The cuff reinflates on its own in 90 seconds (NLM 2016a).

Urinary catheters and intraluminal devices are often confused. Urinary catheters are drainage devices because they drain urine to the outside of the body. These can either be a urethral catheter into the bladder through the natural opening or a suprapubic catheter placed percutaneously above the pubic bone and into the bladder. Intraluminal devices (stents) are used to dilate the ureters. They are not drainage devices because their purpose is not to drain urine to the outside. The intent is to keep the ureter open. In addition, they are completely within the lumen of the ureter, making them intraluminal devices. The same is true if the stent is placed in the urethra. Table 17.2 lists the device values available for coding procedures performed on the urinary system.

Coding Tip

Irrigation or flushing of previously placed drains is coded to the root operation Irrigation of indwelling device in the Administration section of ICD-10-PCS.

Table 17.2. Devices for the Urinary system

Device Value	Devices—Urinary System (T)
0	Drainage Device
2	Monitoring Device
3	Infusion Device
7	Autologous Tissue Substitute
C	Extraluminal Device
D	Intraluminal Device
J	Synthetic Substitute
K	Nonautologous Tissue Substitute
L	Artificial Sphincter
M	Stimulator Lead
Y	Other Device
Z	No Device

Qualifiers for the Urinary System

The qualifiers used to code procedures performed on the urinary system include the information regarding the source of a transplanted kidney. The source of an allogeneic kidney is another human donor. The source of a syngeneic kidney is an identical twin human donor and the source of a zooplastic kidney is an animal donor. The qualifier also identifies the destination of the bypass, or the body part bypassed to, in the root operation Bypass. Urinary system procedures may also use the standard qualifiers of X for Diagnostic and Z for No Qualifier. Table 17.3 lists the qualifier values used to code procedures performed on the Urinary system.

Table 17.3. Qualifiers for the Urinary system

Qualifier Value	Qualifiers—Urinary System (T)
0	Allogeneic
1	Syngeneic
2	Zooplastic
3	Kidney, Pelvis, Right
4	Kidney, Pelvis, Left
6	Ureter, Right
7	Ureter, Left
9	Colocutaneous
A	Ileum
B	Bladder
C	Ileocutaneous
D	Cutaneous
X	Diagnostic
Z	No Qualifier

 Code Building

Case #1:

PROCEDURE STATEMENT: Placement of a urethral stent

ADDITIONAL INFORMATION: The urethra is dilated and a urethral stent is deployed using an endoscope.

ROOT AND INDEX ENTRIES FOR THE STATEMENT: Dilation is the root operation performed in this procedure, defined as expanding an orifice or the lumen of a tubular body part. The Index entry is:

Dilation

    Urethra   0T7D

Code Characters:

Section	Body System	Root Operation	Body Part	Approach	Device	Qualifier
Medical and Surgical	Urinary System	Dilation	Urethra	Via Natural or Artificial Opening Endoscopic	Intraluminal Device	No Qualifier
0	T	7	D	8	D	Z

RATIONALE FOR THE ANSWER: The intent of the procedure is to dilate the urethra, not simply to insert a device into the urethra; therefore, the root operation Dilation is the most appropriate. The urethra stent is an intraluminal device, deployed using the Via Natural or Artificial Opening Endoscopic approach. The correct code assignment is 0T7D8DZ.

Case #2:

PROCEDURE STATEMENT: Percutaneous endoscopic biopsy of right renal pelvis

ADDITIONAL INFORMATION: The right renal pelvis is inspected and an excision of the renal pelvis is performed.

ROOT AND INDEX ENTRIES FOR THE STATEMENT: Excision is the root operation performed in this procedure, defined as cutting out or off, without replacement, a portion of a body part. The Index entry is:

Excision

    Kidney pelvis

       Right   0TB3

Code Characters:

Section	Body System	Root Operation	Body Part	Approach	Device	Qualifier
Medical and Surgical	Urinary System	Excision	Kidney Pelvis, Right	Percutaneous Endoscopic	No Device	Diagnostic
0	T	B	3	4	Z	X

RATIONALE FOR THE ANSWER: If the approach is through the skin, around the base of the kidney, and directly into the renal pelvis, the capsule of the kidney is not entered. This is the percutaneous endoscopic approach. The qualifier X, Diagnostic is assigned because the procedure description states that a biopsy was performed. The correct code assignment is 0TB34ZX.

Code Building Exercises

Work through each case and check your answers using the answer key in appendix B of the textbook before going on to the Check Your Understanding questions that follow.

Exercise 1:

PREOPERATIVE DIAGNOSIS: Left Ureteral Calculus, weak urinary stream

POSTOPERATIVE DIAGNOSIS: Same. Bladder Neck Contracture

OPERATION: Cystoscopy, Dilation of bladder neck contracture, with insertion of left ureteral stent, shock wave lithotripsy, left ureter

Pre-op KUB x-ray was taken and reviewed. The patient was placed in the lithotomy position and prepped and draped in the usual manner after satisfactory general anesthesia. A 22 scope was passed per urethra. He was noted to have a bladder neck contracture, from previous prostatic surgery, requiring attention. The transurethral incision of the bladder neck was performed and bladder entered. The bladder appeared normal.

A .035 glide wire was passed up the left ureteral orifice to the left renal pelvis. A 6 × 26 Fr ureteral stent was advanced over the wire and using the pusher, the stent was delivered into the bladder and the stent was pushed into adequate position under fluoroscopic guidance. The glide wire was removed and the distal coil formed in the bladder and proximal coil formed adequately in the left renal pelvis.

Following this, the patient was taken to the Lithotripsy suite, placed in the gantry, and positioned. Fluoroscopy was used to localize the stone in the left proximal ureter measuring 6 mm in size. A total of 2400 shocks were delivered to a maximum of 20 KV. Fluoroscopy was used intermittently and ultimately determined good fragmentation of the stone.

Questions:

1.1. How many procedures are represented in this report? What are they?

1.2. Which group of root operations would be used to select the root operation(s) for the procedure(s)?

1.3. Which root operation(s) is(are) assigned for the procedure(s)?

1.4. Is the insertion of the ureteral stent coded separately?

1.5. What code(s) should be assigned? (Do not code the fluoroscopy for this operative report.)

Exercise 2:

PREOPERATIVE DIAGNOSIS: Right renal mass

POSTOPERATIVE DIAGNOSIS: Right renal mass

PROCEDURE: Robotic-assisted laparoscopic right radical nephrectomy

INDICATIONS: This 84-year-old male was being worked up for his chronic kidney disease when a CT scan was done and a 9-cm central right renal mass was noted. The patient elected for surgical management.

DESCRIPTION OF PROCEDURE: Under general anesthesia, pneumoperitoneum was achieved with the Veress needle and brought to 15 mmHg. A 15-mm trocar was then placed lateral to the umbilicus and, under direct visualization, a 12-mm port, two robotic ports, and a 5-mm liver retractor port were placed. The robot was docked and the operation proceeded. The plane between Gerota's fascia and the right colon was then taken down with the combination of cautery and cutting. I dissected down and lifted the inferior portion of the kidney. The ureter was easily identified and we began tracking up to the hilum. The gonadal vein was then dissected out at the level of the vena cava and secured at the level of the vena cava with two Weck clips.

The solitary right renal artery was taken with a 45-mm vascular stapler. I then came across the renal vein with a 45-mm load vascular stapler. The superior and lateral aspects of the kidney were freed up using cautery. The remaining ureter was then taken with a series of staplers. The resection bed was irrigated. The pneumo-peritoneum was brought down to 8 mmHg and the patient's blood pressure was brought up to 140 systolic. There was no evidence of bleeding. Next, using Surgicel and Evicel, the resection bed was coated. The robot was undocked.

Next, the ports were removed and two of the port sites were connected. The incision was made larger to remove the large size kidney and finish the full inspection. This was done without difficulty. The fascia was closed with a #1 PDS in a running manner ×2. The subcutaneous layers were all closed with 3-0 Vicryl suture and the skin was closed with 4-0 Monocryl.

Questions:

2.1. Which guideline is useful in determining the approach value for this procedure?

_____

2.2. In addition to the code for the robotic assistance procedure (8E0W4CZ—Robotic Assisted Procedure of Trunk Region, Percutaneous Endoscopic Approach), what code(s) would be assigned?

_____

 Check Your Understanding

Coding Knowledge Check

1. Ablation of a renal tumor is performed. Which root operation is coded to describe the intent of this procedure?
    a. Destruction
    b. Excision
    c. Extraction
    d. Resection

2. Code 0T2BX0Z describes the procedure of changing a _____.

3. The surgeon performs an open urinary diversion of the left ureter using ileal conduit to skin and a laser removal of a left ureteral lesion. How is this coded?
    a. 0T170ZD, 0T570ZZ
    b. 0T570ZZ
    c. 0T170ZC, 0T570ZZ
    d. 0T180ZD

4. A Marshall-Marchetti-Krantz urethral suspension operation is coded with the root operation of

    _____.

5. A suprapubic aspiration of the bladder is performed. Which approach value is assigned?_____.

Procedure Statement Coding

Assign ICD-10-PCS codes to the following procedure statements and scenarios. List the root operation selected and the code assigned.

1. The patient underwent an exploratory laparotomy after presentation with severe urinary hemorrhage. The procedure found an extensive adenocarcinoma of the left kidney with metastasis to the left lower lobe of the lung, great vessels, and lateral diaphragm. The tumor could not be removed, and, therefore, the left ureter was surgically ligated to prevent further urinary hemorrhage.

    _____

2. A patient with recurrent urethral strictures was taken to the operating room, where a meatotomy was performed due to stricture. A scope was advanced through the urethra into the bladder, where a bladder neck contracture was found. The contracture was incised.

    _____

3. Extracorporeal shock wave lithotripsy of large bladder stone

4. Right kidney transplant from matched donor

5. Suturing of bladder laceration, open

6. Destruction of urethral tumor, endoscopic

7. Change of ureterostomy tube

8. Open adhesiolysis of left ureter

9. Open insertion of inflatable bladder neck sphincter for stress incontinence

10. Paraurethral bladder neck suspension utilizing Pereyra suture, open

Case Studies
Assign ICD-10-PCS codes to the following case studies.

1. Operative Report

PREOPERATIVE DIAGNOSIS: Glanular hypospadias

POSTOPERATIVE DIAGNOSIS: Glanular hypospadias

PROCEDURE: Hypospadias repair

INDICATION FOR PROCEDURE: An 11-month-old with glanular hypospadias. He has already been circumcised. Parents are requesting hypospadias repair, which is performed today without contraindication.

OPERATIVE FINDINGS: A simple meatal advancement was able to be performed. No glanuloplasty had to be performed.

OPERATIVE NOTE: Informed consent was obtained. The patient was brought to the operating room and placed supine on the procedure table, given general anesthetic and prepped and draped per protocol. Surgical verification and patient verification were performed. Intravenous antibiotics were administered and a penile block was administered as dictated above, using 9.5 mL of 0.25 percent Marcaine without epinephrine in order to assist with postoperative analgesia. Prolene suture was placed through the glans penis and the meatus was opened utilizing a hypospadias pickup. A deep back plate incision was made after a tourniquet was applied and the urothelium was advanced to the epithelium of the glans with interrupted 7-0 Vicryl sutures. The corners were then placed with small clamps for stay sutures and then the back plate was then incised thoroughly. The urethral mucosa was then advanced to the epithelium in the midline and then on either side with interrupted

7-0 Vicryl sutures such that the entire bridge of tissue had been obliterated and the urethra was in the normal glanular position. Hemostasis was meticulous. The tourniquet was removed. Bacitracin was applied. The patient was then awakened and transferred to the recovery room in stable condition. There were no complications. At the end of the case, the sponge and needle count were correct ×3.

2. Operative Report

PREOPERATIVE DIAGNOSIS:	Bladder tumor
POSTOPERATIVE DIAGNOSIS:	Bladder tumor
OPERATION:	Transurethral resection of a 3-cm bladder tumor
SPECIMENS:	Sessile bladder tumor and tumor base
FINDINGS:	A 3-cm high-grade appearing tumor, thought to be transitional cell carcinoma, right posterior bladder wall
INDICATION:	A 62-year-old patient with hematuria with bladder tumor identified on CT of the pelvis

DESCRIPTION OF PROCEDURE: The patient was brought to the operating room. General anesthesia was induced. The patient was placed in lithotomy and genitalia was prepped and draped in the usual manner. The patient was identified and the procedure was confirmed. Resectoscope passed. Tumor visualized, right posterior bladder wall, approximately 3 cm in greatest dimension. It is very sessile in nature, quite red, and angry-appearing. There were some papillary areas. Overall, the tumor had a very high-grade appearance to it. It was near but did not involve the right ureteral orifice.

The tumor was resected and the biopsy specimen sent for permanent section. Separate biopsies were taken of the tumor base to rule out deep muscle invasion. The area was thoroughly cauterized with loop electrode. No bleeding was seen with the bladder decompressed. No other abnormalities were noted. Scope removed. The patient tolerated the procedure well.

3. Operative Report

PREOPERATIVE DIAGNOSIS:	A large bladder stone
POSTOPERATIVE DIAGNOSIS:	A large bladder stone
PROCEDURE:	Suprapubic removal of a bladder stone

PROCEDURE: Under general anesthesia, an incision was made in the suprapubic area. The incision was carried down to the subcutaneous tissue. The fascia was nicked using the knife, and the incision was carried up and down using the Mayo scissors. The rectus muscle was then separated in the midline. The area over the bladder was identified. The #27 gauge syringe was then inserted into the bladder, and the bladder was irrigated to properly identify it. There was an incision made in the bladder area. The incision was thickened by a previous inflammatory reaction. Incision was carried down through and into the bladder. The bladder was found with great difficulty. The bladder was opened, and there was a very large bladder stone found which appeared to be attached to a foreign body. The stone was removed. The bladder was inspected for any other foreign bodies and/or stones. The bladder was then closed in two layers with 2-0 chromic, which the first layer was running, and the second layer was an interrupted layer. All bleeding around the bladder was then identified and cauterized. A Jackson-Pratt drain was then placed in the retropubic space and brought out through all layers. The wound was closed in the following manner. The muscle was closed using 2-0 chromic suture. The rectus fascia was closed using #1 Vicryl in a running fashion. The subcutaneous layer was closed using 3-0 plain suture in an interrupted fashion. The skin was closed using the skin staples. The drain was anchored to the skin using 2-0 silk suture. A fluffy dressing was applied to the wound, and the patient was taken to the recovery room in good condition.

4. Operative Report

PREOPERATIVE DIAGNOSIS: Right renal calculus

POSTOPERATIVE DIAGNOSIS: Right renal calculus

PROCEDURE: Right extracorporeal shock wave lithotripsy

PROCEDURE DESCRIPTION: The patient was placed in the supine position and in the F2 focus of the MSL 5000 lithotriptor, shock wave lithotripsy was begun at 17 kV and progressed to 23. A total of 3,000 shocks were given to the stone with resultant fragmentation of the calculus in the right renal pelvis. No complications were noted. The patient tolerated the procedure well and was taken to recovery in satisfactory condition.

5. Operative Report

PREOPERATIVE DIAGNOSIS: Left grade III vesicoureteral reflux

POSTOPERATIVE DIAGNOSIS: Left grade III vesicoureteral reflux

OPERATION: Cystoscopy with bilateral subureteric injection of Deflux

INDICATIONS: History of left grade III vesicoureteral reflux and voiding dysfunction including nocturnal enuresis and accidents. Informed consent was obtained.

FINDINGS: Normal urethra, bladder mucosa with multiple trabeculations and large capacity, capacious left ureteral orifice with a very laterally displaced location, orthotopic right ureteral orifice.

DESCRIPTION OF PROCEDURE: Under general anesthesia, the patient was placed in a dorsal lithotomy position and her external genitalia were prepped and draped in the usual sterile fashion. A rigid cystoscope was passed per urethra into the urinary bladder under direct vision. Pancystoscopy was performed, revealing a very wide-open left ureteral orifice, which was laterally displaced.

A 20-gauge endoscopic needle was passed via the working port of the cystoscope and 1.1 cc of Deflux was placed in the left subureteric space, using the hydrodistention-implantation technique (HIT). Then, 0.8 cc of Deflux was placed in the right subureteric space. The bladder was then drained with no obvious signs of bleeding, and 10 cc of 2 percent lidocaine gel was inserted into the urethral meatus. The patient was gently awakened from anesthesia, transferred to a stretcher, and taken to recovery without incident.

6. Operative Report

PREOPERATIVE DIAGNOSIS: Left ureteral stone

POSTOPERATIVE DIAGNOSIS: Left ureteral stone

PROCEDURES:
1. Left ureteral stone manipulation
2. Left ureteroscopic stone fragmentation
3. Stent placement

INDICATIONS FOR SURGERY: The patient is a 65-year-old white male who has had left flank pain. He was found to have a left mid ureteral stone measured at about 5 mm. He was therefore taken to the operating room for stent placement and possible stone removal. He understood that the stent will give him discomfort and there is no guarantee that the stone can be removed.

PROCEDURE IN DETAIL: After laryngeal mask anesthesia was induced, the patient was placed in lithotomy position. His external genitalia was prepped and draped in sterile fashion. A 22-French cystoscope with 30-degree lens was inserted into the bladder. A full inspection was made. The prostate was not obstructive; however, he had a fairly high bladder neck. Both ureteral orifices were identified. No bladder tumor or stones were found. The left ureteral orifice was cannulated with 0.035 sensor guidewire, which was advanced all the way to the renal pelvis under fluoroscopic guidance. A fluoroscopic inspection identified a radiopacity in the proximal ureter. A semi-rigid ureteroscope was then inserted into the ureter and advanced all the way distal to the stone. The stone was fairly large, and it was impacted into the mucosa. The stone was manipulated so that it migrated slightly proximally into the open dilated ureter. The stone was then engaged with a grasping forceps. It turns out that the stone was fairly soft and therefore it was breaking easily with this grasper. The stone was fragmented into many pieces. The largest piece, however, was about half of the size of the original stone. At this point we could not further fragment the stone with the grasper. Then, a Gemini stone basket was used to engage the fragment and the fragment was extracted. No other large fragments were found. A 6-French / 28 cm left ureteral double-J stent was passed over the wire under fluoroscopic guidance. It formed adequate coils on both ends. The cystoscope was reinserted into the bladder. The bladder was drained. There was some mild bleeding from the bladder neck. After the bladder was drained, the scope was removed. The patient was then brought to the recovery room in satisfactory condition.

Chapter 18

Male Reproductive System

The major function of the reproductive systems, both male and female, is to produce offspring and maintain the species. The 2nd character value for the Male Reproductive body system is V.

Functions of the Male Reproductive System

The function of the male reproductive system is to produce gamete cells (called sperm), to transport and sustain these cells, and to produce hormones (Applegate 2011, 421).

Organization of the Male Reproductive System

The male reproductive system in ICD-10-PCS contains the prostate, seminal vesicle, scrotum, tunica vaginalis, testis, spermatic cord, epididymis, vas deferens, penis, and prepuce. The primary reproductive organ in the male is the testes. All other structures in this system are considered secondary reproductive organs. Figure 18.1 displays the structures of the male reproductive system.

The two testes, or testicles, are located within the scrotum and are approximately 5 cm in length × 2.5 cm in diameter. The scrotum is a skin-covered sac between the thighs that provides a protective outer covering for both the testes (McKinley et al. 2017, 855). On the inside of the scrotum, the tunica vaginalis surrounds

Figure 18.1. Male Reproductive system

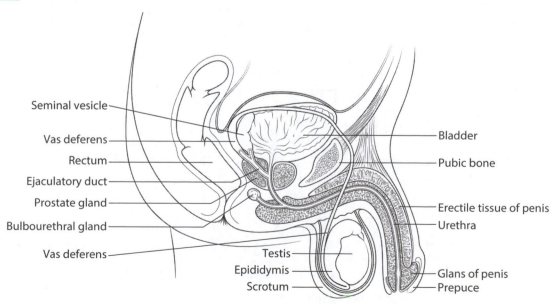

© AHIMA 2019

each testicle. Beneath the tunica vaginalis is a covering of dense white fibrous connective tissue called the tunica albuginea that extends inward to form septa that divide the testis into lobules (Rizzo 2016, 454).

Sperm develop in each testicle and travel through the small ducts that empty into the epididymis, a compact set of dense tubules at the top of each testicle. From the epididymis, the sperm travel to the vas deferens, or ductus deferens, which loops over the urinary bladder and goes toward the prostate gland on the posterior side of the bladder. The proximal portion of the vas deferens is a part of the spermatic cord, which contains vascular and neural structures that supply the testes. The spermatic cord passes through the deep inguinal ring and contains the vas deferens, testicular artery and vein, lymph vessels, testicular nerve, cremaster muscle, and a connective tissue covering (Applegate 2011, 424).

The seminal vesicle ducts join the vas deferens and empty into the urethra. The seminal fluid produced by the vesicle helps sperm movement. The prostate gland, which surrounds the base of the urethra, and the bulbo-urethral glands also provide additional fluid to help with sperm movement.

The penis is the male organ for delivery of sperm and is found at the anterior of the scrotum. It is formed of erectile tissue and has a root, body, and glans penis. The glans penis is covered by a loose fold of protective skin called the prepuce (Applegate 2011, 425). The male urethra is common to the reproductive and urinary systems and is categorized in the Urinary system in ICD-10-PCS. Figure 18.2 is a detailed drawing of the male reproductive structures that form the reproductive ductal system.

Figure 18.2.   **Detailed male anatomy**

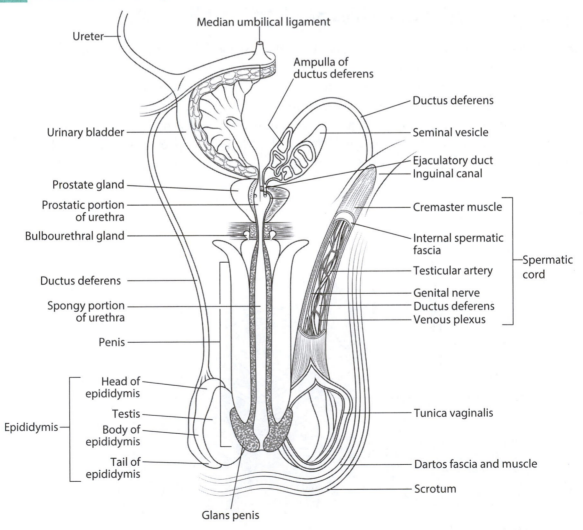

Common Root Operations Used in Coding Procedures on the Male Reproductive System

Circumcision surgically removes the prepuce from the glans penis and is coded with the root operation Resection because the entire prepuce body part is removed. The intent of the vasectomy procedure is to occlude the vas deferens tubes to prevent sperm from passing out of the body, and it is coded to the root operation Occlusion. The method used to occlude the tube does not matter, just that the final result is occlusion.

Reposition is used to code the relocation of undescended testes into the scrotum, or the procedure called orchiopexy. Documentation should be read carefully to determine the extent of procedures performed on the prostate. Prostatectomy typically describes complete resection of the prostate. Transurethral resection of the prostate (TURP), however, rarely means complete resection as ICD-10-PCS defines the procedure but is instead an excision of a portion of the prostate. Laser prostatectomy is destruction of some, or all, of the prostate and is coded to the root operation Destruction.

Testes that have been removed, either for disease or prophylactically, can be replaced with a synthetic substitute. As with any Replacement procedure, if the native body part is removed at the same operative session, the Excision or Resection is not coded separately.

The prepuce, or foreskin, is an excellent source of skin for reconstruction of the penile shaft or the urethra. The foreskin can be transferred to the shaft of the penis after surgeries such as detethering the penis or release of chordee. The foreskin is still attached to the vascular and nervous supply and takes over the function of the missing skin following these procedures. The foreskin can also be used to reconstruct a missing urethra. See the discussion of hypospadias in chapter 17. These foreskin transfers are coded in the male reproductive system because the body part value is the tissue being transferred. The destination of both of these transfers is identified in the qualifier value.

Be sure to research any procedure that is unfamiliar to ensure correct coding. If the documentation includes an eponym (procedure named for a person) and the intent of the procedure is unclear, query the physician for specifics.

Body Part Values for the Male Reproductive System

Procedures performed on the male urethra will be coded within the urinary body system because both the male and female urethra are classified in the urinary system with the body part value D in ICD-10-PCS. Body part value D, Testis, is available for use in coding procedures using the root operations of Change, Insertion, Inspection, Removal, and Revision where lateral specificity is not required.

Body part values for some combined structures, such as prostate and seminal vesicles, scrotum and tunica vaginalis, and epididymis and spermatic cord are also available to use in coding these same root operations (Change, Insertion, Inspection, Removal, and Revision) when devices or inspection are involved. The body part values for combined structures are not available for use with any other root operations. Table 18.1 lists the body part values associated with the male reproductive system. If the documentation includes specific body part names that are not included in this list, refer to the body part key for other body part synonyms and alternative terms.

Table 18.1. Body parts in the Male Reproductive system

Body Part Value	Body Parts—Male Reproductive System (V)
0	Prostate
1	Seminal Vesicle, Right
2	Seminal Vesicle, Left
3	Seminal Vesicles, Bilateral
4	Prostate and Seminal Vesicles

(Continued)

Body Part Value	Body Parts—Male Reproductive System (V)
5	Scrotum
6	Tunica Vaginalis, Right
7	Tunica Vaginalis, Left
8	Scrotum and Tunica Vaginalis
9	Testis, Right
B	Testis, Left
C	Testes, Bilateral
D	Testis
F	Spermatic Cord, Right
G	Spermatic Cord, Left
H	Spermatic Cords, Bilateral
J	Epididymis, Right
K	Epididymis, Left
L	Epididymis, Bilateral
M	Epididymis and Spermatic Cord
N	Vas Deferens, Right
P	Vas Deferens, Left
Q	Vas Deferens, Bilateral
R	Vas Deferens
S	Penis
T	Prepuce

Table 18.1. Body parts in the Male Reproductive system (continued)

Coding Tip

The male urethra is part of the reproductive organ of the penis but is a shared structure between the male reproductive system and the urinary system. Both the male and female urethra are classified in the urinary system as body part value D in ICD-10-PCS.

Approaches Used in the Male Reproductive System

Prostatectomies are performed using various anatomical approaches, such as perineal, suprapubic, and retropubic. All of these approaches are considered approach value 0, Open in ICD-10-PCS because they involve cutting through body layers to expose the site of the procedure. Other prostatectomies can be performed using a cystoscope and approaching the prostate through the urethral wall. This approach value is 8, Via Natural or Artificial Opening Endoscopic. Procedures performed on the external male genitalia can be coded using approach value X, External.

Devices Common to the Male Reproductive System

The devices utilized in procedures performed on the male reproductive system are the typical devices that are inserted for drainage, delivery of radiation therapy, and infusions. Device values are also available for occlusion of tubular body parts, such as extraluminal devices and intraluminal devices. Device values available for the root operations Bypass, Supplement, Removal, and Revision include autologous tissue substitute, synthetic substitute, and nonautologous tissue substitute. The standard values for other device and no device are also available. Table 18.2 lists the device values available for coding procedures performed on the Male Reproductive system.

Table 18.2.	Devices for the Male Reproductive system
Device Value	**Devices—Male Reproductive System (V)**
0	Drainage Device
1	Radioactive Element
3	Infusion Device
7	Autologous Tissue Substitute
C	Extraluminal Device
D	Intraluminal Device
J	Synthetic Substitute
K	Nonautologous Tissue Substitute
Y	Other Device
Z	No Device

Qualifiers for the Male Reproductive System

Qualifiers are used in the male reproductive system to describe the destination in the root operations of Bypass and Transfer. Male reproductive system procedures may also use the standard qualifiers of X for Diagnostic and Z for No Qualifier. Table 18.3 lists the qualifier values available for coding procedures performed on the Male Reproductive system.

Table 18.3.	Qualifiers for the Male Reproductive system
Qualifier Value	**Qualifiers—Male Reproductive System (V)**
D	Urethra
J	Epididymis, Right
K	Epididymis, Left
N	Vas Deferens, Right
P	Vas Deferens, Left
S	Penis
X	Diagnostic
Z	No Qualifier

 Code Building

Case #1:

PROCEDURE STATEMENT: Excision of right spermatocele

ADDITIONAL INFORMATION: The spermatocele is a cyst in the scrotum, within the epididymis, that contains fluid, blood, and/or dead sperm. This additional fluid causes pressure and pain and, when large enough, needs surgical removal through the wall of the scrotum (Pais 2016). In this case, the cystic sac and the contents are removed from the epididymis. The cystic structure is not drained.

ROOT AND INDEX ENTRIES FOR THE STATEMENT: Excision is the root operation performed in this procedure, defined as cutting out or off, without replacement, a portion of a body part. The Index entry is:

Excision

    Epididymis

      Right   0VBJ

Code Characters:

Section	Body System	Root Operation	Body Part	Approach	Device	Qualifier
Medical and Surgical	Male Reproductive System	Excision	Epididymis, Right	Open	No Device	No Qualifier
0	V	B	J	0	Z	Z

RATIONALE FOR THE ANSWER: The root operation Excision is used because a portion of the epididymis is removed. If the documentation stated that the spermatocele was in any location other than the epididymis, the documented body part would have been coded instead. The open approach is used because the epididymis is accessed through the scrotal wall. The correct code assignment is 0VBJ0ZZ.

Case #2:

PROCEDURE STATEMENT: Aspiration biopsy of prostatic abscess

ADDITIONAL INFORMATION: The prostatic abscess is drained after failed attempts to clear the infection using antibiotics. The procedure is performed transurethrally using an endoscope. This aspiration is specifically stated as a biopsy of the fluid.

ROOT AND INDEX ENTRIES FOR THE STATEMENT: Drainage is the root operation performed in this procedure, defined as taking or letting out fluids and/or gases from a body part. The Index entry is:

Drainage

    Prostate   0V90

Code Characters:

Section	Body System	Root Operation	Body Part	Approach	Device	Qualifier
Medical and Surgical	Male Reproductive System	Drainage	Prostate	Via Natural or Artificial Opening Endoscopic	No Device	Diagnostic
0	V	9	0	8	Z	X

RATIONALE FOR THE ANSWER: The root operation Drainage describes the procedure of aspiration of fluid from a body part. The prostate is drained via a natural opening and using an endoscope for the Approach value of 8. Because the documentation states that it was a biopsy, the qualifier of X, Diagnostic is assigned. The correct code assignment is 0V908ZX.

Case #3:

PROCEDURE STATEMENT: Placement of bilateral testicular prostheses following bilateral orchiectomy

ADDITIONAL INFORMATION: None.

ROOT AND INDEX ENTRIES FOR THE STATEMENT: Replacement is the root operation performed in this procedure, defined as putting in or on biological or synthetic material that physically takes the place and/or function of all or a portion of a body part. The Index entry is:

Replacement

    Testis

        Bilateral   0VRC0JZ

Code Characters:

Section	Body System	Root Operation	Body Part	Approach	Device	Qualifier
Medical and Surgical	Male Reproductive System	Replacement	Testes, Bilateral	Open	Synthetic Substitute	No Qualifier
0	V	R	C	0	J	Z

RATIONALE FOR THE ANSWER: The root operation Replacement is appropriate because the testes are removed and prosthetic testes are placed into the scrotum. The orchiectomy is not coded separately because resection of the native body part is included in the root operation Replacement. The approach value is 0, Open. The correct code assignment is 0VRC0JZ.

Code Building Exercises

Work through each case and check your answers using the answer key in appendix B of the textbook before going on to the Check Your Understanding questions that follow.

Exercise 1:

PREOPERATIVE DIAGNOSIS: Right testicular torsion

POSTOPERATIVE DIAGNOSES: Right in-utero testicular torsion and necrotic right testicle

PROCEDURES PERFORMED: Right inguinal and scrotal exploration with right orchiectomy

SPECIMENS: Right testicle

INDICATION FOR OPERATION: Initial newborn examination of this 36-week gestation, preterm infant demonstrated a normal appearing scrotum, but on repeat examination this morning, the right testicle was found to be firm, enlarged, and discolored, very concerning for testicular torsion. Ultrasound of the scrotum confirmed no significant Doppler flow within it. Emergent exploration was warranted. Parents understand and agree, and the patient was taken emergently to the OR.

PROCEDURE IN DETAIL: After an adequate general anesthesia was established, his bilateral groins, penis, and scrotum were then prepped and draped in the usual sterile fashion. An incision was made along a skin crease overlying the right inguinal canal sharply. This was carried down through the layers. The spermatic cord was noted to be clearly twisted as it entered the scrotum. The testicle was too firm and swollen to be delivered through the inguinal incision. The right hemiscrotum was then carefully entered in an attempt to free up the testicle. The testicle was detorsed but was clearly necrotic in appearance with no significant change in its appearance noted 5 minutes after detorsion. Doppler did not identify flow signal in the testicle itself. For confirmation, a vertical incision was made in the testicle itself. It was frankly necrotic tissue without any viable tissue present. Therefore, an inguinal orchiectomy was performed. The cord was then transected sharply and the testicle was passed off the field as a specimen. The external oblique was then reapproximated using a running Vicryl suture. The inguinal wound was closed in layers. The scrotal incision was closed using interrupted chromic sutures. The scrotal incision was dressed with Bacitracin and the inguinal incision was dressed with a Steri-Strip. Overall, the patient tolerated the procedure well and there were no intraoperative complications.

Questions:

1.1. What was the intent of this procedure?

_____

1.2. Is the exploration coded separately?

_____

1.3. What code(s) would be assigned?

_____

Exercise 2:

PREOPERATIVE DIAGNOSES: Acute urinary retention and severe phimosis

POSTOPERATIVE DIAGNOSES: Acute urinary retention, severe phimosis, and meatal/urethral stricture

PROCEDURES: Extensive lysis of foreskin adhesions and meatal and urethral dilation

INDICATIONS: This is a 56-year-old gentleman who presented to the emergency department in acute urinary retention. After reviewing his findings and options, he elected to proceed with dorsal slit, cystoscopy, possible placement of suprapubic tube and related procedures. An informed consent was obtained.

DESCRIPTION OF OPERATION: After successful induction of general anesthesia, he was then placed in modified dorsal lithotomy position. His external genitalia was prepped and draped in the usual sterile fashion including the suprapubic area. There was evidence of severe phimosis with a pinpoint opening on the foreskin. Unsuccessful attempt was made to reduce the foreskin. A dorsal slit was then carried out. There were severe foreskin adhesions on the glans penis and using fine Metzenbaums and fine mosquito, both the dorsal slit and extensive lysis of foreskin adhesions were carried out. The glans penis appeared to be edematous from chronic balanoposthitis. The external meatus was finally identified following dorsal slit and lysis of adhesions.

Upon inspection, it was obvious that the external urethral meatus appeared to be stenotic as well. At this time, using gradual male sounds, the external meatus as well as the extremely stenotic urethra was calibrated and then dilated using graduated male sound dilators. The dilation was carried up to 24 French and then using a 22 French, 30-degree lens scope under direct visualization using video camera, cystoscopy was carried out. The proximal urethra appeared to be patent without any evidence of stricture. The prostate appeared to be mildly enlarged without significant obstruction. The bladder was entered without difficulty. Bladder mucosa appeared to be diffusely inflamed due to chronic urinary retention. However, there were no obvious suspicious lesions, tumors, or stones in the bladder. Both ureteric orifices were identified, and they appeared to have clear efflux and away from the bladder neck. At this time, the cystoscope was removed and the 22 French Foley catheter was placed to maintain the dilation. The balloon was inflated and the catheter was connected to a drainage bag. The dorsal slit edges were then reapproximated using 3-0 chromic in a running fashion, and the wound site was covered by bacitracin ointment, sterile Telfa, and Coban dressing. The patient tolerated the procedure and was transferred to recovery room in satisfactory condition.

Questions:

2.1. How many procedures that require coding are represented in this report? What are they?

_____

2.2. What body part is being released to treat the phimosis?

_____

2.3. Why is the Foley catheter inserted at the end of this procedure? What device value would you assign for the Foley catheter?

_____

2.4. What code(s) should be assigned?

_____

✓ Check Your Understanding

Coding Knowledge Check

1. The spermatic cord contains which of the following structures?
   a. Seminal vesicle
   b. Dartos fascia
   c. Vas deferens
   d. Epididymis

2. True or false? The male urethra is classified as a body part in the male reproductive system in ICD-10-PCS. _____

3. Laser prostatectomy is coded with the root operation _____.

4. Qualifier values other than X and Z are assigned to which type of procedure in this section of ICD-10-PCS?
   a. Alteration
   b. Bypass
   c. Creation
   d. Repair

5. A circumcision is the surgical removal of the _____ body part.

Procedure Statement Coding

Assign ICD-10-PCS codes to the following procedure statements and scenarios. List the root operation selected and the code assigned.

   1. Retropubic total prostatectomy

_____

(Continued)

2. Open reduction of left testicular torsion

_____

3. The patient's semirigid penile prosthesis had been causing problems. It was removed and a Duraphase II penile prosthesis was inserted using an open approach.

_____

4. Puncture aspiration of left hydrocele of vas deferens

_____

5. Right testicular biopsy, open approach

_____

6. Percutaneous drainage of abscess of right epididymis

_____

7. Removal of foreign body from scrotum, open approach

_____

8. Right orchiopexy via scrotal incision for undescended testicle

_____

9. Surgical removal of left epididymis for chronic epididymitis, open approach

_____

10. Bilateral vasovasostomy for vasectomy reversal, open approach

_____

Case Studies

Assign ICD-10-PCS codes to the following case studies.

1. Operative Report

PREOPERATIVE DIAGNOSIS: Desired sterilization

POSTOPERATIVE DIAGNOSIS: Desired sterilization

FINDINGS: Normal male anatomy

INDICATIONS FOR PROCEDURE: The patient has two healthy children and has been married for 26 years. He and his spouse desire a permanent form of birth control. After the alternatives, potential risks, and complications were discussed with the patient, an informed consent was obtained. He understands that he will not be considered sterile until confirmed by a negative semen analysis at approximately 8 weeks from now.

PROCEDURE: The patient was taken to the procedure room, where he was placed in a supine position, prepped, and draped for scrotal surgery. The right vas deferens was identified and isolated. Local anesthesia was infiltrated using 1 percent Xylocaine without epinephrine. The vas was fixed in position with a towel clip. An incision was made overlying the vas. The vas was identified and brought through the incision. A 2.5-cm segment of the vas deferens was excised between hemostats. Hemostasis was achieved with Bovie electrocautery. The distal end was suture ligated and folded back on itself with 3-0 chromic. The proximal end was suture ligated and folded back upon itself and sutured in place with a separate 2-0 chromic. The distal end was then buried in the adventitia with 3-0 chromic. Hemostasis was verified.

Then, attention was directed to the left, where an identical procedure was done in mirror-image fashion. Hemostasis was again verified and both vas were returned to the scrotum in their normal positions. The skin and dartos layers were closed using interrupted sutures of 3-0 chromic. The patient was returned to the recovery room in good condition.

2. Operative Report

PREOPERATIVE DIAGNOSIS: Benign prostatic hyperplasia with lower urinary tract symptoms including nocturia

POSTOPERATIVE DIAGNOSIS: Same

OPERATION: Partial prostatectomy

FINDINGS: Regrowth of obstructing hyperplasia of the prostate, particularly in the anterior lobe

INDICATION FOR PROCEDURE: Patient with prior history of TURP but well over two decades ago. Has had progressive worsening of LUTS including nocturia. Recent cystoscopy showed significant regrowth of obstructing hyperplasia of the prostate. He presents for prostatectomy.

DESCRIPTION OF PROCEDURE: The patient was brought to the operating room. Spinal anesthetic was placed. Patient was placed in the lithotomy position. Genitalia was prepped and draped in the usual manner. The patient was identified and procedure confirmed. The resecting cystoscope was introduced. The prostate was resected to create a wide-open urine passage. Resection carried to the level of but not beyond the verumontanum distally. The scope was removed. The patient tolerated the procedure well and was returned to the recovery room in satisfactory condition.

3. Operative Report

PREOPERATIVE DIAGNOSIS: Metastatic prostate cancer

POSTOPERATIVE DIAGNOSIS: Metastatic prostate cancer

PROCEDURE PERFORMED: Bilateral orchiectomy

INDICATIONS: This 71-year-old white male developed leg swelling, and a CT scan revealed retroperitoneal lymphadenopathy. Biopsy of these lymph nodes was positive for adenocarcinoma, PSA positive, suggesting prostate cancer. His PSA was 105 nanograms.

The options of treatment were discussed with the patient. He was advised to have bilateral orchiectomy. He has been started on Casodex. The patient agreed to surgery.

After satisfactory general anesthesia, the patient was prepped and draped in supine position. Incision was made in the median raphe of the scrotum. The testicular tunics were incised on the left side and the left testicle delivered from the wound. Spermatic cord was doubly clamped and excised. The spermatic cord was controlled with a proximal tie of #1 chromic catgut and a distal suture ligature of #1 chromic catgut. In similar fashion, the right testicle was removed. No complications were encountered. Wound was closed routinely in layers and sterile dressings were applied as well as a scrotal support. The patient was taken to the recovery room in good condition.

4. Operative Report

PREOPERATIVE DIAGNOSIS:	Benign prostatic hypertrophy
POSTOPERATIVE DIAGNOSIS:	Benign prostatic hypertrophy
PROCEDURES PERFORMED:	1. Cystoscopy
	2. EVOLVE laser transurethral resection of the prostate
	3. Electrosurgical transurethral resection of the prostate
SPECIMENS:	Prostate chips

INDICATIONS: This is a 66-year-old gentleman with a long-standing history of lower urinary tract symptoms linked to benign prostatic hypertrophy. He has undergone a trial of medical therapy without substantial improvement in symptoms. He presents for definitive treatment of the same.

DETAILS OF PROCEDURE: Informed consent was obtained, during which the risks, benefits, and alternatives to the procedure were explained in detail. The patient agreed to proceed.

The patient was taken to the operating room, where general anesthesia was induced. He was placed in the dorsal lithotomy position and prepped and draped in the usual standard sterile fashion. A 22-French cystoscope sheath with obturator was lubricated and inserted into the urethral meatus. The 30-degree lens with laser bridge was inserted through the scope and the prostate was inspected. It was notable for a large protruding median lobe in addition to bilateral lobar coaptation. Both ureteral orifices were identified in the bladder and were noted to be normal in appearance. There were no bladder mucosal lesions.

The EVOLVE laser fiber was advanced through the port, and using an energy of 180 watts, the prostate was photocoagulated in a systematic fashion. This was first done on the median lobe and then we proceeded to the patient's left and right lobes. We took extreme care to avoid damage to the ureteral orifices and did not extend our margin of resection further distal than the demarcation of the verumontanum. At the conclusion of the case, there seemed to be some degree of excess median lobar tissue remaining. Therefore, we elected to perform conventional transurethral resection on this portion of the prostate. A 24-French resectoscope sheath with obturator was inserted into the urethra, and a 24-French resectoscope loop was used to resect several swipes of the median lobe. These were then evacuated using a Toomey syringe and coagulated using the coagulation current. The patient was hemostatic at the conclusion of the case. The specimen was sent for permanent section pathology. The cystoscope was then removed. The patient tolerated the procedure well, and there were no complications.

5. Operative Report

PREOPERATIVE DIAGNOSIS:	History of recurrent foreskin infection
POSTOPERATIVE DIAGNOSIS:	Same
PROCEDURE:	Circumcision

INDICATIONS: The patient has had some evidence of recurrent foreskin infection, and his wife has had recurrent infections. Her gynecologist has recommended that the patient undergo circumcision. The patient presented at this time to complete that recommendation.

OPERATIVE PROCEDURE: The patient was taken to the operating room and placed in the supine position. General anesthetic was initiated. After good anesthesia was achieved the patient's penis was prepped and draped in the appropriate fashion. A straight hemostat was used to crush the foreskin on the dorsal aspect first. After it was placed for a period of time, the hemostat was released and the crushed segment was then divided. A similar action was performed on the ventral side. This was done down to the desired site of the circumcision. Then, a 3-0 chromic suture was placed on the dorsum ventral side connecting the cut ends of tissue. Then, curved hemostats were used circumferentially around the penis on the right side to the desired length of the circumcision. After the tissue was crushed, it was divided and then the excess foreskin was removed. Good hemostasis was achieved using the Bovie, and the remaining cut ends of the tissue were reapproximated using interrupted 3-0 chromic suture. Next, a similar action was done on the left side using curved hemostats around the side of the penis to crush the foreskin. The foreskin was divided at the crush point. Good hemostasis was achieved using the Bovie and 4-0 chromic ties. Then, the remaining cut edges of the tissue were reapproximated using interrupted 3-0 chromic suture. Next, Vaseline gauze was placed at the suture line followed by dry gauze. The patient tolerated the procedure well. There were no complications. The patient left the operating room in stable condition.

6. Operative Report

NOTE: Do not code the introduction of local anesthesia on this case.

PREOPERATIVE DIAGNOSIS: Redundant preputial skin, urethral meatal stenosis

POSTOPERATIVE DIAGNOSIS: Redundant preputial skin, urethral meatal stenosis

PROCEDURE PERFORMED: Circumcision revision, urethral meatoplasty

INDICATIONS: The patient is a 13-month-old male who was seen in consultation for circumcision concerns. After outpatient counseling, he presents for operative intervention accompanied by his family.

DESCRIPTION OF PROCEDURE: The patient was identified, brought to the operative room, and placed supine on the operative room table. After induction of adequate general anesthesia, the patient was prepped and draped in the usual sterile fashion. A surgical timeout was taken to identify the patient and planned procedures. The obstructing lower lip of the urethral meatus was crushed and incised. The mucosa was advanced and everted to the glans skin with interrupted 7-0 PDS. A vertical 5-0 Monocryl glans holding suture was placed. Two circumferential incisions were marked and made. Redundant prepuce was excised. There was no bleeding. The incision was aligned and closed with layers of Dermabond. There was excellent cosmesis. A 0.25 percent Marcaine dorsal penile block and ring block at the base of the penis were injected for postoperative analgesia. The glans holding suture was removed. The counts were correct. The patient tolerated the procedure well and was taken to the recovery room in stable condition.

Female Reproductive System

The major function of the reproductive systems, both male and female, is to produce offspring and maintain the species. The 2nd character value for the Female Reproductive body system is U.

Functions of the Female Reproductive System

The functions of the female reproductive system are to produce gamete cells, called eggs or ova; to transport and sustain these cells; to nurture the developing offspring; and to produce hormones (Applegate 2011, 421). The primary reproductive organ in the female is the ovary. All other structures are considered secondary reproductive organs.

Organization of the Female Reproductive System

The female reproductive system in ICD-10-PCS contains the ovaries, uterine supporting structures, fallopian tubes, uterus, endometrium, cervix, cul-de-sac, vagina, clitoris, hymen, vestibular glands, vulva, and ova. Each ovary is a small, solid structure that is found on either side of the uterus and held in place by peritoneal ligaments. The ovaries produce ova in an ovarian follicle. Once the egg is released, the follicle enlarges and becomes a corpus luteum that secretes hormones until it is no longer needed. If the egg is fertilized, the corpus luteum continues to produce hormones until the placenta is developed sufficiently to secrete the required hormones (Applegate 2011, 428).

The released egg is caught by the fimbriae at the end of the fallopian tube and transported toward the uterus. If fertilization occurs, the egg is classified as a Product of Conception in ICD-10-PCS. The fertilized egg implants into the endometrium of the uterus and develops into a fetus. Additional information on this process is found in chapter 20 of this text.

The uterus is a muscular structure that is located in the pelvic cavity between the rectum and the urinary bladder and is held in place by a series of ligaments (Rizzo 2016, 466) called the uterine supporting structures. The uterine supporting structures include the broad ligaments, infundibulopelvic ligaments, ovarian ligaments, and the round ligaments, based on the ICD-10-PCS body part key.

The cul-de-sac is a blind pouch closed at one end and is also known as the rectouterine pouch (*Mosby's* 2017, 472). Together the Skene's glands and the Bartholin's glands are known as the vestibular glands, because they surround the vaginal vestibule (Rizzo 2016, 469). The endometrium is the inner lining of the uterus. Figure 19.1 shows the structures of the female reproductive system.

Anatomy Alert

The uterine supporting structures include the broad, infundibulopelvic, ovarian, and round ligaments.

Figure 19.1.   Female reproductive system

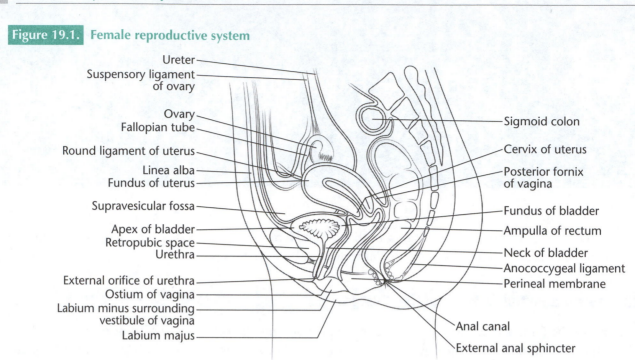

© AHIMA 2019

The vulva collectively includes the external female genitalia of the mons pubis, labia majora, labia minora, clitoris, urethral and vaginal openings, and the vestibular glands. The hymen encloses the distal end of the vagina until ruptured during the first sexual intercourse (Rizzo 2016, 469). Figure 19.2 displays the structures of the external female genitalia.

Figure 19.2.   External female genitalia

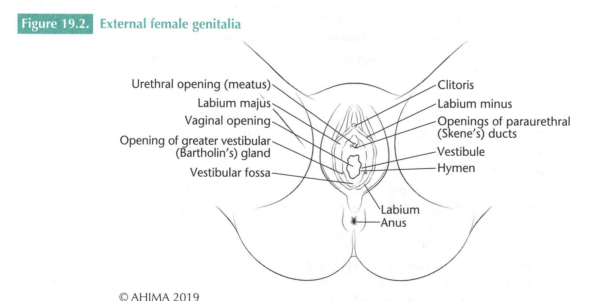

© AHIMA 2019

Common Root Operations Used in Coding Procedures on the Female Reproductive System

Sterilization is a common procedure performed on the female reproductive system. In ICD-10-PCS, the root operation assigned is Occlusion, based on the intent of the procedure to eliminate passage of eggs to the uterus. For example, sterilization can be accomplished by occluding the fallopian tubes by sutures, clips, or rings, by excising a small portion of tube, or by burning the fallopian tubes with electrocautery. Regardless of the method used, the root operation is Occlusion. Division of the tubular body part prior to closing it is an integral part of the Occlusion procedure (CMS 2016b, 61). The root operation Resection may also be coded if the method used is the complete removal of the fallopian tubes.

Coding Tip

Sterilization procedures are coded to the root operation of Occlusion, regardless of the method used to accomplish the occlusion.

Reversal of a previous tubal ligation procedure is called tubotubal anastomosis and is coded with the root operation Repair. In this procedure, the physician removes the blocked or previously ligated portion of the tube and sutures the excised edges together to form the anastomosis.

Colporrhaphy is the operation of suturing the pelvic fascia surrounding the vagina (*Mosby's* 2017, 405) because either the rectum or the bladder prolapsed into the vagina through a rupture. An anterior colporrhaphy is the repair of the rupture in the front of the vagina with involvement of the bladder, which may be called a cystocele repair. A posterior colporrhaphy is the repair of the rupture in the back of the vagina with involvement of the rectum, which may be called a rectocele repair. Either of these ruptures may be associated with fistulas between the organs. The root operation Repair is used to code the procedure colporrhaphy of the fascia to eliminate the rupture or fistulas. If the colporrhaphy is performed with the use of mesh, the root operation Supplement would be used to code the procedure.

Colpocleisis is a procedure performed to surgically close the vaginal canal (NLM 2018). This is performed to treat uterine or vaginal vault prolapse in patients who are typically elderly, unable to undergo more extensive fixation procedures, and are no longer sexually active. The root operation Occlusion describes the process of closing the vaginal vault and introitus permanently, using the vaginal approach. To treat uterine or vaginal vault prolapse with fixation and maintain the vaginal introitus, uteropexy and/or colpopexy are performed. The root operation Reposition is coded for these fixation procedures.

Cervical conization, also called cold knife cone biopsy, is used to treat very early stages of cervical cancer. A small cone-shaped sample of tissue is excised from the cervix and examined under a microscope for any signs of cancer. This biopsy may also be the treatment if the doctor removes all of the diseased tissue (NLM 2016b). This procedure can also be performed using a loop electrode to remove the tissue, called a loop electrosurgical excision procedure, or LEEP, or using a laser to circumscribe the tissue to be removed. The root operation Excision is used to code this procedure, and when performed as a biopsy, the qualifier of X, Diagnostic is assigned.

When the cervix is not strong enough to maintain closure during a pregnancy, a cervical cerclage procedure is performed to place a strong suture or wire around the cervix, making the opening smaller and stronger during pregnancy. Even though the patient is pregnant, this procedure is coded in the female reproductive body system because it is performed on the female anatomy and not on the products of conception (see chapter 20 for more information on the Obstetrical System). The root operation Restriction is used to code the cervical cerclage procedure.

The root operation Destruction is used to code endometrial ablation procedures performed either by thermal ablation (heat) or by cryoablation (cold) because the intent of the procedure is to destroy the proliferative function of the endometrium. The root operation Extraction is coded when an endometrial biopsy or uterine curettage are performed.

Coding Tip

An endometrial biopsy is not coded to the root operation Excision. The procedure is coded to Extraction, with the qualifier of Diagnostic.

The Bartholin's gland, one of the vestibular glands, can form recurring cysts or infections. To prevent this, marsupialization of the gland is performed by draining the cyst and then excising the cystic sac. Both the root operations Drainage and Excision can be coded if documentation supports that both procedures were performed.

The root operation Transplantation is available for coding procedures on the Female Reproductive body system and involves the transplantation of the ovary, either right or left, and the uterus. With a uterus transplant, In Vitro fertilization can be performed to achieve pregnancy. Be sure to research any procedure that is unfamiliar to ensure correct coding. If the documentation includes an eponym (procedure named for a person) and the intent of the procedure is unclear, query the physician for specific information.

C2. Procedures performed following a delivery or abortion for curettage of the endometrium or evacuation of retained products of conception are all coded in the Obstetrics section, to the root operation Extraction and the body part Products of Conception, Retained. Diagnostic or therapeutic dilation and curettage performed during times other than the postpartum or post-abortion period are all coded in the Medical and Surgical section, to the root operation Extraction and the body part Endometrium.

Body Part Values for the Female Reproductive System

The body part values within the Female Reproductive body system are specific to the individual structure. The term "total hysterectomy" is the removal of both the uterus and the cervix. The term "subtotal hysterectomy," also called a supracervical hysterectomy, means that only the uterus is removed and the cervix remains intact (Medicine Net 2016). Subtotal hysterectomies are coded using the root operation Resection with the qualifier value of L, Supracervical to indicate that only the uterus was resected. A total abdominal hysterectomy with a bilateral salpingo-oophorectomy (TAH-BSO) requires four codes in ICD-10-PCS because of the specificity of the body part values. One code is required to describe each of the resections performed: uterus, cervix, bilateral ovaries, and bilateral fallopian tubes. In this case, the resection of the uterus is coded with the qualifier of Z, No Qualifier because the cervix was resected.

Coding Tip

A total abdominal hysterectomy with a bilateral salpingo-oophorectomy (TAH-BSO) requires four codes in ICD-10-PCS because of the specificity of the body part values. One code is required to describe each of the resections performed: the uterus, cervix, bilateral ovaries, and bilateral fallopian tubes.

Body part values are available for the individual ovaries and fallopian tubes, as well as for bilateral ovaries and fallopian tubes. If procedures are performed bilaterally, the bilateral body part value should be used rather than coding the left and right body part values separately.

B4.3. Bilateral body part values are available for a limited number of body parts. If the identical procedure is performed on contralateral body parts, and a bilateral body part value exists for that body part, a single procedure is coded using the bilateral body part value. If no bilateral body part value exists, each procedure is coded separately using the appropriate body part value.

Example: The identical procedure performed on both fallopian tubes is coded once using the body part value Fallopian Tube, Bilateral. The identical procedure performed on both knee joints is coded twice using the body part values Knee Joint, Right, and Knee Joint, Left.

Body part values for some combined structures, such as uterus and cervix or vagina and cul-de-sac, are available for use in coding the root operations that involve devices or inspection (Change, Insertion, Inspection, Removal, and Revision). The body part values for combined structures are not available for use with any other root operations used in this system.

Note that the female perineum is not coded within the female reproductive system. The body part value for female perineum is found in the anatomical regions, general body system. Repair of perineal lacerations due to delivery will be discussed in chapter 20.

Table 19.1 lists the body part values available for coding procedures performed on the female reproductive system. If the documentation includes specific body part names that are not included in this list, refer to the body part key for other body part synonyms and alternative terms.

Table 19.1.   Body parts in the Female Reproductive system

Body Part Value	Body Parts—Female Reproductive System (U)
0	Ovary, Right
1	Ovary, Left
2	Ovaries, Bilateral
3	Ovary
4	Uterine Supporting Structure
5	Fallopian Tube, Right
6	Fallopian Tube, Left
7	Fallopian Tubes, Bilateral
8	Fallopian Tube
9	Uterus
B	Endometrium
C	Cervix
D	Uterus and Cervix
F	Cul-de-sac
G	Vagina
H	Vagina and Cul-de-sac
J	Clitoris
K	Hymen
L	Vestibular Gland
M	Vulva
N	Ova

Approaches Used in the Female Reproductive System

The female reproductive system allows the approach value F, Via Natural or Artificial Opening with percutaneous endoscopic assistance for one of the hysterectomy procedures. The hysterectomy procedure (root operation Resection) can be performed using four different variations, each coded with different approaches in ICD-10-PCS. They are as follows:

- Open
  - All organs disconnected from the internal attachments and removed through an incision in the abdomen and often referred to as an abdominal hysterectomy (approach 0, Open)
- Vaginal
  - All organs disconnected from the internal attachments and removed through the vaginal opening (approach 7, Via Natural or Artificial Opening)

- Laparoscopic
  - All organs disconnected from the internal attachments using laparoscopic tools. This includes the cervix, which is dissected from the abdominal side using the laparoscopic tools. All organs are removed through either the laparoscopic ports or through the opening in the vagina made during the cervical dissection (approach 4, Percutaneous Endoscopic)
- Laparoscopic-assisted vaginal
  - Uterus (plus tubes and ovaries, if involved) disconnected from the internal attachments using laparoscopic tools. Cervix directly dissected from the vaginal vault through the vaginal route and all organs removed through the vaginal opening (approach F, Via Natural or Artificial Opening with percutaneous endoscopic assistance for the uterus, tubes, and ovaries and approach 7, Via Natural or Artificial Opening for the cervix). In this procedure, the resection of the cervix is coded separately because it is resected through a different approach. The laparoscopic-assisted vaginal hysterectomy is pictured in figure 1.6 in chapter 1.

The female reproductive system has all of the seven approach values available for coding procedures performed on this system.

Devices Common to the Female Reproductive System

Device value G, Intraluminal Device, Pessary is a device unique to this system. This device is pictured in chapter 1 as figure 1.8. The pessary is "a device inserted into the vagina to treat uterine prolapse, uterine retroversion or cervical incompetence" (*Mosby's* 2017, 1377). The pessary must be fitted to the patient by a healthcare provider.

Device value H, Contraceptive Device, typically refers to an intrauterine device (IUD) for contraception in this body system. IUDs must be inserted and removed by a healthcare provider. The Open approach is available to describe the placement of an IUD at the time of a cesarean section delivery. Table 19.2 lists the device values available for coding procedures performed on the female reproductive system.

Table 19.2. Devices for the Female Reproductive system

Device Value	Devices—Female Reproductive System (U)
0	Drainage Device
1	Radioactive Element
3	Infusion Device
7	Autologous Tissue Substitute
C	Extraluminal Device
D	Intraluminal Device
G	Intraluminal Device, Pessary
H	Contraceptive Device
J	Synthetic Substitute
K	Nonautologous Tissue Substitute
Y	Other Device
Z	No Device

Qualifiers for the Female Reproductive System

The root operation Transplantation can be used in the female reproductive system to describe the process of transplanting either the right or the left ovary. Because of this, qualifier values are available to describe the source of the transplanted organs as Allogeneic, Syngeneic, or Zooplastic. Female reproductive system procedures may also use the standard qualifiers of X for Diagnostic and Z for No Qualifier. Table 19.3 lists the qualifier values available for use in coding procedures performed on the female reproductive system.

Table 19.3. Qualifiers for the Female Reproductive system

Qualifier Value	Qualifiers—Female Reproductive System (U)
0	Allogeneic
1	Syngeneic
2	Zooplastic
5	Fallopian Tube, Right
6	Fallopian Tube, Left
9	Uterus
L	Supracervical
X	Diagnostic
Z	No Qualifier

 Code Building

Case #1:

PROCEDURE STATEMENT: Laparoscopic lysis of intrauterine synechiae

ADDITIONAL INFORMATION: The patient has multiple adhesions extending from endometrial wall to endometrial wall inside the uterine cavity. The surgeon excises and removes them using a hysteroscope.

ROOT AND INDEX ENTRIES FOR THE STATEMENT: Release is the root operation performed in this procedure, defined as freeing a body part from an abnormal physical constraint. The Index entry is:

Release

    Uterus   0UN9

Code Characters:

Section	Body System	Root Operation	Body Part	Approach	Device	Qualifier
Medical and Surgical	Female Reproductive System	Release	Uterus	Via Natural or Artificial Opening Endoscopic	No Device	No Qualifier
0	U	N	9	8	Z	Z

RATIONALE FOR THE ANSWER: The root operation Release is coded because the walls of the uterus are abnormally constrained by adhesions, also called synechiae. The abnormal constraint that is released can either be inside the body part or outside the body part. The procedure is performed using a hysteroscope, making the approach value 8, Via Natural or Artificial Opening Endoscopic the appropriate approach. No devices or qualifiers are appropriate for this code. The correct code assignment is 0UN98ZZ.

Case #2:

PROCEDURE STATEMENT: Tubal ligation using electrocautery, open

ADDITIONAL INFORMATION: The physician makes a midline incision in the abdomen and then transects each fallopian tube using electrocautery.

ROOT AND INDEX ENTRIES FOR THE STATEMENT: Occlusion is the root operation performed in this procedure, defined as completely closing an orifice or the lumen of a tubular body part. The Index entry is:

Occlusion

    Fallopian Tube

        Left   0UL6

        Right   0UL5

    Fallopian Tubes, Bilateral   0UL7

Code Characters:

Section	Body System	Root Operation	Body Part	Approach	Device	Qualifier
Medical and Surgical	Female Reproductive System	Occlusion	Fallopian Tubes, Bilateral	Open	No Device	No Qualifier
0	U	L	7	0	Z	Z

RATIONALE FOR THE ANSWER: The root operation Occlusion is used because the intent of the procedure is to completely close the lumen of the fallopian tubes. The body part value of 7, Fallopian Tubes, Bilateral is used because both tubes were ligated with electrocautery. The approach was stated as open and no devices or qualifiers are appropriate for this code. The correct code assignment is 0UL70ZZ.

Case #3:

PROCEDURE STATEMENT: Colpopexy

ADDITIONAL INFORMATION: The patient has a prolapsed vagina which is repaired by suturing the sacrospinous ligament to the apex of the vagina using an open approach.

ROOT AND INDEX ENTRIES FOR THE STATEMENT: Reposition is the root operation performed in this procedure, defined as moving to its normal location or other suitable location all or a portion of a body part. The Index entry is:

Reposition

    Vagina 0USG

Code Characters:

Section	Body System	Root Operation	Body Part	Approach	Device	Qualifier
Medical and Surgical	Female Reproductive System	Reposition	Vagina	Open	No Device	No Qualifier
0	U	S	G	0	Z	Z

RATIONALE FOR THE ANSWER: The root operation Reposition is coded when body parts are repositioned into their normal position after prolapse. This procedure is also called a vaginal suspension procedure. The approach is documented as an open procedure, defined as cutting through the skin or mucous membrane and any other body layers necessary to expose the site of the procedure. No device or qualifier values are appropriate for this code. The correct code assignment is 0USG0ZZ.

Code Building Exercises

Work through each case and check your answers using the answer key in appendix B of the textbook before going on to the Check Your Understanding questions that follow.

Exercise 1:

DIAGNOSIS: Vaginal bleeding, prolapsing graft, status post vaginal prolapse surgery with mesh 2 weeks ago

OPERATION PERFORMED:
1. Examination under anesthesia
2. Excision of prolapsing graft pieces
3. Repair of anterior vaginal wall dehiscence

DESCRIPTION OF OPERATION: Following satisfactory induction of anesthesia, the patient was positioned in the dorsolithotomy position, was prepped in the usual fashion. Foley catheter was inserted. Examination revealed intact posterior vaginal wall with evidence of opening of the anterior vaginal wall incision with prolapse of the remnants of the graft and sutures. The graft was trimmed, and ends that were prolapsing were removed. The incision was thoroughly irrigated, excess suture removed, and the vaginal edges were freshened. The anterior vaginal wound was brought together with running 0 Vicryl suture. Additional hemostatic sutures were placed as needed. Vaginal packing was put in place and patient left for the recovery room in satisfactory condition.

Questions:

1.1. Which root operation would be assigned for the trimming of the graft material?

1.2. Which body part value is assigned for the repair of the dehiscence?

1.3. What code(s) would be assigned?

Exercise 2:

PREOPERATIVE DIAGNOSIS: Symptomatic vaginal prolapse

POSTOPERATIVE DIAGNOSIS: Symptomatic vaginal prolapse and rectocele

OPERATION PERFORMED: Bilateral sacrospinous suspension, posterior repair

DESCRIPTION OF OPERATION: The patient was taken to the operating room where spinal anesthesia was achieved without difficulty, and prepped and draped in normal sterile fashion. Examination under anesthesia was performed. Foley was introduced. A Lone Star retractor was introduced. A midline incision was made and undermined with Metzenbaum. The incision was continued posteriorly and perirectal spaces were opened and entered. Sacrospinous ligaments were palpated bilaterally and cleared off of overlying loose tissue. With Capio device, a suture was placed bilaterally into the ligament. Good placement was assured. SurgiSIS graft was threaded bilaterally. The base was sutured to the cervix. After securing the sutures bilaterally on the ligament, the apex was lifted and vaginal suspension was completed using the graft arms.

Then, attention was turned to the posterior repair portion of the surgery where the posterior vaginal mucosa was injected with a mixture of lidocaine, normal saline, and vasopressin, and a cut of the introitus was made. The cut portion of the vaginal mucosa was lifted with two Allis', and vaginal mucosa was undermined and cut in the midline and dissected off of underlying rectocele. This was repaired with additional SurgiSIS graft material. Three figure-of-eights were placed to reinforce the pelvic fascia, which was closed after FloSeal application for good hemostasis. Vagina was packed with Premarin cream. All instrument and lap counts were correct ×2. The patient was awakened and taken to the recovery room in stable condition.

Questions:

2.1. How many procedures that require coding are represented in this report? What are they?

_____

2.2. What root operations are assigned for these procedures?

_____

2.3. Research SurgiSIS. What device value will be assigned for the use of this material?

_____

2.4. What code(s) would be assigned?

_____

✓ Check Your Understanding

Coding Knowledge Check

1. True or false? The vulva is a combination of internal female reproductive body parts. _____
   _____.

2. A hysteroscopy, performed without any additional procedures, is coded to the root operation of _____ and an approach value of _____.

3. A subtotal hysterectomy removes which of the following body parts?
   a. Vagina
   b. Cervix
   c. Uterus
   d. Uterus and cervix

4. A cone biopsy of the cervix is coded to the root operation of _____.

5. Combination body part values, such as vagina and cul-de-sac, can be used with which of the following root operations?
   a. Bypass
   b. Destruction
   c. Excision
   d. Inspection

Procedure Statement Coding

Assign ICD-10-PCS codes to the following procedure statements and scenarios. List the root operation selected and the code assigned.

1. Vulvar biopsy of the labia majora

   _____

2. Bilateral tubal ligation by Falope Ring, laparoscopic

   _____

3. Harvesting of ova for InVitro fertilization, percutaneous approach

   _____

4. Supracervical laparoscopic hysterectomy

   _____

5. Colpocleisis for vaginal vault prolapse

   _____

6. Hysteroscopy

   _____

7. Endometrial ablation

   _____

8. Percutaneous right ovarian biopsy

   _____

9. Surgical drainage of Skene's gland abscess without a drainage device

   _____

10. A bivalve speculum was placed in the vagina and the cervix was prepped with Betadine solution. The uterine cavity was sounded at 7 cm. The endometrial cavity was curetted for tissue sampling. Specimen was sent to pathology. The patient tolerated the procedure well and left the operating suite in good condition.

    _____

Case Studies

Assign ICD-10-PCS codes to the following case studies.

1. Procedure Report

PREOPERATIVE DIAGNOSES:	Large fibroid uterus with menometrorrhagia
POSTOPERATIVE DIAGNOSES:	Large fibroid uterus with menometrorrhagia
PROCEDURES PERFORMED:	Total laparoscopic hysterectomy with bilateral salpingo-oophorectomy
SPECIMENS:	Complete uterus, fallopian tubes and ovaries

DESCRIPTION OF PROCEDURE: Under general anesthesia, the patient was prepped and draped in usual manner for a vaginal and abdominal procedure, a uterine manipulator was placed within the uterine cavity with the cup seated against the cervix and secured. This was then followed by placement of a Veress needle with CO_2 insufflation. An 8-mm port was placed above the umbilicus and the laparoscope was inserted. Left and right 8-mm ports were placed and a left upper quadrant assistant port was then placed. The patient was placed in steep Trendelenburg. Hysterectomy was then started by incision into the round ligaments bilaterally and then the utero-ovarian ligaments and fallopian tube. This freed the uterus for manipulation towards the vascular pedicles. The vascular pedicles were then able to be cauterized and cut on each side using the VasoSeal device. The manipulator ring was then used as a guide to dissect the vaginal cuff and incised the colpotomy. The fallopian tubes and ovaries on each side were able to be excised, performing bilateral salpingo-oophorectomy. The tubes, ovaries, uterus, and cervix were pulled into the vagina for removal. The vaginal cuff was then closed with a running locking stitch of V-Loc suture. Adequate hemostasis was achieved. Suction irrigation was performed following cuff closure and all fluid removed. The ports were then used to express the CO_2. All instruments were removed. Port sites were closed with 0 Vicryl suture on the fascia. Subcutaneous closure was done using 4-0 Monocryl. Port sites were infiltrated with 0.25% Marcaine. The vaginal vault was examined and the vaginal cuff was found to be well closed with no bleeding.

2. Procedure Report

PREOPERATIVE DIAGNOSIS: Recurrent ovarian cancer

POSTOPERATIVE DIAGNOSIS: Recurrent ovarian cancer

PROCEDURE: Examination under anesthesia, exploratory laparotomy with planned cytoreductive surgery

DESCRIPTION OF PROCEDURE: Under general anesthesia, she was placed into a frogleg position. Exam under anesthesia was then performed. There was a large mass in the left upper quadrant measuring 20 × 20 cm. There were multiple nodules of tumor in the subcutaneous tissues of the mid portion of the abdomen underneath her midline vertical incision. This exam was consistent with her having recurrent widespread ovarian cancer. The old scar was excised and the abdomen was entered through a midline vertical incision.

Examination of the left paracolic gutter was normal. There was a 15 × 15 cm tumor mass at the splenic flexure involving the spleen and the splenic flexure of the colon. There was a 20 × 20 cm mass involving the lesser sac, the transverse colon, and the inferior portion of the stomach, this mass felt to me to be into the porta hepatis. There was 12 × 12 cm mass on the mesenteric surface of the medial portion of the ascending colon. Examination of the pelvis revealed a large tumor mass incorporating the rectosigmoid, the undersurface of the bladder, the vagina, and appeared to be growing into the right and left retroperitoneal spaces. It was apparent that this tumor was adherent to the bladder, rectosigmoid, retroperitoneum, and in my opinion was unresectable. Based on this, it was my impression that cytoreductive surgery was impossible. It was also my opinion that we were unable to provide any sort of palliative procedure, which would allow the patient to urinate. Finally, it was my impression that pursuing further surgery was likely to result in significant blood loss, would require multiple bowel anastomoses and a significant operative injury. Based on all of this, I elected to abandon the procedure. The fascia was then closed with a running, nonlocking suture of #1 PDS. Subcutaneous tissues were reapproximated with 2-0 Vicryl. The skin was closed using staples. The patient tolerated the procedure well and left the suite in good condition.

3. Operative Report

OPERATION: Transabdominal cervical cerclage with broad Mersilene tape

INDICATION: Cervical incompetence

PROCEDURE: Under general anesthesia, the abdomen was opened using a transverse suprapubic incision. The vesical peritoneum overlying the lower uterine segment was divided transversely. The bladder and paravesical tissues were pushed caudally until the supravaginal cervix could be seen and palpated in the midline with good exposure laterally. The uterine vessels were displaced laterally, opening the paracervical connective tissue space. The needle was passed anteroposteriorly above the paracervical vessels immediately adjacent to the cervix at the level of the cervicoisthmic junction superior to the medial insertions of the uterosacral ligaments, care being taken to retract the uterine vessels laterally and to guide the needle tip with fingers behind the broad ligament. Before being pulled through completely, the band width of the tape was verified as being flush with the anterior cervicoisthmic tissues. The knot was then tied in the posterior.

4. Operative Report

PREOPERATIVE DIAGNOSIS: Cystic solid left ovarian mass

POSTOPERATIVE DIAGNOSIS: Cystic solid left ovarian mass

NAME OF PROCEDURE: 1. Diagnostic laparoscopy
                                   2. Excision of left ovarian solid fibroma

SPECIMEN SENT: Solid fibroma from left ovary

DESCRIPTION OF OPERATION: After adequate general anesthesia, the patient was placed in modified dorsal lithotomy position using Allen stirrups. She did have a hysterectomy prior to this. She was sterilely prepped and draped in the usual fashion. We did place a stick sponge in the vagina. I then changed gloves. We passed the Veress needle into the peritoneal cavity confirming its position using a saline drop test. The patient was then insufflated with 2 liters of CO_2 gas. The Veress needle was removed and a 10 mm laparoscopic trocar and sleeve was placed. I then placed a 5-mm suprapubic port. With the aid of Trendelenburg positioning and a probe, we were able to squeeze the bowel superiorly. We then swept the valve superiorly. The left ovary was identified. The right ovary was identified as well. The right ovary appeared completely normal. The left ovary was slightly enlarged, but did have two obvious cystic structures about 2 cm each in diameter. We used unipolar cautery to open the cortex. Deep within the ovary we could feel a solid, fibrous structure that appeared round and appeared to be a fibroma. We were able to incise the ovary around most of this structure and then remove the fibroma in one piece in toto. We then increased the size of the midline suprapubic port to 12 mm and placed an Endosac. We were able to remove the mass with the Endosac through the abdominal wall. We then used irrigation. There was slight oozing from the left ovary, and this was made hemostatic with Kleppinger bipolar cautery. The left fallopian tube appeared normal. We had no sign of any injury. We inspected the ovary and pelvic structures several times. We allowed the abdomen to deflate through the laparoscopic sleeve. We closed the midline suprapubic incision with 0-0 Vicryl suture by placing two interrupted sutures in the fascia and then closed the remaining port incisions with 4-0 undyed Vicryl. The stick sponge was removed. Instrument, needle, and sponge count were correct.

5. Operative Report

PREOPERATIVE DIAGNOSIS: Post-menopausal bleeding and endometriosis

POSTOPERATIVE DIAGNOSIS: Post-menopausal bleeding and endometriosis

PROCEDURE PERFORMED: Laparoscopic-assisted vaginal hysterectomy and bilateral salpingo-oophorectomy

PROCEDURE DESCRIPTION: Under general anesthesia, the patient was then prepped and draped in the standard sterile manner in the dorsal lithotomy position with stirrups. A Rubin cannula was placed in the cervix. The Veress needle was introduced with proper placement verified by saline drop test and an opening pressure of 3 mm Hg. The abdomen was insufflated. Two towel clips were then placed to elevate the skin of the abdomen. The pelvis was examined and noted to be generally normal. Two additional 10 mm trocar locations were placed in the left and right lower quadrants under direct visualization.

The pelvis was again examined and the uterus was found to be grossly normal and retroverted. The tubes and ovaries appeared normal bilaterally. The left infundibulopelvic ligament was clamped and verification was made that the ureter was not within the clamp. The ligament was ligated with the Endostapler. The broad ligament was then cut through with the stapling device, after verification of the location of the ureter. The right side was transected in a similar manner using the stapler. The bladder was then elevated and the peritoneum above the bladder was transected with the Endoshears. Our attention then turned to the vagina. The patient was changed to high Allen stirrups. A weighted speculum was placed in the posterior vagina and a Deaver retractor in the anterior vagina. The cervix was grasped with two clamps and the mucosa of the cervix was dissected circumferentially with Bovie from the vaginal vault and removed. The bladder was dissected off the lower uterine segment and the peritoneum was entered. The remaining uterine connections were then clamped on each side, transected and suture-ligated with 0 Vicryl. The uterus, tubes, and ovaries were then easily removed through the vagina. The vaginal cuff and perineum were closed together using a 2-0 Vicryl from the 12 o'clock to 6 o'clock position, tied in the midline. The uterosacral ligament pedicles had been tagged and were tied in the midline and reattached to the vaginal cuff. The vaginal cuff had good hemostasis after the sutures were placed. All instruments were removed.

6. Operative Report

PREOPERATIVE DIAGNOSIS: Severe right-sided pelvic pain and hemorrhagic right ovarian cyst

POSTOPERATIVE DIAGNOSIS: Severe right-sided pelvic pain and hemorrhagic right ovarian cyst

OPERATION: Operative laparoscopy with right ovarian cystectomy

OPERATIVE FINDINGS: Roughly 4 cm appearing hemorrhagic right ovarian cyst. Evidence of endometric implant on the right ovarian capsule. Bilateral tubes appeared normal. Uterus appeared normal. The rest of the pelvis appeared normal. Upper abdominal survey appeared normal.

PROCEDURE: Under general anesthesia, a bivalve speculum was placed in the patient's vagina. The anterior lip of the cervix was grasped with a single toothed tenaculum. An acorn uterine manipulator was then placed. Gloves were changed and an infraumbilical skin incision was made 1 cm in length. A Veress needle with the step attached was advanced. Intra-abdominal placement was confirmed using a water-filled syringe. A 10-mm blunt-tipped trocar was then advanced through the step. The patient was then placed in the Trendelenburg position on the left side. A 5-mm Versaport trocar was then advanced under direct visualization directly contralateral on the right and left side. The pelvic and other findings were noted above. The endometriotic implant on the right ovarian capsule was coagulated with cautery. The thin-appearing side of the ovarian capsule was entered with the harmonic scalpel. Serous fluid was noted to escape with rupture of the cyst. Parts of the cyst wall were removed by grasping with a dissector. The thin part of the ovarian capsule was excised using the harmonic scalpel and retrieved. The inner part of the ovarian cortex was oozing, and hemostasis was obtained using the needle-tip cautery. The pelvis and abdomen were copiously irrigated with normal saline. All fluid was suctioned. The patient was placed in the supine position. The two side ports were removed under direct visualization. Gas was released from the patient's abdomen and the infraumbilical port was also removed. The skin incisions were closed using 4-0 Vicryl in interrupted subcuticular fashion and Dermabond. The Acorn manipulator and tenaculum were removed.

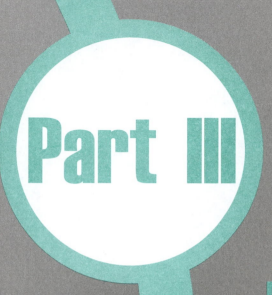

Part III

Medical and Surgical-related Sections

20

Obstetrics

The 1st character value for obstetrics is 1. The 2nd character value for obstetrics is always 0, Pregnancy.

Character 1	Character 2	Character 3	Character 4	Character 5	Character 6	Character 7
Section	Body System	Root Operation	Body Part	Approach	Device	Qualifier

Products of Conception

This section of ICD-10-PCS classifies only procedures performed on the products of conception. Products of conception are defined as the intrauterine tissue that results from the fertilization of an ovum with sperm, and include the fetus, placenta, amniotic sac, amniotic fluid, and umbilical cord. Any of these products of conception can also be referred to as the "conceptus." If the body part belongs to a female when she is not pregnant, the body part is not a product of conception. If the procedure is performed on a body part other than a product of conception, even during pregnancy or delivery, the procedure is coded to the appropriate body part value in the medical and surgical section. Figure 20.1 displays the products of conception in relationship to the female reproductive organs.

Figure 20.1. Products of conception

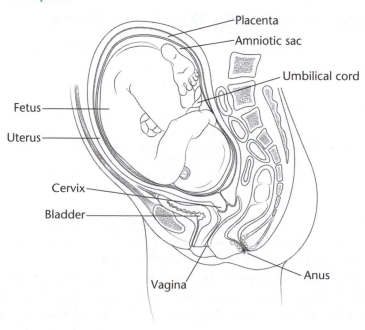

@ AHIMA 2019

Products of conception can be in the normal position, inside the uterus. The embryo is meant to implant in the nutrient-rich endometrial lining. When it implants anywhere else in the body, it is called ectopic. "An ectopic pregnancy occurs when a fertilized egg implants somewhere other than the main cavity of the uterus. Pregnancy begins with a fertilized egg. Normally, the fertilized egg attaches itself to the lining of the uterus" (Mayo Clinic 2015a).

Types of ectopic pregnancies are named based on their implanted location. The names frequently documented for locations are abdominal (anywhere within the abdominal cavity), interstitial (within the wall of the uterus), isthmic (approximately midtube), ampular (at the enlarged, distal end of the tube), and fimbrial (in the fimbriae of the fallopian tube). The locations of implantation for ectopic pregnancies within the fallopian tube are displayed in figure 20.2.

Figure 20.2. Ectopic pregnancy

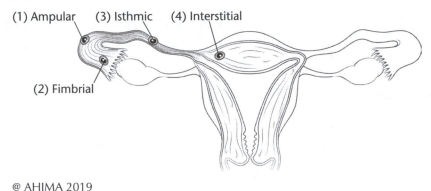

@ AHIMA 2019

The term "retained products of conception" (RPOC) means that placental or fetal tissue is not completely expelled from the uterus following a spontaneous abortion (miscarriage), surgical abortion, or delivery. Incomplete abortion or miscarriage is the presence of RPOC. Complete abortion or miscarriage is complete expulsion of all products of conception.

Common Root Operations Used in Coding Obstetrics Procedures

There are two root operations that are unique to the Obstetrics section of ICD-10-PCS. They are Abortion and Delivery.

Root Operation

Abortion (A): Artificially terminating a pregnancy.
Delivery (E): Assisting the passage of the products of conception from the genital canal.

Abortion

The root operation Abortion is assigned, regardless of the method used to terminate the pregnancy, and is subdivided based on whether an additional method is used to accomplish the procedure, such as Laminaria or an abortifacient. Laminaria is inserted vaginally to dilate the cervix and is a species of seaweed, hydroscopic when dry, but dilates three to five times its diameter when wet. A sterilized version of this seaweed is formed into a plug, called a tent, which is placed into the cervix to cause dilation in preparation for invasive uterine surgery such as an abortion or D&C (Mayo Clinic 2015b). An abortifacient is an agent that induces abortion of the products of conception. An abortifacient can be used in the oral form, such as the "abortion pill" pharmaceutical or an herbal substance.

Coding Tip

The root operation Abortion is subdivided according to whether an additional device such as laminaria or an abortifacient is used, and with the approach of Via natural or artificial opening. All other Abortion procedures are those done by mechanical means (the products of conception are physically removed using instrumentation), and the device value is Z, No device

Delivery and Extraction

The root operation Delivery in ICD-10-PCS is specific to passage of the products of conception from the genital canal without instrumentation or incision. When an incision or instrumentation is required, such as forceps or internal version, the root operation Extraction is coded. Internal version is performed when the physician inserts a hand into the uterus to turn the fetus to a more appropriate position. In ICD-10-PCS, this is captured in the qualifier value associated with the root operation Extraction. The physician's hand is used as an instrument to perform the extraction. Cesarean deliveries are coded to the root operation Extraction. Repeat cesarean deliveries are not coded differently in ICD-10-PCS than initial cesarean sections. Both are coded to the root operation Extraction.

Coding Tip

The root operation Delivery applies only to manually assisted, vaginal delivery and is defined as assisting the passage of the products of conception from the genital canal. Cesarean deliveries are coded in this section to the root operation Extraction

C2. Procedures performed following a delivery or abortion for curettage of the endometrium or evacuation of retained products of conception are all coded in the Obstetrics section, to the root operation Extraction and the body part Products of Conception, Retained. Diagnostic or therapeutic dilation and curettage performed during times other than the postpartum or post-abortion period are all coded in the Medical and Surgical section, to the root operation Extraction and the body part Endometrium.

Deliveries of multiple gestation pregnancies are coded with one ICD-10-PCS code when the same method of delivery is used for both fetuses. For example, Twin A and Twin B are both delivered through the same C-section incision. This delivery is coded with one code, assigning the root operation Extraction and a qualifier appropriate for the type of incision. However, Twin A is delivered using low forceps and Twin B was delivered using internal version. Two codes are assigned because the qualifier value is different.

Drainage

When the documentation states that the physician performed an artificial rupture of membranes, or AROM, the root operation of Drainage is assigned from the Obstetrics section and a qualifier of Amniotic fluid, therapeutic is assigned. Drainage is assigned because the intent of the procedure is to remove amniotic fluid. When the cervix is dilated to induce labor, the root operation Dilation is coded in the Female Reproductive system from the Medical and Surgical section because the cervix is not a product of conception. Induction of labor using a hormone infusion, such as Pitocin, is also coded separately. The administration of Pitocin for induction is coded as 3E033VJ in the Administration section of ICD-10-PCS.

Other Root Operations

There are 10 other root operations included in this section that all share a common definition with the same root operations found in the Medical and Surgical section of ICD-10-PCS. The root operation Reposition is used in the Obstetrics section to move the products of conception to a new presentation, also known as external version of the fetus. External version is different from internal version in that manipulation done through the skin to turn a fetus from a breech position (feet-down) or transverse position (sideways) into a vertex (head-down) position before labor begins or the amniotic sac is ruptured. A monitoring electrode may be placed on the fetus before the version procedure is performed. The root operations of Insertion, Change, and Removal are used mainly with the device value 3, Monitoring Electrode, when the monitoring device is used to check the heartbeat of the fetus during delivery or other procedures.

The root operation Repair is used in this section when the repair is performed on the products of conception. This root operation is used with qualifiers to describe the body system of the fetus that is repaired.

In chapter 7, the subject of episiotomy was discussed. The root operation Division in the Anatomical Regions, General body system is used to describe the single procedure of episiotomy, or the division of the female perineum, normally performed at the time of the delivery. An episiorrhaphy, the root operation Repair, is not coded separately when an episiotomy was performed. This is based on Guideline B3.1b, which states that procedural steps necessary to reach the operative site and close the operative site are not coded separately. However, if a perineal laceration takes place during the delivery or if an episiotomy incision tears further, the root operation Repair is used to code the repair of the laceration after the delivery is complete.

In a third degree repair, the anal sphincter must be repaired in addition to the perineal muscle because the anal sphincter is in a different body system. In a fourth degree repair, the tear extends upward in the gastrointestinal system and the rectum must also be repaired. The anal sphincter and the rectum are separate structures and are not covered by Guideline B3.5 regarding overlapping layers of the musculoskeletal system. Therefore, additional codes must be assigned.

Table 20.1 reviews the various codes required for perineal laceration repairs associated with delivery.

Table 20.1. Perineal laceration repair

Laceration Degree	Location and Depth of Laceration	Code(s)
1st Degree	Outermost layer of the perineum and vaginal mucosa	0HQ9XZZ
2nd Degree	Perineal skin, subcutaneous tissue and muscles	0KQM0ZZ
3rd Degree	Perineal skin, subcutaneous tissue, muscles and anal sphincter	0KQM0ZZ 0DQR0ZZ
4th Degree	Perineal skin, subcutaneous tissue, muscles, anal sphincter and rectal mucosa	0KQM0ZZ 0DQR0ZZ 0DQP0ZZ

In Vitro Fertilization

In vitro fertilization involves a series of steps to complete the procedure. Each is performed at a different time and coded with different sections of ICD-10-PCS:

- **Step 1**—Extraction of the eggs from the ovary. This is coded using the 0UD table, with body part value N, Ova. The Open, Percutaneous, or Percutaneous Endoscopic approach can be coded. The Device and Qualifier value are both Z.
- **Step 2**—Fertilization of the eggs outside the body. This is coded as 8E0ZXY1 in the Other Procedures section of ICD-10-PCS.
- **Step 3**—Implantation of the fertilized egg(s) is coded with the root operation Introduction in the Administration section of ICD-10-PCS. Two codes are available for this step
  - ○ 3E0P7Q0 to implant an autologous fertilized ovum
  - ○ 3E0P7Q1 to implant a nonautologous fertilized ovum, such as in a surrogate mother

Be sure to research any procedure that is unfamiliar to ensure correct coding. If the documentation includes an eponym (procedure named for a person) and the intent of the procedure is unclear, query the physician for specifics.

Body Part Values for Obstetrics

There are only three body part values within the Obstetrics section of ICD-10-PCS: Products of Conception; Products of Conception, Retained; and Products of Conception, Ectopic. Procedures performed on body parts associated with the female anatomy are coded in the Medical and Surgical section of ICD-10-PCS as directed by Guideline C1. Table 20.2 lists the body part values for procedures classified to the Obstetrics section.

C1. Procedures performed on the products of conception are coded to the Obstetrics section. Procedures performed on the pregnant female other than the products of conception are coded to the appropriate root operation in the Medical and Surgical section.

Example: Amniocentesis is coded to the products of conception body part in the Obstetrics section. Repair of obstetric urethral laceration is coded to the urethra body part in the Medical and Surgical section.

Table 20.2. Body parts for obstetrics

Body Part Value	Body Parts—Pregnancy (0)
0	Products of Conception
1	Products of Conception, Retained
2	Products of Conception, Ectopic

A.7. It is not required to consult the index first before proceeding to the tables to complete the code. A valid code may be chosen directly from the tables.

Approaches Used in Obstetrics

By definition, cesarean section procedures are open procedures. Other Extraction procedures can be performed vaginally and assigned the approach value of 7, Via Natural or Artificial Opening or 8, Via Natural or Artificial Opening, Endoscopic. Amniocentesis procedures are typically performed percutaneously, approach value 3. Approach value 4, Percutaneous Endoscopic is used with the root Operation Drainage, Abortion, Inspection, Repair, Reposition, Resection, and Transplantation. Approach value X, External is used for the external version procedure and the root operation Reposition, Inspection, and Delivery.

Devices Common to Obstetrics

The device value of 3, Monitoring Electrode is used to describe the monitor that is typically placed on the fetus's scalp. This device value is used with the root operations Change, Insertion, and Removal. The device value of Y, Other device is available for use with the root operations of Insertion, Removal, and Repair. Device value Z, No Device, is available for use when no device remains in place following the completion of the procedure. Table 20.3 lists the available device values for coding Obstetrics procedures.

Table 20.3. Devices for obstetrics

Device Value	Devices—Pregnancy (0)
3	Monitoring Electrode
Y	Other Device
Z	No Device

Qualifiers for Obstetrics

The qualifier values for obstetrics include additional information on the incision type for cesarean section deliveries, the method used for instrument-assisted deliveries, the type of assistance used for inducing an abortion, the fluid drained from the products of conception, and the fetal body systems on which Repair and Transplantation procedures are performed.

For cesarean section deliveries, the incision type is assigned a qualifier value based on the following definitions:

- **High**—A method for surgically delivering a baby through a high vertical or transverse incision of the upper segment of the uterus. For many practitioners this is the fastest method of cesarean delivery. However, it produces a weaker scar, and, because the upper segment is thicker and more vascular, more bleeding occurs during surgery than from the low cesarean section. This can also be documented as a classical or high uterine incision.
- **Low**—A surgical procedure to deliver a baby through a low vertical or transverse incision in the thin supracervical part of the lower uterine segment, behind the bladder and the bladder flap. This incision bleeds less during surgery and heals with a stronger scar than the higher scar, such as a classic cesarean section.
- **Extraperitoneal**—A method for surgically delivering a baby through an incision in the lower uterine segment without entering the peritoneal cavity. The uterus is approached through the paravesical space. This procedure is performed most often to prevent spread of infection from the uterus into the peritoneal cavity. It takes longer to perform than the low cervical or classic cesarean operation. (*Mosby's* 2017, 667)

The American Congress of Obstetricians and Gynecologists (ACOG) provides the following criteria for the types of forceps deliveries completed with instrumentation:

- **Low forceps**—The leading point of the fetal skull is at a station greater than or equal to +2 cm and is not on the pelvic floor; any degree of rotation may be present.
- **Mid forceps**—The station is above +2 cm, but the head is engaged.
- **High forceps**—This is not included in the current ACOG classification. Previous systems classified high-forceps deliveries as procedures performed when the head is not engaged. High-forceps deliveries are not recommended. (ACOG 2000)

When the same root operation is performed on the same body part but different methods or instrumentation are used, as defined by different qualifier values, different procedure codes are assigned to each procedure, such as in the example of the twin delivery discussed earlier in this chapter. Table 20.4 lists the qualifiers available for coding obstetrics procedures.

Table 20.4.   **Qualifiers for Obstetrics**

Qualifier Value	Qualifiers—Pregnancy (0)
0	High
1	Low
2	Extraperitoneal
3	Low Forceps
4	Mid Forceps
5	High Forceps
6	Vacuum
7	Internal Version

(Continued)

Table 20.4. Qualifiers for Obstetrics (continued)

Qualifier Value	Qualifiers—Pregnancy (0)
8	Other
9	Fetal Blood
9	Manual
A	Fetal Cerebrospinal Fluid
B	Fetal Fluid, Other
C	Amniotic Fluid, Therapeutic
D	Fluid, Other
E	Nervous System
F	Cardiovascular System
G	Lymphatics And Hemic
H	Eye
J	Ear, Nose and Sinus
K	Respiratory System
L	Mouth and Throat
M	Gastrointestinal System
N	Hepatobiliary and Pancreas
P	Endocrine System
Q	Skin
R	Musculoskeletal System
S	Urinary System
T	Female Reproductive System
U	Amniotic Fluid, Diagnostic
V	Male Reproductive System
W	Laminaria
X	Abortifacient
Y	Other Body System
Z	No Qualifier

Code Building

Case #1:

PROCEDURE STATEMENT: Spontaneous vaginal delivery

ADDITIONAL INFORMATION: No instrumentation or incision is used in the delivery.

ROOT AND INDEX ENTRIES FOR THE STATEMENT: Delivery is the root operation performed in this procedure, defined as assisting the passage of the products of conception from the genital canal. The Index entry is:

Delivery

    Manually assisted 10E0XZZ

    Products of Conception 10E0XZZ

Code Characters:

Section	Body System	Root Operation	Body Part	Approach	Device	Qualifier
Obstetrics	Pregnancy	Delivery	Products of Conception	External	No Device	No Qualifier
1	0	E	0	X	Z	Z

RATIONALE FOR THE ANSWER: The ICD-10-PCS system contains only one code for spontaneous delivery of products of conception that are manually assisted (no instrumentation or incision required). The correct code assignment is 10E0XZZ.

Case #2:

PROCEDURE STATEMENT: Amniocentesis

ADDITIONAL INFORMATION: Amniotic fluid is collected for diagnostic evaluation of possible intrauterine infection.

ROOT AND INDEX ENTRIES FOR THE STATEMENT: Drainage is the root operation performed in this procedure, defined as taking or letting out fluids and/or gases from a body part. The Index entry is:

Drainage

    Products of Conception

        Amniotic Fluid

            Diagnostic 1090

            Therapeutic 1090

Code Characters:

Section	Body System	Root Operation	Body Part	Approach	Device	Qualifier
Obstetrics	Pregnancy	Drainage	Products of Conception	Percutaneous	No Device	Amniotic Fluid, Diagnostic
1	0	9	0	3	Z	U

RATIONALE FOR THE ANSWER: Centesis is percutaneous drainage of fluid from a body part. The qualifier defines the type of fluid that is being drained and for what purpose. The qualifier value U defines the fluid as amniotic fluid and drained for diagnostic purposes. The correct code assignment is 10903ZU.

Case #3:

PROCEDURE STATEMENT: Vacuum extraction delivery

ADDITIONAL INFORMATION: The documentation states that this is a vaginal delivery.

ROOT AND INDEX ENTRIES FOR THE STATEMENT: Extraction is the root operation performed in this procedure, defined as pulling or stripping out or off all or a portion of a body part by the use of force. The Index entry is:

Extraction

Products of Conception

Vacuum 10D07Z6

Code Characters:

Section	Body System	Root Operation	Body Part	Approach	Device	Qualifier
Obstetrics	Pregnancy	Extraction	Products of Conception	Via Natural or Artificial Opening	No Device	Vacuum
1	0	D	0	7	Z	6

RATIONALE FOR THE ANSWER: The root operation Extraction is used because instrumentation or incision is used to remove the body part. The approach value is 7 because the products of conception are extracted through a natural opening. The qualifier value of 6 identifies the instrumentation as vacuum extraction. The correct code assignment is 10D07Z6.

Code Building Exercises

Work through each case and check your answers using the answer key in appendix B of the textbook before going on to the Check Your Understanding questions that follow.

Exercise 1:

PRE-OP DIAGNOSIS: IUP at 39 weeks, History of cesarean ×3

POST-OP DIAGNOSIS: Same

ANESTHESIA: Spinal, Epidural

PROCEDURES: Repeat low transverse C-Section

FINDINGS: Viable female infant APGARs 8, 9 in left occiput transverse position

INDICATION: This is a 36 yr old G4P3003 at 39 weeks who presents for scheduled repeat cesarean. Patient has history of cesarean ×3.

DESCRIPTION OF PROCEDURE: Following anesthesia, prepping, and draping, a Pfannenstiel skin incision was made and carried through to the underlying layer of fascia. The fascia was incised in midline and the rectus muscles were separated in the midline. The peritoneum was entered bluntly. The vesicouterine peritoneum was identified and entered sharply. The bladder flap created digitally. A low transverse incision was then made on the uterus with the scalpel. Viable female infant was delivered in left occiput transverse position. The cord was double clamped and cut and the infant handed off. Cord gases and blood were collected.

The placenta was expressed. The uterus was exteriorized and cleared of all clots and debris. Tone was noted to be boggy, but bleeding was stable. The hysterotomy was repaired in a running, locked fashion with 0 vicryl. A second layer of the same suture was used to obtain hemostasis. The hysterotomy was inspected and noted to be hemostatic. The wound was repaired in layers.

Addendum: I was called to the recovery unit for treatment of postpartum hemorrhage, secondary to lower uterine segment atony. Hemabate, misoprostol, and methergine were given. I placed a Bakri balloon transvaginally into the uterus, which stopped the bleeding. No further bleeding noted on repeat exam. Balloon was removed after 8 hrs of no recurrent bleeding. Total EBL 1688 cc. Postop Hb 8.4.

Questions:

1.1. What root operation is assigned for this delivery?

_____

1.2. What clue is present in the report to help identify the appropriate qualifier for this procedure?

_____

1.3. Research the Bakri balloon that was placed in the recovery room. Is there a root operation that describes the use of this balloon? If so, what is it?

_____

1.4. What code(s) should be assigned?

_____

Exercise 2:

DIAGNOSES: Intrauterine pregnancy at 39 weeks' gestational age with history of 3 prior cesarean sections, multiple hernias in the anterior abdominal wall

PROCEDURE: Cesarean hysterectomy with bilateral salpingo-oophorectomy and panniculectomy

INDICATIONS FOR THE PROCEDURE: The patient is a 41-year-old G4P3003 at 39 weeks gestational age with a history of 3 prior cesarean sections and morbid obesity.

DESCRIPTION OF PROCEDURE: The patient was brought to the operating room where spinal anesthesia was obtained without difficulty. The patient was prepped and draped in usual sterile fashion. The area of the patient's pannus that was planned to be excised was outlined with a permanent black marker.

A midline skin incision was made and carried down to the underlying layer of fascia, which was incised. The peritoneum was identified, tented up, transilluminated, and entered sharply. The uterus was incised in a vertical fashion. The amniotic fluid sac was identified and entered where the amniotic fluid was clear in nature. The infant was easily, gently brought to the uterine incision and delivered atraumatically without difficulty. The umbilical cord was clamped times 2 and cut. The infant was handed off to awaiting pediatrician. Cord gases and cord blood were collected and sent. The placenta delivered manually. The uterus was exteriorized and cleared of all clots and debris.

The uterine ligaments were all identified, clamped, transected, and suture ligated. The uterine arteries were skeletonized bilaterally, clamped, and suture ligated. The cervix was cross clamped, dissected from the vagina with curved Mayo scissors, and the entire uterus with ovaries and fallopian tubes were removed and sent to pathology for analysis. The vaginal cuff was reapproximated with #2-0 Vicryl. The vaginal cuff was inspected with excellent hemostasis. The abdomen and pelvis were thoroughly irrigated with approximately 4 L of warm normal saline.

The pannus was dissected away from the medial fascial incision using a Bovie with cauterization of bleeders, inclusive of the three fascial defects (a 4-cm umbilical hernia, a 2-cm left inferior periumbilical hernia, and a right superior 3-cm periumbilical hernia) and their respective hernia sacs. The pannus was dissected away along the marker lines and sent to pathology for tissue analysis. The remaining healthy fascial layer was reapproximated with #0 PDS in a running fashion. The subcutaneous tissue and subdermal tissue was reapproximated with #2-0 and #3-0 interrupted Vicryl sutures. The skin was reapproximated with #4-0 Monocryl.

Questions:

2.1. When a C-section is performed through a midline incision, which qualifier value is assigned?

_____

2.2. A panniculectomy is performed on which body part? What body part value is assigned?

_____

2.3. What code(s) should be assigned?

_____

Check Your Understanding

Coding Knowledge Check

1. A cesarean section that involves an incision in the upper segment of the uterus is coded as _____.
   a. 10D00Z0
   b. 10D07Z8
   c. 10D00Z2
   d. 10E0XZZ

2. An abortion completed using a laminaria tent is coded to the qualifier value of _____.

3. True or false? Qualifier values to be coded with the root operations Repair or Transplantation are assigned when the procedure is performed on the associated body systems of the pregnant female. _____

4. An interstitial uterine pregnancy is coded to body part value _____.

5. True or false? Cesarean section delivery of twins requires the assignment of two codes. _____

Procedure Statement Coding

Assign ICD-10-PCS codes to the following procedure statements and scenarios. List the root operation selected and the code assigned.

1. HISTORY: The patient was 23-3/7 weeks' gestation with a fetal demise. The patient delivered the nonviable infant yesterday, along with the placenta. On exam today, heavy bleeding was found from the cervical os. The patient was taken to the operating room, where retained placenta fragments were removed vaginally with banjo curettage.

   _____

2. Fetal scalp blood sampling, vaginal approach

   _____

3. *Do not code the obstetrical ultrasound performed with this case.*

   HISTORY: The patient is a gravida 1, para 0, at 38-5/7 weeks' gestation, based on ultrasound at 21 weeks and last menstrual period. The ultrasound last week revealed a 7 pound, 6 ounce infant in the breech position.

   Today on exam, the infant still remained in the breech position and the patient consented to external cephalic version of the fetus. An IV line was placed and the breech presentation was confirmed again on ultrasound. The patient was given Terbutaline 0.25 mg subcutaneously prior to the procedure. Pressure was placed on the maternal abdomen to do a forward roll of the fetus, with the assistance

(Continued)

of Dr. X. Ultrasound guidance confirmed the successful version. Fetal heart tones were within the normal range throughout.

4. Thoracentesis of fetus, vaginal approach

5. Vaginal delivery with internal version

6. Placement of fetal monitoring device on scalp

7. The patient was admitted in her 39th week, in labor. The fetus is in cephalic position and no rotation is necessary. The labor continues to progress, and 5 hours later she is taken to delivery. During the delivery she was fatigued, so low forceps were required over a midline episiotomy, which was repaired. A single liveborn infant was delivered.

8. Amniocentesis for therapeutic reduction

9. The patient was 3 cm dilated when admitted. The duration of the first stage of labor was 6 hours, second stage was 14 minutes, third stage was 5 minutes. She was given local anesthesia. An episiotomy was performed and repaired. There were no lacerations. A term female infant was delivered spontaneously. The mother and liveborn baby were discharged from the delivery room in good condition.

10. Induced abortion with abortifacient

11. Change of fetal scalp monitoring electrode

12. Removal of retained products of conception from the uterus through the vagina

Case Studies

Assign ICD-10-PCS codes to the following case studies.

1. Operative Report

PREOPERATIVE DIAGNOSIS: 1. Term intrauterine pregnancy at 39-weeks plus 3-days gestational age
2. Polyhydramnios
3. Failure to progress

POSTOPERATIVE DIAGNOSIS: 1. Term intrauterine pregnancy at 39-weeks plus 3-days gestational age
2. Viable male infant. Apgars 8 at 1 minute and 9 at 5 minutes. Birth weight 7 lbs. 10 oz.

OPERATION: Primary Cesarean section with low-cervical uterine incision

DESCRIPTION OF PROCEDURE: The patient was brought to the surgical delivery room suite and anesthesia was administered. The patient was placed in a supine position with left lateral uterine displacement. The abdomen was sterilely prepped and draped in the usual fashion for Cesarean section. After ascertaining the adequacy of the anesthetic level with an Allis test, a Pfannenstiel incision was made approximately three fingerbreadths above the pubic symphysis and carried down to the level of the fascia. The fascia was dissected off of the underlying rectus muscles using both sharp and blunt dissection. The recti were now divided in the midline and the peritoneum was carefully entered. The bladder was retracted inferiorly with a DeLee retractor and then a bladder flap was created. The DeLee retractor was repositioned to further retract the bladder inferiorly.

A transverse curvilinear incision was made in the lower uterine segment and extended upward and laterally using blunt dissection. Fetal membranes were ruptured and a viable male infant was delivered from a vertex presentation in an atraumatic fashion. The oropharynx and nares were suctioned on the operative field. The umbilical cord was doubly clamped and cut. The infant was handed off to the awaiting pediatric personnel.

Cord blood was obtained after a segment of cord was clamped and saved for cord blood gases pending Apgars. The placenta was delivered by manual extraction. The uterus was explored to remove any remaining fragments of membranes. The uterus was exteriorized. The uterine incision was reapproximated with double layered closure using No. 1 chromic suture in a running and locking fashion.

The uterus was returned to the abdominal cavity. The uterine incision was inspected once again for hemostasis. All blood and clots were cleared from the lateral gutters and then a final inspection confirmed hemostasis of the uterine incision. The rectus muscles were brought together with three simple interrupted 2-0 Vicryl sutures. The fascia was reapproximated using two separate 0 Vicryl sutures in a running fashion. The subcutaneous tissues were irrigated and the skin was reapproximated with surgical steel staples. A sterile dressing was applied.

2. Operative Report

PREOPERATIVE DIAGNOSIS:	Suspected right ectopic pregnancy
POSTOPERATIVE DIAGNOSIS:	Ruptured right ectopic pregnancy
PROCEDURES PERFORMED:	Dilation and curettage
	Open laparotomy with a right salpingectomy
FINDINGS:	Ruptured ectopic in the right fallopian tube. Normal appearing ovaries and uterus

PROCEDURE DESCRIPTION: The patient was brought to the operating room and placed in the supine position. General anesthesia was administered. The patient was prepped and draped in the usual sterile fashion for both abdominal and vaginal surgery. Vaginally, a single-tooth tenaculum was placed in the cervix, and the cervix was dilated to allow a #9 vacurette. The uterus was suctioned and the D&C specimen was sent to pathology, which reported the finding of no villi.

An open laparotomy incision was made. The ectopic was excised from the distal end of the tube with an attempt made to spare the fimbria. It was determined that the fimbria were significantly damaged and patency could not be restored. Therefore, the entire right tube was removed by dissecting it off the uterus and placing one 0 Vicryl suture. Hemostasis was ensured. Suctioning was performed, followed by copious irrigation. Hemostasis was again ensured and the fascia was closed using 0 Vicryl suture. The skin was closed with surgical staples. The patient tolerated the procedure well and was taken to the recovery room in good condition.

3. Operative Report

PREOPERATIVE DIAGNOSIS: Term intrauterine pregnancy at 38 weeks plus 5 days gestational age

POSTOPERATIVE DIAGNOSIS:
1. Term intrauterine pregnancy at 38 weeks plus 5 days gestational age
2. Viable female infant. Apgars 7 at 1 minute and 9 at 5 minutes. Birth weight 6 lbs. 14 oz.

PROCEDURE: Vaginal delivery

PROCEDURE DESCRIPTION: The patient progressed to delivery of the head to the perineum. With the patient in a McRoberts position, the patient pushed, without further delivery of the head. Suprapubic pressure was applied by the nurse at this point. With the suprapubic pressure, McRoberts position and gentle traction on the baby's head during the next major push, the baby was delivered. The baby was bulb suctioned. The cord was then clamped, cut, and the baby was given to the awaiting pediatric staff. She delivered a female with 7 and 9 Apgars, weight 6 pounds, 14 ounces over an intact perineum. The placenta was delivered intact with three-vessel cord. Cervix is intact.

4. Operative Report

PREOPERATIVE DIAGNOSIS: Premature rupture of membranes, in labor with twin gestation

POSTOPERATIVE DIAGNOSIS: Premature rupture of membranes, in labor with twin gestation

PROCEDURE PERFORMED: Repeat low-cervical cesarean section and a modified Pomeroy tubal ligation

INDICATION: Prior C-section 32. The patient with premature rupture of membranes in labor. The patient with twin gestation, twin-twin transfusion, twin A being growth restricted.

The patient was prepped and draped under spinal anesthesia in the recumbent position left lateral tilt. Pfannenstiel incision was performed through skin extending through subcutaneous fat, fascia. Rectus muscle was separated in the midline and the uterus was identified after perforating through peritoneal covering. The incision was made through uterus in a low-transverse fashion, penetrating the intrauterine cavity. Chorioamnionic membranes were expressed and the first twin, which was in vertex presentation, was delivered, rupturing the membranes, clear fluid being expressed, and the infant was atraumatically delivered with the head being shelved out of the pelvis and with fundal pressure the baby easily delivered, the cord was double clamped and cut, and delivered to the pediatrician from the NICU, who was in attendance. The second twin was located in the transverse lie. The bag was ruptured and the baby was delivered by breech extraction. This being done the cord was doubly clamped and cut. Once again cord sample was obtained and sent to the laboratory. The baby was delivered to the neonatologist, who was in attendance. Twin A was a male delivered at 5:44; Twin B was also a male, delivered at 5:48. Apgars were not obtained as of this time. Placenta was then manually extracted and sent to surgical pathology. Uterus was herniated out of the peritoneal cavity and uterine cavity cleansed with a dry sponge to remove all residual clots and membranes. The cervix was opened with a long Kelly. The uterus was then closed in the usual fashion with two layers, first layer with running locked 0 chromic suture, second layer also with running locking 0 chromic suture. Both layers being closed hemostasis was noted and the uterus was then subjected to a modified Pomeroy tubal ligation in which the fallopian tube was grasped in the ampullary portion, tented and a knuckle was clamped with a long Kelly and then a suture of 0 chromic suture was passed through in the avascular portion of the mesosalpinx and the loop was isolated and tied with a 0 chromic suture. A second tie was then done more proximal to this first suture. The knuckle of tube was incised and the open ends were coagulated with the Bovie to obtain hemostasis. The same was done to the contralateral side. No complications were encountered. Uterus was replaced back into the peritoneal cavity and then the abdomen was closed in the usual fashion, first closing the fascia with simple running 0 Vicryl sutures. The fascia was closed with simple running 0 Vicryl suture. The fat was not approximated and the skin was closed with staples. The patient was then sent in stable condition to the recovery room. Foley catheter was in place, urine being clear. No complications.

5. Operative Report

PREOPERATIVE DIAGNOSIS: Gravida 1 para 0 female at 38 weeks' gestation; prolonged rupture of membranes; prolonged second stage of labor with failure to descend

POSTOPERATIVE DIAGNOSIS: Same

OPERATION: Primary Cesarean section—classical

COMPLICATIONS: Classical extension of initially low transverse incision

FINDINGS: Viable female infant; complete placenta with three-vessel cord

INDICATIONS: This is a 26-year-old female gravida 1 para 0 who presented at 38 weeks' gestation with complaints of leaking fluid. The patient was approximately 1 cm dilated and 80 percent effaced at that time. She was felt to be having some leaking, although membranes could still be palpated. Therefore, artificial rupture of membranes was performed. The patient progressed very slowly in labor and required Pitocin augmentation. Fetal head was seen with separation of the labia; however, after 3 hours and maternal exhaustion, she made no further progression of the fetal head over the last hour of pushing. The patient was counseled regarding the need for assistance, and forceps assistance versus Cesarean section were offered. The risk and benefits of both were explained, and the patient opted for a Cesarean section.

TECHNIQUE: The patient was taken to the operating room and placed under epidural anesthesia. She was prepped and draped in the normal sterile fashion in dorsal supine position with leftward tilt. Pfannenstiel skin incision was made two fingerbreadths above the symphysis pubis in the midline and carried through the underlying fascia. The rectus muscles were dissected off the fascia using both blunt and sharp dissection. Rectus muscles were then separated in the midline. The peritoneum was entered bluntly and extended superiorly and inferiorly. The bladder blade was inserted. The vesicouterine peritoneum was grasped with pickups and entered with Metzenbaum scissors. The bladder flap was created digitally. The bladder blade was reinserted. The lower uterine segment was incised in a transverse fashion with a scalpel and extended laterally with blunt dissection. The infant's head was very low in the pelvis. Attempt to deliver the fetal head was difficult, and we were unable to reduce the fetal head from the vaginal canal. An attempt was made to retract on the shoulders of the infant in order to dislodge the fetal head from the vaginal canal, but again this was unsuccessful. For this reason, the uterine incision was extended vertically in a classical fashion, and the feet were grasped and pulled to the uterine incision. The feet were then delivered, and the infant was delivered in a breech fashion. Nose and mouth were suctioned and cord was clamped and cut. The infant was then handed off to the waiting pediatrician.

Cord gas was obtained. The cord blood was inadvertently not obtained. The placenta was removed. The uterus was cleared of clots and debris. The uterus was exteriorized for better visualization; 0 Vicryl sutures were used to close the vertical incision in the uterus in several layers. Two layers were done initially, then the transverse portion of the incision was closed. There was a cervical extension distally, and this was also closed with 0 Vicryl sutures. Once the transverse portion of the incision was closed, attention was again turned back to the vertical incision. The uterus was returned to the abdomen and inspection of the incision appeared to be hemostatic. With all the layers being closed and the sponge, lap, and needle counts were correct ×2. The patient tolerated the procedure well and was taken to the recovery room in stable condition.

Chapter 21

Placement, Administration, Measurement, and Monitoring

The first character values for these sections are:

2—Placement
3—Administration
4—Measurement and Monitoring

Types of Procedures Included in these Sections

These sections include codes for a variety of procedures, such as the following:

- Epidural injection
- Intraoperative central nervous system monitoring
- Application of a plaster cast
- Cervical traction with traction apparatus
- Voiding pressure studies associated with a cystometrogram
- Interrogation of an indwelling cardiac pacemaker

Character Definition for the Placement Section (2)

Character 1	Character 2	Character 3	Character 4	Character 5	Character 6	Character 7
Section	Body System	Root Operation	Body Region	Approach	Device	Qualifier

Common Root Operations Used in the Placement Section

The second character values for the Placement section uses two body system values:

W—Anatomical regions
Y—Anatomical orifices

Within these two divisions, seven root operations are used to describe procedures, two of which have the same definition as found in the Medical and Surgical section, Change and Removal. The definition of each root operation is as follows.

Root Operation

Change (0): Taking out or off a device from a body region and putting back an identical or similar device in or on the same body region without cutting or puncturing the skin or a mucous membrane.

Example: Changing a cast on a non-displaced fractured arm

Compression (1): Putting pressure on a body region.

Example: Application of compression stockings to increase circulation

Dressing (2): Putting material on a body region for protection.

Example: Application of a burn dressing

Immobilization (3): Limiting or preventing motion of a body region.

Example: Placement of a cast on a sprained ankle

Packing (4): Putting material in a body region.

Example: Packing the nasal cavity to control epistaxis

Removal (5): Taking out or off a device from a body region.

Example: Removal of a urinary catheter

Traction (6): Exerting a pulling force on a body region in a distal direction.

Example: Placement of cervical traction apparatus

Body Regions for Placement

Character 4, Body Regions, has values that describe general regions of the body, such as neck, chest wall, and lower extremity. There are also values for the natural orifices of the body, including the mouth and pharynx, nose, ear, anorectal canal, female genital tract, and urethra. Table 21.1 lists the body region values for procedures coded in the Placement section.

Table 21.1. Body region values

Body Region Value	Body Regions—Placement, Anatomical Regions (W)	Body Region Value	Body Regions—Placement, Anatomical Orifices (Y)
0	Head	0	Mouth and Pharynx
1	Face	1	Nasal
2	Neck	2	Ear
3	Abdominal Wall	3	Anorectal
4	Chest Wall	4	Female Genital Tract
5	Back	5	Urethra
6	Inguinal Region, Right		
7	Inguinal Region, Left		
8	Upper Extremity, Right		
9	Upper Extremity, Left		
A	Upper Arm, Right		
B	Upper Arm, Left		
C	Lower Arm, Right		

(Continued)

Table 21.1. Body region values (continued)

Body Region Value	Body Regions—Placement, Anatomical Regions (W)
D	Lower Arm, Left
E	Hand, Right
F	Hand, Left
G	Thumb, Right
H	Thumb, Left
J	Finger, Right
K	Finger, Left
L	Lower Extremity, Right
M	Lower Extremity, Left
N	Upper Leg, Right
P	Upper Leg, Left
Q	Lower Leg, Right
R	Lower Leg, Left
S	Foot, Right
T	Foot, Left
U	Toe, Right
V	Toe, Left

Coding Tip

The root operation Traction in this section includes only the task performed using a mechanical traction apparatus. Manual traction performed by a physical therapist is coded to Manual Therapy Techniques in section F, Physical Rehabilitation and Diagnostic Audiology.

Approaches Used for the Placement Section

For placement, the approach is always X, for External.

Devices Common to the Placement Section

Devices in the Placement section

- specify the material or device in the placement procedure (such as splint, traction apparatus, pressure dressing, bandage),
- include casts for nondisplaced fractures and dislocations, and
- are off the shelf and do not require any extensive design, fabrication, or fitting.

If a cast, splint, or brace is the only treatment for a nondisplaced fracture, the application of those devices is coded to the root operation Immobilization in the Placement section.

In the Placement section, Anatomical Orifices body system, the device is always value 5, Packing Material. Table 21.2 displays the devices used in coding procedures performed within anatomical regions.

Table 21.2.	Devices for Placement section
Device Value	**Devices—Placement (W and Y)**
0	Traction Apparatus
1	Splint
2	Cast
3	Brace
4	Bandage
5	Packing Material
6	Pressure Dressing
7	Intermittent Pressure Device
9	Wire
Y	Other Device

Coding Tip

The procedures to fit a device, such as splints and braces, as described in F0DZ6EZ and F0DZ7EZ, apply only to the rehabilitation setting. Splints and braces placed in other inpatient settings are coded to Immobilization, ICD-10-PCS table 2W3 in the Placement section.

Qualifiers Used in the Placement Section

For placement, the qualifier is always Z, No Qualifier. Table 21.3 displays this qualifier value.

Table 21.3.	Qualifier for Placement section
Qualifier Value	**Qualifier—Placement (W and Y)**
Z	No Qualifier

Character Definition for the Administration Section (3)

Character 1	Character 2	Character 3	Character 4	Character 5	Character 6	Character 7
Section	Body System (General Type)	Root Operation	Body System/Region (Specific System)	Approach	Substance	Qualifier

Common Root Operations Used in the Administration Section

The second character values for the Administration section uses three general type body system values:

    0—Circulatory
    C—Indwelling device
    E—Physiological systems and anatomical regions

Within these three divisions in the Administration section, three root operations are used to describe procedures. The definition of each root operation is as follows.

Root Operation

Introduction (0): Putting in or on a therapeutic, diagnostic, nutritional, physiological, or prophylactic substance, except blood or blood products.

Example: Injection of an antibiotic

Irrigation (1): Putting in or on a cleansing substance.

Example: Irrigating an infected joint

Transfusion (2): Putting in blood or blood products.

Example: Transfusing whole blood into a peripheral vein

B6.2. Procedures performed on a device only and not on a body part are specified in the root operations Change, Irrigation, Removal, and Revision and are coded to the procedure performed.

Example: Irrigation of percutaneous nephrostomy tube is coded to the root operation Irrigation of indwelling device in the Administration section.

Body Systems and Regions for Administration Section

The Circulatory body system and region contains body parts that are arteries and veins, as well as the circulatory system of the products of conception. The Indwelling Device body system and region does not differentiate between body parts. The only body part value in this system is Z, None. The Physiological Systems and Regions include body parts for arteries and veins, the products of conception, and the major body systems. Table 21.4 lists the body system and region values for the Administration section.

Coding Tip

Based on guidance from the body part key, procedures performed on the epidural space within the spinal column are coded to the body part value R, Spinal Canal. Procedures performed on the cranial epidural space are coded to the body part value S, Epidural Space.

Approaches Used for the Administration Section

The approaches for the Administration section are Open, Percutaneous, Via Natural or Artificial Opening (both with and without an endoscope), and External.

Substance Values for the Administration Section

ICD-10-PCS differentiates between devices, substances, and equipment based on the three key factors of procedural objective, location, and removability. Substances are generally liquid or blood components that are central to the accomplishment of the procedural objective. They are not placed into a fixed position and are intended to be absorbed, dispersed, or incorporated into the body. Substances are identified by the fact that once they are absorbed or dispersed, they are not removable. The substance values for the Administration section include blood and blood products for the root operation Transfusion, irrigation substance for the root operation Irrigation, and a variety of substances for the root operation Introduction. The substances include the major categories of medication, dialysate for dialysis, stem cells, contrast material, anesthetic, destructive agents, gas, adhesion barriers (such as SepraFilm) and such.

Table 21.4.   Body systems and regions values for Administration section

Body System/Region Value	Body Systems and Regions—Administration, Circulatory (0)	Body System/Region Value	Body Systems and Regions—Administration, Indwelling Device (C)	Body System/Region Value	Body Systems and Regions—Administration, Physiological Systems and Regions (E)
3	Peripheral Vein	Z	None	0	Skin and Mucous Membranes
4	Central Vein			1	Subcutaneous Tissue
5	Peripheral Artery			2	Muscle
6	Central Artery			3	Peripheral Vein
7	Products of Conception, Circulatory			4	Central Vein
8	Vein			5	Peripheral Artery
				6	Central Artery
				7	Coronary Artery
				8	Heart
				9	Nose
				A	Bone Marrow
				B	Ear
				C	Eye
				D	Mouth and Pharynx
				E	Products of Conception
				F	Respiratory Tract
				G	Upper GI
				H	Lower GI
				J	Biliary and Pancreatic Tract
				K	Genitourinary Tract
				L	Pleural Cavity
				M	Peritoneal Cavity
				N	Male Reproductive
				P	Female Reproductive
				Q	Cranial Cavity and Brain
				R	Spinal Canal
				S	Epidural Space
				T	Peripheral Nerves and Plexi
				U	Joints
				V	Bones
				W	Lymphatics
				X	Cranial Nerves
				Y	Pericardial Cavity

Refer to table 1.13 in chapter 1 to review the differences between the classifications of devices, substances, and equipment in ICD-10-PCS. The concept of Equipment will be explored more in chapters 22 and 25. Table 21.5 lists the substance values available for coding procedures in the Administration section.

Table 21.5.   Substance values for Administration section

Substance Value	Substances— Administration, Circulatory (0)	Substance Value	Substances— Indwelling Device (C)	Substance Value	Substances— Physiological Systems and Regions (E)
A	Stem Cells, Embryonic	8	Irrigating Substance	0	Antineoplastic
B	4-Factor Prothrombin Complex Concentrate			1	Thrombolytic
				2	Anti-infective
G	Bone Marrow			3	Anti-inflammatory
H	Whole Blood			4	Serum, Toxoid and Vaccine
J	Serum Albumin			5	Adhesion Barrier
K	Frozen Plasma			6	Nutritional Substance
L	Fresh Plasma			7	Electrolytic and Water Balance Substance
M	Plasma Cryoprecipitate			8	Irrigating Substance
N	Red Blood Cells			9	Dialysate
P	Frozen Red Cells			A	Stem Cells, Embryonic
Q	White Cells			B	Anesthetic Agent
R	Platelets			E	Stem Cells, Somatic
S	Globulin			F	Intracirculatory Anesthetic
T	Fibrinogen			G	Other Therapeutic Substance
V	Antihemophilic Factors			H	Radioactive Substance
W	Factor IX			K	Other Diagnostic Substance
X	Stem Cells, Cord Blood			L	Sperm
Y	Stem Cells, Hematopoietic			M	Pigment
				N	Analgesics, Hypnotics, Sedatives
				P	Platelet Inhibitor
				Q	Fertilized Ovum
				R	Antiarrhythmic
				S	Gas
				T	Destructive Agent
				U	Pancreatic Islet Cells
				V	Hormone
				W	Immunotherapeutic
				X	Vasopressor
				Y	Pericardial Cavity

Coding Tip

Botulinum toxin is a paralyzing agent with temporary effects; it does not destroy the nerve and is coded to substance value G, Other therapeutic substance.

Qualifiers Used in the Administration Section

The qualifiers in the Administration section describe autologous versus nonautologous sources and specific medication types. Table 21.6 lists the qualifier values available for coding procedures in the Administration section.

Table 21.6. Qualifiers for Administration section

Qualifier Value	Qualifier— Circulatory (0)
0	Autologous
1	Nonautologous
2	Allogeneic, Related
3	Allogeneic, Unrelated
4	Allogeneic, Unspecified
Z	No Qualifier

Qualifier Value	Qualifiers— Indwelling Device (C)
Z	No Qualifier

Qualifier Value	Qualifiers—Physiological Systems and Regions (E)
0	Autologous
0	Influenza Vaccine
1	Nonautologous
2	Highdose Interleukin-2
3	Low-dose Interleukin-2
4	Liquid Brachytherapy Radioisotope
5	Other Antineoplastic
6	Recombinant Human Activated Protein C
7	Other Thrombolytic
8	Oxazolidinones
9	Other Anti-infective
A	Anti-infective Envelope
B	Recombinant Bone Morphogenetic Protein
C	Other Substance
D	Nitric Oxide
F	Other Gas
G	Insulin
H	Human B-type Natriuretic Peptide
J	Other Hormone
K	Immunostimulator
L	Immunosuppressive
M	Monoclonal Antibody
N	Blood Brain Barrier Disruption
P	Clofarabine
Q	Glucarpidase
X	Diagnostic
Z	No Qualifier

Character Definition for the Measurement and Monitoring Section (4)

Character 1	Character 2	Character 3	Character 4	Character 5	Character 6	Character 7
Section	Body System (General Type)	Root Operation	Body System (Specific System)	Approach	Function/ Device	Qualifier

Common Root Operations Used in the Measurement and Monitoring Section

The first character value for Measurement and Monitoring is 4. The second character values for the Measurement and Monitoring section use two body system values indicating the general type of system:

A—Physiological Systems
B—Physiological Devices

This character differentiates between measurement and monitoring of a naturally occurring body function and measurement and monitoring of a previously placed device that performs a function. Within these two divisions, two root operations are used to describe procedures.

Root Operation

Measurement (0): Determining the level of a physiological or physical function at a point in time.

Example: Sampling and pressure measurement in the left heart done via catheterization. Determining cardiac electrical activity with an EKG. Manometry of an organ (pressure measurement).

Monitoring (1): Determining the level of a physiological or physical function repetitively over a period of time.

Example: Fetal heart monitoring. Gastrointestinal motility monitoring.

Coding Tip

Measurement describes a single level taken, while monitoring describes a series of levels obtained at intervals. Examples: A single temperature reading is considered Measurement. Temperature taken every half hour for 8 hours is considered Monitoring.

Body Systems for the Measurement and Monitoring Section

The 4th character in Measurement and Monitoring indicates the specific body system upon which the measurement or monitoring takes place. Refer to chapter 11 for a discussion of cardiac measurement and cardiac catheterization procedures. Table 21.7 lists the body system values for the 4th character.

Table 21.7. Body system values for Measurement and Monitoring section

Body System Value	Body Systems—Measurement and Monitoring (4)
0	Central Nervous
1	Peripheral Nervous
2	Cardiac
3	Arterial
4	Venous

(Continued)

Table 21.7. Body system values for Measurement and Monitoring section (continued)

Body System Value	Body Systems—Measurement and Monitoring (4)
5	Circulatory
6	Lymphatic
7	Visual
8	Olfactory
9	Respiratory
B	Gastrointestinal
C	Biliary
D	Urinary
F	Musculoskeletal
G	Skin and Breast
H	Products of Conception, Cardiac
J	Products of Conception, Nervous
Z	None

Approaches Used for the Measurement and Monitoring Section

The approaches for the Measurement and Monitoring section are Open, Percutaneous, Via Natural or Artificial Opening (both with and without an endoscope), and External.

Function and Device Values for the Measurement and Monitoring Section

The function and device values for the Measurement and Monitoring section describe the body functions, such as movement, flow, electricity, metabolism, pressure, and temperature. The devices include the stimulator, pacemaker, and defibrillator. Table 21.8 lists the function and device values for the Measurement and Monitoring section.

Table 21.8. Functions and devices for Measurement and Monitoring section

Function/Device Value	Functions and Devices—Measurement and Monitoring (4)
0	Acuity
1	Capacity
2	Conductivity
3	Contractility
4	Electrical Activity
5	Flow
6	Metabolism
8	Motility
9	Output
B	Pressure
C	Rate
D	Resistance
F	Rhythm

(Continued)

Table 21.8. Functions and devices for Measurement and Monitoring section (continued)

Function/Device Value	Functions and Devices—Measurement and Monitoring (4)
G	Secretion
H	Sound
J	Pulse
K	Temperature
L	Volume
M	Total Activity
N	Sampling and Pressure
P	Action Currents
Q	Sleep
R	Saturation
S	Pacemaker
S	Vascular Perfusion
T	Defibrillator
V	Stimulator

Qualifiers Used in the Measurement and Monitoring Section

Table 21.9 lists the qualifiers for the Measurement and Monitoring section that provide additional information for procedures coded in this section.

Table 21.9. Qualifiers for Measurement and Monitoring section

Qualifier Value	Qualifier—Measurement and Monitoring (4)
0	Central
1	Peripheral
2	Portal
3	Pulmonary
4	Stress
5	Ambulatory
6	Right Heart
7	Left Heart
8	Bilateral
9	Sensory
A	Guidance
B	Motor
C	Coronary
D	Intracranial
F	Other Thoracic
G	Intraoperative
H	Indocyanine Green Dye
Z	No Qualifier

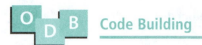

Code Building

Case #1:

PROCEDURE STATEMENT: Injection of left sacroiliac joint

ADDITIONAL INFORMATION: Anesthetic and steroid are injected using ultrasound guidance.

ROOT AND INDEX ENTRIES FOR THE STATEMENT: Introduction is the root operation performed in this procedure, defined as putting in or on a therapeutic, diagnostic, nutritional, physiological, or prophylactic substance, except blood or blood products. The Index entry is:

Introduction

    Joint   3E0U

        Analgesics   3E0U3NZ

        Anesthetic agent   3E0U3BZ

        Anti-infective   3E0U32

        Anti-inflammatory   3E0U33Z

Code Characters for Steroid Injection:

Section	Body System	Root Operation	Body Part	Approach	Device	Qualifier
Administration	Physiological Systems and Anatomical Regions	Introduction	Joints	Percutaneous	Anti-inflammatory	No Qualifier
3	E	0	U	3	3	Z

Code Characters for Anesthetic Agent:

Section	Body System	Root Operation	Body Part	Approach	Device	Qualifier
Administration	Physiological Systems and Anatomical Regions	Introduction	Joints	Percutaneous	Anesthetic agent	No Qualifier
3	E	0	U	3	B	Z

RATIONALE FOR THE ANSWER: The root operation Introduction is used to code this procedure. The injection is a mixture of steroid and local anesthetic for pain control. This is coded to the substance value 3, Anti-inflammatory. The anesthetic is substance value B, Anesthetic Agent. The approach is percutaneous and no qualifier value is appropriate for either code. The correct code assignment is 3E0U33Z and 3E0U3BZ.

Case #2:

PROCEDURE STATEMENT: Fetal heart monitoring

ADDITIONAL INFORMATION: The physician orders a fetal heart monitor to monitor the baby's heart rate during labor. Internal monitoring is performed.

ROOT AND INDEX ENTRIES FOR THE STATEMENT: Monitoring is the root operation performed in this procedure, defined as determining the level of a physiological or physical function repetitively over a period of time. The Index entry is:

Monitoring

    Products of conception

        Cardiac

        Electrical activity   4A1H

        Rate   4A1H

        Rhythm   4A1H

        Sound   4A1H

Code Characters:

Section	Body System	Root Operation	Body Part	Approach	Device	Qualifier
Measurement and Monitoring	Physiological Systems	Monitoring	Products of Conception, Cardiac	Via Natural or Artificial Opening	Rate	No Qualifier
4	A	1	H	7	C	Z

RATIONALE FOR THE ANSWER: The root operation Monitoring is used to code this procedure. The body part value is H, Products of Conception, Cardiac. The approach value is 7, Via Natural or Artificial Opening because internal monitoring was performed. (External monitoring can also be performed through the abdominal wall.) The function being monitored is value C, Rate. No qualifier value is appropriate for this code. The correct code assignment is 4A1H7CZ.

Check Your Understanding

Coding Knowledge Check

1. What procedure is described by ICD-10-PCS code 3E1M39Z?
2. Substance value _____ is assigned when recombinant bone morphogenic protein is placed into the femur.
3. Interrogating a previously installed pacemaker is coded as _____.
   a. 4A12X45
   b. 4B02XSZ
   c. 4B02XTZ
   d. 4B0FXV2
4. True or false? Irrigation of a previously placed indwelling device has only one possible code in ICD-10-PCS.
5. Urinary manometry is coded with the root operation _____ as code _____.

Procedure Statement Coding

Assign ICD-10-PCS codes to the following procedure statements and scenarios. List the root operation selected and the code assigned.

(Continued)

1. Lumbar facet joint injection at L4–L5 on the right using 20 mg of Kenalog

2. Chemical pleurodesis is performed by instilling a slurry of talc through a chest tube to cause adhesion of the parietal and visceral pleura.

3. Administration of a hepatitis B vaccine, IM

4. IV Glucarpidase into a peripheral vein

5. The surgeon performs a craniectomy for an intracranial abscess in the left hemisphere and drains the area, leaving a drain in place. The surgeon creates a burr hole over the right side of the cerebellum and implants an intracranial pressure-recording device into the cranial cavity. An incision is made and a 3 cm × 5 cm fascia graft is obtained from the patient's left thigh and is used to temporarily replace the cranium over the pressure device.

Case Studies

Assign ICD-10-PCS codes to the following case studies.

1. Procedure Report

PREOPERATIVE DIAGNOSIS: Achalasia

POSTOPERATIVE DIAGNOSIS: Achalasia

PROCEDURE: Upper endoscopy with Botox injection

INDICATIONS: The patient is an 83-year-old with achalasia. A previous Botox was performed in December which has been quite effective until this time.

TECHNIQUE: The Olympus video upper endoscope was passed through the upper esophagus and advanced through a very tortuous esophagus. The distal esophagus showed the lower esophageal sphincter in spasm. There was a large hiatal hernia with much of the stomach in the chest. The stomach and duodenum were otherwise negative. Botox injections were performed with 1 mL in 4 quadrants of the esophagus. She tolerated the procedure without discomfort.

IMPRESSION: Achalasia status post Botox injections

2. Operative Report

INDICATION: A 52-year-old man with recent left arm and chest pain that occurred at work while carrying a heaving object. He has hypertension and takes a diuretic daily. No other pertinent medical history.

PROCEDURE: He is exercised by Bruce protocol for a duration of 7 minutes, using the treadmill. Maximum heart rate achieved was 135, 86 percent. Maximum predicted was 137. His blood pressure during the stress test was a maximum of 176/84. He denied any arm pain with this exercise.

Following exercise, he was placed at rest. At 1 minute, he had STT wave depression and T-wave inversion in the interior and V5 and V6 leads. His blood pressure dropped to 76/40 at 5 minutes. During this time, he remained pain free and felt fine. At the 10-minute mark, the T-wave inversion resolved and the STT waves returned to normal.

IMPRESSION: He was advised that a cardiac catheterization would be appropriate to rule out ischemic heart disease, and this is scheduled.

3. Procedure Report

PREOPERATIVE DIAGNOSIS:	Herniated disc at L4–L5, L5–S1, good relief from two previous epidural blocks
POSTOPERATIVE DIAGNOSIS:	Same
PROCEDURE:	Therapeutic epidural block

The patient is kept on the left lateral side. The back is prepped with Betadine solution, and 1 percent Xylocaine is infiltrated at the L5–S1 interspace. Deep infiltration is carried out with a 22-gauge needle, and a 17-gauge Touhy needle is taken and the epidural performed. After careful aspiration, which was negative for blood and cerebrospinal fluid, about 80 mg of Depo-Medrol was injected along with 5 cc of 0.25 percent Marcaine and 1 cc of 50 mcg of Fentanyl. The injection was done in a fractionated dose in a slow fashion. The patient was examined and evaluated following the block and was found to have excellent relief of pain. The patient is advised to continue physical therapy and to come back in one month for further evaluation.

4. Operative Report

IDENTIFYING DATA: The patient is an 18-month-old female who has a history of non-accidental trauma with multiple brain bleeds and seizures at the time of injury. Seizure free since one week post-trauma. This procedure is to assess seizure activity prior to discontinuance of medication.

MEDICATIONS: Keppra

DESCRIPTION: This is a digital electroencephalogram recorded using the 10–20 Electrode Placement System. The recording was performed as a sleep deprived study. The patient is cooperative but unable to participate in the activating procedure of hyperventilation due to age constraints.

FINDINGS: The overall voltage is normal. The tracing is variable, symmetric, and continuous. The posterior basic rhythm of medium voltage, at 7.5–8 Hz, is present over the parietal-occipital regions bilaterally. Reactivity to eye opening and closure was appropriate. At maximum wakefulness, the background consists of mostly posterior alpha with moderate amounts of admixed, higher voltage, polymorphic theta and superimposed faster beta activity within the frontal regions bilaterally. During drowsy and sleep states, there was additional hypersynchronized, diffuse slowing of mostly delta and theta frequency. Sleep features include vertex waves and sleep spindles. Photic stimulation did not result in any appreciable driving response. Hyperventilation was not voluntarily performed due to the patient's age, but a brief period of crying resulted in mild to moderate diffuse slowing that reversed after crying cessation.

IMPRESSION: This is a normal sleep and awake EEG. No epileptiform discharges are noted.

Note: Absence of epileptiform activity does not preclude a clinical diagnosis of epilepsy or seizures.

5. Procedure Report

Chemotherapy Administration
The patient is a 73-year-old woman who arrives today for her scheduled chemotherapy treatment. All injections are sequential. She is being treated for serous papillary ovarian cancer with metastasis to the lungs. Treatment today through her central venous catheter:

   Carboplatin infusion, 50 mg
      Start time 1:30 p.m., End time 2:05 p.m.

   Paclitaxel infusion, 25 mg
      Start time 2:06 p.m., End time 3:10 p.m.

   Ondansetron infusion, 1 mg
      Start time 3:12 p.m., End time 3:32 p.m.

Chapter 22

Extracorporeal or Systemic Assistance, Performance, and Therapies

The 1st character values for these sections are:

5—Extracorporeal or Systemic Assistance and Performance
6—Extracorporeal or Systemic Therapies

Types of Procedures Included in these Sections

These sections include codes for a variety of procedures, such as the following:

- Extracorporeal membrane oxygenation (ECMO)
- Cardiopulmonary bypass procedures
- Mechanical ventilation
- Shock wave therapy to the plantar fascia
- Hyperbaric wound therapy

Character Definition for the Extracorporeal or Systemic Assistance and Performance Section (5)

Character 1	Character 2	Character 3	Character 4	Character 5	Character 6	Character 7
Section	Body System (General Type)	Root Operation	Body System (Specific System)	Duration	Function	Qualifier

Common Root Operations Used in the Extracorporeal or Systemic Assistance and Performance Section

The 2nd character value for the Extracorporeal or Systemic Assistance and Performance section is always A—Physiological Systems. Within this division, three root operations are used to describe procedures. Each root operation is defined as follows.

Root Operation

Assistance (0): Taking over a portion of a physiological function by extracorporeal means.

Coding Tip

Assistance defines procedures that support a physiological function but do not take complete control of it, such as intra-aortic balloon pump to support cardiac output and hyperbaric oxygen treatment.

Performance (1): Completely taking over a physiological function by extracorporeal means.

Coding Tip

Performance defines procedures where complete control is exercised over a physiological function, such as total mechanical ventilation, cardiac pacing, and cardiopulmonary bypass.

Restoration (2): Returning, or attempting to return, a physiological function to its original state by extracorporeal means.

Coding Tip

Restoration defines only external cardioversion and defibrillation procedures. Failed cardioversion procedures are also included in the definition of the root operation Restoration and are coded the same as successful procedures.

Body Systems for Extracorporeal or Systemic Assistance and Performance Section

The 4th character in the Extracorporeal or Systemic Assistance and Performance section is the body system value that describes the specific system that requires assistance or performance of a function. The body system values are limited because the systems that require assistance or performance in this section are very specific areas of the body. Table 22.1 lists the available 4th character body system values for this section.

Table 22.1. Body systems for Extracorporeal or Systemic Assistance and Performance section

Body System Value	Body Systems—Extracorporeal or Systemic Assistance and Performance (5)
2	Cardiac
5	Circulatory
9	Respiratory
C	Biliary
D	Urinary

Duration Values Used for the Extracorporeal or Systemic Assistance and Performance Section

The 5th character in the Extracorporeal or Systemic Assistance and Performance section is the Duration value. This character describes whether the procedure was performed on a single occasion or multiple occasions, or on an intermittent or continuous basis. For respiratory assistance and mechanical ventilation (respiratory performance), the specific time range of consecutive hours is available for coding in the duration value. For urinary filtration (hemodialysis), the specific number of hours per day is available for coding in the duration value.

Mechanical Ventilation

Mechanical ventilation is the process by which gases are moved into and out of the lungs by mechanical means. This service is provided for the patient through endotracheal intubation or through a tracheostomy. The duration value is determined based on the number of consecutive, or uninterrupted, hours that the performance of the respiratory function takes place. The start time for calculating the duration of mechanical ventilation is noted when any of the following take place:

- "Endotracheal intubation and subsequent initiation of mechanical ventilation
- Initiation of mechanical ventilation through a tracheostomy

- Admission of a previously intubated patient or a patient with a tracheostomy who is on mechanical ventilation." (AHA 2014)
- CPAP (continuous positive airway pressure) is delivered through a tracheostomy

Continue counting consecutive hours when:

- The endotracheal tube is immediately replaced with a new tube
- The endotracheal tube is immediately exchanged for a tracheostomy tube
- The patient is being weaned (or trying to be successfully removed from mechanical ventilation) using:
  - A T-tube
  - Intermittent mandatory ventilation (IMV)
  - Pressure support ventilation (PSV)

The end time for consecutive hours of mechanical ventilation is noted when any of the following take place:

- Endotracheal extubation
- Cessation of mechanical ventilation from a patient with a tracheostomy (weaning is complete)
- Discharge or transfer of a patient on mechanical ventilation

Assign the duration value based on the number of consecutive hours of mechanical ventilation performed. If the patient receives mechanical ventilation for more than one period of ventilation, assign separate codes for each period of ventilation, based on the number of consecutive hours in each period. Do not add the number of hours together. Each period counts uninterrupted hours of mechanical ventilation. Note that insertion of the endotracheal tube is coded separately from mechanical ventilation and mechanical ventilation provided to support surgery is not coded separately. If the mechanical ventilation continues for a longer than normal period, the mechanical ventilation should then be calculated from the time the patient was intubated. Query the physician to verify the expected, normal period following surgery, if unsure. Table 22.2 lists the available duration values for this section.

Table 22.2. Duration values for Extracorporeal or Systemic Assistance and Performance section

Duration Value	Durations—Extracorporeal or Systemic Assistance and Performance (5)
0	Single
1	Intermittent
2	Continuous
3	Less than 24 Consecutive Hours
4	24–96 Consecutive Hours
5	Greater than 96 Hours
6	Multiple
7	Intermittent, Less than 6 Hours Per Day
8	Prolonged Intermittent, 6–18 Hours Per Day
9	Continuous, Greater than 18 Hours Per Day

Function Values for the Extracorporeal or Systemic Assistance and Performance Section

The 6th character value in this section is the Function value. The output function is coded with the cardiac system and is used to code the use of cardiopulmonary bypass equipment in open heart surgery. The pacing function is used to code the use of temporary cardiac pacemaker during a procedure. The insertion and removal of pacemaker leads used during the temporary intraoperative pacing are not coded separately. The filtration function is only coded with the Biliary and Urinary body systems. The rhythm function is only coded with the root operation Restoration to describe a single procedure called cardioversion, or restoring the heart to its normal rhythm. Table 22.3 displays the functions performed in extracorporeal or systemic assistance and performance procedures.

Table 22.3.	Function values for Extracorporeal or Systemic Assistance and Performance section
Function Value	**Functions—Extracorporeal or Systemic Assistance and Performance (5)**
0	Filtration
1	Output
2	Oxygenation
3	Pacing
4	Rhythm
5	Ventilation

Coding Tip

Insertion of the endotracheal (ET) tube to be used for a mechanical ventilation procedure is coded in addition to the mechanical ventilation, other than when solely used during a surgical procedure (AHA 2014, 3). The insertion of the ET tube is coded as 0BH17EZ because the tube is inserted with the use of a laryngoscope, not via (through) the laryngoscope.

Qualifiers Used in the Extracorporeal or Systemic Assistance and Performance Section

The qualifiers in the Extracorporeal or Systemic Assistance and Performance section identify the methods or devices used to accomplish assistance or performance. The most common form of balloon pump is the intra-aortic balloon pump, or IABP. The IABP is a polyethylene balloon filled with helium that is inserted with a catheter. "The other end of the catheter attaches to a computer console. This console has a mechanism for inflating and deflating the balloon at the proper time" when the heart beats (Johns Hopkins 2018). With the IABP in place, blood flows more effectively into the coronary arteries with each contraction. The balloon inflates as the heart relaxes and deflates when the heart contracts, allowing the heart to pump with less work. The continuous use of the balloon pump is coded in this section. "Hyperbaric oxygen treatment is used to treat wounds. When you suffer an injury, your tissue needs more oxygen to survive. Chronic wounds develop when the natural healing process is disrupted due to factors like advanced age, infection, low blood flow, poor nutrition, diabetes, and decreased levels of oxygen in the blood. Hyperbaric oxygen therapy (HBO_2) helps chronic wounds heal by increasing the flow of oxygen" (Aurora Health Care 2017).

Pulsatile compression refers to the use of the pneumatic devices on the limbs to pump blood from the extremities back to the heart using alternating compression and release to help move the blood. These devices are used to assist circulation in patients who are having surgery or will be nonmobile for long periods of time.

Continuous positive airway pressure (CPAP) is a treatment that uses mild air pressure to keep one's airways open. CPAP typically is used for people who have breathing problems, such as sleep apnea (NHLBI 2011). In contrast, negative airway pressure was historically called "the iron lung." The current equivalent is a smaller device called a cuirass. "Modern applications of extrathoracic ventilation are best described as Biphasic Cuirass Ventilation (BCV)" (Linton 2005, 22).

Supersaturation is also known as superoxygenation:

SuperOxygenation therapy is designed to improve progressive myocardial necrosis by minimizing microvascular damage in acute myocardial infarction patients after percutaneous coronary artery stent placement. The therapy is performed immediately after the placement of the coronary stent using the guide components already in place for arterial access. The therapy is accomplished by a cartridge-based automated system that withdraws arterial blood from the patient. The blood is then mixed with a small amount of saline and supersaturated with oxygen to create highly oxygen-enriched blood. Using an infusion catheter, the SuperOxygenated blood is delivered directly to the stented coronary artery. (AHA 2008, 162)

An impeller pump is a rotor inside a tube or conduit used to increase the pressure and flow of a fluid. A cavopulmonary impeller pump device raises filling pressures in the heart in patients with a univentricular heart defect. The impeller pump is a catheter-delivered pump that is implanted into the four-way intersection where the inferior and superior vena cavae meet the right and left pulmonary arteries. The pump is then expanded, forming a shape that resembles two cones joined at the base. The device spins at about 10,000 revolutions per minute, connected via a slender cable to a small motor outside of the body (Ostrovsky 2010).

Mechanical ventilation takes place using equipment. Nonmechanical ventilation would be known as mouth-to-mouth resuscitation or artificial respiration. Extracorporeal membrane oxygenation (ECMO) is a process where blood is oxygenated through a membrane in a machine outside the body. Performance of cardiorespiratory or respiratory function using ECMO has three different qualifier options to describe the specific type of ECMO provided. The qualifiers are:

F, Membrane, Central
G, Membrane, Peripheral Veno-Arterial
H, Membrane, Peripheral Veno-Venous

Central veno-arterial (VA) ECMO requires cannulation of a central artery and central vein through a sternotomy. It often is used at the time of open chest surgery. Central VA ECMO is often called "long term CP bypass." In central VA ECMO, blood flows to the ECMO machine through the inferior vena cava, is oxygenated and returns to the body through the ascending aorta to flow through the body. Typical cannulation locations are the inferior vena cava and the ascending aorta. This cannulation completely bypasses both the lungs and the heart, providing both cardiac and pulmonary support.

Peripheral VA ECMO also provides both cardiac and pulmonary support but does not require the use of central vessels and a sternotomy. In peripheral VA ECMO, blood flows to the ECMO machine through the right femoral vein, is oxygenated and returns to the body through the right femoral artery to flow through the body, completely bypassing the heart and the lungs. Typical cannulation locations are the right femoral vein and right femoral artery in patients over age 2. Typical cannulation locations for neonates and infants up to age 2 are in the neck, using the right internal jugular vein and the right common carotid artery.

Peripheral veno-venous (VV) ECMO provides pulmonary support in acute respiratory distress or respiratory failure cases. In peripheral VV ECMO, blood flows to the ECMO machine through the right femoral vein, is oxygenated and returns to the body through the right internal jugular vein to flow through the body. Typical cannulation locations are VV ECMO are the right femoral vein and right internal jugular vein (Harvey 2018).

When coding ECMO, first determine if the cannulation is through a vein and an artery. If so, it is VA ECMO. Then, determine if the veno-arterial cannulations are performed using the central vessels. If so, it is central VA ECMO, coded as 5A1522F. If the vein and artery are not central, it is peripheral VA ECMO, coded as 5A1522G. If the cannulation takes place in two veins, it is VV ECMO, which is only performed peripherally and is coded as 5A1522H. Note that the cannulation or de-cannulation is not being coded. The performance of the function is being coded based on the type of connection to the ECMO machine. Figure 22.1 displays the decision making necessary when coding ECMO.

Figure 22.1.   **Extracorporeal membrane oxygenation (ECMO) coding**

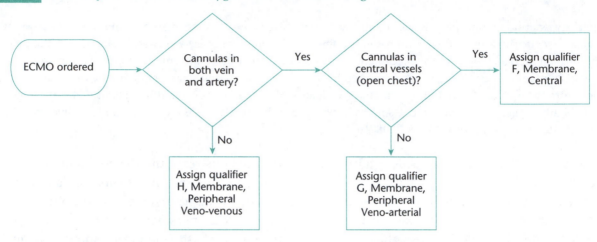

©Kuehn Consulting, LLC. Used with permission.

Table 22.4 lists the qualifier values available for coding Extracorporeal or Systemic Assistance and Performance procedures.

Table 22.4.   **Qualifiers for Extracorporeal or Systemic Assistance and Performance section**

Qualifier Value	Qualifiers—Extracorporeal or Systemic Assistance and Performance (5)
0	Balloon Pump
1	Hyperbaric
2	Manual
4	Nonmechanical
5	Pulsatile Compression
6	Other Pump
7	Continuous Positive Airway Pressure
8	Intermittent Positive Airway Pressure
9	Continuous Negative Airway Pressure
B	Intermittent Negative Airway Pressure
C	Supersaturated
D	Impeller Pump
F	Membrane, Central
G	Membrane, Peripheral Veno-arterial
H	Membrane, Peripheral Veno-venous
Z	No Qualifier

Character Definition for the Extracorporeal or Systemic Therapies Section (6)

Character 1	Character 2	Character 3	Character 4	Character 5	Character 6	Character 7
Section	Body System (General Type)	Root Operation	Body System (Specific System)	Duration	Qualifier	Qualifier

Common Root Operations Used in the Extracorporeal or Systemic Therapies Section

The 2nd character value for the Extracorporeal or Systemic Therapies section is always A, Physiological Systems. Within this division, 11 root operations are used to describe procedures. The definition of each root operation follows.

Root Operation

Atmospheric Control (0): Extracorporeal control of atmospheric pressure and composition.

Decompression (1): Extracorporeal elimination of undissolved gas from body fluids.

Coding Tip

The root operation Decompression describes a single type of procedure—treatment of decompression sickness (the bends) in a hyperbaric chamber.

Electromagnetic Therapy (2): Extracorporeal treatment by electromagnetic rays.

Hyperthermia (3): Extracorporeal raising of body temperature, used to treat temperature imbalance

Coding Tip

The root operation Hyperthermia is used both to treat temperature imbalance and as an adjunct radiation treatment for cancer. When performed to treat temperature imbalance, the procedure is coded to this section. When performed for cancer treatment, whole-body hyperthermia is used to create vasodilation and better oxygenation to improve the cell kill rate (Purdie et al. 2009, 129). Whole-body hyperthermia is classified as a modality qualifier in section D, Radiation Oncology.

Hypothermia (4): Extracorporeal lowering of body temperature.

Pheresis (5): Extracorporeal separation of blood products.

Coding Tip

The root operation Pheresis is used in medical practice for two main purposes: to treat diseases where too much of a blood component is produced, such as leukemia, or to remove a blood product, such as platelets from a donor, for transfusion into a patient who needs them.

Phototherapy (6): Extracorporeal treatment by light rays.

Coding Tip

The root operation Phototherapy to the circulatory system means exposing the blood to light rays outside the body, using a machine that recirculates the blood and returns it to the body after phototherapy.

Ultrasound Therapy (7): Extracorporeal treatment by ultrasound.

Ultraviolet Light Therapy (8): Extracorporeal treatment by ultraviolet light.

Shock Wave Therapy (9): Extracorporeal treatment by shock waves.

Perfusion (B): Extracorporeal treatment by diffusion of therapeutic fluid

Coding Tip

The perfusion process flushes and provides temporary continuous normothermic machine perfusion of donor organs. Note that perfusion is only coded if the perfusion leads to the organ being transplanted into the patient.

Body Systems for Extracorporeal or Systemic Therapies Section

The 4th character in the Extracorporeal or Systemic Therapies section is the body system value that describes the specific system being treated. The body system values are limited because the therapies in this section treat very specific areas of the body. Table 22.5 lists the available 4th character body system values for this section.

Table 22.5. Body system values for Extracorporeal or Systemic Therapies section

Body System Value	Body Systems—Extracorporeal or Systemic Therapies (6)
0	Skin
1	Urinary
2	Central Nervous
3	Musculoskeletal
5	Circulatory
B	Respiratory System
F	Hepatobiliary System and Pancreas
T	Urinary System
Z	None

Duration Values Used for the Extracorporeal or Systemic Therapies Section

The 5th character in the Extracorporeal or Systemic Therapies section is the Duration value. This character describes whether the treatment was provided in a single treatment or multiple treatments. Table 22.6 lists the two available duration values for this section.

Table 22.6. Duration values for Extracorporeal or Systemic Therapies section

Duration Value	Durations—Extracorporeal or Systemic Therapies (6)
0	Single
1	Multiple

6th Character Qualifier Values for the Extracorporeal or Systemic Therapies Section

The 6th character qualifier value for the Extracorporeal or Systemic Therapies section includes the valve of B, Donor Organ for the Perfusion root operation. All other therapies have a 6th character qualifier of Z, No Qualifier. Table 22.7 lists the available 6th character qualifiers for the Extracorporeal or Systemic Therapies section.

Table 22.7. 6th character qualifier values for Extracorporeal or Systemic Therapies section

6th Character Qualifier Value	6th Character Qualifier—Extracorporeal or Systemic Therapies (B)
B	Donor Organ
Z	No Qualifier

7th Character Qualifiers Used in the Extracorporeal or Systemic Therapies Section

The qualifier Hyperbaric is not used in the Extracorporeal or Systemic Therapies section with the root operation Decompression (treatment for the bends, also called decompression sickness), even though the terms are commonly used together in the documentation. In ICD-10-PCS, the qualifier hyperbaric is used with the root operation Assistance in the Extracorporeal or Systemic Assistance and Performance section when the hyperbaric chamber is used to assist with wound healing, also called oxygenation of a wound.

The 7th character qualifiers in this section are used to describe the blood cell type that is separated in the root operation Pheresis and the location of the ultrasound therapy. Table 22.8 lists the available 7th character qualifiers for the Extracorporeal Therapies section.

Table 22.8. 7th character qualifier values for Extracorporeal or Systemic Therapies section

7th Character Qualifier Value	7th Character Qualifiers—Extracorporeal or Systemic Therapies (6)
0	Erythrocytes
1	Leukocytes
2	Platelets
3	Plasma
4	Head and Neck Vessels
5	Heart
6	Peripheral Vessels
7	Other Vessels
T	Stem Cells, Cord Blood
V	Stem Cells, Hematopoietic
Z	No Qualifier

Code Building

Case #1:

PROCEDURE STATEMENT: Mechanical ventilation

ADDITIONAL INFORMATION: The mechanical ventilation was used for 20 consecutive hours.

ROOT AND INDEX ENTRIES FOR THE STATEMENT: Performance is the root operation performed in this procedure, defined as completely taking over a physiological function by extracorporeal means. The Index entry is:

Performance

Respiratory

Less than 24 Consecutive Hours, Ventilation   5A1935Z

Code Characters:

Section	Body System	Root Operation	Body System	Duration	Function	Qualifier
Extracorporeal or Systemic Assistance and Performance	Physiological Systems	Performance	Respiratory	Less than 24 Consecutive Hours	Ventilation	No Qualifier
5	A	1	9	3	5	Z

RATIONALE FOR THE ANSWER: The root operation Performance is used to code this procedure because the mechanical ventilator completely takes over the function for less than 24 consecutive hours. The function value is 5, Ventilation, and there is no qualifier value for this code. The correct code assignment is 5A1935Z.

Case #2:

PROCEDURE STATEMENT: Electromagnetic therapy for treatment of depression

ADDITIONAL INFORMATION: Therapy is performed daily to the brain for seven days

ROOT AND INDEX ENTRIES FOR THE STATEMENT: Electromagnetic therapy is the root operation performed in this procedure, defined as extracorporeal treatment by electromagnetic rays. The Index entry is:

Electromagnetic Therapy

   Central Nervous   6A22

Code Characters:

Section	Body System	Root Operation	Body System	Duration	Qualifier	Qualifier
Extracorporeal or Systemic Therapies	Physiological Systems	Electromagnetic Therapy	Central Nervous	Multiple	No Qualifier	No Qualifier
6	A	2	2	1	Z	Z

RATIONALE FOR THE ANSWER: The root operation Electromagnetic Therapy is used to code this treatment. The treatment was provided to the central nervous system in multiple treatments. There are no 6th and 7th character qualifiers for this code. The correct code assignment is 6A221ZZ.

Case #3:

PROCEDURE STATEMENT: Intermittent Positive Pressure Breathing

ADDITIONAL INFORMATION: The patient has atelectasis and was treated for 37 hours.

ROOT AND INDEX ENTRIES FOR THE STATEMENT: Assistance is the root operation performed in this procedure, defined as taking over a portion of a physiological function by extracorporeal means. The Index entry is:

Assistance

   Respiratory

   24–96 Consecutive Hours

   Intermittent Positive Airway Pressure   5A09458

Code Characters:

Section	Body System	Root Operation	Body System	Duration	Function	Qualifier
Extracorporeal or Systemic Assistance and Performance	Physiological Systems	Assistance	Respiratory	24–96 Consecutive Hours	Ventilation	Intermittent Positive Airway Pressure
5	A	0	9	4	5	8

RATIONALE FOR THE ANSWER: The root operation Assistance is used to code this procedure because the patient can breathe independently, and the procedure is assisting ventilation, not performing it. The duration value is 4, 24 to 96 Consecutive Hours because the patient was treated for 37 hours. The qualifier value is 8, for IPPB. The correct code assignment is 5A09458.

✓ Check Your Understanding

Coding Knowledge Check

1. What procedure is described by the ICD-10-PCS code 5A0221D? _____

2. Use of compression boots during surgery is coded to which body system value and function value? _____

3. Peripheral veno-venous extracorporeal membrane oxygenation (also commonly called ECMO) is coded as _____.
   a. 5A02216
   b. 5A1522G
   c. 5A1522H
   d. 6A151ZZ

4. The only procedure coded with the root operation Restoration is _____

5. True or false? Mouth-to-mouth resuscitation is considered nonmechanical ventilation and is coded as 5A19054. _____

Procedure Statement Coding

Assign ICD-10-PCS codes to the following procedure statements and scenarios. List the root operation selected and the code assigned.

1. CPAP daily, overnight for sleep apnea

   _____

2. Whole-body hypothermia for treatment of hypoxic ischemic encephalopathy, single treatment

   _____

3. Hemodialysis, prolonged intermittent duration

   _____

4. Hyperbaric chamber decompression, multiple treatments

   _____

5. Extracorporeal perfusion of donor lungs from an unrelated donor, with successful bilateral lung transplantation

   _____

6. Plasmapheresis for chronic inflammatory demyelinating polyneuropathy, single treatment

   _____

7. Extracorporeal shock wave therapy to Achilles tendon, single session

   _____

(Continued)

8. External chest compressions in cardiopulmonary resuscitation

9. Ventilator management for over 96 hours

10. Replacement of mitral valve with a synthetic substitute using cardiopulmonary bypass

Case Studies

Assign ICD-10-PCS codes to the following case studies.

1. Operative Report

NOTE: Do not code coronary angiography on this case.

PROCEDURE: Intra-aortic balloon pump placement

INDICATION: Cardiogenic shock

DESCRIPTION OF PROCEDURE: After diagnostic angiography was discontinued due to impending cardiogenic shock during the procedure, the decision was made to proceed with intra-aortic balloon pump placement from the left groin. The left groin had already been prepped. Lidocaine was given and an 8-French intra-aortic balloon pump sheath was placed over a guidewire. An intra-aortic balloon pump was then placed in the thoracic aorta and one-to-one counterpulsation begun. Patient's chest pain improved after intra-aortic balloon pump placement and his hemodynamics also improved.

CONCLUSION: Successful intra-aortic balloon pump placement after discontinued diagnostic angiography via left groin for cardiogenic shock.

2. Procedure Report

HBOT DETAILS

DIAGNOSIS: Chronic refractory osteomyelitis

TREATMENT COURSE NUMBER: 2 of 30

TREATMENT LENGTH: 120 minutes

CHAMBER TYPE: Monoplace

HBO DIVE LOG: 1190 and 1191

TREATMENT PROTOCOL: 2.5 ATA × 90 minutes w/100 percent oxygen and two 5-minute air breaks

TREATMENT DETAILS:

Chamber Pressure	Time	Action	BP	Pulse	Resp	Temp	Capillary Glucose	Pulse Ox
1 ATA	13:22	Compression begins	102/64	67	20	96.6	93	96
2.5 ATA	13:37	Treatment pressure reached						
2.5 ATA	14:07	Break						
2.5 ATA	14:12							
2.5 ATA	14:38	Break						
2.5 ATA	14:44							
2.5 ATA	15:50	Decompression begins						
1 ATA	16:00	Decompression ends	107/69	71	20	96	75	100

EAR EVALUATION: Left Teed Scale: Grade II   Right Teed Scale: Grade III

ADVERSE EVENTS: No

TREATMENT ABSORBED: No

3. Operative Report

PREOPERATIVE DIAGNOSIS: Coronary artery disease

POSTOPERATIVE DIAGNOSIS: Coronary artery disease

OPERATION PERFORMED:

1. Coronary artery bypass ×5 with: left mammary artery to left anterior descending right mammary artery T-graft off the left mammary to the first and third obtuse marginals, sequential saphenous vein graft to the posterior descending artery #1 and #2, which was the true posterior descending.
2. Endoscopic vein harvest.

FINDINGS: The patient is a 49-year-old man with history of recent onset of angina and discovery of multivessel coronary disease. He was recommended to have multi-vessel bypass.

TECHNIQUE: Under general anesthesia was induced. The chest was prepped with ChloraPrep and draped in sterile fashion. The saphenous vein was endoscopically harvested from the left leg and distended with heparinized Plasmalyte solution. The incisions were closed with 3-0 Vicryl subcutaneous suture and 4-0 Monocryl subcuticular suture and the chest was opened through a median sternotomy. The two mammaries were taken as skeletonized, isolated grafts. The right mammary was detached after heparinization and attached to the left with continuous 7-0 Prolene as a T-graft. The patient was heparinized and cannulated with #20 DLP aortic cannula and a two-stage cannula in the right atrial appendage.

The patient was placed on cardiopulmonary bypass and cooled to 32 degrees. The heart was arrested with del Nido cardioplegia given 700 mL antegrade and 300 mL retrograde, and then the grafts were performed. The saphenous graft was sewn first to the posterior descending #2 end-to-side with continuous 7-0 Prolene and then with a side-to-side graft to the posterior descending artery #1 with continuous 7-0 Prolene.

The aortotomy was made with a 4.8 mm punch and the proximal saphenous was anastomosed with continuous 6-0 Prolene. The right mammary T-graft was spatulated distally and then implanted end to side to the third obtuse marginal using continuous 7-0 Prolene and then the same graft was grafted side to side to the first obtuse marginal with continuous 7-0 Prolene. The left mammary was grafted end-to-side to the left anterior descending.

The heart was reperfused and returned to sinus rhythm. The patient was rewarmed and weaned from cardiopulmonary bypass without difficulty. The prime was reinfused and protamine was given to reverse the heparin. All surgical sites were again carefully checked and reinforced as needed and good hemostasis was obtained throughout all surgical areas. The chest was drained with #24 Blake drain in the posterior pericardium. The retrosternal drain was a #28 Blake and the right chest was drained to the base with a #28 Axiom tube. The pericardial defect was closed with continuous 4-0 Prolene. Hemostasis was carefully obtained throughout and then the chest was closed.

The wounds were dressed with Dermabond. The patient was returned to CCU in stable condition.

4. Operative Report

DIAGNOSIS: Atrial fibrillation

TECHNIQUE: After reviewing the risks of the procedure, informed consent was obtained. After appropriate conscious sedation, 100 joules of synchronized biphasic shock was delivered with successful restoration of normal sinus rhythm. The patient tolerated the procedure well.

IMPRESSION: Successful electrical cardioversion for atrial fibrillation.

5. Operative Report

PREOPERATIVE DIAGNOSIS: Coronary occlusive disease

POSTOPERATIVE DIAGNOSIS: Coronary occlusive disease

OPERATION PROCEDURE: Coronary bypass graft ×2 utilizing left internal mammary artery to the left anterior descending, with reverse autologous saphenous vein graft to the obtuse marginal. Total cardiopulmonary bypass, cold-blood potassium cardioplegia, antegrade for myocardial protection.

INDICATION FOR THE PROCEDURE: The patient was a 71-year-old female transferred from an outside facility with the left main, proximal left anterior descending, and proximal circumflex severe coronary occlusive disease, ejection fraction about 40 percent.

DESCRIPTION OF PROCEDURE: The patient was brought to the operating room and placed in the supine position. The patient was induced with general endotracheal anesthesia. Appropriate monitoring devices were placed. The chest, abdomen, and legs were prepped and draped in the sterile fashion. The right saphenous vein was harvested and prepared by two interrupted skin incisions and by ligating all branches with 4-0 Surgilon and flushed with heparinized blood. Hemostasis was achieved in the legs and closed with running 2-0 Dexon in the subcutaneous tissue and running 3-0 Dexon subcuticular in the skin.

Median sternotomy incision was made and the left mammary artery was dissected free from its takeoff of the subclavian to its bifurcation at the diaphragm and surrounded with papaverine-soaked gauze. The pericardium was opened. The pericardial cradle was created. The patient was fully heparinized and cannulated with a single aortic and single venous cannula and bypass was instituted. A retrograde cardioplegic cannula was placed with a pursestring suture of 4-0 Prolene suture in the right atrial wall into the coronary sinus and tied to a Rumel tourniquet. An antegrade cardioplegic needle sump combination was placed in the ascending aorta and tied in place with 4-0 Prolene. Cardiopulmonary bypass was instituted and the ascending aorta was crossclamped. Antegrade cardioplegia was given at a total of 5 mL per kg through the aortic route. This was followed by retrograde cardioplegia through the coronary sinus at a total of 5 mL per kg.

The obtuse marginal coronary was identified and opened. End-to-side anastomosis to the saphenous vein was performed with a running 7-0 Prolene suture. Cold antegrade and retrograde potassium cardioplegia were given. The internal mammary artery was clipped distally, divided and spatulated for anastomosis. The anterior descending was identified and opened. End-to-side anastomosis was performed with running 8-0 Prolene suture and the warm blood potassium cardioplegia was given antegrade and retrograde, and the aortic crossclamp was removed. The partial occlusion clamp was placed. Aortotomy was made. The vein was cut to fit and sutured in place with running 5-0 Prolene suture. A partial occlusion clamp was removed. All anastomoses were inspected and noted to be patent and dry. Ventilation was commenced. The patient was fully warm and was then weaned from cardiopulmonary bypass. The patient was decannulated in routine fashion. Protamine was given. Good hemostasis was noted. A single mediastinal chest tube and bilateral pleural Blake drains were placed. The sternum was closed with figure-of-eight stainless steel wire. The linea alba was closed with figure-of-eight of #1 Vicryl, the sternal fascia closed with running #1 Vicryl, the subcutaneous closed with running 2-0 Dexon, skin with running 4-0 Dexon subcuticular stitch. The patient tolerated the procedure well.

Osteopathic, Other Procedures, and Chiropractic Sections

The 1st character values for these sections are:

7—Osteopathic
8—Other Procedures
9—Chiropractic

Types of Procedures Included in these Sections

These sections include codes for a variety of procedures, such as the following:

- Acupuncture
- Osteopathic treatment
- Chiropractic manipulation
- Therapeutic massage
- Collection of bodily fluids
- Robotic assisted surgery
- Computer assisted surgery

The Other Procedures section contains codes for procedures not included in the other Medical and Surgical-related sections. There are relatively few procedures coded in this section. Whole body therapies, including acupuncture and meditation, are included in this section as well as codes for robotic assisted procedures and computer assisted procedures.

Character Definition for the Osteopathic Section (7)

Character 1	Character 2	Character 3	Character 4	Character 5	Character 6	Character 7
Section	Body System	Root Operation	Body Region	Approach	Method	Qualifier

Common Root Operations Used in the Osteopathic Section

The 1st character value for the Osteopathic section is 7. The 2nd character value for the Osteopathic section is always W—Anatomical Regions. Within that general body system, there is only one root operation.

Root Operation

Treatment (0): Manual treatment to eliminate or alleviate somatic dysfunction and related disorders.

Osteopathic treatment is a form of manual medicine used to treat structural restrictions (somatic dysfunction) and improve the level of health. Some treatments are aimed primarily at joints, others at membranes or fluids, and still others at even deeper levels. The osteopathic philosophy believes that by applying seemingly innocuous forces in a very precise manner, the body's own healing can be enhanced to release strains and patterns imprinted on the body from trauma and stresses of life (AACOM 2015a).

Osteopathic treatment is used to lengthen hypertonic muscles and connective tissue, help joint surfaces glide more normally in physiologic motion, decrease pressure on sensitive small vessels and lymphatics, and decrease level of sympathetic nervous system activation (AACOM 2015b).

Body Regions for Osteopathic Section

The body regions used to classify procedures in the Osteopathic section of ICD-10-PCS use general musculoskeletal and soft tissue regions of the body. Table 23.1 lists the body region values available for coding procedures in the section.

Table 23.1. Body region values

Body Region Value	Body Regions—Osteopathic (7)
0	Head
1	Cervical
2	Thoracic
3	Lumbar
4	Sacrum
5	Pelvis
6	Lower Extremities
7	Upper Extremities
8	Rib Cage
9	Abdomen

Approaches Used for the Osteopathic Section

For Osteopathic, the approach is always X, External.

Method Values for the Osteopathic Section

Table 23.2 displays the method values used in coding procedures performed within anatomical regions. The methods of osteopathic treatment classified in ICD-10-PCS are the following:

Table 23.2. Methods for Osteopathic section

Method Value	Methods—Osteopathic (7)
0	Articulatory-raising
1	Fascial Release
2	General Mobilization
3	High velocity–Low Amplitude
4	Indirect

(Continued)

Table 23.2.	Methods for Osteopathic section (continued)
Method Value	**Methods—Osteopathic (7)**
5	Low velocity–High Amplitude
6	Lymphatic Pump
7	Muscle Energy, Isometric
8	Muscle Energy, Isotonic
9	Other Method

- **Articulatory-raising**—A direct technique of rib raising designed to articulate the rib heads by lifting and rotating them and, through the fascial attachments, to beneficially affect the sympathetic innervations at the chain ganglia (DiGiovanna et al. 2005, 396).
- **Fascial release**—A technique to treat fascial restrictions using palpatory (hands-on) feedback to restore soft tissue mobility.
- **General mobilization**—Joint and tissue mobilization to relieve tension.
- **High velocity–low amplitude (HVLA)**—High velocity–low amplitude treatment uses forces quickly applied to a discrete area. Commonly known as a thrusting or "popping" technique.
- **Indirect**—Counterstrain is a common indirect technique that uses tender points (discrete tender areas that are caused by structural problems) to locate a problem. The body is positioned in such a fashion as to relieve the tenderness at this point and is held until the body reacts.
- **Low velocity–high amplitude**—Gentle, larger mobilization movements used to relieve tension.
- **Lymphatic pump**—Treatment used to increase the rate of lymph flow in order to help fight infection.
- **Muscle energy, isometric**—Muscle energy that uses the force of the patient's voluntarily directed muscle contractions for treatment. Isometric means using equal force or measurement.
- **Muscle energy, isotonic**—Muscle energy that uses the force of the patient's voluntarily directed muscle contractions for treatment. Isotonic means using resistance.
- **Other method**—Other treatment techniques are balanced tension, lateral fluctuation, CV4/EV4 and percussion (AACOM 2015b).

Qualifiers Used in the Osteopathic Section

The qualifier for the Osteopathic section is always Z, None.

Character Definition for the Other Procedures Section (8)

Character 1	Character 2	Character 3	Character 4	Character 5	Character 6	Character 7
Section	Body System	Root Operation	Body Region	Approach	Method	Qualifier

Common Root Operations Used in the Other Procedures Section

The 1st character value for the Other Procedures section is 8. The 2nd character values for the Other Procedures section are:

C—Indwelling device
E—Physiological systems and anatomical regions

Within these two body systems, only one root operation is used to describe procedures.

Root Operation

Other Procedures (0): Methodologies that attempt to remediate or cure a disorder or disease.

Body Regions for Other Procedures Section

The body regions used to classify procedures in the Other Procedures section of ICD-10-PCS use general musculoskeletal and soft tissue regions of the body. Table 23.3 lists the body region values available for coding procedures in this section.

Table 23.3. Body regions values for Other Procedures section

Body Region Value	Body Regions—Other Procedures (8)
1	Nervous System
2	Circulatory System
9	Head and Neck Region
H	Integumentary System and Breast
K	Musculoskeletal System
U	Female Reproductive System
V	Male Reproductive System
W	Trunk Region
X	Upper Extremity
Y	Lower Extremity
Z	None

Approaches Used for the Other Procedures Section

The approach values for the Other Procedures section of ICD-10-PCS are six of the seven approaches used within the Medical and Surgical section of ICD-10-PCS and retain the same definitions used within that section.

Method Values for the Other Procedures Section

The methods values used to code in this section are

- **Acupuncture**—Describes a family of procedures involving the stimulation of anatomical points on the body using a variety of techniques, involving penetrating the skin with thin, solid, metallic needles that are manipulated by the hands or by electrical stimulation (NIH 2016).
- **Therapeutic massage**—(Also called reflexology) Manipulation of the muscles and tissues of the body to prevent and alleviate pain, discomfort, and stress.
- **Collection**—Obtaining a specimen that does not require draining the specimen from a body part. Fluids collected directly from a body part are coded in the Medical and Surgical section using the root operation Drainage. In the Other Procedures section, collection is used to obtain a specimen of bodily fluids from an indwelling device or to collect two bodily fluids that do not require drainage—breast milk and sperm.
- **Computer assisted procedure**—Used for preoperative planning, surgical navigation, and to assist in performing surgical procedures (FDA 2015).

- **Robotic assisted procedure**—Procedure performed using small incisions to introduce miniaturized wristed instruments and a high-definition 3D camera. Seated at the console, the surgeon views a magnified, high-resolution 3D image of the surgical site. The robotic and computer technologies scale, filter, and seamlessly translate the surgeon's hand movements into precise micro-movements of the robotic instruments. The system cannot be programmed. It requires that every surgical maneuver be performed with direct input from the surgeon (Intuitive Surgical, Inc. 2015). One of the manufacturers of robotic surgical equipment is DaVinci, which describes its product's use as minimally invasive robotic assisted surgery, using small instruments through very small incisions. The approach for these procedures is approach value 4, Percutaneous Endoscopic.
- **Near infrared spectroscopy**—NIRS is a noninvasive technique that estimates cerebral blood flow in the human brain and can assess changes in the concentration of oxyhemoglobin (oxy-Hb), deoxyhemoglobin (deoxy-Hb), and total hemoglobin (total-Hb) as an index of neural activity (NIPS 2010).
- **Other method**—Includes the methods identified in the qualifier value as Examination, Suture Removal, Piercing, In Vitro Fertilization, Yoga Therapy, Meditation, and Isolation.

Table 23.4 displays the method values used in coding procedures classified to the Other Procedures section of ICD-10-PCS.

Coding Tip

Computer assisted procedures and robotic assisted procedures are coded in addition to other procedures. The primary procedure is coded separately.

Qualifiers Used in the Other Procedures Section

The qualifiers in the Other Procedures section describe a variety of different pieces of information. They describe bodily fluids (breast milk and sperm), more detail about the methods (anesthesia and with fluoroscopy), and body parts (prostate and rectum). The qualifier provides additional information that cannot be conveniently classified in other characters. Table 23.5 lists the qualifier values used to code procedures in the Other Procedures section.

Table 23.4. Method values for Other Procedures section

Method Value	Methods—Other Procedures (8)
0	Acupuncture
1	Therapeutic massage
6	Collection
B	Computer assisted procedure
C	Robotic assisted procedure
D	Near infrared spectroscopy
Y	Other Method

Table 23.5. Qualifiers for Other Procedures section

Qualifier Value	Qualifiers—Other Procedures (8)
0	Anesthesia
1	In Vitro Fertilization
2	Breast Milk
3	Sperm

(Continued)

Table 23.5. Qualifiers for Other Procedures section (continued)

Qualifier Value	Qualifiers—Other Procedures (8)
4	Yoga Therapy
5	Meditation
6	Isolation
7	Examination
8	Suture Removal
9	Piercing
C	Prostate
D	Rectum
F	With Fluoroscopy
G	With Computerized Tomography
H	With Magnetic Resonance Imaging
J	Cerebrospinal Fluid
K	Blood
L	Other Fluid

Character Definition for the Chiropractic Section (9)

Character 1	Character 2	Character 3	Character 4	Character 5	Character 6	Character 7
Section	Body System	Root Operation	Body Region	Approach	Method	Qualifier

Common Root Operations Used in the Chiropractic Section

The 1st character value for the Chiropractic section is 9. The 2nd character value for the Chiropractic section is always W—Anatomical Regions. Within this body system, one root operation is used to describe procedures.

Root Operation

Manipulation (B): Manual procedure that involves a directed thrust to move a joint past the physiological range of motion, without exceeding the anatomical limit

Chiropractic is a healthcare profession that focuses on disorders of the musculoskeletal system and the nervous system and the effects of these disorders on general health. Chiropractic care is used most often to treat neuromusculoskeletal complaints, including but not limited to back pain, neck pain, pain in the joints of the arms or legs, and headaches. Chiropractic adjustment or manipulation is a manual procedure where the chiropractor uses his or her hands—or an instrument—to manipulate the joints of the body, particularly the spine, in order to restore or enhance joint function. This often helps resolve joint inflammation and reduces the patient's pain. Chiropractic manipulation is a highly controlled procedure that rarely causes discomfort (ACA 2017).

Body Regions for the Chiropractic Section

The body regions used to classify procedures in the Chiropractic section of ICD-10-PCS use general musculoskeletal and soft tissue regions of the body. Table 23.6 lists the body region values available for coding procedures in the section.

Table 23.6. Body regions values for Chiropractic section

Body Region Value	Body Regions—Chiropractic Section (9)
0	Head
1	Cervical
2	Thoracic
3	Lumbar
4	Sacrum
5	Pelvis
6	Lower Extremities
7	Upper Extremities
8	Rib Cage
9	Abdomen

Approaches Used for the Chiropractic Section

The approach value for the Chiropractic section is always X, External.

Method Values for the Chiropractic Section

Table 23.7 lists the methods values available for use in coding Chiropractic procedures. The definitions of the methods values used to code in this section are as follows:

Table 23.7. Method values for Chiropractic section

Method Value	Methods—Chiropractic (9)
B	Non-manual
C	Indirect Visceral
D	Extra-articular
F	Direct Visceral
G	Long Lever Specific Contact
H	Short Lever Specific Contact
J	Long and Short Lever Specific Contact
K	Mechanically Assisted
L	Other Method

- **Non-manual**—These methods include heat and ice, ultrasound, electrical stimulation, rehabilitative exercise, and magnetic therapy.
- **Indirect visceral**—Visceral manipulation is a gentle way of working with mobile organs of the cranium, chest, abdomen, and pelvis to normalize their physiology. Utilizing this non-invasive, manual approach, viscera can be stimulated to restore mobility, circulation, and motility, thus treating internal organ dysfunction. The indirect technique means moving to create slack or reduce tension in an organ or structure.
- **Extra-articular**—Manipulation directed toward areas other than the joints of the body.
- **Direct visceral**—Visceral manipulation, as defined above, but using the direct technique on the structure to stretch or break up an adhesion or tension.

- **Long lever specific contact**—Long-lever manipulation uses the femur, shoulder, head, or pelvis to affect larger sections of the spine.
- **Short lever specific contact**—Specific short lever dynamic thrusts utilize a specific contact on a transverse spinous process of vertebra, muscle, or ligament.
- **Long and short lever specific contact**—Combination of both the above methods (Meeker and Haldeman 2002, 216).

Qualifiers Used in the Chiropractic Section

The qualifier value for the Chiropractic section is always Z, None.

 Code Building

Case #1:

PROCEDURE STATEMENT: Articulatory raising of rib cage

ADDITIONAL INFORMATION: This is an osteopathic method to relieve rib pain.

ROOT AND INDEX ENTRIES FOR THE STATEMENT: Treatment (Osteopathic Treatment) is the root operation performed in this procedure, defined as manual treatment to eliminate or alleviate somatic dysfunction and related disorders. The Index entry is:

Osteopathic Treatment

   Rib cage   7W08X

Code Characters:

Section	Body System	Root Operation	Body Region	Approach	Method	Qualifier
Osteopathic	Anatomical Regions	Treatment	Rib Cage	External	Articulatory-Raising	No Qualifier
7	W	0	8	X	0	Z

RATIONALE FOR THE ANSWER: The root operation Treatment is used to code this procedure. The main term in the index is Osteopathic treatment. The body region value is 8, Rib Cage. The approach for all osteopathic procedures is X, External. The method value is 0, Articulatory-Raising, and there is no qualifier in this code. The correct code assignment is 7W08X0Z.

Case #2:

PROCEDURE STATEMENT: Acupuncture

ADDITIONAL INFORMATION: The reason for this acupuncture procedure is anesthesia for a skin procedure.

ROOT AND INDEX ENTRIES FOR THE STATEMENT: Acupuncture is the index term for this procedure. The Index entry is:

Acupuncture

Integumentary System

Anesthesia   8E0H300

Code Characters:

Section	Body System	Root Operation	Body Region	Approach	Method	Qualifier
Other Procedures	Physiological Systems and Anatomical Regions	Other Procedures	Integumentary System and Breast	Percutaneous	Acupuncture	Anesthesia
8	E	0	H	3	0	0

RATIONALE FOR THE ANSWER: The main term in the index is Acupuncture. The index differentiates between acupuncture with no qualifier and acupuncture for anesthesia and then provides all seven characters for the code. The correct code assignment is 8E0H300.

Case #3:

PROCEDURE STATEMENT: Chiropractic manipulation

ADDITIONAL INFORMATION: The lumbar spine is manipulated using the long lever method.

ROOT AND INDEX ENTRIES FOR THE STATEMENT: Manipulation (Chiropractic Manipulation) is the root operation performed in this procedure, defined as a manual procedure that involves a directed thrust to move a joint past the physiological range of motion, without exceeding the anatomical limit. The Index entry is:

Chiropractic Manipulation

Lumbar   9WB3X

Code Characters:

Section	Body System	Root Operation	Body Region	Approach	Method	Qualifier
Chiropractic	Anatomical Regions	Manipulation	Lumbar	External	Long Lever Specific Contact	No Qualifier
9	W	B	3	X	G	Z

RATIONALE FOR THE ANSWER: The main term in the index for this procedure is Chiropractic Manipulation. The body region value is 3, Lumbar, and the approach is always X, External for chiropractic procedures. The method value is G, Long Lever Specific Contact, and there is no qualifier value. The correct code assignment is 9WB3XGZ.

Check Your Understanding

Coding Knowledge Check

1. What procedure is described by the ICD-10-PCS code 8E0ZXY6?

_____

2. The approach for the Osteopathic and Chiropractic sections is always _____.

Match the following terms to the correct definition or example:

3. _____   Manipulation   a. Used to eliminate or alleviate somatic dysfunction and related disorders

4. _____   Non-manual   b. Balanced tension

5. _____   Other Method   c. Procedure performed using a partial 3-dimensional model of the operative site

6. _____   Computer Assisted   d. Heat and ice

7. _____   Treatment   e. Procedure performed using small incisions to introduce miniaturized wristed instruments and a high-definition 3D camera

8. _____   Robotic Assisted   f. Directed toward areas other than the joints of the body

                                        g. Directed thrust to move a joint past the physiological range of motion, without exceeding the anatomical limit

Procedure Statement Coding

Assign ICD-10-PCS codes to the following procedure statements and scenarios. List the root operation selected and the code assigned.

1. Chiropractic short-lever manipulation of the cervical and thoracic spine

_____

2. Collection of CSF from a VP shunt

_____

3. Mechanically assisted manipulation of the thoracic region

_____

4. Fascial release of the cervical region

_____

5. Indirect treatment of pelvis

_____

6. Blood specimen collection from indwelling device

_____

7. Near infrared spectroscopy of cranial vessels

_____

8. Lymphatic pump treatment of lower extremities

_____

9. Stealth-assisted left temporal craniotomy for complete excision of metastatic tumor within the cerebral hemisphere

_____

10. Suture removal from arm

_____

11. CT computer assisted partial removal of pineal gland, open

_____

12. daVinci total hysterectomy

_____

Case Studies

Assign ICD-10-PCS codes to the following case studies.

1. Operative Report

PREOPERATIVE DIAGNOSIS:	Longstanding problem with low back pain
POSTOPERATIVE DIAGNOSIS:	Longstanding problem with low back pain

INDICATION: The patient is here for his fourth electrical acupuncture treatment. He states that his back is doing somewhat better and is looking forward to this treatment. The patient signed an informed consent today.

PROCEDURE: Treatment today is spleen 6, spleen 9, large intestine 4, stomach 36, kidney 3, liver 3, and gallbladder 34. We put ion gold seeds in his ear over shen men for muscle relaxation of thalamus and kidney as well as for liver. We electrically tonified spleen 6 to spleen 9 at 5.5 Hz for 10 minutes. He tolerated this treatment.

2. Operative Report

PREOPERATIVE DIAGNOSIS:	Prostate cancer
POSTOPERATIVE DIAGNOSIS:	Prostate cancer
OPERATION:	1. Robotic bilateral pelvic lymphadenectomy
	2. Open retropubic prostatectomy
ANESTHESIA:	General
ESTIMATED BLOOD LOSS:	300 cc
SPECIMENS:	1. Bilateral pelvic lymphadenectomy
	2. Bladder neck
	3. Radical prostatectomy specimen

INDICATIONS FOR PROCEDURE: The patient is a 73-year-old man with prostate cancer and a PSA of approximately 8. The patient also had a bone scan that was unremarkable, but a CAT scan that showed some pelvic lymphadenopathy. Secondary to the above, the patient decided he wishes to undergo prostatectomy. He does understand the risks and potential complications, including anesthetic and medical complications, infection, bleeding, pain, change in sensation, change in cosmesis, a possibility of incontinence, and the fact that he is already impotent and will continue this way. He also does understand that given his Gleason score of 9 and the possibility of pelvic lymphadenopathy that he could have metastatic disease and require other treatment with progression of his cancer. He does wish to proceed as planned. Preoperative intravenous antibiotics and a modified bowel preparation were given.

PROCEDURE: After proper counseling and consent, the patient was brought to the operating room, where a general anesthetic was given. He had TED hose and compression stockings placed preoperatively and was placed in the padded supine lithotomy position and shaved, prepped, and draped in standard fashion. A Veress insufflation needle was placed above the umbilicus. A 12-mm port was then placed for the camera. A robotic cannula was then placed approximately 10 cm to the left of the umbilicus and a 12-mm accessory port was placed 10 cm beyond this. On the right side, a cannula was placed 10 cm to the right as well as approximately 10 cm to the right of that, a 12-mm accessory port and a 5-mm accessory port. The robot was then docked. Using the bipolar cautery as well as the hook cautery, the umbilical ligaments were taken down, and the retropubic space was developed. The pelvic lymph nodes were sampled from each side and frozen sections obtained, which failed to reveal any metastatic carcinoma. The endopelvic fascia was then taken down at the bladder neck, and the bladder neck was incised. The dorsal venous complex was ligated with 2-0 Vicryl suture in a figure-of-eight. It was found that the patient had a median lobe. The ureteral orifices were identified. Dissection was taken posteriorly, and the seminal vesicles were identified. The pedicles were taken using the bipolar. A non-nerve-sparing procedure was performed since the patient is impotent. Dissection was carried out posteriorly, but secondary to the patient's large amount of intra-abdominal fat as well as the fact that the prostate was quite stuck posteriorly, it was elected to finish the operation open. A midline incision was made, and the Buchwalter retractor was used for exposure. The apex was developed and incised, and the urethra was isolated. The apex was then incised anteriorly and posteriorly. The remaining pedicles were taken down using 2-0 silk suture, and the prostate was removed in its entirety.

A biopsy was taken of the bladder neck. The wound was copiously irrigated and small bleeding points were cauterized. The bladder was closed in a racket handle fashion using two layers of 2-0 chromic suture. The mucosa was everted with 4-0 chromic suture, and the incision was tied with 0 chromic sutures at the 12, 3, 6, and 9 o'clock positions at corresponding points over a 20-French two-way Foley catheter with 15 cc in the balloon. Irrigation had no leakage.

A Jackson-Pratt drain was placed through a separate stab incision in the left lower quadrant and secured to the skin with a 2-0 nylon suture. The wound was closed with a 0 looped PDS intermittently locking suture. The subcutaneous tissue was irrigated and closed with staples. The port sites were closed with either Dermabond or a running 4-0 Monocryl suture. Dressings were placed. The Foley catheter was secured at the patient's leg and was draining clear urine. The patient was transferred to the recovery room in good condition. All sponge and needle counts were correct times three. The patient tolerated the procedure well and was transferred to the recovery room in good condition without apparent complication.

3. Procedure Report

PREOPERATIVE DIAGNOSIS: Degenerative osteoarthritis of the right knee with resulting genu varum deformity

POSTOPERATIVE DIAGNOSIS: Degenerative osteoarthritis of the right knee with resulting genu varum deformity

OPERATION PERFORMED: Computer-assisted navigation right total knee arthroplasty

COMPONENTS USED: Biomet Vanguard metal femur 67.5 mm PS, polyethylene tibial tray 83 mm, 10 mm PS insert

ANESTHESIA: Continuous spinal epidural

DESCRIPTION OF PROCEDURE: The patient was brought to the operating room. After instillation of satisfactory CSE anesthesia and placement of Foley catheter, the right lower extremity was appropriately prepared and draped in the usual sterile fashion. The two tibial trackers were placed into the proximal tibia. Tourniquet was inflated to 300 mm Hg.

A midline incision was made centered over the patella and carried down to the quadriceps mechanism. Median parapatellar incision was fashioned. Subperiosteal dissection of proximal medial plateau of the postero-medial corner was accomplished. Distal femoral trackers were placed. At this point, the registration process was begun. Following the surgical registration with kinematic analysis, the procedure was begun. The distal femoral tracker was navigated into position and pinned in place and confirmed. Distal femoral cut was made and veri-fied. The 2 sizing jig was positioned in the hybrid technique for rotation and was computer navigated. The 67.5 was selected and the anterior, posterior, condylar, and chamber cuts were made. Following this, the remnants of the anterior cruciate ligament and medial and lateral menisci were excised, followed by placement of a Homén retractor to expose the proximal tibia. Anterior tibial osteophyte was resected. The tibial cut block was navi-gated into position and pinned in place. This was confirmed. The proximal tibial cut was made and verified. The 83 sizing plate was positioned and selected.

Extramedullary alignment was used to confirm alignment and was pinned in place. Stem punch was passed. Following this, the posterior cruciate ligament was excised, posterior condylar osteophytes were resected, and posterior capsular release was accomplished. The intercondylar notch guide was placed and the notch cut was made. All components were cemented and the patella tracked well at the conclusion of the procedure.

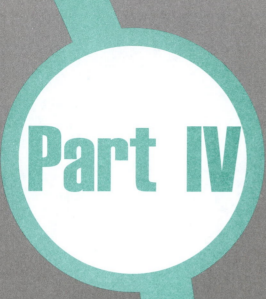

Part IV

Ancillary Sections

Imaging, Nuclear Medicine, and Radiation Therapy

The 1st character values for these sections are:

B—Imaging
C—Nuclear Medicine
D—Radiation Therapy

Types of Procedures Included in these Sections

These sections include codes for a variety of procedures, such as the following:

- Radiology studies, such as plain films, computerized tomography, and magnetic resonance imaging
- Nuclear medicine uptake tests
- Nuclear medicine systemic treatments
- Brachytherapy
- Stereotactic radiosurgery

Character Definition for the Imaging Section (B)

Character 1	Character 2	Character 3	Character 4	Character 5	Character 6	Character 7
Section	Body System	Root Type	Body Part	Contrast	Qualifier	Qualifier

The 1st character value for the Imaging section is B. The 2nd character values for body systems in the Imaging section are similar to the body system values within the Medical and Surgical section of ICD-10-PCS with a few exceptions. The Imaging section splits the musculoskeletal system into the axial and nonaxial skeleton and provides a body system for fetus and obstetrical imaging. The body system values for the Imaging section are listed in table 24.1.

Anatomy Alert

The Imaging section of ICD-10-PCS uses the terms Axial Skeleton and Non-Axial Skeleton rather than the traditional anatomical divisions of axial and appendicular skeleton.

Table 24.1.   Body systems for the Imaging section

Body System Value	Body Systems—Imaging (B)
0	Central Nervous System
2	Heart
3	Upper Arteries
4	Lower Arteries
5	Veins
7	Lymphatic System
8	Eye
9	Ear, Nose, Mouth, and Throat
B	Respiratory System
D	Gastrointestinal System
F	Hepatobiliary System and Pancreas
G	Endocrine System
H	Skin, Subcutaneous Tissue and Breast
L	Connective Tissue
N	Skull and Facial Bones
P	Non-Axial Upper Bones
Q	Non-Axial Lower Bones
R	Axial Skeleton, Except Skull and Facial Bones
T	Urinary System
U	Female Reproductive System
V	Male Reproductive System
W	Anatomical Regions
Y	Fetus and Obstetrical

Common Root Types Used in the Imaging Section

The 3rd character values for the root types in the Imaging section are defined as follows:

Root Type

Plain Radiography (0): Planar display of an image developed from the capture of external ionizing radiation on photographic or photoconductive plate.

Fluoroscopy (1): Single plane or bi-plane real time display of an image developed from the capture of external ionizing radiation on a fluorescent screen. The image may also be stored by either digital or analog means.

Computerized Tomography (CT Scan) (2): Computer-reformatted digital display of multi-planar images developed from the capture of multiple exposures of external ionizing radiation.

Magnetic Resonance Imaging (MRI) (3): Computer-reformatted digital display of multi-planar images developed from the capture of radio-frequency signals emitted by nuclei in a body site excited within a magnetic field.

Ultrasonography (4): Real time display of images of anatomy or flow information developed from the capture of reflected and attenuated high frequency sound waves.

Bone x-rays are coded as the root type Plain Radiography in ICD-10-PCS. Mammography is also coded to the root type Plain Radiography. The other root types have names that are commonly found in medical documentation, such as CT Scan, MRIs, and Ultrasounds.

Coding Tip

Imaging guidance done to assist in the performance of a procedure is coded separately in this section as the root type Fluoroscopy or Ultrasound, with the qualifier value A, Guidance.

A cardiac catheterization is a percutaneous procedure to diagnose cardiac disease. Following the heart catheterization, a series of fluoroscopy images of the heart and great vessels is taken after contrast has been injected using a catheter. The catheter is placed into the heart or vessels, usually via the groin into the femoral artery. The catheter tip is positioned into the vessels requiring imaging and may be moved multiple times during the procedure. A left ventriculogram is often performed along with the coronary angiography. During the procedures, the real-time fluoroscopy images are viewed on the video screen, and the physician will complete the necessary interventions (thrombectomies, dilations, or stent placements) during the same catheterization session. The coronary angiography is coded with the root type Fluoroscopy and the appropriate body part for the number and type of coronary arteries imaged. The ventriculography is coded to the root type Fluoroscopy but is coded with the body part value for the appropriate unilateral or bilateral side of the heart. The interventions are coded based on the root operation performed, such as Extirpation or Dilation. Therefore, the operative session usually includes multiple codes for Measurement, Fluoroscopy, and the interventions performed. Refer to chapter 11 for a discussion of how to code the interventions.

Body Parts for Imaging Section

The body part values within the Imaging section mirror the body parts within the Medical and Surgical section, unique to each body system in character 2. Refer to the complete set of tables in the code set for the descriptions of the body part values available for coding imaging procedures.

Contrast Used for the Imaging Section

Contrast material, or media, is used in computed tomography and other fluoroscopy imaging procedures. This substance changes the appearance of certain structures in the image, which helps with visualization. Two examples of high osmolar contrast media is Diatrizoate for use in gastrointestinal procedures and Cysto-Conray II for use in urinary procedures. The following is a list of low osmolar contrast media:

- Isovue 200, 250, 300, and 370
- Omnipaque 140, 180, 240, 300, and 350
- Optiray 160, 240, 300, 320, and 350
- Oxilan 300 and 350
- Ultravist 150, 240, 300, and 370
- Visipaque 320

Another source of information about whether a contrast is a high or low osmolar contrast media is an annotated (enhanced) version of the Health Care Procedure Coding System (HCPCS), maintained by the Centers for Medicare and Medicaid Services and published by various code book publishers. The code descriptors for Q9951 and Q9965 through Q9967 in the enhanced versions describe low osmolar contrast materials and list common product names. The code descriptors for Q9958 through Q9964 in the enhanced versions describe high osmolar contrast materials and list common product names. Cross-referencing the documented contrast product and the dose will help you determine the type of contrast material if the physician has not documented that information. If the type of contrast media cannot be identified, the provider who performed the Imaging service should be queried. Table 24.2 lists the contrast values available for coding Imaging procedures.

Table 24.2.	Contrast values for Imaging section
Contrast Value	**Contrasts—Imaging (B)**
0	High osmolar
1	Low osmolar
Y	Other contrast
Z	None

6th Character Qualifiers Common to the Imaging Section

"Optical coherence tomography [OCT] is an intravascular imaging technique that may help physicians identify the vulnerable plaques that lead to heart attacks or sudden cardiac death.... By creating extremely high-resolution images from within the artery, OCT can pinpoint the microscopic characteristics of a vulnerable plaque, as opposed to intravascular ultrasound (IVUS), which is more widely used, but has a lower resolution" (MGH 2017). OCT is coded with the 6th character value of 2, Intravascular Optical Coherence.

The 6th character value 0, Unenhanced and enhanced, refers to the use of contrast media and is often described in documentation as "with and without contrast." The 6th character value 1, Laser is used with the 7th character qualifier 0, Intraoperative to describe the process of laser-guided intraoperative fluoroscopy. Table 24.3 lists the available 6th character qualifiers for the Imaging section.

Table 24.3.	6th character qualifiers for Imaging section
6th Character Qualifier Value	**6th Character Qualifiers—Imaging (B)**
0	Unenhanced and Enhanced
1	Laser
2	Intravascular Optical Coherence
Z	None

7th Character Qualifiers Used in the Imaging Section

The 7th character qualifier in the Imaging section provides additional information about the imaging procedure, such as the specific location of intravascular or transesophageal. The 7th character qualifier also identifies that a bone ultrasound was done as a densitometry study or that fluoroscopy or ultrasound were used as guidance for another root operation. Table 24.4 lists the available 7th character qualifier values for the Imaging section.

Table 24.4.	7th character qualifiers for Imaging section
7th Character Qualifier Value	**7th Character Qualifiers—Imaging (B)**
0	Intraoperative
1	Densitometry
3	Intravascular
4	Transesophageal
A	Guidance
Z	None

Character Definition for the Nuclear Medicine Section (C)

Character 1	Character 2	Character 3	Character 4	Character 5	Character 6	Character 7
Section	Body System	Root Type	Body Part	Radionuclide	Qualifier	Qualifier

The 1st character value for the Nuclear Medicine section is C. Nuclear medicine procedures are used for both diagnostic and therapeutic purposes. Diagnostic nuclear medicine uses unstable radioactive elements that have been irradiated with neutrons and become radionuclides. These radionuclide materials are ingested, injected, or infused into the patient. As the radionuclide decays, the gamma photon that is released is detected by a gamma camera and creates a recordable image. Therapeutic nuclear medicine uses radioactive beta particles to kill specific, targeted cells (Ziessman and Rehm 2011, 4, 56).

The 2nd character values for the body systems in the Nuclear Medicine section are similar to the body system values for the major systems of the Medical and Surgical section of ICD-10-PCS. The body system values for the Nuclear Medicine section are listed in table 24.5.

Table 24.5. Body systems for Nuclear Medicine section

Body System Value	Body Systems—Nuclear Medicine (C)
0	Central Nervous System
2	Heart
5	Veins
7	Lymphatic and Hematologic System
8	Eye
9	Ear, Nose, Mouth, and Throat
B	Respiratory System
D	Gastrointestinal System
F	Hepatobiliary System and Pancreas
G	Endocrine System
H	Skin, Subcutaneous Tissue, and Breast
P	Musculoskeletal System
T	Urinary System
V	Male Reproductive System
W	Anatomical Regions

Common Root Types Used in the Nuclear Medicine Section

The root type Systemic Nuclear Medicine Therapy describes the therapeutic form of nuclear medicine and the other root types describe the various types of diagnostic testing done with the use of nuclear medicine technology. Planar nuclear medicine imaging is also referred to as scintigraphy and SPECT (single photon emission computed tomography) is Tomographic Nuclear Medicine Imaging (Mayfield Clinic 2016). The definitions of the root types available in this section are as follows:

Root Type

Nonimaging Nuclear Medicine Assay (6): Introduction of radioactive materials into the body for the study of body fluids and blood elements, by the detection of radioactive emissions.

Root Type

Nonimaging Nuclear Medicine Probe (5): Introduction of radioactive materials into the body for the study of the distribution and fate of certain substances by the detection of radioactive emissions; or, alternatively, measurement of absorption of radioactive emissions from an external source.

Nonimaging Nuclear Medicine Uptake (4): Introduction of radioactive materials into the body for measurements of organ function, from the detection of radioactive emissions.

Planar Nuclear Medicine Imaging (1): Introduction of radioactive materials in to the body for single plane display of images developed from the capture of radioactive emissions.

Positron Emission Tomography (PET) (3): Introduction of radioactive materials into the body for three-dimensional display of images developed from the simultaneous capture, 180 degrees apart, of radioactive emissions.

Systemic Nuclear Medicine Therapy (7): Introduction of unsealed radioactive materials into the body for treatment.

Tomographic Nuclear Medicine Imaging (2): Introduction of radioactive materials into the body for three-dimensional display of images developed from the capture of radioactive emissions.

Body Parts for Nuclear Medicine Section

The body part values within the Nuclear Medicine section mirror the body parts within the Medical and Surgical section, unique to each body system in character 2, in a condensed version. Refer to the complete set of tables in the code set for the descriptions of the body part values available for coding nuclear medicine procedures.

Radionuclides Used for the Nuclear Medicine Section

In ICD-10-PCS, the 5th character in a nuclear medicine code describes the radionuclide used to create the chemical tracer. A tracer is composed of various radionuclides that are bound to a biological marker (chemical, molecule, or cell type) for a specific physiologic function. These tracers give off gamma rays or positrons that can help determine the functioning of organs or the presence of disease. Table 24.6 lists the radionuclide values available for coding nuclear medicine procedures.

Table 24.6. Radionuclides for Nuclear Medicine section

Radionuclide Value	Radionuclides—Nuclear Medicine (C)
1	Technetium 99m (Tc-99m)
7	Cobalt 58 (Co-58)
8	Samarium 153 (Sm-153)
9	Krypton (Kr-81m)
B	Carbon 11 (C-11)
C	Cobalt 57 (Co-57)
D	Indium 111 (In-111)
F	Iodine 123 (I-123)
G	Iodine 131 (I-131)
H	Iodine 125 (I-125)

(Continued)

Table 24.6. Radionuclides for Nuclear Medicine section (continued)

Radionuclide Value	Radionuclides—Nuclear Medicine (C)
K	Fluorine 18 (F-18)
L	Gallium 67 (Ga-67)
M	Oxygen 15 (O-15)
N	Phosphorus 32 (P-32)
P	Strontium 89 (Sr-89)
Q	Rubidium 82 (Rb-82)
R	Nitrogen 13 (N-13)
S	Thallium 201 (Tl-201)
T	Xenon 127 (Xe-127)
V	Xenon 133 (Xe-133)
W	Chromium (Cr-51)
Y	Other radionuclide
Z	None

6th and 7th Character Qualifier Values for the Nuclear Medicine Section

The 6th and 7th character qualifier values for the Nuclear Medicine section are always Z, None.

Character Definition for the Radiation Therapy Section (D)

Character 1	Character 2	Character 3	Character 4	Character 5	Character 6	Character 7
Section	Body System	Root Type (Modality)	Treatment Site	Modality Qualifier	Isotope	Qualifier

The 1st character value for the Radiation Therapy section is D. Radiation therapy is the use of various doses of radiation on a particular schedule to treat and kill tumor cells while systematically sparing the normal tissue (Purdie et al. 2009, 19). Various modalities of treatment are used, based on the type of tumor and the location within the body.

The 2nd character values for body systems in the Radiation Therapy section are similar to the body system values for the major systems of the Medical and Surgical sections of ICD-10-PCS. Table 24.7 displays the body system values for the Radiation Therapy section.

Table 24.7. Body systems for the Radiation Therapy section

Body System Value	Body Systems—Radiation Therapy (D)
0	Central and Peripheral Nervous System
7	Lymphatic and Hematologic System
8	Eye
9	Ear, Nose, Mouth, and Throat
B	Respiratory System
D	Gastrointestinal System
F	Hepatobiliary System and Pancreas

(Continued)

Table 24.7. Body systems for the Radiation Therapy section (continued)

Body System Value	Body Systems—Radiation Therapy (D)
G	Endocrine System
H	Skin
M	Breast
P	Musculoskeletal System
T	Urinary System
U	Female Reproductive System
V	Male Reproductive System
W	Anatomical Regions

Common Root Types (Modalities) Used in the Radiation Therapy Section

The modalities used in Radiation Therapy are as follows:

Root Type

Beam Radiation (0): Beam radiation therapy is a local treatment delivered by equipment that aims the radiation at the specific body part where the tumor is located. The equipment does not touch the patient, but rather sends the radiation beams to the body from many directions (NIH 2011). Also called Teletherapy because it is delivered from "afar."

Brachytherapy (1): Brachy means "near." Brachytherapy delivers treatment at a close proximity, often internally with probes or Palladium seeds, such as to the prostate. Can be termed intracavitary or interstitial brachytherapy, depending on the exact site of delivery (Purdie et al. 2009, 96).

Stereotactic Radiosurgery (2): The practice of using a single treatment of high-dose radiation on tumors with a volume less than 20 cm³. Both gamma knife and linear accelerators (LINAC radiosurgery) are able to perform stereotactic radiosurgery (Purdie et al. 2009, 122).

Other Radiation (Y): Other modalities not identified above.

Treatment Sites for the Radiation Therapy Section

The treatment site values within the Radiation Therapy section mirror the body parts within the Medical and Surgical section, unique to each body system in character 2, in a condensed version. Refer to the complete set of tables in the code set for the descriptions of the treatment site values available for coding radiation therapy procedures.

Modality Qualifiers Used for the Radiation Therapy Section

Radiation therapy works by exposing tumor cells to high levels of energy from a radiation source. This energy damages the genetic material in the tumor cells so they can no longer reproduce. Tumor cells have degenerated from their original form and do not have the mechanism to repair their genetic material (DNA) when it becomes damaged. This makes the tumor cells more susceptible to the effects of the radiation and spares the normal cells that can repair their damaged DNA. Treatment modalities for radiation oncology are chosen to maximize the "cell kill levels" and spare the maximum number of healthy cells. Table 24.8 lists the treatment modality qualifiers used to code radiation oncology procedures. These modalities describe variations in the way the modalities can be delivered, such as at a high or low dose rate, with whole-body hyperthermia or as laser interstitial thermal therapy or LITT.

Table 24.8. Modality qualifiers for Radiation Therapy section

Modality Qualifier Value	Modality Qualifiers—Radiation Therapy (D)
0	Photons < 1 MeV
1	Photons 1–10 MeV
2	Photons > 10 MeV
3	Electrons
4	Heavy Particles (Protons, Ions)
5	Neutrons
6	Neutron Capture
7	Contact Radiation
8	Hyperthermia
9	High Dose Rate (HDR)
B	Low Dose Rate (LDR)
C	Intraoperative Radiation Therapy (IORT)
D	Stereotactic Other Photon Radiosurgery
F	Plaque Radiation
H	Stereotactic Particulate Radiosurgery
J	Stereotactic Gamma Beam Radiosurgery
K	Laser Interstitial Thermal Therapy

Isotope Values for the Radiation Therapy Section

Radioactive isotopes are used in radiation therapy to destroy cancer cells using their radioactive make-up. The isotope is selected based on the type of cancer being treated because cancer cells respond differently to different isotopes. The isotope values used to code radiation therapy procedures are listed in table 24.9.

Coding Tip

The root operation Hyperthermia is used both to treat temperature imbalance and as an adjunct radiation treatment for cancer. When performed to treat temperature imbalance, the procedure is coded to the Extracorporeal Therapies section. When performed for cancer treatment, whole-body hyperthermia is used to create vasodilation and better oxygenation to improve the cell kill rate (Purdie et al. 2009, 129). Whole-body hyperthermia is classified as a modality qualifier in this section.

Table 24.9. Isotopes for Radiation Therapy section

Isotope Value	Isotopes—Radiation Therapy (D)
7	Cesium 137 (Cs-137)
8	Iridium 192 (Ir-192)
9	Iodine 125 (I-125)
B	Palladium 103 (Pd-103)
C	Californium 252 (Cf-252)

(Continued)

Table 24.9. Isotopes for Radiation Therapy section (continued)

Isotope Value	Isotopes—Radiation Therapy (D)
D	Iodine 131 (I-131)
F	Phosphorus 32 (P-32)
G	Strontium 89 (Sr-89)
H	Strontium 90 (Sr-90)
Y	Other Isotope
Z	None

Qualifiers Used in the Radiation Therapy Section

"Use of radiation during surgical oncology procedures is known as intraoperative electron beam therapy (IOEBT). In the operating room the surgeon removes as much tumor bulk as possible. Inaccessible or microscopic tumor beyond the surgical margins may remain despite the surgeon's best effort. The radiation oncologist then uses electron therapy to treat. A single dose is delivered to the open patient on the table" (Purdie et al. 2009, 131). The 7th character qualifier of 0, Intraoperative is coded when this procedure is documented. Table 24.10 lists the available 7th character qualifiers for the Radiation Therapy section.

Table 24.10. Qualifiers for Radiation Therapy section

Qualifier Value	Qualifiers—Radiation Therapy (D)
0	Intraoperative
Z	None

 Code Building

Case #1:

PROCEDURE STATEMENT: CT of abdomen and pelvis, with and without contrast

ADDITIONAL INFORMATION: The contrast used is Omnipaque 140.

ROOT AND INDEX ENTRIES FOR THE STATEMENT: Computerized tomography is the root type performed in this procedure, defined as computer-reformatted digital display of multiplanar images developed from the capture of multiple exposures of external ionizing radiation. The Index entry is:

Computerized Tomography (CT Scan)

Abdomen	BW20
Chest and Pelvis	BW25
Abdomen and Chest	BW24
Abdomen and Pelvis	BW21

Code Characters:

Section	Body System	Root Type	Body Part	Contrast	Qualifier	Qualifier
Imaging	Anatomical Regions	Computerized Tomography (CT Scan)	Abdomen and Pelvis	Low Osmolar	Unenhanced and Enhanced	None
B	W	2	1	1	0	Z

RATIONALE FOR THE ANSWER: The root operation Computerized Tomography is used to code this procedure. The description says the procedure is with and without contrast, 6th character qualifier value, 0, Unenhanced and Enhanced. The contrast media is documented as Omnipaque, which is a common low osmolar contrast media, contrast value 1, Low Osmolar. There is no qualifier for this code. The correct code assignment is BW2110Z.

Case #2:

PROCEDURE STATEMENT: Intraoperative electron beam therapy

ADDITIONAL INFORMATION: The procedure is performed on the shaft of the femur during another surgical procedure.

ROOT AND INDEX ENTRIES FOR THE STATEMENT: Beam Radiation is the root operation performed in this procedure, defined as treatment delivered by equipment that aims the radiation at a specific body part where the tumor is located. The Index entry is:

Beam Radiation

Bone

    Other   DP0C

      Intraoperative   DP0C3Z0

Femur DP09

      Intraoperative   DP093Z0

Code Characters:

Section	Body System	Root Type	Treatment Site	Modality Qualifier	Isotope	Qualifier
Radiation Oncology	Musculoskeletal System	Beam Radiation	Femur	Electrons	None	Intraoperative
D	P	0	9	3	Z	0

RATIONALE FOR THE ANSWER: The treatment modality is Beam Radiation with a modality qualifier of 3, Electrons. The index contains an entry for beam radiation to the bone but also contains a more specific Index entry for femur, which was selected for coding. There is no isotope value for this code, and the 7th character qualifier value is 0, Intraoperative. The correct code assignment is DP093Z0.

Case #3:

PROCEDURE STATEMENT: I-131 therapy for Graves disease and hyperthyroidism

ADDITIONAL INFORMATION: A previous I-123 uptake scan showed increased uptake. The patient was treated with an ingestion of a single capsule of 21.3 mCi of I-131 to treat her thyroid disease.

ROOT AND INDEX ENTRIES FOR THE STATEMENT: Systemic Nuclear Medicine Therapy is the root type performed in this procedure, defined as introduction of unsealed radioactive materials into the body for treatment. The Index entry is:

Systemic Nuclear Medicine Therapy
Abdomen	CW70
Anatomical regions, multiple	CW7YYZZ
Chest	CW73
Thyroid	CW7G
Whole body	CW7N

Code Characters:

Section	Body System	Root Type	Body Part	Radionuclide	Qualifier	Qualifier
Nuclear Medicine	Anatomical Regions	Systemic Nuclear Medicine Therapy	Thyroid	Iodine 131 (I-131)	None	None
C	W	7	G	G	Z	Z

RATIONALE FOR THE ANSWER: The root type Systemic Nuclear Medicine Therapy is used to code this therapy using the radionuclide Iodine 131 or I-131. The body part being treated is the thyroid, body part value G. There are no 6th or 7th character values for this code. The correct code assignment is CW7GGZZ.

✓ **Check Your Understanding**

Coding Knowledge Check

1. Which root type is assigned to a bilateral mammogram procedure?_____

2. Which body system value and body part value are assigned to the following procedure:

   Body system: _____

   Body part: _____

MRI OF THE PELVIS WITHOUT CONTRAST

HISTORY: Vaginal lump in the midline that the patient has noticed for a week

FINDINGS: The uterus is of normal size and demonstrates no obvious mass or leiomyoma involving it. The ovaries are of normal size and demonstrate numerous small follicular cysts within both of them, which is a normal finding. With regard to the vagina, there is no obvious mass or adenopathy noted involving the vagina. There is no definite MRI evidence of a diverticulum of the urethra. The urinary bladder is not well distended with urine, and hence evaluation is somewhat limited. Given this limitation, no definite abnormality of the urinary bladder is seen.

IMPRESSION: MRI evaluation of the pelvis demonstrates normal appearance of the uterus and ovaries. No intravenous mass or cyst impressing on the vagina, nor is there any definite evidence of urethral diverticulum.

3. Positron emission tomography is a procedure in which section of ICD-10-PCS?
   a. Computerized Tomography
   b. Imaging
   c. Nuclear Medicine
   d. Radiation Therapy

4. The one therapeutic nuclear medicine procedure is which root type? _____

5. True or false? The Imaging section of ICD-10-PCS is organized first by body system, with each root type listed within that body system.

_____

Case Studies

Assign ICD-10-PCS codes to the following case studies.

1. Procedure Report

INDICATION FOR PROCEDURE: Renal vascular hypertension

PROCEDURE PERFORMED: Bilateral renal angiograms and right renal angioplasty

REPORT OF RADIOLOGIST: The risks and benefits of the procedure were discussed with the patient and both oral and written consents were obtained. The right groin was prepped and draped in a sterile fashion and a 15 French pigtail catheter was advanced into the aorta to approximately the L1-L2 level. A cut film angiogram was performed followed by a DSA study. These showed a very tight, probably 80–90 percent, stenosis at the junction of the proximal and middle third of the main right renal artery. The artery showed slight nodularity in this area with a second milder lesion of approximately 20 percent stenosis just past the more severe narrowing. This appearance, coupled with the patient's age, makes fibromuscular dysplasia the most likely diagnosis. The patient has single renal arteries on both sides. The left renal artery is normal in appearance. The aorta and proximal iliac arteries are normal.

Next, a 5 French Cobra catheter was used to enter the orifice of the right renal artery, and a TAD wire was inserted through the catheter across the area of tight stenosis. The patient was given 3,000 units of IV heparin just before the stenosis was crossed. Next, a Cobra catheter was advanced through the lesion and the TAD wire was exchanged for a Rosen wire. The Cobra catheter was then exchanged for a 4 mm diameter by 2 cm long low profile Meditech balloon. This balloon was inserted to the area of tight stenosis and it was inflated several times to a maximum of 7 atmospheres. After dilatation, the Rosen wire was exchanged for a 021 straight wire, and the balloon catheter was withdrawn so that it was proximal to the lesion. An angiogram was done through the balloon catheter that showed no complications and dramatic improvement in the degree of stenosis. Next, the wire and the balloon catheter were withdrawn and a 5 French pigtail was reinserted. A repeat DSA angiogram was performed. The final images showed some slight irregularity of the right renal artery in the angioplasty site with minimal residual stenosis measuring approximately 10 percent. No complications were identified.

RADIOLOGIC DIAGNOSIS: Successful angioplasty of very tight lesion in the proximal to mid right renal artery. This lesion is most likely due to fibromuscular dysplasia. After angioplasty there is a mild irregularity of the right renal artery with approximately 10 percent residual stenosis.

2. Procedure Report

PROCEDURE:	1. Right femoral arterial access
	2. Selective coronary angiograms
	3. PTCA/stent 3.0 × 28 mm bare-metal stent proximal RCA for final reference diameter 3.30 mm
	4. PTCA/stent mid RCA with 3.0 × 12 mm bare-metal stent with final reference diameter 3.30 mm
	5. Left heart catheterization
	6. Intra-aortic balloon pump placement
INDICATIONS:	1. Chest pain
	2. STEMI
COMPLICATIONS:	None
ESTIMATED BLOOD LOSS:	Less than 50 mL
FLUOROSCOPY CONTRAST:	Optiray
SEDATION:	Conscious local

DESCRIPTION OF PROCEDURE: Informed consent obtained from the patient. Written informed consent obtained from patient. Provided risk of procedure to include but not limited to bleeding, infection, hematoma, deep venous thrombosis, pulmonary embolism, limb or organ dysfunction, limb loss, kidney failure, permanent dialysis, stroke, arrhythmia, myocardial infarction, allergic reaction, respiratory complication, death. The patient was aware of risk and agreeable to proceed. The patient brought to catheterization laboratory, attached to continuous monitoring oxygen saturation, blood pressure, heart rhythm. The patient prepped sterile fashion. Right groin anesthetized 1 percent Xylocaine. Using modified Seldinger technique, micropuncture kit used to obtain access to right common femoral artery, upsized 7-French sheath, properly aspirated and flushed. JL-4 diagnostic catheter used to engage left coronary artery. Selective angiogram performed. This exchanged over the wire for JR-4 guide catheter 6-French used to engage right coronary. Selective angiogram performed in multiple views as well.

Next, BMW wire was attempted to pass the RCA occlusion; however, this was not possible so this was exchanged for a pilot wire which successfully negotiated past the occlusion. Angiogram performed and wire placement was confirmed. A 2.5 × 12 balloon used to perform inflation in the proximal RCA. This was removed. Subsequent angiograms demonstrated residual stenosis. There was some size discrepancy between the proximal and mid RCA. A 3.0 × 28 mm bare-metal stent, Vision, was deployed at the lesion site and inflated to nominal pressures. TIMI 3 flow was finally obtained. In the mid to distal RCA, there was an eccentric 80 percent stenosis, so the 2.5 × 12 balloon was carefully taken past the proximal stent and positioned. This more distal lesion inflated at nominal pressures. The balloon was then removed and a 3.0 × 12 mm bare-metal stent, Vision, was positioned in the distal RCA and dilated at nominal atmospheres. This stent balloon was then removed. Next, a noncompliant 3.25 × 12 balloon was positioned within the stent margins and was inflated at pressures for a reference diameter 3.30 mm. This balloon was then removed. Next, a 3.25 × 20 noncompliant balloon was positioned within the proximal stent margins and inflated to the rated stent diameter in overlapping fashion. It should be noted the patient was on aspirin, Plavix, and Angiomax for the procedure as well as received nitroglycerin intracoronary at various times throughout the procedure. Pigtail catheter was used to perform left heart catheterization and the LV pressures measured and pullback across the aortic valve recorded. There were acceptable results, so the equipment was removed from the right coronary and sheath upsized to balloon pump sheath. Balloon pump was positioned in the descending aorta appropriately and catheter and balloon pump sutured into place. The patient transferred for further care to ICU.

FINDINGS: Hemodynamic data: Rest AO of 120/78 mm Hg. LV 121/22 mm Hg. No aortic valve gradient. Left ventricular angiogram was not performed due to unknown renal function.

SELECTIVE CORONARY ANGIOGRAM: Left main coronary approximately 8 mm in length before bifurcating left anterior descending artery and left circumflex coronary artery. Left anterior descending artery is a large vessel, reaches the apex. It gives rise to large septal branch and distally the LAD gives off a larger diagonal branch. There are left-to-right collaterals via septal, which are faint. Left circumflex nondominant vessel, large vessel. The AV groove branch is smaller. Large obtuse marginal branch. The left circumflex and its branches angiographically normal. Right coronary artery dominant vessel, large vessel, occluded proximally with TIMI 0 flow. After establishing flow, there is a plaque rupture proximally. The mid RCA has an eccentric 80 percent stenosis TIMI 2 to 3 flow. Distally the RCA has a medium-sized posterolateral ventricular branch with luminal irregularities and large posterior descending artery with mild luminal irregularities. Remainder of the right coronary has mild luminal irregularities. There is an RV branch mid-vessel as well.

CONCLUSION:

1. Successful PTCA/stenting of proximal RCA with reduction of 100 percent occlusion to 0 percent residual stenosis, TIMI 3 flow. No edge dissection. No distal emboli. Using a Vision 3.0 × 28 mm bare-metal stent final reference diameter 3.30 mm.

2. Successful PTCA/stenting of distal right coronary artery with reduction of 80 percent eccentric stenosis to 0 percent with TIMI 3 flow.

RECOMMENDATIONS:

1. Will continue intra-aortic balloon pump and maximize medical therapy.

2. The patient has ICU admission.

3. Procedure Report

PROCEDURE: Left heart catheterization, coronary angiography, left ventriculography, and attempted PTCA of the right posterior lateral branch

INDICATIONS: This is a 29-year-old male who presented to this hospital earlier this morning with evolving acute inferior myocardial infarction. The symptoms improved with morphine and nitrates, aspirin, and thrombolytic therapy earlier today but had no evidence of reperfusion by total EKG or reperfusion arrhythmias. He was still having low-grade arm discomfort when he was transferred for attempted salvage revascularization.

PROCEDURE DETAILS: Informed consent was obtained. He was brought to the cardiac catheterization suite, prepped, and draped in the usual sterile manner. 1 percent Xylocaine was used for local anesthesia. A 6 French sheath was placed in the right femoral artery by the modified Seldinger technique. Coronary angiography was performed with Omnipaque using the Judkins 5 French four curved left angiographic catheters. We then checked the baseline ACT, gave 5,000 units of intra-arterial heparin and subsequent ACT in 2 hours and 50 seconds. A 6 French JR-4 guiding catheter was chosen and a 300-cm, 14 reflux guidewire was used to cross the stenosis in the distal right posterolateral branch with some difficulty.

We performed a total of four inflations with a 2.0 × 20 mm rocket balloon without evidence of restoration of flow. He received 400 mcg of intracoronary nitroglycerin in three divided doses. The symptoms had not changed. He was thought to be clinically stable. This is a small vessel in the distal distribution. It is thought not prudent to warrant further attempted angioplasty. The dilating catheters, the guidewire, and the guiding catheter were removed. A 5 French straight pigtail catheter was advanced to the left ventricle for pressure recordings. Single plain left ventriculogram was performed in the right anterior oblique using power-inducted contrast. Pull-back across the aortic valve revealed no gradient. The sheath was secured. The patient was taken to the holding area in hemodynamically stable condition with intact distal pulses.

RESULTS:

PRESSURES: Aortic pressure 120/70. Left ventricular pressure 120/80.

LEFT VENTRICULOGRAPHY: Single plain left ventriculography reveals inferobasal hypokinesis with an ejection fraction estimated to be 50 percent without mitral regurgitation.

CORONARY ANGIOGRAPHY: Left main: Left main coronary divided into the left anterior descending artery (LAD) and circumflex vessel and is normal.

Left anterior descending artery gives rise to two diagonal branches in the central perforator branch and traverses to an apical recurrent branch. There is a 40 percent tapering at the proximal aspect of the first diagonal branch, otherwise there are no flow-limiting lesions in the LAD, diagonal system.

LEFT CIRCUMFLEX: Left circumflex coronary artery consists of one very high obtuse marginal branch as well as subsequent second and third obtuse marginal branches and atrioventricular groove continuation and is normal.

RIGHT CORONARY: Right coronary artery is a dominant vessel for the posterior circulation giving rise to a posterior descending artery, posterior lateral left ventricular branch, and right ventricular marginal branches as well as atrial branches. There is a 20 percent taper in the proximal right coronary artery and a flush occlusion in the mid to distal segment of the right posterolateral branch with some staining of contrast present there.

POST PTCA OF THE RIGHT POSTERIOR LATERAL BRANCH: There is no significant change with persistent TIMI grade 0 flow in the small distal vessel, which is judged to be approximately 2.0 to 2.2 mm. There is no disruption in the main body of the right coronary artery as a result of procedure.

IMPRESSION:

1. Evolution of acute inferior myocardial infarction secondary to occluded distal right posterior lateral branch with unsuccessful attempted salvage (PTCA after failing thrombolytic therapy)

2. Preserved left ventricular systolic function

3. Family history of heart disease and tobacco use

---

4. Procedure Report

PREOPERATIVE DIAGNOSIS: Unstable progressive angina pectoris, markedly abnormal thallium exercise test, 95 percent circumflex coronary artery stenosis

POSTOPERATIVE DIAGNOSIS: Unstable progressive angina pectoris, markedly abnormal thallium exercise test, 95 percent circumflex coronary artery stenosis

PROCEDURE: PTCA of left circumflex with stent placement

CONTRAST MEDIA: Low osmolar

PROCEDURE DETAILS: Following 1 percent Xylocaine local anesthesia in the left femoral region using the Seldinger technique, 8 French sheaths were inserted in the left femoral artery and vein. A 7 French Swan-Ganz catheter was advanced in antegrade fashion through the right heart chambers and positioned in the pulmonary artery. Selective left coronary angiography was performed with a 8Fr JL4 curved short tipped guiding catheter, after which time a 0.014 inch microglide exchange wire was passed down the length of the circumflex coronary artery and a 2.5 mm Shadow balloon dilatation catheter was advanced over the wire and inflated to a maximum of 9 atmospheres on multiple occasions. This balloon catheter was then removed and a 2.5-mm Cordis CYPHER drug-eluting stent was placed over a 3.0-mm compliant balloon catheter in the circumflex main trunk. This balloon was inflated to 9 atmospheres and kept inflated for 4.0 minutes. This balloon catheter was then removed and selective angiography was performed, which demonstrated excellent flow and run-off in the circumflex and no evidence of occlusive type dissection. At this time, the arterial and venous sheaths were sutured in place and the patient was taken to the holding area of the catheterization laboratory without incident. There were no complications resulting from the procedure.

Physical Rehabilitation and Diagnostic Audiology, Mental Health, Substance Abuse Treatment, and New Technology

The 1st character values for these sections are:

F—Physical Rehabilitation and Diagnostic Audiology
G—Mental Health
H—Substance Abuse Treatment
X—New Technology

Types of Procedures Included in these Sections

The procedures included in this section may not be coded in all facilities. This chapter will introduce the coding concepts necessary to assign codes. Coding professionals who are required by their facility to assign these codes should refer to the tables and the complete definitions in the code set.

These sections include codes for a variety of procedures, such as:

- Motor function assessments
- Device fittings
- Electroconvulsive therapy
- Psychotherapy
- Individual counseling
- Detoxification services
- New technologies

Character Definition for the Physical Rehabilitation Section (F)

Character 1	Character 2	Character 3	Character 4	Character 5	Character 6	Character 7
Section	Section Qualifier	Root Type	Body System and Region	Type Qualifier	Equipment	Qualifier

Section Qualifiers Used in the Physical Rehabilitation and Diagnostic Audiology Section

This section contains codes for a combination of two separate subjects, Physical Rehabilitation and Diagnostic Audiology. Physical Rehabilitation and Diagnostic Audiology section codes should be coded for discharges from long-term acute hospitals and inpatient rehabilitation units, as these codes are an important factor in the assignment of MS-DRGs for these admissions. These subjects are not body systems as described in other sections of ICD-10-PCS. Therefore, the 2nd character has been labeled as a Section

Qualifier to distinguish between these two subjects in the code assignment. The 2nd character values used in the Physical Rehabilitation and Diagnostic Audiology section for the Section Qualifier are:

0 = Rehabilitation
1 = Diagnostic Audiology

Common Root Types Used in the Physical Rehabilitation and Diagnostic Audiology Section

The root types for Physical Rehabilitation and Diagnostic Audiology include root types for both assessment and treatment. The definition of each root operation is as follows:

Root Type

Activities of Daily Living Assessment (2): Measurement of functional level for activities of daily living.

Activities of Daily Living Treatment (8): Exercise or activities to facilitate functional competence for activities of daily living.

Caregiver Training (F): Training in activities to support patient's optimal level of function.

Cochlear Implant Treatment (B): Application of techniques to improve the communication abilities of individuals with cochlear implant.

Device Fitting (D): Fitting of a device designed to facilitate or support achievement of a higher level of function.

Hearing Assessment (3): Measurement of hearing and related functions.

Hearing Aid Assessment (4): Measurement of the appropriateness and/or effectiveness of a hearing device.

Hearing Treatment (9): Application of techniques to improve, augment, or compensate for hearing and related functional impairment.

Motor Treatment (7): Exercise or activities to increase or facilitate motor function.

Motor and/or Nerve Function Assessment (1): Measurement of motor, nerve, and related functions.

Speech Assessment (0): Measurement of speech and related functions.

Speech Treatment (6): Application of techniques to improve, augment, or compensate for speech and related functional impairment.

Vestibular Assessment (5): Measurement of the vestibular system and related functions.

Vestibular Treatment (C): Application of techniques to improve, augment, or compensate for vestibular and related functional impairment.

Coding Tip

The procedures to fit a device, such as splints and braces, as described in F0DZ6EZ and F0DZ7EZ, apply only to the rehabilitation setting. Splints and braces placed in other inpatient settings are coded to Immobilization, table 2W3 in the Placement section.

Body System and Regions for Physical Rehabilitation and Diagnostic Audiology Section

The 4th character value for the Physical Rehabilitation and Diagnostic Audiology sections is called the Body System and Region value. This value is subdivided for the Physical Rehabilitation section qualifier. The groupings divide the body into the Neurological system, Circulatory system, Respiratory system, Integumentary system,

Musculoskeletal system, Genitourinary system, and None (as shown in table 25.1). This value is not defined for the Diagnostic Audiology section qualifier.

Table 25.1. Body system and region values

Body System and Region Value	Body Systems and Regions—Rehabilitation (0)
0	Neurological System—Head and Neck
1	Neurological System—Upper Back/Upper Extremity
2	Neurological System—Lower Back/Lower Extremity
3	Neurological System—Whole Body
4	Circulatory System—Head and Neck
5	Circulatory System—Upper Back/Upper Extremity
6	Circulatory System—Lower Back/Lower Extremity
7	Circulatory System—Whole Body
8	Respiratory System—Head and Neck
9	Respiratory System—Upper Back/Upper Extremity
B	Respiratory System—Lower Back/Lower Extremity
C	Respiratory System—Whole Body
D	Integumentary System—Head and Neck
F	Integumentary System—Upper Back/Upper Extremity
G	Integumentary System—Lower Back/Lower Extremity
H	Integumentary System—Whole Body
J	Musculoskeletal System—Head and Neck
K	Musculoskeletal System—Upper Back/Upper Extremity
L	Musculoskeletal System—Lower Back/Lower Extremity
M	Musculoskeletal System—Whole Body
N	Genitourinary System
Z	None

Body System and Region Value	Body Systems and Regions—Diagnostic Audiology (1)
Z	None

5th Character Type Qualifiers Common to the Physical Rehabilitation and Diagnostic Audiology Section

The 5th character value is the type qualifier in Physical Rehabilitation and Diagnostic Audiology section. This character provides extensive subdivisions for the types of services described in the 3rd character of root type. Summary tables are not provided here because it is best to view the type character values in context with their root type and specific body system/region. Please refer to the tables in Section F of the code set for examples of the different type qualifiers available.

6th Character Equipment Common to the Physical Rehabilitation and Diagnostic Audiology Section

The 6th character value is the equipment used to perform the services and procedures coded in the Physical Rehabilitation and Diagnostic Audiology section. The equipment value is specific to the unique combination of the 3rd, 4th, and 5th characters that precede it. As with the 5th character, summary tables are not provided here because it is best to view the equipment values in context with their root type, specific body system/region, and type qualifier values. Please refer to the tables in Section F of the code set for examples of the different equipment values available.

Qualifiers Used in the Physical Rehabilitation and Diagnostic Audiology Section

For Physical Rehabilitation and Diagnostic Audiology, the 7th character qualifier is always Z, None.

Character Definition for the Mental Health Section (G)

Character 1	Character 2	Character 3	Character 4	Character 5	Character 6	Character 7
Section	Body System	Root Type	Type Qualifier	Qualifier	Qualifier	Qualifier

The Mental Health section of ICD-10-PCS provides codes only for one system, and, therefore, the 2nd character value for the Mental Health section is always Z, None to maintain the code structure.

Common Root Types Used in the Mental Health Section

There are 12 root type values used to describe mental health services. The definition of each root type is discussed in the following section:

Root Type

Biofeedback (C): Provision of information from the monitoring and regulating of physiological processes in conjunction with cognitive-behavioral techniques to improve patient functioning or well-being.

Includes/Examples: Includes EEG, blood pressure, skin temperature or peripheral blood flow, ECG, electroculogram, EMG, respirometry or capnometry, GSR/EDR, perineometry to monitor/regulate bowel/bladder activity, electrogastrogram to monitor/regulate gastric motility.

Counseling (6): The application of psychological methods to treat an individual with normal developmental issues and psychological problems in order to increase function, improve well-being, alleviate distress or maladjustment, or resolve crises.

Crisis Intervention (2): Treatment of a traumatized, acutely disturbed or distressed individual for the purpose of short-term stabilization.

Includes/Examples: Includes defusing, debriefing, counseling, psychotherapy and/or coordination of care with other providers or agencies.

Electroconvulsive Therapy (B): The application of controlled electrical voltages to treat a mental health disorder.

Includes/Examples: Includes appropriate sedation and other preparation of the individual.

Family Psychotherapy (7): Treatment that includes one or more family members of an individual with a mental health disorder by behavioral, cognitive, psychoanalytic, psychodynamic, or psychophysiological means to improve functioning or well-being.

Explanation: Remediation of emotional or behavioral problems presented by one or more family members in cases were psychotherapy with more than one family member is indicated.

Group Psychotherapy (H): Treatment of two or more individuals with a mental health disorder by behavioral, cognitive, psychoanalytic, psychodynamic, or psychophysiological means to improve functioning or well-being.

Hypnosis (F): Induction of a state of heightened suggestibility by auditory, visual, and tactile techniques to elicit an emotional or behavioral response.

Individual Psychotherapy (5): Treatment of an individual with a mental health disorder by behavioral, cognitive, psychoanalytic, psychodynamic, or psychophysiological means to improve functioning or well-being.

Light Therapy (J): Application of specialized light treatments to improve functioning or well-being.

Medication Management (3): Monitoring and adjusting the use of medications for the treatment of a mental health disorder.

Narcosynthesis (G): Administration of intravenous barbiturates in order to release suppressed or repressed thoughts.

Psychological Testing (1): The administration and interpretation of standardized psychological tests and measurement instruments for the assessment of psychological function.

The following are examples of various psychological tests that can be administered and their corresponding character 4 type qualifier value names:

- Developmental test examples
  - Developmental Screening Test II (Denver, DDST II)
  - Early Language Milestone Screen (ELM)
  - Parent Evaluation of Developmental Status (PEDS)
  - Ages and Stages (ASQ)
  - Vanderbilt ADHD Rating Scales
  - Clinical Adaptive Test (CAT)
  - Clinical Linguistic and Auditory Milestone Scales (CLAMS)
  - Bayley Scales of Infant Development
  - Mullen Scales of Early Learning
  - Peabody Picture Vocabulary Test (PPVT)
  - Vineland Adaptive Behavior Scales
- Personality and behavioral test examples
  - Minnesota Multiphasic Personality Inventory (MMPI)
  - Personality Assessment Inventory (PAI)
- Intellectual and psychoeducational test examples
  - Wechsler Adult Intelligence Scale (WAIS)
  - Wechsler Intelligence Scale for Children (WISC)
  - Shipley Scale
- Neuropsychological test examples
  - Halstead-Reitan Neuropsychological Battery
  - Wechsler Memory Scales
  - Wisconsin Card Sorting Test
- Neurobehavioral and cognitive status test example
  - Neurobehavioral Cognitive Status Exam (NCSE) (Kuehn 2011)

Type Qualifiers Used in the Mental Health Section

Behavioral	Primarily to modify behavior. *Includes/Examples*: Includes modeling and role playing, positive reinforcement of target behaviors, response cost, and training of self-management skills.
Cognitive	Primarily to correct cognitive distortions and errors.

Cognitive-behavioral	Combining cognitive and behavioral treatment strategies to improve functioning. *Explanation*: Maladaptive responses are examined to determine how cognitions relate to behavior patterns in response to an event. Uses learning principles and information-processing models.
Developmental	Age-normed developmental status of cognitive, social, and adaptive behavior skills.
Intellectual and psycho-educational	Intellectual abilities, academic achievement, and learning capabilities (including behaviors and emotional factors affecting learning).
Interactive	Uses primarily physical aids and other forms of non-oral interaction with a patient who is physically, psychologically, or developmentally unable to use ordinary language for communication. *Includes/Examples*: Includes the use of toys in symbolic play.
Interpersonal	Helps an individual make changes in interpersonal behaviors to reduce psychological dysfunction. *Includes/Examples*: Includes exploratory techniques, encouragement of affective expression, clarification of patient statements, analysis of communication patterns, use of therapy relationship, and behavior change techniques.
Neurobehavioral and cognitive status	Includes neurobehavioral status exam, interview(s), and observation for the clinical assessment of thinking, reasoning and judgment, acquired knowledge, attention, memory, visual spatial abilities, language functions, and planning.
Neuropsychological	Thinking, reasoning, and judgment, acquired knowledge, attention, memory, visual spatial abilities, language functions, and planning.
Personality and behavioral	Mood, emotion, behavior, social functioning, psychopathological conditions, personality traits, and characteristics.
Psychoanalysis	Methods of obtaining a detailed account of past and present mental and emotional experiences to determine the source and eliminate or diminish the undesirable effects of unconscious conflicts. *Explanation*: Accomplished by making the individual aware of the existence, origin, and inappropriate expression of emotions and behavior.
Psychodynamic	Exploration of past and present emotional experiences to understand motives and drives using insight-oriented techniques to reduce the undesirable effects of internal conflicts on emotions and behavior. *Explanation*: Techniques include empathetic listening, clarifying self-defeating behavior patterns, and exploring adaptive alternatives.
Psychophysiological	Monitoring and alteration of physiological processes to help the individual associate physiological reactions combined with cognitive and behavioral strategies to gain improved control of these processes to help the individual cope more effectively.
Supportive	Formation of therapeutic relationship primarily for providing emotional support to prevent further deterioration in functioning during periods of particular stress. *Explanation*: Often used in conjunction with other therapeutic approaches.
Vocational	Exploration of vocational interests, aptitudes, and required adaptive behavior skills to develop and carry out a plan for achieving a successful vocational placement. *Includes/Examples*: Includes enhancing work-related adjustment and/or pursuing viable options in training education or preparation.

Table 25.2 and table 25.3 list the type qualifier values available for specific root types for coding within the Mental Health section of ICD-10-PCS. The type qualifier value for the root types of Crisis intervention, Hypnosis, Medication management, Narcosynthesis, Group Psychotherapy, and Light Therapy is Z, None.

Table 25.2. Type qualifier values for Psychological Testing, Psychotherapy, and Counseling

Type Qualifier Value	Mental Health—Psychological Tests (1)
0	Developmental
1	Personality and Behavioral
2	Intellectual and Psychoeducational
3	Neuropsychological
4	Neurobehavioral and Cognitive Status

Type Qualifier Value	Mental Health—Counseling (6)
0	Educational
1	Vocational
3	Other Counseling

Type Qualifier Value	Mental Health—Individual Psychotherapy (5)
0	Interactive
1	Behavioral
2	Cognitive
3	Interpersonal
4	Psychoanalysis
5	Psychodynamic
6	Supportive
8	Cognitive-behavioral
9	Psychophysiological

Table 25.3. Type qualifier values for Family Psychotherapy, Electroconvulsive Therapy, and Biofeedback

Type Qualifier Value	Mental Health—Family Psychotherapy (7)
2	Other Family Psychotherapy

Type Qualifier Value	Mental Health—Biofeedback (C)
9	Other Biofeedback

Type Qualifier Value	Mental Health—Electroconvulsive Therapy (B)
0	Unilateral-single Seizure
1	Unilateral-multiple Seizure
2	Bilateral-single Seizure
3	Bilateral-multiple Seizure
4	Other Electroconvulsive Therapy

5th, 6th, and 7th Character Qualifiers Used in the Mental Health Section

The 5th character through the 7th character of a Mental Health section code is not currently defined and is reported using the qualifier value Z, None.

Character Definition for the Substance Abuse Treatment Section (H)

Character 1	Character 2	Character 3	Character 4	Character 5	Character 6	Character 7
Section	Body System	Root Type	Type Qualifier	Qualifier	Qualifier	Qualifier

The Substance Abuse Treatment section of ICD-10-PCS provides codes only for one system, and, therefore, the 2nd character value for this section is always Z, None to maintain the code structure.

Common Root Types Used in the Substance Abuse Treatment Section

There are seven root type values used to describe substance abuse treatment services. The definition of each root type is as follows:

Detoxification Services (2): Detoxification from alcohol and/or drugs:

Explanation: Not a treatment modality, but helps the patient stabilize physically and psychologically until the body becomes free of drugs and the effects of alcohol

Individual Counseling (3): The application of psychological methods to treat an individual with addictive behavior:

Explanation: Comprised of several different techniques, which apply various strategies to address drug addiction

Group Counseling (4): The application of psychological methods to treat two or more individuals with addictive behavior:

Explanation: Provides structured group counseling sessions and healing power through the connection with others

Individual Psychotherapy (5): Treatment of an individual with addictive behavior by behavioral, cognitive, psychoanalytic, psychodynamic or psychophysiological means

Family Counseling (6): The application of psychological methods that includes one or more family members to treat an individual with addictive behavior:

Explanation: Provides support and education for family members of addicted individuals. Family members' participation is seen as a critical area of substance abuse treatment

Medication Management (8): Monitoring and adjusting the use of replacement medications for the treatment of addiction

Pharmacotherapy (9): The use of replacement medications for the treatment of addiction

Type Qualifiers for the Substance Abuse Treatment Section

Table 25.4 and table 25.5 list the type qualifier values available for specific root types for coding within the Substance Abuse Treatment section of ICD-10-PCS. The type qualifier value for the root type Detoxification (2) is always Z, None.

Table 25.4. Type qualifier values for Individual/Group Counseling/Individual Psychotherapy

Type Qualifier Value	Substance Abuse Treatment— Individual Counseling (3) and Group Counseling (4)	Type Qualifier Value	Substance Abuse Treatment— Individual Psychotherapy (5)
0	Cognitive	0	Cognitive
1	Behavioral	1	Behavioral
2	Cognitive-Behavioral	2	Cognitive-Behavioral
3	12-Step	3	12-Step
4	Interpersonal	4	Interpersonal
5	Vocational	5	Interactive
6	Psychoeducation	6	Psychoeducation
7	Motivational Enhancement	7	Motivational Enhancement
8	Confrontational	8	Confrontational
9	Continuing Care	9	Supportive
B	Spiritual	B	Psychoanalysis
C	Pre/Post-Test Infectious Disease	C	Psychodynamic
		D	Psychophysiological

Table 25.5. Type qualifier values for Family Counseling/Medication Management/Pharmacotherapy

Type Qualifier Value	Substance Abuse Treatment—Family Counseling (6)		Type Qualifier Value	Substance Abuse Treatment—Medication Management (8) and Pharmacotherapy (9)
3	Other Family Counseling		0	Nicotine Replacement
			1	Methadone Maintenance
			2	Levo-alpha-acetyl-methadol (LAAM)
			3	Antabuse
			4	Naltrexone
			5	Naloxone
			6	Clonidine
			7	Bupropion
			8	Psychiatric Medication
			9	Other Replacement Medication

5th, 6th, and 7th Qualifier Characters Used in the Substance Abuse Treatment Section

The 5th character through the 7th character of a substance abuse treatment code is not currently defined and is reported using the qualifier value of Z, None.

Character Definition for the New Technology Section (X)

Character 1	Character 2	Character 3	Character 4	Character 5	Character 6	Character 7
Section	Body System/Region	Root Operation	Body Part	Approach	Device/Substance/Technology	Qualifier

The New Technology section contains codes for services that are new to ICD-10-PCS or that capture services not routinely captured in ICD-10-PCS that have been presented for public comment at a Coordination and Maintenance Committee Meeting. These codes may be deleted in future years, after they have served their purpose, and may or may not be recreated into the body of ICD-10-PCS at a later date. These codes are meant to describe the procedure without the need for additional codes from another section. For example, XV508A4, which describes robotic water ablation, does not require an additional code from Section 8, Other Procedures for the use of the robot because this new technology service is only performed with the use of the robot and it is included in the Device/Substance/Technology character description.

Body Systems and Regions for New Technology Section

The 2nd character describes the body systems on which the New Technology operations can be performed. Table 25.6 displays the body systems included in this section.

Root Operations for New Technology Section

The third character contains the root operations appropriate for the New Technology section. They retain the same definition as found within the main body of ICD-10-PCS. Table 25.7 displays the root operations for New Technology.

Table 25.6. Body systems in the New Technology section

Body System Value	Body Systems
2	Cardiovascular System
H	Skin, Subcutaneous Tissue, Fascia and Breast
K	Muscles, Tendons, Bursae And Ligaments
N	Bones
R	Joints
V	Male Reproductive
W	Anatomical Regions
Y	Extracorporeal

Table 25.7. Root operations in the New Technology section

Root Operation Value	Root Operations—New Technology (X)
0	Introduction
2	Monitoring
5	Destruction
A	Assistance
C	Extirpation
G	Fusion
R	Replacement
S	Reposition

Approach Character for New Technology Section

The fifth character describes the approaches used to reach the body part for the procedure. Open, Percutaneous, Percutaneous Endoscopic, Via Natural or Artificial Opening Endoscopic and External are the approaches identified for procedures coded in this section. All of these approaches use the same definition used within the remainder of ICD-10-PCS.

Device/Substance/Technology Character for New Technology Section

The sixth character describes the devices, substances, or technologies identified in the code. This character describes devices that are used in the procedure or substances that are introduced into the body part. Table 25.8 displays these values in the New Technology section.

Table 25.8. Device/substance/technology values for New Technology section

Device/Substance/Technology Value	Device/Substance/Technology—New Technology (X)
0	Concentrated Bone Marrow Aspirate
1	Cerebral Embolic Filtration, Dual Filter
2	Ceftazidime-Avibactam Anti-infective
2	Intraoperative Knee Replacement Sensor
3	Idarucizumab, Dabigatran Reversal Agent
3	Magnetically Controlled Growth Rod(S)
3	Zooplastic Tissue, Rapid Deployment Technique
4	Isavuconazole Anti-infective
5	Blinatumomab Antineoplastic Immunotherapy
6	Orbital Atherectomy Technology
7	Andexanet Alfa, Factor Xa Inhibitor Reversal Agent
8	Endothelial Damage Inhibitor
8	Uridine Triacetate
9	Interbody Fusion Device, Nanotextured Surface
9	Defibrotide Sodium Anticoagulant

(Continued)

Table 25.8. Device/substance/technology values for New Technology section (continued)

Device/Substance/Technology Value	Device/Substance/Technology—New Technology (X)
A	Bezlotoxumab Monoclonal Antibody
A	Robotic Waterjet Ablation
B	Cytarabine and Daunorubicin Liposome Antineoplastic
C	Engineered Autologous Chimeric Antigen Receptor T-cell Immunotherapy
F	Interbody Fusion Device, Radiolucent Porous
F	Other New Technology Therapeutic Substance
G	Plazomicin Anti-infective
H	Synthetic Human Angiotensin II
L	Skin Substitute, Porcine Liver Derived

Qualifiers Used in the New Technology Section

As new codes are added to this section, the qualifier value will describe the group in which the technology was added to this system. "For example, Section X codes added for the first year have the seventh character value 1, New Technology Group 1, and the next year that Section X codes are added have the seventh character value 2, New Technology Group 2, and so on" (CMS 2016b).

 Code Building

Case #1:

PROCEDURE STATEMENT: Speech therapy for aphasia

ADDITIONAL INFORMATION: The therapist assists the patient with learning to use a communication board technique.

ROOT AND TABLE LOCATION FOR THE STATEMENT: Speech treatment is the root type used to code this procedure, defined as application of techniques to improve, augment, or compensate for speech and related functional impairment. The table location is:

Physical Rehabilitation and Diagnostic Audiology (F)

> Rehabilitation (0)
>
> > Speech Treatment (6)
> >
> > None (Z)

Code Characters:

Section	Section Qualifier	Root Type	Body System and Region	Type Qualifier	Equipment	Qualifier
Physical Rehabilitation and Diagnostic Audiology	Rehabilitation	Speech Treatment	None	Aphasia	Augmentative/ Alternative Communication	None
F	0	6	Z	3	M	Z

RATIONALE FOR THE ANSWER: The root type Speech Treatment is used to code this procedure. This root type is found in the Rehabilitation subsection of the Physical Rehabilitation and Diagnostic Audiology section of ICD-10-PCS. The communication board is augmentative/alternative communication equipment. The correct code assignment is F06Z3MZ.

Case #2:

PROCEDURE STATEMENT: Pharmacotherapy for substance abuse

ADDITIONAL INFORMATION: The patient is treated with methadone maintenance for heroin dependency.

ROOT AND INDEX ENTRIES FOR THE STATEMENT: Pharmacotherapy is the root type used to code this procedure, defined as the use of replacement medications for the treatment of addiction. The Index entry is:

Pharmacotherapy, for substance abuse

Methadone Maintenance HZ91ZZZ

Code Characters:

Section	Body System	Root Type	Type Qualifier	Qualifier	Qualifier	Qualifier
Substance Abuse Treatment	None	Pharmaco-therapy	Methadone Maintenance	None	None	None
H	Z	9	1	Z	Z	Z

RATIONALE FOR THE ANSWER: Methadone maintenance works on the same opioid receptors as the heroin that the patient is dependent on. The root type Pharmacotherapy is used to code the procedure of treating the dependence with the methadone substitute. The correct code assignment is HZ91ZZZ.

Case #3:

PROCEDURE STATEMENT: Hypnotherapy

ADDITIONAL INFORMATION: The patient is undergoing hypnosis to treat anxiety attacks.

ROOT AND INDEX ENTRIES FOR THE STATEMENT: Hypnosis is the root type used to code this procedure, defined as induction of a state of heightened suggestibility by auditory, visual, and tactile techniques to elicit an emotional or behavioral response. The Index entry is:

Hypnosis GZFZZZZ

Code Characters:

Section	Body System	Root Type	Type Qualifier	Qualifier	Qualifier	Qualifier
Mental Health	None	Hypnosis	None	None	None	None
G	Z	F	Z	Z	Z	Z

RATIONALE FOR THE ANSWER: Hypnosis is the root type used to code this procedure and is the main term in the index. The index lists the entire 7-character code. The correct code assignment is GZFZZZZ.

Check Your Understanding

Coding Knowledge Check

1. Adjustment of a cochlear implant is coded to which root type?_____

2. All of the procedures in the Mental Health section end in which three values? _____, _____,
   _____

Match each of the following terms to the correct definition:

3. _____ Vestibular treatment   a. Monitoring and adjusting the use of replacement medications for the treatment of addiction

4. _____ Crisis intervention   b. Application of psychological methods to treat an individual with addictive behavior

5. _____ Caregiver training   c. Application of techniques to improve, augment, or compensate for vestibular and related functional impairment

6. _____ Narcosynthesis   d. Application of specialized light treatments to improve functioning or well-being

7. _____ Individual counseling   e. Treatment of a traumatized, acutely disturbed, or distressed individual for the purpose of short-term stabilization

8. _____ Light therapy   f. Administration of intravenous barbiturates in order to release suppressed or repressed thoughts

   g. Training in activities to support patient's optimal level of function

9. The use of the rapid deployment technique to place a zooplastic heart valve is coded to the root operation of _____.

10. Procedure code XRGB092 describes fusion using what special technology?_____
    _____

Procedure Statement Coding

Assign ICD-10-PCS codes to the following procedure statements and scenarios. List the root operation selected and the code assigned.

1. Bilateral electroshock therapy creating a single seizure

2. Custom fabrication and fitting of a static ankle orthesis

3. Admission for acute alcohol intoxication with detox

4. Group counseling on interpersonal relationships for those with substance addiction

(Continued)

5. Open placement of magnetically controlled growth rods on both sides of the thoracic spine to straighten the spine due to scoliosis

6. Training in exercises to strengthen neck muscles following a whiplash injury

7. Administration of WAIS testing

8. Atherectomy performed on two coronary artery sites using percutaneous orbital technology

9. Therapy for motor skill improvement with transfers using adaptive techniques

10. Introduction of Andexant Alfa Factor Xa Inhibitor Reverse Agent into a peripheral IV line to treat a life-threatening bleed from Xarelto.

Case Studies

Assign ICD-10-PCS codes to the following case studies.

1. Operative Report

DIAGNOSES: Spinal stenosis of cervical region

PROCEDURES: 1. C4-C5 arthrodesis anterior interbody including discectomy with COHERE
2. Anterior instrumentation two vertebral segments

IMPLANTS: 1. COHERE polyetheretherketone (PEEK) radiolucent, porous 6 mm cage
2. Hyper-C anterior cervical plate
3. Bone allograft

OPERATION: The patient was taken to the Operating Room and placed in the supine position. General endotracheal anesthesia was obtained. The patient had the usual monitors placed. The patient was then positioned with shoulder roll and neck gently extended. The patient then had the left side of her neck marked with an incision at the level of the cricoid cartilage. She was prepped and draped in a sterile fashion. Timeout was done per protocol confirming the correct patient and all equipment needed was present and correct procedure was confirmed. The patient then had the incision injected with local and then opened. Dissection was carried down through the platysma, which was undermined and hemostasis was obtained using bipolar cautery and Bovie. The plane between the sternocleidomastoid muscle and the strap muscles was developed with salvage of the external jugular vein. Once the area was exposed, the omohyoid muscle was bisected. This allowed entry into the prevertebral space, which was opened and the disc space was identified at C4-C5. The disc space was cauterized and then the longus colli muscles were mobilized bilaterally.

The discectomy was begun using a #15 blade scalpel and pituitary rongeurs and curettes, and then the approach was made from the right side and the distracting pins were placed in the vertebral bodies of

C4 and C5. The microscope and the drill were used to decorticate the endplates all way back to the posterior longitudinal ligament, which was lifted up and incised and then removed. Nerve roots were free in the foramen, without osteophytes. The patient then had the sizers used and the 6 mm trial was felt to be appropriate for C4-C5, and the patient had this assessed using fluoroscopy and it was noted to be in good position. The bone allograft was hydrated. The trial was removed and the bone graft was impacted into place with Grafton Putty superiorly and inferiorly, and then their position was checked using fluoroscopy and noted to be good. The patient was taken out of extension and then the Hyper-C anterior cervical plate was chosen and was secured using holding pins and this showed that the plate appeared to have good alignment and good trajectory. The screws were then placed and again the trajectory was checked and adjusted as needed. All the final tightening was done. The wound was irrigated out and the drain was brought out through a separate stab wound. The wound was closed in multiple layers over the drain and the patient had the wound dressed and was then brought back to the recovery room in a cervical collar, extubated, and moving all extremities.

2. Operative Report

DIAGNOSIS: Nonhealing ischemic ulcer

OPERATION: Debridement of soft tissue of the right first metatarsophalangeal head area wound with application of MIRODERM

OPERATIVE FINDINGS: Fibrotic wound base noted to the right foot first metatarsophalangeal joint wound, some bleeding noted upon debridement. No underlying purulence noted.

INDICATION FOR PROCEDURE: This is an 86-year-old female with history of peripheral vascular disease and nonhealing ischemic ulcer to the right first metatarsophalangeal head area. The wound developed from previous failed primary closure and the patient has been receiving local wound care without significant improvement of wound. Wound has no signs of infection. Debridement of wound with application of MIRODERM, a new porcine liver derived product, has been discussed in detail with the patient. The patient understands all the risks and benefits of surgery including being increased bleeding, increased pain, increased numbness, infection, nonhealing surgical wound and possibility of further procedures. Consent signed.

PROCEDURE IN DETAIL: The patient was brought into the operating room and placed on the operating table in supine position. Upon IV sedation, local anesthesia was brought about the patient's right lower extremity using 12 mL of 1:1 mixture of 1% lidocaine and 0.5% Marcaine. The right foot was then prepped and draped in usual aseptic manner. No tourniquet was used. Attention was then directed to the right foot at the first metatarsophalangeal joint where a fibrotic wound approximately 6 × 4 cm was noted. Using a rongeur, the wound was debrided to bleeding and granular tissue. The wound was irrigated with copious amount of double antibiotic solution. MIRODERM was then applied to the first metatarsophalangeal head wound site. Using a staple gun, the wound matrix was secured onto the skin into the wound. The wound was then covered with a layer of Adaptic. The patient tolerated the procedure well and was transferred back to the post-anesthesia care unit under the care of the anesthesiologist in apparent stable condition. All sponge count and needle count were accounted for at the end of the case.

3. Procedure Summary

Findings:

1. Acute NSTEMI.
2. Proximal left circumflex mild disease mid segment.
3. Two small obtuse marginal branches are patent.
4. Large ramus branch has mild disease mid segment.
5. LAD calcified proximal severe disease, mid 85-90% culprit lesion. Patent diagonal branches but small in size.
6. Proximal RCA 20%, mid discrete lesions.
7. Normal left ventricular systolic function. No mitral regurgitation.
8. LVEF 60%.

Recommendations: Aspirin and Plavix. May need RCA stenting in the future.

Procedure Type:

Diagnostic procedure:	Left Heart Catheterization, Left ventriculography, Coronary Angiogram, multiple arteries
PCI procedure:	Orbital atherectomy and drug eluting coronary stent

Procedure Data:

Diagnostic Cath Status:	Emergency
Interventional Cath Status:	Emergency
Indications:	Abnormal enzymes and Abnormal ECG.
Entry Locations:	Percutaneous access was performed through the Right Femoral artery. A 6 Fr sheath was inserted. Hemostasis was successfully obtained using Angio-Seal.

Diagnostic Catheters:

6 French Right side Cordis 6Fr JL4 Dx Cath was used for Left coronary angiography.

6 French Right side Cordis 6Fr JR4 Dx Cath was used for Right coronary angiography.

6 French Right side Cordis 6Fr Angled Pigtail Catheter was used for Left ventriculography.

Estimated Blood Loss:	10 ml.
Complications:	No Complications.
Contrast Material:	Omnipaque 200 ml
Fluoroscopy Time:	Diagnostic: 1:30 minutes. PCI: 9:00 minutes. Total: 10:30 minutes.

Angiographic Findings. Cardiac Arteries and Lesion

LAD: Lesion on Prox LAC: Mid subsection. 95% stenosis. Pre procedure TIMI 0 flow was noted. Post Procedure TIMI III flow was present. The lesion was diagnosed as High Risk (C). The lesion was heavily calcified. The lesion showed favorable near total occlusion.

Treatment results:	Interventional treatment was successful.

Devices used:

6Fr EBU 3.75 Guide Cath.

Viperwire.

Diamondback 360 orbital atherectomy catheter

Emerge RX 2.0 × 15mm. 1 inflation(s) to a max pressure of 12 atm.

Xience Expedition 2.5 × 15mm. Diameter: 2.5 mm. Length: 15 mm. 2 inflation(s) to a max pressure of: 14 atm.

NC Quantum Apex RX 2.5 × 12mm. 2 inflation(s) to a max pressure of: 15 atm.

RCA: Lesion on Prox RCA: Mid subsection. 20% stenosis.

Hemodynamics at Rest:

O_2 Consumption: Estimated: 216.56   Heart Rate: 67 bpm

Pressures:

Site	Pressure
AO	118/63 (86)
AO	118/67 (89)
LV	114/9, 19
LV	114/10, 18

4. Operative Report

PREOPERATIVE AND POSTOPERATIVE DIAGNOSIS: Benign prostatic hypertrophy

PROCEDURE: Transurethral Aquabeam robotic-assisted ablation of the prostate

INDICATIONS: The patient is a 68-year-old gentleman with benign prostatic hypertrophy who has had LUTS of urinary retention treated multiple times in the past. Following complete descriptions of the treatment options, the patient selected Aquabeam robotic-assisted ablation. He is aware that complications may include incontinence, bleeding, infection, impotence and urethral strictures. Consent was signed.

PROCEDURE DESCRIPTION: Under general anesthesia, prophylactic antibiotics were administered. The patient was then prepped and draped in typical sterile fashion was cystoscopy procedures. Cystoscopy was then performed by using the Aquabeam cystoscope. The prostatic urethra appeared to be significantly hypertrophied due to the hypertrophy of the lateral lobes. The median lobe is also enlarged. The anterior urethra was normal. The bladder was normal. Photographs were obtained. The ultrasound wand was placed into the rectum. Ultrasound images of the prostate were obtained and fed into the robotic console. The robot determined the treatment zones and delivered the Aquabeam saline ablation to the lateral lobes and median lobe. Bleeders were then laser coagulated. A #24-French Foley catheter was then inserted atraumatically with blood tinged urine flowing freely. The patient tolerated the procedure well without apparent complications.

5. Operative Report

PREOPERATIVE DIAGNOSIS: Thoracogenic progressive scoliosis of thoracic spine.

POSTOPERATIVE DIAGNOSIS: Thoracogenic progressive scoliosis of thoracic spine.

NAME OF PROCEDURE: Magnetically-controlled growing rod construct T2 to L2.

INDICATIONS: The patient is a 12-year-old female with a complex medical history of tetralogy of Fallot status post repair, as well as transient complete heart block with pacemaker in place. She has progressive thoracogenic scoliosis, possibly secondary to her previous thoracic procedures. There is concern that it may start affecting lung function, especially as she goes through her rapid growth spurt at this time. She is a very immature 12-year-old female. She would not be able to tolerate a brace due to her pulmonary issues. She would also not tolerate repeated anesthesia for traditional growing rods. Risks and benefits of magnetic growing rod construct were discussed with the family, and they wished to proceed. Consent was signed. The site was marked. The risks including bleeding, infection, neurologic injury, rod breakage, implant failure and pulling away from the bone were all discussed.

DESCRIPTION OF PROCEDURE: Under general anesthesia by the anesthesia team, she was placed prone on the Jackson table after MMPs and SSEPs were obtained. Dr. X was in charge of neuromonitoring. The back was prepped and draped in the usual sterile fashion. Timeout was documented. Antibiotics was administered.

We used C-arm to localize the spinous process of T1 and T2 as well as L1 and L2. We then dissected down through the skin and then left the midline structures intact and went paraspinal reflecting the muscles away from the bone. Once I was down on the pedicle on the right side, we x-rayed again to confirm the level and made our dissection out to the transverse processes from T1 and T2, as well as L1 and L2, leaving the adjacent joints intact.

We began implanting in the lumbar spine. MAGEC rod system was used. Vertebral hook was placed over L2 and secured in place on the right side first. We then measured the length of the right rod. We used a chest tube and a tonsil to tunnel through the muscle to get from the thoracic wound to the lumbar wound. We passed the rod within the chest tube to protect it from going to the chest wall. I then connected the thoracic end of the rod with the appropriate thoracic kyphosis into the connector. I oriented the magnetic controller appropriately to the posterior and tested the orientation. The left sided rod was measured and placed in the same fashion. Once I had the rods on both sides placed, tested and reduced, we then did x-rays. The lung films showed the implants in good position and the curve was slightly improved. Again, I did not try to distract beyond what the bones could handle.

We attempted the wake-up test, however, the patient never got to the point where she was awake enough to follow commands, despite being able to follow commands in the preop holding area for Dr. X. MMPs and SSEPs had never changed throughout. The decision was made at that time to wake the patient completely. We are comfortable that no injury was had on the spinal cord. Superficial drains were placed above the fascia. Closed the skin in layered fashion, dry dressings applied.

PLAN: The patient will be admitted to the Pediatric Intensive Care Unit. She will likely need a PCA for a day or two. No running, jumping, or sports. I anticipate discharge in 3 to 5 days. Must have bowel movement before discharge and mobilizing well. Likely follow up at 6 weeks for clinical check in the office and have the first magnetic distraction.

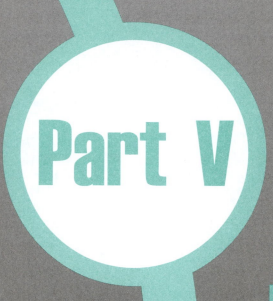

Part V

Review Exercises and Case Studies

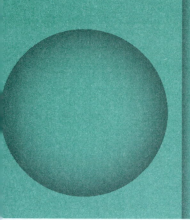

Exercises and Case Studies

Exercises

Assign ICD-10-PCS codes to the following procedure statements and scenarios. List the root operation selected and the code assigned.

1. Stereotactic gamma beam radiosurgery for eradication of a pituitary tumor

2. Laparoscopic placement of a gastric band for morbid obesity

3. High energy extracorporeal shockwave treatment to humeral epicondyle, multiple treatments

4. Coblator reduction of inferior turbinates through nares

5. Percutaneous insertion of posterior spinous process decompression device, L2–L3

6. Reduction of prominent forehead, open approach

7. Gastric manometry via nasal catheter

8. Thoracic multiple level intercostal nerve block with fluoroscopic guidance at T5–T8

9. Insertion of external limb lengthening devices on right tibia and fibula, open approach

10. Radiofrequency facet denervation of the right L2–L3, L3–L4 by rhizotomy, open approach

11. Posterior occipitocervical arthrodesis and C1-C4 arthrodesis with posterior stabilization hardware and autograft bone, open

12. Transthoracic complete thymectomy

13. Patient has Hodgkin's sarcoma disease, confirmed by previous lymph node biopsy of the cervical chain. Megavoltage radiotherapy with 4 MeV was performed.

_____

14. Intracranial neuroendoscopy with excision of pituitary tumor

_____

15. Anterior lumbar arthrodesis (L1-L3) through a posterior approach, posterior arthrodesis (L1-L3), posterior lumbar segmental instrumentation (L1-L3), bone graft from right rib, through an Open approach

_____

16. Hysteroscopy with intraluminal lithotripsy of left fallopian tube calcification

_____

17. Insertion of inflatable penile prosthesis

_____

18. Percutaneous biopsy of left submaxillary gland

_____

19. Radiofrequency ablation of liver tumor of the left lobe, open approach

_____

20. Heart-bilateral lung transplant with recipient cardiectomy-pneumonectomy from a matched donor

_____

21. Remodeling of a pectus excavatum deformity with internal fixation bar (Nuss procedure), percutaneous endoscopic

_____

22. Denervation of hip joint, intrapelvic branch of sciatic nerve, percutaneously using neurolytic agent

_____

23. Mullen Scales of Early Learning tests are administered.

_____

24. Transfusion of whole blood into a peripheral vein from a matched donor

_____

25. Insertion of tissue expander into soft tissue of scalp, open

_____

26. Cystoscopy, bilateral retrograde pyelograms with Omnipaque and right ureteral stent placement

_____

27. Transposition of great vessels (Jatene procedure), pulmonary trunk for thoracic aorta

_____

28. Pharmacotherapy using Clonidine for patient with drug addiction

_____

29. Removal of intrauterine device (IUD) without the use of an endoscope

_____

30. MRI of brain without contrast to assess acute confusion and headache

31. Removal of segmental pedicle screw instrumentation from T6-T9, exploration of thoracic fusion, posterior refusion of T7-T8, placement of pedicle screw fixation from T6-T9, placement of bone morphogenetic protein, and autograft bone from left iliac crest

32. Arthroscopic anterior capsulorrhaphy of right shoulder with labral repair

33. Phenol injection for destruction of the infraorbital branch of the trigeminal nerve

34. Biopsy of right carotid body growth, open approach

35. This asthmatic patient was diagnosed with carbon monoxide poisoning from the household furnace. CO_2 level in the ED was 2.2. Treated with a single treatment of 2 hours, 53 minutes of multiplace HBO and admitted for continuing asthma management.

Case Studies

1.   Operative Report

PREOPERATIVE DIAGNOSIS:	Chronic lumbar pain syndrome
POSTOPERATIVE DIAGNOSIS:	Chronic lumbar pain syndrome
PROCEDURE:	Laminotomy, T10-T11 with placement of a single neurostimulator paddle electrode and placement of subcutaneous neurostimulator generator, right back

INDICATIONS FOR PROCEDURE: This 39-year-old female presented with a complex history of chronic low back and lower extremity pain. She has undergone multiple previous lumbar spine procedures including decompressions and fusions. The patient was evaluated by the Pain Service for a spinal cord neurostimulator. Surgery is undertaken at this time in an attempt to bring her some relief of her chronic pain syndrome. Risks and complications, including failure to relieve her symptoms, chronic back pain, paralysis, and death were discussed.

DESCRIPTION OF PROCEDURE: The patient was brought to the OR and general endotracheal anesthesia was induced. The patient was positioned in the prone position on the O.S.I. table. The thoracolumbar spine and the right lateral lower back were sterilely prepped with alcohol followed by iodine solution and appropriately draped employing a steri-drape. Under C-arm fluoroscopy guidance, a 2-inch incision was made over the T10-T11 area. The incision was carried down through subcutaneous tissue. Soft tissue and muscle attachments of the posterior elements were dissected free and mobilized and the self-retractor placed. The interspinous ligament was incised and laminotomy performed at T10-T11 entering the epidural space without difficulty. Paddle electrode, 16-lead type, was placed on the dorsum of the epidural space over the spinal cord and directed under fluoroscopy into the midline position. Position confirmed with fluoroscopy. Wires secured.

Attention was then directed to the right lateral lower back. Through a transverse 4-cm incision, a subcutaneous pocket was developed and tunneling was performed from the pocket to the spinal wound. Wire electrodes were tunneled to the pocket on the right back and the wires were inserted into the battery-stimulator. The impedance was checked and noted to be normal for all leads. The wounds were irrigated with antibiotic solution and closed in layers. The spinal wound fascia was closed with interrupted sutures of 0 Vicryl, subcutaneous tissue with interrupted sutures of 2-0 Vicryl. The skin was closed with staples. The subcutaneous pocket was closed with subcutaneous sutures of 2-0 Vicryl and staples. The patient tolerated the procedure well without complications.

Postoperative plan includes programming of device on postoperative day 1.

---

2. Operative Report

PREOPERATIVE DIAGNOSIS: End stage renal disease secondary to dysplasia

POSTOPERATIVE DIAGNOSIS: End stage renal disease secondary to dysplasia

OPERATIONS:
  1. Living, related donor renal transplant
  2. Removal of peritoneal dialysis catheter

INDICATIONS FOR OPERATION: This patient is a 3-year-old male who has been on peritoneal dialysis for over a year-and-a-half due to renal dysplasia. His father came forward as a live donor. After workup of both the recipient and the donor, the patient is taken to the operating room for elective living, related kidney transplantation.

DONOR INFORMATION: A left kidney was used from the father with a single artery, vein, and ureter.

PROCEDURE DESCRIPTION: The ABO verification sheet was signed and the patient was identified, brought to the operating room, and placed in the supine position. He was administered a general endotracheal anesthetic. The patient was explored through a midline incision in the linea alba from the pubic tubercle to just short of the sternal notch. The peritoneal dialysis infusion catheter cuff was noted in the linea alba. It was dissected from the linea alba and removed. The intraperitoneal portion of the catheter was wrapped around omentum, which required a single lysis of adhesions to remove it. The right colon was taken off its lateral attachments, fully exposing the retroperitoneal portion of the inferior vena cava and the distal aorta. The distal inferior vena cava was skeletonized of its surrounding structures. Small lumbar veins were ligated between 4-0 silk ties and transected. The right gonadal vein was also ligated between 2-0 silk ties and transected. The distal aorta was then skeletonized of its surrounding structures. The left common iliac artery was controlled with a vessel loop. Dissection over the distal aorta and right common iliac artery was performed.

The donor kidney was procured in a separate procedure. It was transported to the recipient room by me and placed into a cold bath of heparin-containing Ringer's solution. The staple line over the renal vein was removed, the staple line over the renal artery was removed, and the kidney was flushed with approximately 300 cc of the cold heparin-containing lactated Ringer's solution. It flushed quite easily. The staples were removed from the renal vein and replaced with 2-0 silk ties. The renal vein was then skeletonized toward the hilum of the kidney. The adrenal vein was ligated between 2-0 silk ties and transected as well. The renal artery was then skeletonized toward the hilum of the kidney. Perinephric fat was removed. The kidney remained in cold storage.

The patient was then systemically heparinized with 1000 units intravenously. After three minutes, crossclamps were placed on the distal cava and the aorta. A cavotomy was created to the appropriate length, and an end renal vein to side distal inferior vena caval anastomosis was created with running 5-0 prolene. The anastomosis was flushed with heparinized saline. Next, an arteriotomy was made in the distal aorta. A 4.4-mm aortic punch was used and an end renal artery to side distal aorta anastomosis was created with running 6-0 PDS. Again, the anastomosis was flushed with the heparinized saline. The crossclamps were removed and the kidney reperfused nicely. The bladder was then dissected out from the surrounding structures, and an anterior cystotomy was created. The ureter was brought through a stab incision in the right lateral dome of the bladder. The ureter was then cut to the appropriate length and spatulated, and a Leadbetter-Politano type neoureterocystostomy was created with interrupted 5-0 chromic. The ureter had a good vascular supply and there was no tension on the anastomosis. The bladder was irrigated with saline. The Foley was also irrigated. Hemostasis was noted within the hilum of the kidney, the capsule of the kidney, and along the anastomotic lines. The right colon was then placed back into the right lower quadrant. The incision was then closed in three layers using 2-0 prolene in the fascial layer, 3-0 Vicryl in the subcutaneous layer and a 4-0 Monocryl running stitch. The skin was also reinforced with Dermabond.

3. Operative Report

PREOPERATIVE DIAGNOSIS: Obliterative arterial disease with ischemic right foot

POSTOPERATIVE DIAGNOSIS: Obliterative arterial disease with ischemic right foot

PROCEDURE PERFORMED: Right femoral to posterior tibial with greater saphenous bypass

HISTORY: This 67-year-old white male has had ischemia of the right foot. Cardiac work-up was positive and he has undergone coronary artery bypass grafting. He now presents to the OR for right femoral to posterior tibial in situ bypass.

OPERATIVE SUMMARY: After placement of an epidural catheter for spinal anesthesia, the patient was taken to the operating room, placed on the table in the supine position. The right leg and groin were prepped and draped in the usual sterile fashion.

A two team approach was used to open the right groin and the femoral vessels were all dissected out and controlled individually. The saphenofemoral junction was dissected out and multiple tributaries to the saphenous vein were divided between 2-0 or 4-0 silk ties. The medial right calf was opened. An excellent saphenous vein was dissected out. Multiple side branches were divided between 2-0 or 4-0 silk ties. We then deepened the incision, pulled the gastroc and psoas posteriorly, identified the posterior tibial artery, and encircled it for a length with vessel loops.

We then gave the patient 2000 units of intravenous heparin. After waiting three minutes, we occluded the posterior tibial artery and opened it up with an 11 blade knife and Potts scissors to make sure we had an adequate lumen, which we did. We also flushed with heparinized saline in both directions. We then divided the vein distally and ligated it with 2-0 silk. We occluded the saphenofemoral junction, amputated the vein off, closed the femoral venotomy with 5-0 Prolene, and excised the proximal valve under direct vision with fine spring scissors.

We then controlled the femoral vessels and made an arteriotomy across the origin of the SFA. We brought the vein graft over and sewed an anastomosis with 5-0 Prolene from the heel around the toe and tied on the side. We flushed everything down the vein. We broke the valves with #2 and then a #3 Gore-Tex valvulotome, had excellent inflow. We back flushed with heparinized saline, controlled the graft with a disposable gray bulldog clamp. We then cut the vein graft to match the posterior tibial artery and sewed a 6-0 Prolene anastomosis from the heel around the toe and tied on the side after flushing in all directions. We removed all the clamps. We had excellent Doppler signals and we had a restoration of the posterior tibial pulse at the ankle. We needed a couple of additional ties on the side branches on the vein of 4-0 silk, irrigated with antibiotic solution to both wounds. We listened with the Doppler and could not demonstrate any side branches to the leg so we left Surgicel over the anastomosis, closed with layers of 2-0 and 3-0 Vicryl and then 4-0 Vicryl on the skin, subcuticular stitch, Benzoin and Steri-strips. The patient tolerated the procedure well, went to PACU in good condition. All sponge, needle, and instrument counts were correct at the end of the case. Estimated blood loss was 50 cc.

4.   Operative Report

PREOPERATIVE DIAGNOSIS: Chronic otitis

POSTOPERATIVE DIAGNOSIS: Chronic otitis

OPERATION: Ventilation tube placement

PROCEDURE DESCRIPTION: The patient was induced under general anesthesia in the supine position via a face mask. Her right tympanic membrane was visualized. There was tympanosclerosis on the entire eardrum except for an area anterior and inferiorly. This was incised, thin fluid was sucked from the middle ear space, and a ventilation tube was placed. In a similar fashion, the left tympanic membrane was visualized, incised, drained, and tubed. The patient was awakened and brought to the recovery room in good condition.

5.   Operative Report

Do not code imaging in this case.

PREOPERATIVE DIAGNOSIS: Peripheral vascular disease and ischemic right foot

POSTOPERATIVE DIAGNOSIS: Peripheral vascular disease and ischemic right foot

PROCEDURES PERFORMED:
1. Right lower extremity angiogram with interpretation
2. Exposure of the right popliteal artery and a popliteal, anterior tibial and posterior tibial artery embolectomy
3. Infusion of tPA with patch repair of the popliteal artery with reverse saphenous vein graft
4. Endoscopic harvesting of left saphenous vein

INDICATION: The patient has a severely ischemic right leg and foot with no feeling on the plantar dorsal aspect of the right foot.

PROCEDURE: Under general anesthesia, right leg was prepped and draped in the usual manner. The left foot looked good, had an excellent Doppler and a pulse. On the right side, there were no signals in the foot and it was still quite pale.

    At this point, I placed a micropuncture needle and wire into the superficial femoral artery, proximally directed. Angiogram showed that the popliteal below the knee was occluded at the origin of all of the tibial vessels. I opened the popliteal artery and performed embolectomy down to the anterior tibial artery. I patched the popliteal artery with greater saphenous vein patch from the left leg.

I opened the posterior tibial artery at the popliteal junction and retrieved a 2 cm long plug of organized thrombus. A palpable pulse was finally felt after this. Both of these wounds were irrigated, backbled and closed. During this time, the right foot finally demonstrated signals and started to look better. I closed the outer layers of the groin incisions. Sterile dressings were applied to the wounds.

6. Operative Report

PREOPERATIVE DIAGNOSIS: Gangrene of the left foot

POSTOPERATIVE DIAGNOSIS: Gangrene of the left foot

OPERATION: Left below-knee amputation

INDICATIONS FOR SURGERY: This is an 86-year-old male who has a history of vasculitis, and peripheral vascular disease, who presents with gangrene of the left foot. He has developed gangrene of his left foot. Angiogram showed most disease in the distal vessels and surgical treatment is not an option for these vessels. The gangrene continues to progress and our recommendation is below-knee amputation, to which the patient agrees.

DESCRIPTION OF PROCEDURE: After general anesthesia was initiated and regional nerve blocks were performed, the patient was placed supine on the table and his entire left lower extremity was prepped and draped in a sterile fashion.

Fish-mouth incisions were made around the entire circumference of the lower calf region. Dissection was completed through the subcutaneous and fascia layers. The posterior flap was created including both the gastrocnemius and the soleus muscles. The posterior tibial vessels were tied and transected. Following this, the muscles of the anterior and lateral compartments were transected with the cautery. The anterior tibial vessels were tied and transected. The tibia was then cut at mid calf with a bone saw. The fibula was also cut at mid calf with the bone saw. The peroneal vessels were tied and transected. The remaining muscles were transected and the specimen was sent to Pathology. After hemostasis was achieved, the wound was irrigated and hemostasis checked again. The wound was closed in layers over the bone using 0 chromic to form the stump. The fascia was closed with 2-0 Vicryl in interrupted fashion. The skin was closed with staples and the stump was splinted. The patient tolerated the procedure well and was sent to PACU in stable condition.

7. Operative Report

PREOPERATIVE DIAGNOSIS: Malfunctioning peritoneal dialysis catheter

POSTOPERATIVE DIAGNOSIS: Malfunctioning peritoneal dialysis catheter

OPERATION: Repositioning of peritoneal dialysis catheter via laparoscopic technique

INDICATION: A 52-year-old female patient who has end-stage renal disease who had a peritoneal dialysis catheter placed a little over a year ago. She was admitted early yesterday when it became obvious that it was not malfunctioning. Hemodialysis used in the interim. She is now stable and ready for the operating room to reposition the peritoneal dialysis catheter and repair or revise this access.

PROCEDURE DETAILS: Under general anesthesia, the patient was placed in the supine position and prepped and draped for lap surgery. An incision was made in the infraumbilical area using the Hassan technique. The fascia was opened and peritoneum was then entered. The small 5 mm port was then passed into the peritoneal cavity followed by a 5-mm camera. CO_2 was insufflated into the abdomen. A 5 mm port was then passed under direct vision on the right and the left side of the abdomen. A total of 3 ports were used, the center port with the camera.

Under direct visualization the laparoscopic arms were placed on either side with a long 2 to 3 cm length grabbers. Using these laparoscopic grabbers, the small intestine was gently moved aside and the second grabber was used to reposition the curled peritoneal dialysis catheter from the left lower quadrant down into the cul-de-sac behind the uterus and anterior to the rectum. The small intestine was allowed to pass on top of the catheter. The catheter was tested multiple times. About 100 cc to 200 cc was injected initially and drained very well. Care was taken to avoid placing the catheter too high on the left side to avoid some scar tissue on the left from a previous surgery, but there was no bleeding encountered on the left. At this point, the catheter was then successfully tested again after the laparoscopic ports were removed. The openings were closed with nylon. The midline incision was closed with figure-of-eight 2-0 Vicryl sutures and then the catheter was then tested again with 100 cc of saline which drained briskly and no impediment of flow was encountered. The new extension tubing was placed on the peritoneal dialysis catheter. The midline was closed with Vicryl and a running subcuticular 4-0 PDS. Sterile dressings were applied.

---

8.   Operative Report

PREOPERATIVE DIAGNOSIS: Nasal septal deviation and bilateral inferior turbinate hypertrophy causing nasal airway obstruction

POSTOPERATIVE DIAGNOSIS: Nasal septal deviation and bilateral inferior turbinate hypertrophy causing nasal airway obstruction

OPERATION: Nasal septoplasty, bilateral inferior turbinate submucous resection

OPERATIVE INDICATIONS: This patient is a 34-year-old man with a lifelong history of nasal airway obstruction, which has been unremitting in spite of nasal spray and oral decongestants. Operative findings included a very tortuous septum. He has obstructed airway related to his septum bilaterally. He had extremely large turbinates as well.

OPERATIVE PROCEDURE: The patient was brought to the operating suite and placed in a semi-Fowler position on the operating table. He was given one gram of Ancef prior to the initiation of the procedure. A total of 15 cc of 1 percent Xylocaine with 1:100,000 epinephrine was injected in divided doses during the case. A total of 2 cc of 10 percent cocaine was placed topically on pledgets in the nose.

The patient was prepped and draped in a sterile fashion. A left hemitransfixion incision was created, and mucoperichondrial and mucoperiosteal flaps were elevated. A 1 cm caudal strut was left in position. The quadrilateral cartilage was separated inferiorly from the maxillary crest and posteriorly from the perpendicular plate of the ethmoid. The quadrilateral cartilage was morselized to help straighten it. An inferior piece of quadrilateral cartilage was removed from the inferior portion. Once this was done, the septum was markedly improved. A small drainage hole was placed in the posterior portion of the right inferior flap. A piece of morselized quadrilateral cartilage was placed between the mucoperiosteal flaps posteriorly. The hemitransfixion incision was closed with interrupted sutures of 5-0 chromic.

At this point, the left inferior turbinate submucous resection was done. The inferior turbinate was outfractured. An incision was made along the inferior border of the turbinate. The bone was dissected free from the lateral mucosal flap. This was done in the anterior one third of the inferior turbinate. The free edge was cauterized. The same procedure was carried out on the other side. The free edges were then cauterized with cautery. This created an excellent nasal airway. The free edges of the inferior turbinates were packed with two pieces of bacitracin-impregnated Gelfoam. Doyle nasal splints impregnated with bacitracin ointment were also placed in the nose and secured with a single transseptal suture of 2-0 silk.

9. Operative Report

PREOPERATIVE DIAGNOSIS: Direct and indirect right inguinal hernia

POSTOPERATIVE DIAGNOSIS: Direct and indirect right inguinal hernia

OPERATION: Inguinal herniorrhaphy

FINDINGS: A huge defect was noted from the level of the internal inguinal ring which was a combination of a sliding hernia with some chronic incarceration of properitoneal fat down to the scrotal area. There was a weakness medial to the epigastric vessels and adjacent to the lacunar ligament, where there was a small bulge of fat protruding through, consistent with a direct hernia as well.

PROCEDURE DESCRIPTION: The patient was prepped and draped in the usual fashion, infiltrated with 2 percent Xylocaine with epinephrine and 0.5 percent Marcaine with epinephrine. An incision was made in the inguinal area and carried through subcutaneous tissue. Bleeders were clamped, ligated, and cauterized. Scarpa's fascia was divided, and the aponeurosis of the external oblique was identified. This was then divided parallel to the fibers, following which the cord was encircled with a rubber drain. The sac at this point was opened, allowing us to reduce the chronically incarcerated adipose tissue and placing it back within the abdominal cavity. The sac was dissected from the associated vessels in the pampiniform plexus. At the level of the internal inguinal ring, it was internally sutured with 0 Surgilon.

Following this, repair was performed utilizing 0 Surgilon from the shelving edge of Poupart's ligament to the transversalis and conjoined tendon medially. This was done from the level of the symphysis pubis and extended up to the internal inguinal ring where I was allowed to place my distal index finger through this canal area. Following this, an onlay of Marlex mesh was placed. The lower end was secured with 0 Surgilon, following which both medial and lateral areas were sutured, the lateralmost to the inguinal ligament utilizing 2-0 Prolene from the level of the symphysis up to a point above the level of the internal inguinal ring. On the medial portion, it was sewn to the conjoined tendon and transversalis fascia medially. A small keyhole was made within the Marlex to allow the cord to extend through this, and the Marlex was brought to a level above the level of the ring. Vicryl 3-0 was utilized for approximation of the external oblique aponeurosis as well as for approximation of Scarpa's fascia. Subcuticular 4-0 Vicryl was utilized for approximation of the skin. Steri-Strips and a pressure dressing were applied.

10. Operative Report

PREOPERATIVE DIAGNOSIS: Obstructing sigmoid colon cancer

POSTOPERATIVE DIAGNOSIS: Metastatic colon cancer to the liver with obstructing sigmoid colon tumor

PROCEDURES:	Exploratory laparotomy
	Liver biopsy
SPECIMEN:	Entire sigmoid colon

INDICATIONS FOR PROCEDURE: This is a 70-year-old female with a history of severe chronic obstructive pulmonary disease, who presented with an obstructing sigmoid colon tumor. This was found to be at 20 cm and was proven on biopsy to be adenocarcinoma. The patient also has a palpable mass in the left lateral segment of the liver on exam. The patient was able to tolerate the bowel prep slowly over 2 to 3 days and got improved control of her COPD with stress dose steroids in preparation for surgery. Given this high risk procedure with this woman on steroids for severe COPD, the potential for colostomy or loop ileostomy was discussed with the patient. She understood and wished to proceed.

The patient was identified, brought to the operating room, and placed in the supine position. She was intubated and placed under general anesthesia. She was placed on a split-leg table, positioned, appropriately padded, secured to the table, and prepped and draped in the usual sterile fashion. We began with an open lower umbilical incision. The abdomen was entered under direct vision. There was an obvious thickened area of sigmoid colon that was densely adherent to the base of the small bowel mesentery. We then placed her in Trendelenburg position, packed off the small bowel, and began mobilizing the sigmoid colon, taking down the white line of Toldt. The left ureter was clearly identified and preserved. The descending colon was mobilized to get adequate mobilization. The sigmoid colon was completely resected under direct vision. At this point, we divided the rectum proximally with an IOA-75 stapler. We had excellent blood supply to our remnant area; in fact, we had both a pulse and an excellent Doppler signal right to the staple line. After carefully mobilizing off the small bowel mesentery, we were able to take the mesentery of the colon, taking the superior hemorrhoidal, and getting into the presacral space. After entering the space, we were able to get excellent mobilization of the rectum. In order to gain adequate margins, we took our resection plane down just to the peritoneal reflection. We then came across the rectum with a cutting TA stapler, and the specimen was passed off the field. At that point, we passed rectal dilators. She was easily able to accommodate a 33 Hegar dilator. At that point, we cleaned off the proximal colon and opened it. There was some liquid stool present, but there had been a fairly decent bowel prep. We put a 2-0 prolene pursestring on the proximal bowel and placed the anvil in that. We then performed our anastomosis under direct vision after bringing the anvil transanally, right out through the staple line. This was approximately 9 cm from the anal verge. The staple line was fired for the end-to-end anastomosis, and both doughnuts were inspected and were complete. We then oversewed the anterior and lateral aspects of our staple line with several 3-0 silks and tested the anastomosis under water. There were no air bubbles. Our attention was then turned to the liver. She had a small, hard nodule in the left lateral segment. This was biopsied, and frozen section came back as metastatic colon cancer. We then copiously irrigated the abdomen and obtained meticulous hemostasis. We then closed the fascia with #1 PDS and placed several interrupted #2 Vicryl internal retention sutures. The wound was irrigated, and hemostasis was achieved. The skin was closed with staples. At this point, the patient was awakened from anesthesia and taken to the intensive care unit in stable condition.

11. Operative Report

| PREOPERATIVE DIAGNOSIS: | Intractable epilepsy. |
| POSTOPERATIVE DIAGNOSIS: | Intractable epilepsy. |

PROCEDURE PERFORMED: Craniotomy and anterior 2/3 corpus callosotomy
Use of neuronavigation, Brainlab
Use of intraoperative microscope

INDICATIONS: The patient is a 12-year-old with intractable epilepsy and drop seizures despite multiple antiepileptic drugs. The above procedure was indicated. Informed consent was obtained both verbally and in writing.

DESCRIPTION OF PROCEDURE: The patient was brought to the operating room. She was intubated and sedated in the usual fashion. Intravenous lines were obtained by Anesthesia. The patient was then affixed to the Mayfield head holder, affixed to the table and placed in the supine position. All pressure points were padded. We then registered the patient's scalp fiducials to the Brainlab neuronavigation system. We then prepped and draped the patient in the usual fashion. We made a transverse incision just anterior to the coronal suture, crossing over the midline to the left side approximately 3 cm. We then dissected down to the skull. We then performed a craniotomy with 2 burr holes on the midline and 1 laterally on the right side. We then, using a curette, dissected away the dura from the skull. We then used the craniotome to perform a craniotomy flap, with the flap being 2/3 anterior to the coronal suture and 1/3 posterior. We then opened the dura in a U fashion and reflected the dura medially. We then brought in the microscope. We used the Greenberg retractor system to dissect down to the cingulate gyrus. We then dissected the adhesions connecting the cingulate gyri together. We then saw the pericallosal arteries. We then put our retractors in between them. We then identified the midline and performed an anterior 2/3 corpus callosotomy under microscopic magnification. After we had satisfactory disconnection, we performed intraoperative MRI, which confirmed our disconnection. We then copiously irrigated the wound and closed the dura and placed DuraGen on top of this. We then replaced the bone flap and the bone dust in the edges of the bone flap. We then placed titanium plates and screws. We then closed the scalp in layers using 3-0 Vicryl sutures and running 4-0 Monocryl and removed the Mayfield head holder and wrapped the head with Kerlix.

12. Operative Report

PREOPERATIVE DIAGNOSES: 1. Severe lumbar stenosis with associated neurogenic claudication secondary to a midline synovial cyst with severe thecal sac compression.
2. Spondylolisthesis at L4-L5.

POSTOPERATIVE DIAGNOSES: Same

PROCEDURE: 1. Left L4-L5 lamimotomy with bilateral decompression of the thecal sac and removal of extradural non-neoplastic mass - synovial cyst.
2. Fusion using posterior transverse process technique on the left at L4-L5.
3. Utilization of bone allograft using Trinity bone substrate.

INDICATIONS: This patient is a 56-year-old woman who presents with left leg radicular pain. She also has some low back pain. Imaging studies showed a large synovial cyst with compression of the thecal sac as well as a spondylolisthesis at L4-L5. Surgical intervention is appropriate and was discussed at length with her. She was not very eager for pedicle screws. We elected to proceed with a unilateral approach with a bilateral decompression with the hope that the unilateral approach would minimize any progressive subluxation. We also plan a posterior transverse process onlay fusion. The patient also understood the need for possible further surgery.

PROCEDURE DETAILS: Under endotracheal anesthesia, was positioned prone on the Jackson table. All bony prominences were well padded. Lumbar region was prepped and draped in routine fashion. C-arm fluoroscopy was then used to localize the area of the incision. Midline vertical incision was then made extending from L3-L5 down through the subcutaneous tissues. Subperiosteal dissection was then carried out on the left side and I exposed the lamina of L4, L5 as well as the posterior aspect of the transverse process of L4 and L5. Self-retaining retractors were then inserted.

Having confirmed the level, I used a coarse diamond bur to remove the left L4 lamina and most of the left L5 lamina. The laminotomy was associated with some mesial facetectomies, particularly over the left L5 nerve root. As I explored to the midline, I could appreciate a large synovial cyst. Using loupe magnification headlight, I gently teased the cyst off of the dura and completely removed the cyst. The thecal sac was had been quite compressed and when I removed the cyst, the thecal sac was decompressed nicely. I did perform a left foramino-tomy over the L4 and L5 nerve roots.

At this point, I felt the thecal sac was nicely decompressed. I therefore turned my attention towards the arthrod-esis. I decorticated the posterior aspect of the transverse process of L4 and L5. I then packed this area using local bone from the laminotomy. At this point, attention was turned towards closure. Retractors were removed, hemostasis was obtained. The wound was closed in multiple layers. The patient tolerated the procedures well. The patient was sent to the recovery room in good condition. There were no apparent complications.

13. Operative Report

PREOPERATIVE DIAGNOSIS:	Dysphagia
POSTOPERATIVE DIAGNOSIS:	Esophageal stricture
OPERATION:	Upper endoscopy with balloon dilation of esophagus
MEDICAL HISTORY:	The patient is an 86-year-old who presents with progressive dysphagia and spontaneously passed meat impactions.

PROCEDURE: The Olympus video upper endoscope was passed into the upper esophagus. There was a stricture in the distal esophagus. Endoscopic photographs were taken. The scope would not pass. A balloon dilation was performed in gradations from 36 French to 45 French. The balloon was inflated for 60 seconds. Visualization showed appropriate mucosal dilation. The stomach and duodenum were otherwise normal on endoscopic exam. The patient will take Omeprazole 20 mg q day and have a repeat balloon dilation to 48 French in one month.

14. Operative Report

PREOPERATIVE DIAGNOSIS:	Left ureteral calculus
POSTOPERATIVE DIAGNOSIS:	Same
OPERATION:	Cystoscopy, bilateral retrograde pyelograms, left ureteroscopy with electrohy-draulic lithotripsy, and basket extraction of calculi

PROCEDURE: The patient is brought to the cystoscopy suite, where general anesthesia is induced and maintained in the usual fashion without difficulty. The patient then is placed in the dorsal lithotomy position, and the external genitalia are prepped and draped in a routine fashion. A 21-French ACMI panendoscope is assembled and inserted into the patient's bladder without difficulty. Inspection revealed the prostate to be mildly enlarged, but not particularly obstructed. The bladder itself is unremarkable. The ureteral orifices are normal. There is no efflux at all from the left side, a clear efflux from the right. Bilateral retrograde pyelograms are taken using low osmolar contrast media. On the left side, an obvious large stone is obstructing the middle third of the ureter. On the right side, the retrograde pyelogram is normal.

A guide wire is passed into the left ureteral orifice under fluoroscopy and can go past the stone into the renal pelvis. The guide wire is left in place. A cystoscope is now removed, and a ureteroscope is passed alongside the guide wire up to the midureter. There is some mild difficulty in passage but this is accomplished. A large stone was fragmented with lithotripsy. A total of only about 30 shocks are needed to fragment the stone quite easily. At this point, the surgeon was able to basket the large remaining fragments, and stone extraction was completed. Very tiny fragments remain in the ureter but will pass safely.

After ureteroscopy with basket extraction is completed, a cystoscope is reinserted over the guide wire into the bladder. A 7-French, 26 cm double J stent is then passed under fluoroscopy into the renal pelvis, where a good coil forms. The guide wire is then carefully removed. Good positioning of the stent is verified. The procedure is completed.

15. Operative Report

PREPROCEDURE DIAGNOSIS: Emergent airway

POSTPROCEDURE DIAGNOSIS: Emergent airway

PROCEDURE PERFORMED: Cricothyroidotomy

INDICATION: I was called stat to the emergency room to establish an airway on a 53-year-old female who was undergoing cardiopulmonary resuscitation. The patient has morbid obesity.

DESCRIPTION OF THE PROCEDURE: The patient's neck was prepped with Betadine. I made a longitudinal incision overlying what was felt to be the thyroid cartilage. After multiple attempts, I was able to access the trachea just below the thyroid cartilage with a needle. A wire passed through the needle and a cricothyroidotomy tube was passed over the wire in a Seldinger technique.

The patient had adequate breath sounds after placement of the airway. CPR was ongoing. The tube was secured.

16. Operative Report

PREOPERATIVE DIAGNOSIS: Ductal carcinoma in situ, right breast, status post biopsy

POSTOPERATIVE DIAGNOSIS: Ductal carcinoma in situ, right breast, status post biopsy

OPERATION: Lumpectomy and sentinel node biopsy

INDICATIONS: This is a 57-year-old woman who had a routine mammogram performed two weeks ago. A lump was noted on the mammogram about 1.2 cm in size. A needle localization breast biopsy was performed last week which revealed ductal carcinoma in situ. Since this is a ductal carcinoma in situ, lumpectomy will now be performed and sentinel node dissection will be carried out. The patient understands the situation very well and agrees to proceed with surgery.

PROCEDURE: After obtaining the informed consent, the patient was brought into the operating room and placed on the table in the supine position. General anesthesia with laryngeal intubation was conducted smoothly. The skin over the right chest and right arm was prepped and draped in the usual sterile manner. The intended incision line was marked with a marking pen. The blue dye for the sentinel node dissection was injected. The breast tissue was massaged. Five minutes were then allowed to pass before the incision was made.

The incision was made with excision of the previous incisional biopsy scar. The axillary lymphatics were identified and dissected. The suspicious sentinel nodes were biopsied. Then the lumpectomy was performed with upper and lower skin flaps. The dissection of the breast tissue and subcutaneous tissue to raise the two flaps was conducted smoothly. A large lump was dissected and the dissection carried to the pectoralis muscles and was removed completely. Hemostasis was confirmed by cauterization. The wound was then irrigated with copious amounts of warm water solution. The specimen was sent to pathology and the sentinel nodes were sent separately to pathology. The wound was then closed in layers using 2-0 Vicryl for the deeper layer, 3-0 Vicryl for the subcutaneous tissue, and 4-0 Vicryl for the skin. The patient tolerated the whole procedure very well and was sent to the recovery room in stable condition after extubation. Blood loss was minimal. Sponge and needle counts were correct. No drain was left. The specimens were sent to pathology.

17. Operative Report

Do not code the imaging in this case.

PRE-CATHETERIZATION DIAGNOSIS: Atrial septal defect with mild to moderate right ventricular volume overload, static dimension by transthoracic echocardiogram was 9 × 11 mm.

POST-CATHETERIZATION DIAGNOSIS:
1. Secundum atrial septal defect, relatively centrally located, somewhat small retroaortic rim. Static dimension by transesophageal echo at 7 mm.
2. Left-to-right shunt of 1.6:1 with normal pulmonary vascular resistance at 1.3 Woods units.
3. Stop flow technique/balloon stretch diameter of 13 to 14 mm.
4. Successful closure with a 14-mm Amplatzer septal occluder in the Cath Lab today.

NAME OF PROCEDURE: Transesophageal echocardiogram, general anesthesia, and right heart and transseptal left heart catheterization through existing septal opening, transcatheter closure of septal defect.

DESCRIPTION OF PROCEDURE: The patient was brought to the Cardiac Cath Lab and intubated uneventfully. A transesophageal echo probe was placed. Access to the right femoral vein was obtained with the use of a SonoSite.

Through the 6-French sheath placed in the right femoral vein, a 6-French wedge catheter was used to sample saturations and pressures in the SVC, RA, RV, RPA, LPA, RP wedge, LPA wedge, and LA positions. A Rosen wire was positioned in the left upper pulmonary vein. Over the Rosen wire, an 18-mm sizing balloon was advanced to perform a stretch diameter. Leaving the Rosen wire in place, a 7-French long ASD closure sheath was advanced according to routine. The dilator and wire were withdrawn with a continuously held positive pressure breath to allow adequate bleed back. The sheath was advanced into the left atrium and the 14-mm Amplatzer septal occluder was advanced according to routine. The distal disk was delivered, brought against the septum, followed by the proximal disk. Traction and pressure were applied to the delivery cable and the device was continuously assessed by transesophageal echocardiogram. Satisfied with its position, the device was released and again reassessed both by echo and fluoroscopy. The procedure was then terminated and hemostasis was obtained uneventfully. I should note that a single dose of 5000 units of heparin was administered, as well as a single dose of antibiotics.

RESULTS:

1. Saturations: SVC 79, RA 77, RV 85, RPA 86, LP 84, RPV assumed 97, AO assumed at 97.
2. PRESSURES: RA was 7, RV was 30/5, LPA was 28/8/14, LPA wedge was 9, RPA was 20/8/12, RP wedge was 8, LA was 9.

ANGIOGRAPHY: None. However, documentation of balloon stretch diameter revealed a balloon stretch diameter of approximately 13 mm.

18. Operative Report

Do not code imaging in this case.

DIAGNOSIS:	NSTEMI
PROCEDURES PERFORMED:	1. Thrombectomy of the left circumflex artery
	2. Stenting angioplasty of the left circumflex artery
	3. Stenting angioplasty of the LAD
	4. Stenting angioplasty of the RCA
	5. Coronary angiography

DESCRIPTION OF PROCEDURE: The patient arrived to the cardiac catheterization lab with evidence of posterior wall myocardial infarction. The right groin was prepped in normal sterilization technique. A 6-French introducer catheter was placed in the right femoral artery using Seldinger technique. Judkins technique was used for coronary angiography.

CORONARY ANGIOGRAPHY: Left main bifurcates into LAD and left circumflex. The left main is extremely short. The left circumflex is occluded. The LAD has a tight hazy-looking lesion in the range about 85%–90%. Right coronary artery is dominant with an 85% mid lesion.

ANGIOPLASTY OF THE LEFT CIRCUMFLEX ARTERY: The guide was an XB 3.5 guide. I started the procedure by putting it in the left main and I started with the angioplasty immediately. The wire was pushed across the left circumflex artery, which is a very large vessel, with a huge obtuse marginal. Thrombectomy was done in the circumflex utilizing the aspiration catheter. TIMI-3 flow was established. After which, a drug-coated Xience stent was placed, achieving a 0% residual stenosis and excellent flow. After that, attention was taken into the LAD. The lesion of the LAD seems to be very proximal hazy 85%–90%. I was worried that it is a ruptured plaque. So, I kept the wire in the left circumflex artery and I advanced another wire into the LAD. I kept the wire in the left circumflex to keep anchoring the guide particularly with a very short left main, afterward direct stenting with Vision stent achieving a 0% residual stenosis and excellent TIMI-3 flow into the LAD.

The right coronary was then evaluated. The lesion was in the mid RCA. The wire was pushed across and a drug-coated Xience stent was placed, achieving a 0% residual stenosis and excellent flow. All wires were removed. Final images were obtained.

19. Operative Report

PREOPERATIVE DIAGNOSIS:	Post-obstructive pneumonia, not resolving for over 6 months
POSTOPERATIVE DIAGNOSES:	Post-obstructive pneumonia, not resolving for over 6 months. Mucus plugging, right upper lobe bronchus.
PROCEDURES PERFORMED:	Bronchoscopy with transbronchial biopsy, endobronchial biopsy and removal of mucus plug

HISTORY: The patient is a 48-year-old male who has been followed since January for pneumonia with waxing and waning improvement and inconsistent follow up. On CT scan, ordered by the Emergency Department today, he demonstrated dense consolidation of the right upper lobe and possible calcifications in the bronchial lumen with multiple pulmonary granulomas present. There were no masses noted. He is still short of breath and sweats easily. He has smoked 2 packs per day for 31 years, although he has cut down considerably in the past months.

PROCEDURE IN DETAIL: The patient was taken to the endoscopy suite and placed on the fluoroscopy table. Four percent nebulized Lidocaine via hand-held nebulizer was utilized to anesthetize the pharynx and larynx. Neo-Synephrine was placed into both nostrils to help dilate the nasal passages. Lidocaine jelly was utilized to anesthetize the right nostril. He was sedated with 10 mg of Versed and appeared to be awake during the entire procedure.

An Olympus 1T40 bronchoscope was passed through the right nostril into the lower airways without difficulty. Upper and lower airways were further anesthetized with 2 percent Xylocaine. Visualization of the right and left bronchial trees were performed. Upper airways and vocal cords were normal. Trachea was unremarkable. Right upper lobe anterior segment demonstrated erythema and swelling with obstructing mucus plug. There was no endobronchial lesion noted. There was no bleeding or purulent mucus. The right middle lobe and right lower lobe were without endobronchial lesions, swelling, erythema, purulent mucus, or bleeding. All segments and subsegments were otherwise patent. Left main stem, left upper lobe lingula, and left lower lobe were without endobronchial lesion noted. There was no bleeding or purulent mucus. All segments and subsegments were patent.

A transbronchial biopsy was obtained percutaneously from the right upper lobe anterior segment and an endobronchial biopsy was obtained from in the right upper bronchus. The mucus plug was suctioned free from the right upper bronchus. The patient tolerated the procedure well without evidence of complication.

20. Operative Report

PREOPERATIVE DIAGNOSIS: Deep laceration, left hand with extensive tendon disruption of the fourth and fifth digits, secondarily of the third digit, middle finger

POSTOPERATIVE DIAGNOSIS: Deep laceration, left hand with extensive tendon disruption of the fourth and fifth digits, secondarily of the third digit, middle finger

OPERATION: Extensive tendon repair, fourth and fifth digits, third digit longitudinally, index finger second digit with extensor hood

The patient was brought to the operating theater and anesthetized with a Bier block. We explored the wounds, and the joint capsule to fourth and fifth was excised into the joint. The tendon of the extensor indices communis to the fifth digit was lacerated. The extensor indices proprius ulnarly was still intact. The extensor hood over the MCP joint of #4 was torn, as was the capsule. The extensor tendon along the central hood of the third digit was torn longitudinally, and the point was spared. The index finger had a longitudinal tear of the extensor hood in the central portion of the midphalanx. The wounds were copiously irrigated with bacitracin saline with a pulsatile lavage. The joint surface of the fourth and fifth were irrigated.

We then began the definitive repairs. We sutured the MCP joint capsule of the fourth and fifth with a 4-0 Vicryl continuous. We sutured the extensor digitorum communis tendon to #5 with 5-0 Prolene and to #4 over the central hood, over the MCP joint with a 5-0 Prolene continuous. The extensor tendon of the third or middle finger was sutured longitudinally, and a lateral band on the radial side was repaired with a 5-0 Vicryl. The longitudinal tear, which was really a split or a double split, was sutured with over-and-over 5-0 Vicryl as well. We then incised in an S-shaped fashion over the index finger to expose the central hood, which was torn. The main extensor hood was repaired with 5-0 Prolene simple sutures. We then irrigated again with a liter of bacitracin pulsatile lavage and closed the skin with figure-of-eight mattress sutures, alternating with simple sutures. A bulky dressing was then applied, with a volar slab, with the hand in the position of function, extension of the wrist, extension of the MCP joint, flexion of the PIP, and DIP of 30 degrees. The patient then had the tourniquet deflated fully and was sent to the recovery room in good condition.

21. Operative Report

PREOPERATIVE DIAGNOSIS: Chronic headache and neck pain

POSTOPERATIVE DIAGNOSIS: Chronic headache and neck pain

INDICATION: The patient also has chronic myalgias in various areas of the body. An informed consent was signed today. The patient states that the first 2 acupuncture treatments did not do much for her and that she is more achy than in the past.

PROCEDURE: We elected to put gold seeds over shen men, muscle relaxation, kidney, liver, and thalamus. We also decided to put in spleen 6, liver 3, gallbladder 34, kidney 3 and bladder 62. Based on her response to these, we will determine whether to treat her back shu points next time or continue with this plan.

22. Operative Report

PREOPERATIVE DIAGNOSES: 1. Retained primary tooth
2. Ankylosed teeth

POSTOPERATIVE DIAGNOSES: Same

OPERATION: 1. Simple extraction of teeth #A, #8 and #32
2. Surgical exposure of teeth #18 and #31

PROCEDURE: He was transferred to the operating table and laid in supine position. After a smooth induction, an endotracheal tube was placed and secured. A brief time out was held with the operating room team to verify the patient and the procedure.

Attention was directed to the patient's maxillary right quadrant, where tooth #A was extracted using elevator and forceps without complication. The surgical site was then irrigated, tissues reapproximated and closed using 3-0 chromic gut. Attention was then directed to the patient's mandibular right quadrant, where a sulcular incision was created around tooth #31. The surgical site was then irrigated and inspected. Tissues were reapproximated and closed using 3-0 chromic gut. Tooth #32 was identified. It was removed in its entirety.

Attention was directed to the patient's maxillary anterior, where tooth #8 was identified. It was noted on previous CT scan to have no root development. It was also noted to have essentially no follicular space. For these reasons, the decision was made to remove this tooth, given extremely poor prognosis. The tooth was removed in its entirely, clinically confirming the radiographic findings. The tooth indeed had no viable root.

Attention was directed to the patient's mandibular left quadrant, where a sulcular incision was created around tooth #18 and carried along the alveolar ridge with a distobuccal hockey-stick releasing incision. The tissues were reflected. Bone was removed using a rotary handpiece under copious amounts of irrigation to identify tooth #18, which was released from the bone. The surgical sites were then all irrigated: tissues reapproximated and closed using 3-0 chromic gut. This concluded the procedure for this patient. The oropharynx was thoroughly irrigated and suctioned, the throat pack was removed. He was turned over to the anesthesia team, where he was extubated without complication and taken to the PACU in good condition with vital signs stable.

23. Operative Report

PRECATHETERIZATION DIAGNOSIS: Palpitations and arrythmia

POSTCATHETERIZATION DIAGNOSIS: Palpitations and arrythmia

NAME OF PROCEDURE: EP study, ablation, coronary angiogram, balloon angioplasty and stenting

DESCRIPTION OF PROCEDURE: The patient was taken to the cardiac catheterization laboratory for ablation. The patient was prepped and draped in a sterile fashion and a time out was performed. Local anesthetic was given in bilateral groins and access was obtained using a modified Seldinger technique. Catheters were placed under fluoroscopic guidance without difficulty. An EPS was performed demonstrating no inducible supraventricular tachycardia. The AP ERP was 600/350 and 400/320 with AVN ERP as well some time before this. SPERRI was 450 msec.

A 4 mm tip D/F curve Biosense catheter was used to map. Mapping in atrial pacing and sinus showed earliest antegrade activation in a right posteroseptal location along the anterior rim of the CS ostium. With multiple lesions, there was loss of preexcitation but then would come back within a minute. Stability was a question so the catheter was exchanged for a D/F 3.5 mm tip ThermoCool SmarTouch catheter. With 30 W of power and contact of 15-20 g of force, there was loss of preexcitation at 5 seconds. A second lesion was placed and following the placement of a second lesion, there was noted to be change in surface QRS with ST elevation. With serial ECG, there was resolution of the changes within 10 minutes back to normal. The blood pressure is completely stable 100 to 110 range. Given this, we proceeded to evaluate the coronary arteries.

Using the right femoral artery access, a 4 French 1.5 JL catheter was utilized and angiograms were taken in the left coronary artery and right coronary artery with 4 French 1.5 JR catheter. We did selective coronary angiography and this demonstrated a near occlusion of the left circumflex not previously identified. At this point we intervened on the left circumflex coronary using 1.5, 1.75, 2, 2.25 coronary balloons and a bare metal stent. Post stent placement angiogram demonstrates normal flow in the circumflex artery with no evidence of thrombi noticed. There is a normal perfusion distally with no evidence of extravasation of contrast or dissection of the coronary artery noted. No hemodynamic data was obtained. Total Omnipaque contrast utilized: 64 mL.

24. Operative Report

PRE-OP DIAGNOSIS: Retained hardware (nonfunctioning bilateral thoracic column neurostimulator generators) with possible infection on the right

POST-OP DIAGNOSIS: Same

PROCEDURE: Removal of bilateral thoracic column stimulator generators

TECHNIQUE: Under general anesthesia, the patient was placed into the side-lying position with the left hip up. The previous site for the left thoracic column stimulator was identified. The stimulator was palpated and an incision was made at the previous incision site. This was carried down to the subcutaneous tissue. The wires were brought into the field and cut. The stimulator generator was removed. The incision was then closed with 2-0 Vicryl suture for the subq layer and 3-0 nylon for skin. Sterile dressing was applied over this area.

The patient was placed back into the supine position and then repositioned with the right hip up. The area was prepped and draped. In the area of the right stimulator, I palpated a large area of ecchymosis. Using the previous incision, which was about 1.5 cm above the margin of the erythema, I opened the pocket down to the soft tissues and then identified the cables. These were brought out of the wound and cut. They appeared clean and normal. They were then retracted wall back into the tissue. This area was then closed off utilizing Vicryl suture. I then made a small incision directly over the stimulator generator. There was no fluid or abnormal tissue noted around the generator. I removed it completely and examined the pocket. I then irrigated the pocket and found the opening to the ecchymosis, evacuated it and irrigated again with antibiotic solution. I placed a catheter for a drain into the pocket and closed around the catheter with 2-0 Vicryl for the subq tissue and 3-0 nylon for the skin. The patient tolerated the procedure well.

25. Operative Report

PREOPERATIVE DIAGNOSIS: Intradural combination of intramedullary extramedullary T12-L1 mass compatible with ependymoma.

POSTOPERATIVE DIAGNOSIS: Intradural combination of intramedullary extramedullary T12-L1 mass compatible with ependymoma.

NAME OF OPERATION: T12-L1 laminectomy, excision of the intradural mix, intramedullary and extramedullary mass compatible with ependymoma. Pedicle screws and rods.

TECHNIQUE: The patient admitted to the operating room. The patient had CT of thoracolumbar spine. The patient received 1 g SoluMedrol and also 2 g Ancef. Under general anesthesia, A-line and Foley catheter was inserted. The patient was hooked up to somatosensory, evoked small motor response and also anal muscle sensor. The patient was turned over to the Allen table in the prone position. Thoracolumbar spine widely prepped and draped. Local Marcaine was administered between the T1-L1 spinous processes.

X-ray was done, position marker appreciated. The incision was marked between spinous process at T11-L3. Incision opened and subcutaneous bleeding controlled with bipolar. Thoracolumbar fascia opened from spinous process and lamina of the T12, L1, L2, and L3. Muscle retracted with cerebral retractor. Marcaine administered to the L1 lamina and lateral x-ray was done. Dissection was done superiorly to expose the lamina of T12, transverse process of the T12, and the pars of the L1. Then, using the drill, first two pedicle screws applied to the pedicle of T12 and pedicle of L1.

Then, we tried to do a lumbar puncture through the interspace between L2-L3 but were not successful. It looks like due to this tumor was no CSF at this level due to the blockage, so this was abandoned.

Then, the spinous process at T12-L1 was removed. Using the 4 mm cutting bur, lower half of lamina of the T12 and lamina of L1 were removed. The yellow ligament between T12-L1 and L1-L2 removed. At this time, the ultrasound was brought to the field. Location of mass was confirmed. At this time, microscope brought to the field and the rest of the operation was done under microscope. The dura opened in vertical fashion with of #15 blade and nerve hook. The dura tagged to upward with a 4-0 Nurolon.

Then, we encountered very large hemorrhagic mass. It essentially occupied whole posterior aspect of the spinal canal. Then, the arachnoid over the mass opened. Then, we tried to tilt the arachnoid upward but were not successful due to size of mass.

I was able to get to the most superior aspect of the mass and it was attached to the conus. Dissection proceeded laterally to the inferior aspect of tumor. Ultimately, I was able to get the distal part of the tumor and elevated it. All of the nerve roots distal to the mass and around the mass meticulously dissected and pushed aside to keep them away from the mass. Then, many small, medial feeders going to tumor were coagulated with bipolar cautery. The filum terminalis was cut and the tumor was elevated and extended all the way to the tip of the conus. Total resection of tumor obtained. Meticulous hemostasis was done and the wound was irrigated. There was much improvement in motor function appreciated. No any sensory function change appreciated. There was sufficient dura to close with a running 5-0 Vicryl.

Attention was directed to the pedicle screws. The proper rod brought to the field, to the mild kyphotic applied to the T12-L1. The screws were capped and locked. Then, dura was covered with DuraSeal and 1 Gram vancomycin. The thoracolumbar fascia was closed with 1-0 Ethibond. A subQ Jackson-Pratt was inserted and brought through a different stab and secured with subcuticular Vicryl and standard Steri-Strips. The patient tolerated well. After applying dressing, the patient transferred to recovery in good condition. Electrodiagnostic tests were improved.

26. Operative Report

PREOPERATIVE DIAGNOSIS: Acquired absence of right breast from previous skin reduction mastectomy for carcinoma.

POSTOPERATIVE DIAGNOSIS: Acquired absence of right breast from previous skin reduction mastectomy for carcinoma.

NAME OF PROCEDURE: Reconstruction of right breast with latissimus dorsi myocutaneous flap and replacement with 300 mL silicone gel implant.

DESCRIPTION OF OPERATION: Under general anesthetic, the chest wall and arm were prepped and draped in the usual fashion. An 8 × 18 cm transverse ellipse of skin was outlined along the posterior bra line preoperatively and the lower skin incision was made to elevate a sub-Scarpa's flap inferiorly for around 10 cm. The upper incision was then made and the flap raised superiorly, identifying the upper border of the latissimus dorsi muscle and undermining deep muscle to free up the flap. Here the intercostal perforators were secured with Hemoclips and the muscle was separated from the lumbodorsal fascia. An incision was made along the anterior chest wall mastectomy scar to create a subcutaneous tunnel. The flap was tunneled and delivered into the anterior chest wall. Closure of the back defect was completed with interrupted 0 Vicryl and Dermabond. The patient was repositioned in the supine position. The medial horizontal scar was then incised and undermined to accommodate the myocutaneous flap. The upper border of the right latissimus muscle was then anchored in place. Using a balloon sizer, we decided to use a 300 mL silicone gel implant. The sizer was removed. Hemostasis established and a #15 Blake drain placed and anchored. A 300 mL silicone gel permanent breast implant was placed in the breast pocket and tacked with a single stitch to prevent the implant from migrating laterally. The distal 3 cm of the flap was de-epithelialized and buried beneath the sternal skin. The skin was closed and suture lines were covered with Dermabond.

27. Operative Report

PREOPERATIVE DIAGNOSES:
1. Multivessel coronary artery disease with angina
2. Small coronary arteries
3. Diabetes mellitus

POSTOPERATIVE DIAGNOSES: Same

OPERATION PERFORMED:
1. Coronary artery bypass times two, one arterial graft, one venous graft (left internal mammary pedicle to left anterior descending, saphenous vein graft to posterior descending artery)
2. Transmyocardial laser revascularization
3. Xenograft implantation to repair pericardium using CorMatrix.
4. Endoscopic vein harvest

ANESTHESIA: General endotracheal

INDICATIONS: This is a 61-year-old male who presented with angina. He has a history of coronary artery disease dating back many years and has had a stent placed. Coronary angiogram showed severe multivessel coronary artery disease with very small coronary arteries, especially the left-sided system. Hence, the patient will benefit from transmyocardial laser revascularization.

DESCRIPTION OF OPERATION: The patient was brought to the operating room and placed in the supine position. After the appropriate monitoring lines were placed by anesthesia, he was given a general endotracheal anesthetic. A transesophageal probe was placed. The TEE showed left ventricular function of about 60% with mild mitral regurgitation. The neck, chest, abdomen, and bilateral lower extremities were then prepped and draped sterilely. The chest was entered through a median sternotomy incision. The left internal mammary was harvested as a pedicle graft. Simultaneously, the left saphenous vein was harvested endoscopically. The leg wound was then closed in layers with Vicryl. The pericardium was opened along the midline. Systemic heparin was already given. The aorta was cannulated with an 18 French arterial cannula and the right atrium with a two-stage venous cannula. A retrograde catheter was placed into the coronary sinus and an antegrade cannula into the ascending aorta. We then went on cardiopulmonary bypass. The aorta was cross clamped. One liter of cold blood antegrade cardioplegia was given, followed by another 500 mL retrograde. Intermittent cardioplegia was given in roughly fifteen minute intervals. A transmyocardial laser revascularization was performed first. Using the PMI probe, I placed in total 22 two channels along the anterior wall and lateral wall over the left ventricle. After this, the heart was arrested.

Coronary revascularization was performed. I used a segment of the vein graft and anastomosed the posterior descending artery which is a 2 mm vessel. The posterior lateral artery is a very small vessel measuring 1 mm or less. Hence, I could not graft this vessel. There were no vessels more than 1 mm on the lateral wall selected on graft and the vessels there. The left anterior descending artery was opened and was found to be about 1.5 mm. Hence, I grafted the left internal mammary to the LAD. The aortic cross-clamp was then removed. The vein graft was anastomosed to the ascending aorta with a partial aortic clamp in place. The vein graft was deaired. After the patient was fully rewarmed and resuscitated, we came off bypass. The retrograde catheter and venous cannula were then removed. Protamine was administered. The aortic cannula was removed last. Two mediastinal and one right pleural chest tubes were placed. I decided to close the pericardium using a sheet of CorMatrix. The CorMatrix was sewn to the pericardial edge with a running 3-0 Prolene. I left one chest tube below and one above the CorMatrix. The sternum was then closed with interrupted steel wires followed by running Vicryl for the fascia and subdermal layers. The skin was then closed with a subcuticular 3-0 Monocryl.

28. Operative Report

PREOPERATIVE DIAGNOSIS: Epigastric and right upper quadrant abdominal pain. Irritable bowel syndrome.

POSTOPERATIVE DIAGNOSIS: Two 2-mm hyperplastic-appearing rectal polyps, status post forceps polypectomy, normal appearing colonic mucosa, status post biopsies in the sigmoid and descending colon to evaluate for microscopic colitis

PROCEDURE: Colonoscopy with polypectomy and biopsy

PROCEDURE DESCRIPTION: After informed consent was obtained, the patient was sedated and placed in the left lateral decubitus position. Perianal and digital rectal examination were unremarkable. A well-lubricated adult colonoscope was placed in the rectum and successfully advanced to the cecum. The ileocecal valve and appendiceal orifice were well visualized. The terminal ileum was intubated and appeared normal. The colonoscope was then slowly withdrawn. The entire colonic mucosa and vascular pattern appeared unremarkable. Biopsies were obtained in the descending and sigmoid colon to evaluate for microscopic colitis. The retroflexed examination of the two 2-mm hyperplastic-appearing polyps in the rectum, which were resected using cold forceps. The colon was decompressed and the scope was completely withdrawn. There were no immediate complications.

29. Operative Report

PREOPERATIVE DIAGNOSIS: Obstructive sleep apnea with upper airway obstruction

POSTOPERATIVE DIAGNOSIS: Obstructive sleep apnea with upper airway obstruction

PROCEDURE: Adenoidectomy, lingual tonsillectomy

INDICATION FOR PROCEDURE: The patient is a 9-year-old male with a history of obstructive sleep apnea. He is currently maintained on BiPAP. He also has some lingual tonsillary hypertrophy as well as a large adenoid pad. He presents today for surgical management of the above.

PROCEDURE DESCRIPTION: After the patient was correctly identified in the holding area, he was taken to the operating room and general endotracheal anesthesia was administered. A time-out was performed. A Crowe-Davis mouth gag was inserted and a mirror was used to visualize the adenoid pad. The adenoid pad was reduced on a Bovie setting of 36.

At this point, anesthesia switched his oral tube for a nasal tube. His tongue was grasped and a suture was placed for retraction. A Jennings mouth gag was used to open his mouth. Under this visualization, the patient's base of tongue was still somewhat difficult to visualize but Bovie was used on a setting of 20 to destroy some of the lingual tonsillar tissue. The lingual surface of the epiglottis was kept free of the Bovie. A mild to moderate amount of lingual tonsillar tissue was removed in this fashion. There was minimal bleeding. The contents of the stomach and esophagus were suctioned. The patient was awakened and taken to recovery in good condition.

30. Operative Report

PREOPERATIVE DIAGNOSIS: Left knee medial gonarthrosis

POSTOPERATIVE DIAGNOSIS: Left knee medial gonarthrosis

PROCEDURE PERFORMED: Left knee unicompartmental arthroplasty, Zimmer, cemented.

PROCEDURE DESCRIPTION: Spinal anesthesia with a femoral block was placed in the holding area. She was then taken to the operating room. After an adequate level of anesthesia was obtained, the patient's left leg had a tourniquet placed on the upper thigh. It was then placed in a leg holder. The foot of the table was bent. The leg was then prepped and draped in the usual sterile fashion. It was then elevated, Esmarch and the tourniquet was inflated to 300 pounds. A median parapatellar incision was then made and carried down sharply through the subcutaneous tissue down to the medial retinaculum. The medial retinaculum was then incised with a direct skin incision from the VMO, not through it, to just medical to the insertion of patellar tendon to the anterior tibial tubercle. Findings revealed bone-on-bone changes over the medial joint line with significant distal femoral and proximal tibial sparing. The ACL was intact. The MCL was intact. The lateral joint line was normal for as far as we could see, and there was no more than grade 1 to 2 changes in the patellofemoral joint. Osteophytes were then removed off the medial side. The tibial cutting guide was put in place, making sure we were parallel to the tibia in both AP and lateral plane. The sagittal cut was sparing the fibers of the anterior cruciate and in the direction of the femur. The depth of the cut was 3 mm deep to the depressed aspect of the tibial plateau. We were easily able then to insert a 10 mm spacer into the tibia in flexion as well as in extension. The 10 mm spacer was then used for the distal femoral cut. This sized to a size C. The C cutting guide was then put in place. Chamfer cuts were then made. We sized to a 3 on the tibia. This was pinned into place. Drill holes were then made and we trialed up to a 10. The 10 seemed to track well. There was no impingement and there was a 2 mm space in both flexion as well as extension. All trials were removed. The wound was irrigated copiously with large-bore suction irrigation. The meniscal remnants were removed. The cement was then pressurized in the tibia and the tibial component put in place, making sure all excess was removed, especially from the posterior aspect of the joint. The same was done on the femur. A 10 mm trial polyethylene insert was then put in place and the cement was allowed to dry in extension. After the cement dried, we then removed all excess cement posteriorly and made sure that the range of motion was as dictated above. The local irrigating solution was then instilled through the posterior capsule, coming around the meniscal rim, and in through the medial retinaculum. The tourniquet was then released after approximately 38 minutes. All visible bleeders were electrocauterized. The implantable polyethylene insert was then put in place and snapped in, making sure it was stable and the range of motion was as dictated above. The retinaculum was then reapproximated with a #1 Vicryl in figure-of-8 interrupted-type sutures. The subcutaneous tissue was then closed with 2-0 Vicryl and the skin was closed with staples. A sterile dressing was then applied. A drain had been placed in the wound and brought out through a separate stab wound superolaterally prior to the closure. The estimated blood loss was approximately 15 mL. The counts were all correct. The patient was awake and taken back to recovery in stable condition.

31. Operative Report

PROCEDURE: Placement of a dual chamber implantable pacing cardioverter-defibrillator

INDICATIONS: Patient with moderate ischemic cardiomyopathy, prior infarct and stent

PROCEDURE DESCRIPTION: After informed consent, the patient is brought to the lab. The procedure was done under conscious sedation fluoroscopic guidance. One percent Lidocaine was used to anesthetize the skin under the left clavicle, and a skin incision was made. A pocket was made for the ICD generator and leads securing good hemostasis. The left subclavian vein was easily cannulated twice using a pediatric set, which was up-sized to regular 037 wires, the position of which was checked under fluoro. I then dilated the access volt with 9-French dilators and used 7-French access sheaths through which a 7-French right ventricular lead was advanced and placed under fluoroscopic guidance with Omnipaque. It was an active fixation lead. The numbers looked good and the lead was sutured down. There was no diaphragmatic stimulation.

A 7-French lead was then advanced under fluoroscopic guidance and placed in the right atrial appendage. The numbers looked good. There was no diaphragmatic stimulation, and the lead was sutured down. The leads were then attached to the generator, which was tested and sutured down in the pocket. Wound closed in layers. The patient tolerated the procedure well, without any complications. The wound was irrigated several times with antibiotics during and at the end of the case.

IMPRESSION: Successful dual chamber ICD as noted above. The patient will be admitted overnight, will get an additional dose of antibiotics and a chest x-ray, and if stable, will be discharged home in the morning.

32. Operative Report

PREOPERATIVE DIAGNOSIS: Displaced left femoral neck fracture

POSTOPERATIVE DIAGNOSIS: Displaced left femoral neck fracture

PROCEDURE PERFORMED: Left hip hemiarthroplasty

INDICATIONS: This 96-year-old male sustained a fall earlier today. He was an independent ambulator at home and had a mechanical fall. He had demonstrated a fracture and a hemiarthroplasty on the contralateral side and understood the expectations, the risk of infection, dislocation, tissue injury, anesthetic risks, DVT were understood and the patient and family wished to proceed. The potential for needing transfusion was also understood.

PROCEDURE DETAILS: Following IV antibiotics of Ancef 2 grams, he was brought to the OR and placed in a lateral position. A spinal anesthetic was administered. He was then positioned on a bean bag positioner. A surgical time-out was called confirming the correct patient and appropriate extremity. The patient was then prepped and draped and an Ioban dressing sealing off the area was placed. An incision was made sharply through the skin and subcutaneous tissue. Hemostasis was obtained using electrocautery. Dissection continued down to the fascia layer which was incised and divided. Charnley retractor was placed. Bursal tissue was resected and reflected. A Kober retractor was placed beneath the abductors. The piriformis was tagged and reflected. The capsular tissue had a T incision made and the corners of the capsule were tagged with Ethibond suture. The femoral head was then dislocated using Chandler retractor. The neck was then evaluated. The neck cut was completed using the oscillating saw with retractors placed. Subsequently the canal preparation was undertaken. The patient had a contralateral hemiarthroplasty previously using a 52 size head. This was trialed and found to be appropriate. Axial reamers were then used down the femoral canal up to a size #8. The broach was used up to a size #7, which was chosen. The canal was then prepared with antibiotic irrigation and distal cement was placed. Osteonics #7 cement sten was placed into the canal. This was held in place and position until the cement cured. Excess cement was removed. We then trialed a #0 neck 52 head, which was appropriate. Therefore, we placed a 26 mm metal head with #0 neck 52 head on the #7 prosthesis stem. The hip was then reduced and taken through range of motion and was stable throughout. We irrigated with antibiotics again and closed the capsule in layers with Ethibond suture. Piriformis was then tacked into the trochanteric area. The fascial layers reapproximated with #1 Vicryl suture. Subcutaneous layer was closed with 2-0 Vicryl and skin was closed with staples. The hip abduction pillow was placed with the patient in the supine position. There were no complications.

33. Operative Report

PREOPERATIVE DIAGNOSIS: End-stage renal disease

POSTOPERATIVE DIAGNOSIS: End-stage renal disease

PROCEDURE: Creation of a left brachiocephalic AV fistula

Insertion of a right internal jugular Perm-A-Cath under ultrasound and fluoroscopic guidance.

ANESTHESIA: Left supraclavicular nerve block and local anesthetic using 1% Xylocaine plain.

INDICATIONS FOR SURGERY: This is a 31-year-old female who has a recent of history of end-stage renal disease and presents for permanent access.

DESCRIPTION OF PROCEDURE: After adequate left supraclavicular nerve block, the patient was placed in the supine position, and her entire left upper extremity was prepped with Betadine scrub and solution, and she was draped in a sterile fashion. Ultrasound was performed on the left arm, and it appeared that the cephalic vein at the wrist level was absent but the cephalic vein in the arm was patent and appeared to measure about 3 mm in diameter.

Because of this, it was decided to perform a brachiocephalic fistula. A transverse incision was made just above the antecubital fossa, and dissection was carried down through the subcutaneous tissue, and the cephalic vein was identified and isolated around its entire circumference for about a 2 cm length. The dissection continued down to the bifurcation of the cephalic vein and both branches were isolated. The fascia was then incised, and the brachial artery was identified. The artery was isolated for about a 1.5 cm length. The artery was found to be soft and of sufficient diameter.

The patient was then administered 3000 units of IV heparin sulfate. After 5 minutes had elapsed, the vein was ligated distally and transected. A #3 dilator was inserted up the vein without difficulty. The artery was then occluded proximally and distally and an arteriotomy was made. The vein was cut to the desired length and shape, and the anastomosis was performed using 6-0 Prolene in a running fashion. The clamps were removed, and there was a good thrill present within the vein. The wound was then irrigated and bleeders were cauterized. The wound was closed with 3-0 Vicryl in a running fashion for the subcutaneous tissue and 5-0 Monocryl in a running subcuticular fashion for the skin.

Attention was next turned toward insertion of the Perm-A-Cath. The right chest and neck were sterilely prepped and draped. Xylocaine 1% plain was injected into the subcutaneous tissue of the right neck. Under ultrasound guidance, the internal jugular vein was identified, and this was punctured with a 19-gauge needle. A guidewire was threaded without difficulty. The needle was removed, and a site was selected on the chest wall for the insertion site of the catheter. This area was injected with 1% Xylocaine plain, as was the tract from this area up to the guidewire site. A nick was made in the skin over the chest wall and also the guidewire site. A subcutaneous tunnel was then created from one wound to the other using a tunneling device. The catheter was pulled through the subcutaneous tunnel, and the antimicrobial cuff was lodged in the tissues.

Dilators were then placed over the guidewire, followed by the introducer and the peel-away sheath. The introducer and the guidewire were removed, and the catheter was slipped into the peel-away sheath. The peel-away sheath was then removed. There was good blood return through both ports, and the catheter was then flushed with saline, followed by heparin 1000 units per cc. The positioning of the catheter was checked under fluoroscopy, and it appeared that the tip was in the superior vena cava, and there was no kinking or twisting of the catheter. The catheter was stitched into place with a 3-0 nylon stitch. The neck wound was closed with 5-0 Monocryl interrupted subcuticular stitches. The patient tolerated the procedure well without complications.

34. Operative Report

FINDINGS: There was a 1.6 × 1.5 cm defect of the right nasal sidewall, remaining after a previous repair following a dog bite. It did extend slightly onto the cheek.

PROCEDURE: After obtaining informed consent, the patient was taken into the operating room and placed in a supine position on the operating table. General anesthesia was induced via endotracheal intubation without difficulty. Approximately 2 mL of 1 percent lidocaine with 1:100,000 epinephrine was injected into the right conchal bowl and the right postauricular region. The face was prepped and draped in a sterile fashion. A surgical pause was performed to confirm the patient's identity and site of surgery. A skin incision was made in the pinna on the right-hand side, and a piece of conchal bowl cartilage measuring approximately 1 × 1.5 cm was harvested and placed in saline to be used as a strut along the right lateral nasal sidewall. This incision was closed using 6-0 fast-absorbing gut.

A piece of foil was used to create a template of the defect in the nose. A full-thickness skin graft matching to the shape of a template was harvested from the right postauricular region of the upper neck. The recipient site was prepared on the right side of the nose. The cartilage was then placed along the lateral sidewall and secured in place with a single through-and-through fast-absorbing gut suture. The central portion of the full-thickness skin graft was also secured with a fast-absorbing gut suture to the central portion of the nasal defect. The perimeter of the graft was then sutured to the nose using interrupted 6-0 nylon suture.

Once the graft had been sutured in place, the harvested site in the postauricular region was expanded into an elliptical-shaped defect by removing some skin superior and inferior to the harvest site itself. Undermining was performed primarily in the posterior direction of the skin under the hairline. Minimal undermining was done of the skin anteriorly toward the pinna of the ear. Hemostasis was obtained after the undermining, and this harvest site incision was closed using 4-0 Vicryl and 5-0 nylon. A small pressure dressing was applied to the right side of the nose, and a Glasscock mastoid dressing was placed on the right ear. The patient was then awakened from the anesthetic, extubated, and transported to the recovery room with stable vital signs and no evidence of stridor.

35. Operative Report

PREOPERATIVE DIAGNOSIS: Four vessel coronary artery disease

POSTOPERATIVE DIAGNOSIS: Four vessel coronary artery disease

PROCEDURES PERFORMED:
1. Left internal mammary artery to left anterior descending artery
2. Reversed saphenous vein graft to obtuse marginal artery, posterior descending artery and posterolateral arteries

OPERATIVE PROCEDURE AND FINDINGS: The patient was taken to the operating room and placed in the supine position under suitable general endotracheal anesthesia and was prepared and draped in the usual sterile fashion. The left greater saphenous vein was procured through several skin incisions. The leg was closed in layers of Vicryl. Simultaneously, the chest was entered through a midline sternotomy incision and the left internal mammary artery taken down as a pedicled, skeletonized graft. It was an excellent conduit. After heparin was administered, it was divided distally and noted to have brisk, pulsatile flow. The left internal mammary artery was anastomosed to the left anterior descending artery.

Epiaortic ultrasound of the ascending aorta was performed to guide cannula placement. 5 separate views were obtained, 3 transverse and 2 longitudinal. Large atheromas over 5 mm were identified in the distal ascending aortic segment (Katz Grade IV). As a result of this study, we elected to perform surgery with the heart on bypass, beating, without crossclamp, to avoid manipulation of the aorta. Simple movement of the heart resulted in hemodynamic compromise, so off-pump techniques were precluded.

The patient was cannulated for bypass with a metal-tipped aortic Sarns line in the ascending aorta where it was soft and free of palpable disease. A 2-stage venous catheter was positioned through the right atrium. The Cardica PasPort proximal anastomotic device was used to anastomose three vein segments to sites on the aorta that the epiaortic ultrasound had demonstrated to be free of atheroma. Good inflow for each was demonstrated. Bypass was instituted and the target vessels were identified. The Medtronic Octopus system was used to stabilize the vessels sequentially to perform the distal anastomoses. The distal vessels described were opened and the anastomoses created with running 7-0 Prolene suture. The patient was weaned from cardiopulmonary bypass on an infusion of nitrates and the contents of the pump oxygenator were returned to the patient. Excellent biphasic Doppler signals and pulses were obtained in all grafts. After decannulation, protamine was used to reverse the effects of heparin. The chest was drained with Blake drains. The pericardium was not closed. The chest was re-approximated in layers with 8 sternal wires and 3 layers of Vicryl to the soft tissues, with Dermabond and a dry sterile dressing to all skin incisions. The sponge, needle, and instrument counts were reported correct by the circulating nurse and the patient was prepared for transfer to the intensive care unit.

36. Operative Report

PREOPERATIVE DIAGNOSIS: Advanced right knee arthrosis

POSTOPERATIVE DIAGNOSIS: Advanced right knee arthrosis

PROCEDURE: Right total knee replacement, cemented posterior cruciate

COMPONENTS USED:

Femoral component: size #7, cemented cruciate sacrificing material: Oxinium Oxidized Zirconium

Tibial component: cemented size #6, Cobalt Chromium

Polyethylene insert: 13 rum, deep dish design

Patellar component: 35 rum diameter, anatomic design, polyethylene

Cement: Antibiotic Simplex P cement

INDICATIONS: The patient presented with severe right knee pain. Preoperative clinical evaluation and x-rays revealed advanced arthritic changes of the knee. After failing conservative management consisting of pain medications and activity modifications, surgical treatment was recommended.

DESCRIPTION OF PROCEDURE: Following successful induction of adequate general anesthesia, the lower extremity was prepped and draped in sterile fashion with the extremity free and the tourniquet at the proximal thigh. Following exsanguination, the tourniquet was inflated to a pressure of 350 mm Hg.

A straight anterior skin incision was centered over the knee and a full thickness subcutaneous flap created to allow a medial parapatellar arthrotomy, performed in partial flexion. The patella was everted or subluxated, and the knee flexed. The anterior cruciate ligament was resected and intercondylar osteophytes were removed.

Access to the medullary canal of the femur and tibia was gained. The femoral intramedullary guide was set at 6 degrees of distal valgus femoral cut. A distal femoral resection was made using the slotted guide and oscillating saw. Appropriate anterior/posterior and chamfer osteotomies were made.

The tibia was stabilized in an anterior subluxation position. Medial and lateral meniscectomies were completed. An intramedullary tibial cutting guide was used to osteotomize the proximal tibial perpendicular to the mechanical axis of the tibia. Measured resection technique was utilized to position the tibial cutting block height. The osteotomy was completed with the proximal tibial cutting block and oscillating saw. A central tibial keel hole was made with primary and secondary punches.

Trial components were inserted. Appropriate prosthetic fit, position, alignment, and flexion/extension ligamentous balance were confirmed using the appropriate tibial polyethylene trial component. The knee was taken through a full range of motion and was found to have good coronal and sagittal plane balancing. Patellar osteophytes were removed, and a transverse patellar osteotomy was performed. Appropriate patellar thickness was confirmed with a caliper. Appropriate patellar component template size was selected. Peg holes were made with the template and drill, medialized so as to reproduce patellar ridge anatomy. Patellar tracking without subluxation with "no thumb" technique and patellar contact with both condyles in 90 degrees flexion was noted.

The patellar and tibial bone surfaces were then prepared for cement using 1/8-inch drill holes for sclerotic bone, saline pulsatile lavage, antibiotic lavage, and gauze drying. Patellar, femoral, and tibial tray components were fixed in place using vacuum-mixed methylmethacrylate delivered with a cement gun. Excess cement was removed. Antibiotic Simplex P cement was used.

The tibial polyethylene component was impacted into place and reduced beneath the femur with the knee flexed to 90 degrees. Appropriate component fixation and position, and patellar tracking were confirmed.

A Hemovac drain was placed. The arthrotomy was closed with the knee in flexion with interrupted #1 suture, and subcutaneous tissue was closed in two layers with interrupted 0 and 2-0 Vicryl suture. The skin apposition and eversion was assured with skin staples. The tourniquet was let down.

37. Operative Report

PREOPERATIVE DIAGNOSIS:	Mitral insufficiency
POST PROCEDURE DIAGNOSIS:	Mitral insufficiency, intra-atrial septal defect
OPERATION PERFORMED:	1. Minimally invasive mitral valve repair, posterior leaflet resection
	2. Medtronics 3D future annuloplasty
	3. Primary closure atrial septal defect

TECHNIQUE: The patient induced to general anesthesia, positioned, draped, and prepped sterile with right chest extended. A right intercostal submammary incision was made within the approximately 3rd interspace, and the patient demonstrated significant elevation of the right hemidiaphragm. The patient was systemically heparinized, cannulated through the right femoral vessels and cardiopulmonary bypass initiated with systemic cooling, which facilitated pericardiotomy anterior to the phrenic. The patient demonstrated extensive mediastinal fat. Transthoracic aorta clamp placed. Antegrade cold blood cardioplegia delivered and with the heart arrested, intra-atrial groove developed, left atriotomy performed. The patient demonstrated evidence of an Amplatz closure device within the intra-atrial septum, with communication to the right atrium. Prolene suture was used to close the intra-atrial septal defect. Evaluation of the mitral valve revealed ruptured chordae of the P2 segment. This was repaired in triangular fashion using interrupted CV5 Gore-Tex suture. Leaflet repair was performed primarily using 2-0 non-pledgeted suture. A 3D future ring annuloplasty seated. With left heart de-aired, facilitated the use of CO_2 insufflation and atriotomy closed with running 3-0 Prolene. The patient systemically warmed, weaned from bypass. Single right pleural chest tube inserted. Pericardiotomy closed within the mid aspect with 5-0 Prolene and with hemostasis achieved and chest closure over #2 Vicryl, fascia, subcutaneous skin closed with running Vicryl. The patient tolerated the procedure, transferred to intensive care stable.

38. Operative Report

PREOPERATIVE DIAGNOSIS(ES):	T3 grade 3 transitional cell carcinoma of the bladder with transitional cell carcinoma of prostate infiltrating prostatic stroma
POSTOPERATIVE DIAGNOSIS(ES):	T3 grade 3 transitional cell carcinoma of the bladder with transitional cell carcinoma of prostate infiltrating prostatic stroma
PROCEDURE(S) PERFORMED:	Radical cystectomy, bilateral pelvic lymphadenectomy, and ileoconduit urinary diversion

DETAILS OF PROCEDURE: Under anesthesia, the patient was placed in the supine position with leg spread on the spreader bars, where his genitalia and lower abdomen were washed with pHisoHex, prepped with Betadine, sterile drapes applied, and sterile catheter placed.

An incision was made from the pubis to a point midway between the umbilicus and xiphisternum, deepened down into the peritoneum. We then separated the bladder from the anterior leaf from the muscular bony pelvis and incised the peritoneum just lateral to the obliterated umbilical vessel from the point just below the umbilicus superiorly down to the femoral canal distally. We found the vas and traced them down to their entrance into the ampulla of vas on each side, thereby making a plane between the rectum and the bladder. We then found both ureters, and with this anatomy and retracting the viscera and placing the patient in Trendelenburg position, we were able to divide the neurovascular pedicle of the bladder from cephalad to cauhad. We did this on each side, and in the inferior portion of the dissection, we found that the rectum was still stuck to the prostate, and with blunt and sharp dissection, we removed the rectum from the prostate and avoided transmural injury of the rectum.

The dorsal vein complex tissue was cut, and the urethra was divided. The catheter was removed and we placed a 24-French Foley catheter with a 30 cc balloon in pelvis and inflated it to 60 cc and placed it on traction.

After the bladder was removed, we then did a bilateral pelvic lymphadenectomy with the margin being the bifurcation, the common iliac artery superiorly, tissue medial to the general femoral nerve laterally, the obturator nerve posteriorly, and the femoral canal distally. Hemostasis was achieved, and the surgeon's gloves, gowns, and instruments were changed.

We removed a 20 cm section of terminal ileum from a point that was about 30 cm distal to the ileocecal valve. The small bowel continuity was re-established using a running continuous layer of 3-0 chromic and an interrupted layer of 3-0 silk, and as the last part of the operation, we closed the mesenteric defect. The butt end of the loop was closed with 3-0 chromic continuous layer in two layers and reinforced by interrupted layers of 3-0 silk. We brought the left ureter beneath the mucosigmoid and incised the posterior parietal peritoneum where the ureter was brought beneath the mesosigmoid. We then sutured the butt end of the loop to the cut end of the mesenteric defect. We then did an end-to-side anastomosis between ends to the left and then right ureter to side of the ileum over diversionary stents using interrupted 5-0 chromic sutures and reinforcing this with 5-0 silk sutures.

All the instruments were removed from the abdomen. We then excised a circle of tissue from skin of the anterior abdominal wall, divided the subcutaneous tissue, excised a circle of fascia, divided the muscle, and in a cruciate incision divided the posterior parietal peritoneum. Two of the surgeon's fingers could be put through his aperture, without distention. We brought the distal end of the ileum through this and anastomosed it to the skin in a nippled fashion. We sutured the diversionary stents before doing anything. We then closed the abdominal wall with 0 Maxon doubled on the fascia, 3-0 Dexon in the subcutaneous tissue, and a subcuticular stitch on the skin. He was returned to the recovery room in satisfactory condition.

39. Operative Report

PREOPERATIVE DIAGNOSIS: Status post transurethral resection of bladder tumor with clot retention

POSTOPERATIVE DIAGNOSIS: Status post transurethral resection of bladder tumor with clot retention

PROCEDURES:
1. Cystoscopy
2. Clot evacuation
3. Fulguration of bleeders

DESCRIPTION OF OPERATION: Following induction of an adequate level of general anesthesia, the patient was placed in the lithotomy position. His penis and surrounding areas were prepared with Betadine and he was draped in a sterile manner.

A 24 French resectoscope sheath was inserted using the obturator without difficulty. The bladder was then inspected using a 12 degree lens. There was a large amount of old clot within the bladder. This was evacuated using a piston syringe. The area of the previous resection appeared to have some small punctuate bleeders, which were fulgurated. When hemostasis was obtained, the bladder was left distended. The resectoscope sheath was removed. A 24 French three-way Foley catheter was inserted. The patient tolerated the procedure well and was sent to the recovery room.

40. Operative Report

PREOPERATIVE DIAGNOSIS: Persistent rejection and failed renal allograft with allograft nephropathy resulting in end-stage renal disease

POSTOPERATIVE DIAGNOSIS: Persistent rejection and failed renal allograft with allograft nephropathy resulting in end-stage renal disease

OPERATION: Transplant nephrectomy

SPECIMENS: Kidney

INDICATIONS: The patient is a 25-year-old female who underwent a kidney transplant that subsequently failed due to persistent rejection. She had met end-stage criteria and is now being dialyzed, however, continues to suffer persistent rejection despite triple immunosuppression. For this reason, she presents to the OR for elective nephrectomy to eliminate the above issues and allow her to discontinue immunosuppressive drugs.

PROCEDURE: The patient was identified and brought to the operating room and placed in the supine position and administered general endotracheal anesthetic. Her entire abdomen was shaved, prepped, and draped in a sterile fashion. She was explored through her previous right hockey stick incision. An incision was carried through the layers of the right abdominal wall with care to avoid entrance into the peritoneal cavity. The kidney transplant was identified. The capsule was separated, freeing the kidney circumferentially down to its vascular pedicle. Large vascular clamps were placed both from a superior and inferior position and crossclamped. The femoral artery pulse was checked and found to be 2+. The kidney was then amputated off its vascular pedicle above the clamps and vessels were secured with two rows of running 3-0 Prolene. Crossclamps were removed and hemostasis was noted with no significant blood loss. The femoral artery was checked again and it still had a 2+ pulse. Sutures were secured. Hemostasis was noted. The retroperitoneum was irrigated. Again, hemostasis was noted. A JP drain was placed subfascially through a right lower quadrant stab incision and secured to the skin with 2-0 nylon. The fascia was then closed in 1 layer using looped #1 PDS. The subcutaneous tissue was closed with 3-0 Vicryl and the skin was closed with staples. A sterile dressing was applied and the patient was extubated and transported to the recovery room in stable condition, having tolerated the procedure without event.

41. Operative Report

PREOPERATIVE DIAGNOSIS: Left partial staghorn calculus

POSTOPERATIVE DIAGNOSIS: Left partial staghorn calculus

| OPERATION: | Left open pyelolithotomy |
| SPECIMENS: | Calculi |

INDICATIONS: The patient is a 50-year-old patient with a history of recurrent urinary tract infections. Workup revealed a large partial staghorn renal calculus. After discussing the options, he has elected to proceed with left open pyelolithotomy.

PROCEDURE: The patient was brought to the operating room. General anesthesia induced. The patient placed in the left-side-up decubitus position. All pressure points padded and supported appropriately. Flank then prepped and draped in the usual manner. Patient identified and procedure confirmed prior to making the incision.

Skin incised over the 12th rib and carried down to the 12th rib. Rib excised sharply sweeping the neurovascular bundle inferiorly. The remaining abdominal wall musculature was then opened using electrocautery and the retroperitoneal space was opened.

It was immediately apparent that the stone had been present for quite some time with ongoing chronic inflammation and infection. I traced the ureter superiorly to find the renal pelvis and the stone. The renal pelvis was exposed as best as possible. Once this was accomplished the renal pelvis was opened by making a stab incision with an 11 blade and then making a U-shaped incision in the renal pelvis itself. Grossly cloudy urine was expelled from the renal pelvis. This was irrigated free, and prior to any further manipulation the wound and retroperitoneum was irrigated copiously with antibiotic solution. I also gave him additional doses of 2 g ampicillin and 80 mg gentamicin.

Using Lowsley stone forceps, the stone was gently worked free from the renal pelvis. Once extracted it was passed off for specimen. A guidewire was then passed down to the bladder and a 6 × 26 double J ureter stent passed over the wire into the bladder. The proximal curl was placed in the renal pelvis. The renal pelvis was closed using a running 3-0 chromic suture. The kidney was placed back into position. The wound was irrigated once again with antibiotic solution, followed by normal saline. Hemostasis assured with clips. Electrocautery as needed. JP drain placed around the area of the renal pelvis closure. The fascia was closed in two layers using a running #1 PDS suture. The subcutaneous tissue was closed with interrupted 3-0 Vicryl. Skin closed with running subcuticular 4-0 Vicryl. Drain secured with 2-0 silk and placed to gravity suction. Dermabond applied to the incision. Dressing applied to the JP. Tolerated well. Returned to the recovery area in good condition.

---

42. Operative Report

PREOPERATIVE DIAGNOSIS:	Left femoral neck fracture
POSTOPERATIVE DIAGNOSIS:	Left femoral neck fracture
OPERATION:	Internal fixation of left femoral neck fracture
IMPLANTS:	Synthes 7.3 cannulated screw ×3

INDICATIONS: The patient is a 63-year-old male who had a fall, sustaining a left femoral neck fracture. He was admitted to the medicine service and after a lengthy, extensive discussion regarding different treatment options, including surgical and nonsurgical management, he wished to proceed to the operating room for pinning and internal fixation of his left femoral neck fracture. All his questions were answered, and no guarantees were given.

PROCEDURE: After proper informed consent was obtained, the patient was brought to the preoperative holding area. The proper extremity was identified and marked for surgery. The patient was then taken to the operating room, where anesthesia induced a spinal anesthetic. TED hoses were placed on both lower extremities. After an appropriate time-out had been performed, the left lower extremity was then placed under traction to align the bone while padding the right lower extremity. A fluoroscopy unit was brought to the field and the hip was identified and was found to have acceptable reduction in the area following traction.

The left lower extremity was then prepped and draped in sterile fashion. After an additional time-out had been performed, an incision was made over the lateral part of the left hip. Sharp and blunt dissection were carried down to the proximal portion of the femur and using a synthes set, three cannulated guidewires were then placed across the fracture while correcting for his rotation and alignment of the proximal femur. All pins were found to have acceptable position and appropriate-size screws. They were then drilled and placed under fluoroscopic assistance. At the completion of the procedure, radiographs were obtained confirming acceptable placement of all hardware without penetration into the joint and all screw heads were past the fracture area. The screws were inserted until they were flush and had appropriate purchase. The images were saved for the patient's chart. The wounds were irrigated with antibiotic solution. The deep fascial layer was closed with #1 Vicryl suture followed by subcutaneous skin closure with a 2-0 Vicryl suture, and skin closure with staples. The patient was taken to the recovery room in stable condition after application of a sterile dressing. The patient will return back to the floor for DVT prophylaxis, gait training, and antibiotics.

43. Operative Report

PREOPERATIVE DIAGNOSIS: Phimosis, hidden penis, penoscrotal tethering, penile torsion

POSTOPERATIVE DIAGNOSIS: Phimosis, hidden penis, penoscrotal tethering, penile torsion

PROCEDURE PERFORMED: Circumcision with release of penoscrotal tethering and hidden penis

INDICATIONS: The patient is a 15-month-old toddler who was seen in consultation for phimosis. After outpatient counseling, he presents for operative intervention, accompanied by his family.

DESCRIPTION OF PROCEDURE: The patient was identified and brought to the operating room and placed supine on the operating table. After induction of adequate general anesthesia, the patient was prepped and draped in the usual sterile fashion. A surgical time-out was taken to identify the patient and the planned procedure. Phimotic foreskin was dilated. A vertical 5-0 Prolene glans holding suture was placed. There was a congenital phimosis of the urethral meatus. The glans was incised to advance the meatus to the proper location. A distal circumferential incision was marked with preservation of a mucosa collar. The penis was degloved to release the angulation that was burying the proximal shaft of the penis within the penopubic fat and to release the penoscrotal tethering. A dorsal and ventral slit were made. The penile skin was secured to the mucosal collar with 6-0 PDS suture.

The penis was marked for circumcision. The prepuce was resected. The circumcision was closed with interrupted 6-0 PDS suture. There was excellent cosmesis. There was no active bleeding. The incision was dressed with benzoin and Tegaderm. A Marcaine dorsal penile block and ring block at the base of the penis were injected for post-operative analgesia. All counts were correct. The patient tolerated the procedure well and was transported to the recovery room in stable condition.

44. Operative Report

PREOPERATIVE DIAGNOSIS: Mastoiditis with suspected advancement to intracranial cavity

POSTOPERATIVE DIAGNOSIS: Mastoiditis with advancement to intracranial cavity

PROCEDURE: Left mastoidectomy and biopsy

INDICATIONS FOR PROCEDURE: The patient presented with acute mastoiditis with suspected spread of the infection. The patient and family were informed of the risks and benefits of the procedure. They understood and wished to proceed with the procedure.

FINDINGS: No frank purulence noted in the mastoid mucosa. Middle ear space was free of fluid or masses. Ossicles were intact and mobile. There was a central dehiscence of the tegmen above the mastoid, less than 1 cm in size. This area was evaluated intraoperatively and pathologic specimens were taken from the mastoid cavity and the dura for evaluation.

OPERATION: The patient was brought to the operating suite and general endotracheal anesthesia was induced. The bed was rotated 90 degrees. Three ccs of local anesthesia were placed in the postauricular sulcus area. The patient was then prepped and draped in the usual sterile manner. A postauricular incision was made and then developed a periosteal PALVA flap was created in a cruciate fashion. The periosteum of the mastoid was then elevated both anteriorly and posteriorly, as well as superiorly underlying the temporalis muscle. After this, care was taken not to enter either the ear canal or the middle ear space through the external auditory canal to avoid any possible communication with CSF. At this point, I then began drilling out the lateral cortex of the mastoid. Once the lateral cortex of the mastoid was entered, we noted that there was no frank purulence or obvious infected contents of the mastoid itself. I then began performing a standard wide mastoidectomy. This was carried down into the antrum, and the position of the incus was verified. The incus itself was mobile and the ossicles were intact. There was no evidence of any fluid inside the middle ear space, and the tissue encountered was normal. There was some moderately inflamed tissue lining the mastoid air cells superiorly and near the dura. The area along the tegmen superiorly was skeletonized, and an area of tegmen dehiscence approximately 0.5 cm was noted in the central portion of the mastoid cavity. Once a wide smooth mastoid cavity was obtained, the dura was inspected and there was no evidence of CSF leak. There were no signs of any obvious infection or purulence. I excised the dura in the area of the dehiscence for dural biopsy and sent these for specimen. The dura was then repaired. There continued to be no signs of CSF leak. I filled the area with Gelfoam soaked in Floxin to help hold this in place and to provide antibiotic coverage. I then closed the wound in layers, including the periosteum, dermis, and then the skin with Dermabond. The ear canal was inspected after closure and there were no signs of any communication with the ear canal itself. The patient was then placed in the standard mastoid head wrap and returned to the PACU in good condition. The estimated blood loss was less than 30 cc. There were no complications.

45. Operative Report

PREOPERATIVE DIAGNOSIS: Persistent menorrhagia, leiomyoma of uterus

POSTOPERATIVE DIAGNOSIS: Persistent menorrhagia, leiomyoma of uterus

OPERATION: Total abdominal hysterectomy and bilateral salpingo-oophorectomy

PROCEDURE DESCRIPTION: Under satisfactory general anesthesia, the patient was placed in the supine position. Her abdomen was prepped and draped in the usual manner for hysterectomy procedure. A Pfannenstiel incision was made through the subcutaneous fascia to the rectal fascia. The fascia was opened transversely with curved Mayo scissors. The recti muscles were separated and partially divided with LigaSure. The abdominal peritoneum was entered. The bowel was then packed to the upper abdomen and the retractor was placed properly. Pelvic findings were as follows: There were multiple small fibroid tumors at the fundus of the uterus. The whole uterus was enlarged to approximately 12 to 13 weeks gestational size. Both ovaries appeared to be normal. There were small follicular cysts noted at the left ovary. Both fallopian tubes were normal. There were no endometrial implantations noted elsewhere in the pelvis or on the surface of the ovaries.

Bilateral round ligaments were clamped with LigaSure, coagulated, and divided. The anterior bladder flap was entered. The bladder peritoneum was pushed away from the lower segment of the uterus and bilateral infundibulopelvic ligaments were clamped with Liga-Sure, coagulated, and divided. Both fallopian tubes and ovaries were intended to be removed. Both side broad ligaments were skeletonized. The tissue surrounding the uterine vessels were identified and also skeletonized. Both side uterine vessels were clamped with curved Heaney, cut and tied with 0 Vicryl sutures. Both sides cardinal ligaments were clamped with straight Heaney and tied with 0 Vicryl sutures. The junction between the cervix and vagina was entered and the uterine body along with fallopian tubes and ovaries from both sides were removed. Next, cornual sutures were placed which included the anterior and posterior vaginal cuff, the pedicles of the uterosacral ligament, and this was then tied with 0 Vicryl. The remaining vaginal cuff was closed with interrupted 0 Vicryl sutures. The uterosacral ligament was then suspended to the vaginal cuff. After hemostasis was checked, the pelvic cavity was thoroughly irrigated with warm, normal saline. After hemostasis was again checked, the cuff was sprayed with Avitene powder for further hemostasis. After needle, sponge and instrument counts were all correct, the abdominal fascia was closed with continuous #1 Vicryl. The skin was approximated and closed with metal staples. Estimated blood loss was approximately 450 mL. The patient tolerated the surgery well and left the operating room in good condition.

46. Operative Report

PREOPERATIVE DIAGNOSIS:	Right ear conductive hearing loss
POSTOPERATIVE DIAGNOSIS:	Right ear Otosclerosis
OPERATION:	Right ear stapedectomy
FINDINGS:	Markedly thickened stapes footplate, intact Eustachian tube, and normal mobility of malleus and incus.

PROCEDURE: The patient was prepared and draped in the normal sterile fashion, and injections were made with 1 percent lidocaine with 1:100,000 parts epinephrine into the external auditory canal wall. The tympanomeatal flap was elevated from 10 o'clock to 6 o'clock in a counterclockwise fashion, using a vertical rolling knife for incision and a duckbill for elevation. The middle ear was entered at 2 o'clock, the chorda tympani nerve identified, and the annulus lifted out of the tympanic sulcus. After elevating the tympanomeatal flap anteriorly, the ossicles were palpated. The malleus and incus moved freely, and the stapes was fixed. The posterior superior canal wall was curetted down after mobilizing the chorda tympani nerve, which was left intact. The stapes footplate was visualized easily and found to be markedly thickened. The pyramidal process was identified and the stapes tendon cut. An IS joint knife was used to dislocate the joint between the incus and stapes. Next, small and large Buckingham mirrors were used, along with a drill, to drill out the stapes footplate. After this was done, a 6 mm × 4 mm Schuknecht piston prosthesis was placed in position. Crimping was achieved, and there was an excellent fit. The stapes footplate area then was packed with small pieces of Gelfoam. The tympanomeatal flap was put back in proper position and the middle ear packed with rayon strips of Cortisporin with a cotton ball in the middle to form a rosette. The patient was awakened in the operating room and transferred to recovery in no apparent distress.

47. Operative Report

PREOPERATIVE DIAGNOSIS:	Bilateral ptosis interfering with vision
POSTOPERATIVE DIAGNOSIS:	Bilateral ptosis interfering with vision
OPERATION:	Bilateral levator resection

PROCEDURE DESCRIPTION: Under intravenous sedation, a 50/50 mixture of 2 percent Xylocaine with 1:100,000 epinephrine and Wydase, 0.5 percent Marcaine with 1:200,000 epinephrine and sodium bicarbonate was injected into the area of the right and left upper lids via the skin surface. The patient was then prepped and draped in the usual sterile fashion.

Attention was first directed to the upper eyelids, where a marking pen and caliper were used to mark the intended skin incision. Then 0.5 Cassidys and Brown-Adson forceps were used to delineate the skin to be excised. Curved Stevens scissors were used to excise the skin and orbicularis. Hemostasis was maintained with monopolar cautery. A 4-0 silk suture was placed in the lid margin, and the lid was placed on downward tension. The orbital septum was incised and opened for the full horizontal length of the eyelid. Then, the levator palpebrae superioris muscle was reflected from its insertion on the underlying tarsus and dissected from underlying Muller's muscle. Multiple interrupted 5-0 Dexon sutures on a 01 needle were then positioned to fashion the tarsus and brought up the levator so that the appropriate height and contour of the eyelid were achieved. The excess levator was excised. The wound was closed with a running 6-0 mild chromic suture. A combination corticosteroid and antibiotic ointment was placed in the patient's eye and the wounds, and ice packs were applied. Surgery was performed on the right and left eyes simultaneously to ensure symmetry. The patient left the operating room for the recovery room in good condition, fully awake.

48. Operative Report

PRE-OPERATIVE DIAGNOSIS:	Pregnancy, 37w2d, Previous cesarean section, Active Labor
POST-OPERATIVE DIAGNOSIS:	Pregnancy, 37w2d, Previous cesarean section, Active Labor
PROCEDURE: DELIVERY TYPE:	Repeat Low Transverse C-Section
INDICATIONS FOR C-SECTION:	Repeat C-S with VBAC not attempted
RUPTURE TYPE:	INTACT
EBL (ML):	400

PROCEDURE DETAILS: The risks, benefits, complications, treatment options, and expected outcomes were discussed with the patient. The patient concurred with the proposed plan, giving informed consent. The site of surgery properly noted/marked. Preoperative antibiotics have been infused as ordered. The patient was taken to operating room #1, identified and the procedure verified as C-section delivery. A time out was held and the above information confirmed.

After induction of anesthesia, the patient was draped and prepped in the usual sterile manner. A Pfannenstiel incision was made and carried down through the subcutaneous tissue to the fascia. Fascial incision was made and extended transversely. The fascia was separated from the underlying rectus tissue superiorly and inferiorly. The peritoneum was identified and entered. Peritoneal incision was extended longitudinally. Balfore self-retaining retractors were placed in the usual manner. The utero-vesical peritoneal reflection was incised transversely and the bladder flap was bluntly freed from the lower uterine segment. A low transverse uterine incision was made atraumatically, with modest uterine pressure and after the bladder blade was removed. The infant's head was delivered from footling breech presentation. The nose and mouth were suctioned with the DeLee suction trap prior to shoulder delivery. The delivered infant was a 3,883 gram female with Apgar scores of 9 at one minute and 9 at five minutes. After the umbilical cord was clamped and cut cord blood was obtained for evaluation. Cord gas was not sent. The placenta was manually removed, was intact and appeared normal. The uterine outline, tubes and ovaries appeared normal. The uterine incision was closed in the usual fashion. The first layer with running locked. The second layer imbricating with 0-Vicryl. Hemostasis was observed. Lavage was carried out until clear. The peritoneum was closed with running 3-0 Vicryl. The muscle was approximated with the 3-0 Vicryl. The fascia was then reapproximated with running sutures of 1 PDS. The skin was reapproximated with subcuticular sutures and subcutaneous sutures. Instrument, sponge, and needle counts were correct prior the abdominal closure and at the conclusion of the case.

GESTATIONAL AGE:	37w2d
PLACENTA REMOVAL:	Manual Removal
PLACENTA APPEARANCE:	Intact
CORD VESSELS:	3 Vessels
CORD COMPLICATIONS:	None

49. Operative Report

PREOPERATIVE DIAGNOSES:	1. Left anterior cruciate ligament tear
	2. Posterior horn lateral meniscal tear
POSTOPERATIVE DIAGNOSES:	1. Left anterior cruciate ligament tear
	2. Posterior horn lateral meniscal tear
OPERATION:	1. Examination left knee under anesthesia
	2. Partial lateral meniscectomy
	3. Anterior cruciate ligament reconstruction using bone-patellar tendon-bone autograft with Arthrex 8 × 25 mm titanium screw in the femur and Arthrex 10 × 20 mm titanium screw in the tibia.

PROCEDURE: Patient is a 24-year-old right-hand dominant female who sustained the above-named left knee injury while playing volleyball. The various treatment options were reviewed and she agreed with the patellar tendon autograft reconstruction.

DETAILS: Patient was brought to the operating room. General anesthesia was obtained. The left knee was examined under anesthesia, found to have full range of motion with positive Lachman, positive pivot shift. No varus or valgus laxity. The extremity was then prepped and draped in the usual sterile manner. The limb was exsanguinated and the tourniquet inflated to 250 mmHg. The arthroscopy was then begun through the usual ports. The patellofemoral joint was normal. The medial and lateral gutters were normal. The lateral compartment revealed a bucket-handle tear of the central aspect of the lateral meniscus in the white-white zone. This was trimmed back to a smooth and stable rim using mechanical motorized cutters. The remainder of this compartment was normal. The notch revealed the complete tear of the ACL off the femoral region. The PCL was intact. A longitudinal incision was then made from the inferior pole of the patella to the tibial tubercle through skin and subcutaneous. The paratenon was incised longitudinally and dissected medially and laterally. The patellar tendon measured approximately 31 mm in width and the central 10 mm was taken with the corresponding 2.5 cm bone plug from the patella and 2.5 cm bone plug from the tibia. The bone plugs were fashioned to fit through the 10 mm tunnel. They were drilled and #5 Ethibond sutures were placed through the holes in the bone plugs. The graft was then soaked in antibiotic solution. The ACL remnant was then debrided using a motorized shaver and a notchplasty was performed using the motorized shaver and bur. The tibial tunnel guide was then placed through the inferomedial arthroscopy portal, centered between the tibial spines. The guide was set at 45 degrees, drilled and found to be in excellent position. It was overreamed using a 10 mm cannulated reamer. The guidewire was then placed through the tunnel to the spot on the femur at the 2 o'clock position. The edges of the tunnel were chamfered smooth. The two-pin passer was then placed and the graft was then pulled through the tunnel without difficulty. An 8 × 25 mm Arthrex titanium femoral screw was placed into the bone plug and the femur and tested. With the knee flexed to 30 degrees and tension on the graft, a 10 × 25 mm Arthrex titanium screw was placed through the tunnel and into the bone plug and the tibia. The knee was again tested with a negative Lachman clinically. The knee was copiously lavaged and drained. All the incisions were irrigated with antibiotic solution. The patellar defect was cleaned and the paratenon was closed using #1 Vicryl. Subcutaneous was closed using 3-0 Vicryl and all skin incisions were closed using staples.

50. Operative Report

PREOPERATIVE DIAGNOSIS: Diaphragmatic hernia

POSTOPERATIVE DIAGNOSIS: Diaphragmatic hernia

INDICATION: The patient is a 66-year-old female who was sent for evaluation of acute onset of hematemesis. Endoscopy was performed and revealed a significant portion of the patient's upper stomach in her chest. A nasojejunal feeding tube was placed at the time of the endoscopy to maintain enteral feeds. The options of laparoscopic versus open repair of the diaphragmatic hernia were discussed with the patient as well as the risks, benefits, and potential complications of the procedure, and she elected to undergo the laparoscopic repair.

PROCEDURE: After consent was obtained, the patient was taken to the operating room and placed supine on the operating table. After adequate general endotracheal anesthesia, the patient's abdomen was prepped and draped in the standard surgical fashion. Initial entry was gained through an infraumbilical elliptical incision. Cut down technique was used. A 5.0-mm trocars was inserted. A pneumoperitoneum was then obtained. Two additional

5.0-mm trocars were placed, one in the left epigastric region and one in the left upper quadrant. A lateral left upper quadrant 5.0-mm trocars was placed as well. The left upper quadrant 5.0-mm trocars was replaced with the 12-mm trocars. A 10-mm 30-degree scope was used throughout the procedure for visualization. The stomach was then grasped with the soft bowel grasper and reduced from the chest in a hand over hand fashion. There were dense attachments of the stomach to the superior portion of the hernia sac in the chest. These were carefully taken down with harmonic shears. This allowed for good mobilization of the stomach and its return to the abdomen. There was an approximately 6.0-cm diaphragmatic hernia to the left of the esophagus, which was repaired with implantation of Prolene mesh patch. The abdomen was then inspected for hemostasis and noted to be pristine. The trocars were removed and the CO_2 insufflation was released. The patient tolerated the procedure well. She was awakened, extubated, and taken to the recovery room in satisfactory condition.

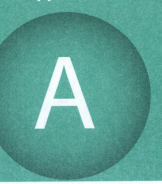
Roots and Approaches

Section 0			Medical and Surgical
0	Alteration	Definition:	Modifying the natural anatomic structure of a body part without affecting the function of the body part Principal purpose is to improve appearance. Face lift, breast augmentation
		Explanation:	Principal purpose is to improve appearance.
		Examples:	Face lift, breast augmentation
1	Bypass	Definition:	Altering the route of passage of the contents of a tubular body part
		Explanation:	Rerouting contents of a body part to a downstream area of the normal route, to a similar route and body part, or to an abnormal route and dissimilar body part. Includes one or more anastomoses, with or without the use of a device.
		Examples:	Coronary artery bypass, colostomy formation
2	Change	Definition:	Taking out or off a device from a body part and putting back an identical or similar device in or on the same body part without cutting or puncturing the skin or a mucous membrane
		Explanation:	All Change procedures are coded using the approach External.
		Examples:	Urinary catheter change, gastrostomy tube change
3	Control	Definition:	Stopping, or attempting to stop, post-procedural or other acute bleeding
		Explanation:	The site of the bleeding is coded as an anatomical region and not to a specific body part.
		Examples:	Control of post-prostatectomy hemorrhage, control of intracranial subdural hemorrhage, control of bleeding duodenal ulcer, control of retroperitoneal hemorrhage.
4	Creation	Definition:	Putting in or on biological or synthetic material to form a new body part that to the extent possible replicates the anatomic structure or function of an absent body part
		Explanation:	Used for gender reassignment surgery and corrective procedure in individuals with congenital anomalies
		Examples:	Creation of vagina in a male, creation of right and left atrioventricular valve from common atrioventricular valve
5	Destruction	Definition:	Physical eradication of all or a portion of a body part by the direct use of energy, force, or a destructive agent
		Explanation:	None of the body part is physically taken out.
		Examples:	Fulguration of rectal polyp, cautery of skin lesion
6	Detachment	Definition:	Cutting off all or part of the upper or lower extremities

Section 0		Medical and Surgical	
		Explanation:	The body part value is the site of the detachment, with a qualifier if applicable to further specify the level where the extremity is detached.
		Examples:	Below-knee amputation, disarticulation of shoulder
7	Dilation	Definition:	Expanding an orifice or the lumen of a tubular body part
		Explanation:	The orifice can be a natural orifice or an artificially created orifice. Accomplished by stretching a tubular body part using Intraluminal pressure or by cutting part of the orifice or wall of the tubular body part.
		Examples:	Percutaneous transluminal angioplasty, internal urethrotomy
8	Division	Definition:	Cutting into a body part without draining fluids and/or gases from the body part in order to separate or transect the body part
		Explanation:	All or a portion of the body part is separated into two or more portions.
		Examples:	Spinal cordotomy, osteotomy
9	Drainage	Definition:	Taking or letting out fluids and/or gases from a body part
		Explanation:	The qualifier diagnostic is used to identify drainage procedures that are biopsies.
		Examples:	Thoracentesis, incision and drainage
B	Excision	Definition:	Cutting out or off, without replacement, a portion of a body part
		Explanation:	The qualifier diagnostic is used to identify excision procedures that are biopsies.
		Examples:	Partial nephrectomy, liver biopsy
C	Extirpation	Definition:	Taking or cutting out solid matter from a body part
		Explanation:	The solid matter may be an abnormal byproduct of a biological function or a foreign body; it may be imbedded in a body part or in the lumen of a tubular body part. The solid matter may or may not have been previously broken into pieces.
		Examples:	Thrombectomy, choledocholithotomy
D	Extraction	Definition:	Pulling or stripping out or off all or a portion of a body part by the use of force
		Explanation:	The qualifier diagnostic is used to identify extractions that are biopsies.
		Examples:	Dilation and curettage, vein stripping
F	Fragmentation	Definition:	Breaking solid matter in a body part into pieces
		Explanation:	Physical force (e.g., manual, ultrasonic) applied directly or indirectly through intervening body parts are used to break the solid matter into pieces. The solid matter may be an abnormal by-product of a biological function or a foreign body. The pieces of solid matter are not taken out, but are eliminated or absorbed through normal biological functions.
		Examples:	Extracorporeal shockwave lithotripsy, transurethral lithotripsy
G	Fusion	Definition:	Joining together portions of an articular body part, rendering the articular body part immobile
		Explanation:	The body part is joined together by fixation device, bone graft, or other means.
		Examples:	Spinal fusion, ankle arthrodesis
H	Insertion	Definition:	Putting in a non-biological appliance that monitors, assists, performs, or prevents a physiological function but does not physically take the place of a body part
		Examples:	Insertion of radioactive implant, insertion of central venous catheter
J	Inspection	Definition:	Visually and/or manually exploring a body part

Section 0		Medical and Surgical	
		Explanation:	Visual exploration may be performed with or without optical instrumentation. Manual exploration may be performed directly or through intervening body layers.
		Examples:	Diagnostic arthroscopy, exploratory laparotomy
K	Map	Definition:	Locating the route of passage of electrical impulses and/or locating functional areas in a body part
		Explanation:	Applicable only to cardiac conduction mechanism and the central nervous system
		Examples:	Cardiac mapping, cortical mapping
L	Occlusion	Definition:	Completely closing an orifice or lumen of a tubular body part
		Explanation:	The orifice can be a natural orifice or an artificially created orifice.
		Examples:	Fallopian tube ligation, ligation of inferior vena cava
M	Reattachment	Definition:	Putting back in or on all or a portion of a separated body part to its normal location or other suitable location
		Explanation:	Vascular circulation and nervous pathways may or may not be reestablished.
		Examples:	Reattachment of hand, reattachment of avulsed kidney
N	Release	Definition:	Freeing a body part from an abnormal physical constraint
		Explanation:	Some of the restraining tissue may be taken out but none of the body part is taken out.
		Examples:	Adhesiolysis, carpel tunnel release
P	Removal	Definition:	Taking out or off a device from a body part
		Explanation:	If a device is taken out and a similar device put in without cutting or puncturing the skin or mucous membrane, the procedure is coded to the root operation Change. Otherwise, the procedure for taking out the device is coded to the root operation Removal, and the procedure for putting in the new device is coded to the root operation that is performed.
		Examples:	Drainage tube removal, cardiac pacemaker removal
Q	Repair	Definition:	Restoring, to the extent possible, a body part to its normal anatomic structure and function
		Explanation:	Used only when the method to accomplish the repair is not one of the other root operations.
		Examples:	Colostomy takedown, herniorrhaphy, suture of laceration
R	Replacement	Definition:	Putting in or on a biological or synthetic material that physically takes the place and/or function of all or a portion of a body part
		Explanation:	The body part may have been taken out or replaced, or may be taken out, physically eradicated, or rendered nonfunctional during the replacement procedure. A removal procedure is coded for taking out the device used in a previous replacement procedure.
		Examples:	Total hip replacement, free skin graft
S	Reposition	Definition:	Moving to its normal location or other suitable location all or a portion of a body part
		Explanation:	The body part is moved to a new location from an abnormal location, or from a normal location where it is not functioning correctly. The body part may or may not be cut out or off to be moved to the new location.
		Examples:	Reposition of undescended testis, fracture reduction

(Continued)

	Section 0	**Medical and Surgical**	
T	Resection	Definition:	Cutting out or off, without replacement, all of a body part
		Examples:	Total nephrectomy, total lobectomy of lung
V	Restriction	Definition:	Partially closing an orifice or the lumen of a tubular body part
		Explanation:	The orifice can be a natural orifice or an artificially created orifice.
		Examples:	Esophagogastric fundoplication, cervical cerclage
W	Revision	Definition:	Correcting, to the extent possible, a portion of a malfunctioning device or the position of a displaced device
		Explanation:	Revision can include correcting a malfunctioning or displaced device by taking out or putting in components of the device, such as a screw or pin.
		Examples:	Adjustment of pacemaker lead, adjust of hip prosthesis
U	Supplement	Definition:	Putting in or on biological or synthetic material that physically reinforces and/or augments the function of a portion of a body part
		Explanation:	The biological material is non-living, or is living and from the same individual. The body part may have been previously replaced, and the supplement procedure is performed to physically reinforce and/or augment the function of the replaced body part.
		Examples:	Herniorrhaphy using mesh, free nerve graft, mitral valve ring annuloplasty, put a new acetabular liner in a previous hip replacement
X	Transfer	Definition:	Moving, without taking out, all or a portion of a body part to another location to take over the function of all or a portion of a body part
		Explanation:	The body part transferred remains connected to its vascular and nervous supply.
		Examples:	Tendon transfer, skin pedicle flap transfer
Y	Transplantation	Definition:	Putting in or on all or a portion of a living body part taken from another individual or animal to physically take the place and/or function of all or a portion of a smaller body part
		Explanation:	The native body part may or may not be taken out, and the transplanted body part may take over all or a portion of its function.
		Examples:	Kidney transplant, heart transplant

	Section 1	**Obstetrics**	
A	Abortion	Definition:	Artificially terminating a pregnancy
		Explanation:	Subdivided according to whether an additional device such as a laminaria or abortifacient is used, or whether the abortion is performed by mechanical means
		Examples:	Transvaginal abortion using vacuum aspiration technique
E	Delivery	Definition:	Assisting the passage of the products of conception from the genital canal
		Explanation:	Applies only to manually assisted, vaginal delivery
		Examples:	Manually assisted delivery

	Section 2	Placement	
0	Change	Definition:	Taking out or off a device from a body region and putting back an identical or similar device in or on the same body region without cutting or puncturing the skin or a mucous membrane
		Explanation:	Procedures performed without making an incision or a puncture
		Examples:	Change of vaginal packing
1	Compression	Definition:	Putting pressure on a body region
		Explanation:	Procedures performed without making an incision or a puncture
		Examples:	Placement of pressure dressing on abdominal wall
2	Dressing	Definition:	Putting material on a body region for protection
		Explanation:	Procedures performed without making an incision or a puncture
		Examples:	Application of a sterile dressing to head wound
3	Immobilization	Definition:	Limiting or preventing motion of a body region
		Explanation:	Procedures to fit a device, such as splints and braces, as described in F0DZ7EZ, apply only to the rehabilitation setting.
		Examples:	Placement of a splint on left finger
4	Packing	Definition:	Putting material in a body region or orifice
		Explanation:	Procedures performed without making an incision or puncture
		Examples:	Placement of nasal packing
5	Removal	Definition:	Taking out or off a device from a body region
		Explanation:	Procedures performed without making an incision or puncture
		Examples:	Removal of stereotactic head frame
6	Traction	Definition:	Exerting a pulling force on a body region in a distal direction
		Explanation:	Traction in this section includes only the task performed using a mechanical traction apparatus.
		Examples:	Lumbar traction using motorized split-traction table

	Section 3	Administration	
0	Introduction	Definition:	Putting in or on a therapeutic, diagnostic, nutritional, physiological, or prophylactic substance except blood or blood products
		Explanation:	All other substances administered, such as antineoplastic substance
		Examples:	Nerve block injection to median nerve
1	Irrigation	Definition:	Putting in or on a cleansing solution
		Explanation:	Substance given is a cleansing substance or dialysate
		Examples:	Flushing of eye
2	Transfusion	Definition:	Putting in blood or blood products
		Explanation:	Substance given is a blood product or a stem cell substance
		Examples:	Transfusion of cell saver red cells into central venous line

Section 4		Measurement and Monitoring	
0	Measurement	Definition:	Determining the level of a physiological or physical function at a point in time
		Explanation:	A single temperature reading is considered measurement.
		Examples:	External electrocardiogram (EKG), single reading
1	Monitoring	Definition:	Determining the level of a physiological or physical function repetitively over a period of time
		Explanation:	Temperature taken every half hour for eight hours is considered monitoring
		Examples:	Urinary pressure monitoring

Section 5		Extracorporeal or Systemic Assistance and Performance	
0	Assistance	Definition:	Taking over a portion of a physiological function by extracorporeal means
		Explanation:	Procedures that support a physiological function but do not take complete control over it, such as intra-aortic balloon pump to support cardiac output and hyperbaric oxygen treatment
		Examples:	Hyperbaric oxygenation of a wound
1	Performance	Definition:	Completely taking over a physiological function by extracorporeal means
		Explanation:	Procedures in which complete control is exercised over a physiological function, such as total mechanical ventilation, cardiac pacing, and cardiopulmonary bypass
		Examples:	Cardiopulmonary bypass in conjunction with CABG
2	Restoration	Definition:	Returning, or attempting to return, a physiological function to its original state by extracorporeal means
		Explanation:	Only external cardioversion and defibrillation procedures.
			Failed cardioversion procedures are also included in the definition of restoration, and are coded the same as successful procedures.
		Examples:	Attempted cardiac defibrillation, unsuccessful

Section 6		Extracorporeal or Systemic Therapies	
0	Atmospheric Control	Definition:	Extracorporeal control of atmospheric pressure and composition
		Examples:	Antigen-free air conditioning, series treatment
1	Decompression	Definition:	Extracorporeal elimination of undissolved gas from body fluids
		Explanation:	A single type of procedure-treatment for decompression sickness (the bends) in a hyperbaric chamber
		Examples:	Hyperbaric decompression treatment, single
2	Electromagnetic Therapy	Definition:	Extracorporeal treatment by electromagnetic rays
		Examples:	TMS (transcranial magnetic stimulation), series treatment
3	Hyperthermia	Definition:	Extracorporeal raising of body temperature
		Explanation:	To treat temperature imbalance, and as an adjunct radiation treatment for cancer. When performed to treat temperature imbalance, the procedure is coded in this section. When performed for cancer treatment, whole-body hyperthermia is classified as a modality qualifier in Section D, Radiation Oncology.

	Section 6		Extracorporeal or Systemic Therapies
4	Hypothermia	Definition:	Extracorporeal lowering of body temperature
		Examples:	Whole body hypothermia treatment for temperature imbalances, series
5	Pheresis	Definition:	Extracorporeal separation of blood products
		Explanation:	Used in medical practice for two main purposes: to treat diseases where too much of a blood component is produced, such as leukemia, or to remove a blood product, such as platelets, from a donor, for transfusion into a patient who needs them
		Examples:	Therapeutic leukapheresis, single treatment
6	Phototherapy	Definition:	Extracorporeal treatment by light rays
		Explanation:	Phototherapy to the circulatory system means exposing the blood to light rays outside the body, using a machine that recirculates the blood and returns it to the body after phototherapy.
		Examples:	Phototherapy of circulatory system, series treatment
7	Ultrasound Therapy	Definition:	Extracorporeal treatment by ultrasound
		Examples:	Therapeutic ultrasound of peripheral vessels, single treatment
8	Ultraviolet Therapy	Definition:	Extracorporeal treatment by ultraviolet light
		Examples:	Ultraviolet light phototherapy, series treatment
9	Shock Wave Therapy	Definition:	Extracorporeal treatment by shockwaves
		Examples:	Shockwave therapy of plantar fascia, single treatment
B	Perfusion	Definition:	Extracorporeal treatment by diffusion of therapeutic fluid
		Examples:	Perfusion of donor lungs prior to successful transplantation

	Section 7		Osteopathic
0	Treatment	Definition:	Manual treatment to eliminate or alleviate somatic dysfunction and related disorders
		Examples:	Fascial release of abdomen, osteopathic treatment

	Section 8		Other Procedures
0	Other Procedures	Definition:	Methodologies that attempt to remediate or cure a disorder or disease
		Explanation:	For nontraditional, whole-body therapies including acupuncture and meditation
		Examples:	Acupuncture

	Section 9		Chiropractic
B	Manipulation	Definition:	Manual procedure that involves a directed thrust to move a joint past the physiological range of motion, without exceeding the anatomical limit
		Examples:	Chiropractic treatment of cervical spine, short lever specific contact

	Section B	Imaging	
0	Plain Radiography	Definition:	Planar display of an image developed from the capture of external ionizing radiation on photographic or photoconductive plate
1	Fluoroscopy	Definition:	Single plane or bi-plane real time display of an image developed from the capture of external ionizing radiation on a fluorescent screen. The image may also be stored by either digital or analog means
2	CT scan	Definition:	Computer-reformatted digital display of multi-planar images developed from the capture of multiple exposures of external ionizing radiation
3	MRI	Definition:	Computer-reformatted digital display of multi-planar images developed from the capture of radio-frequency signals emitted by nuclei in a body site excited within a magnetic field
4	Ultrasonography	Definition:	Real time display of images of anatomy or flow information developed from the capture of reflected and attenuated high-frequency sound waves

	Section C	Nuclear Medicine	
1	Planar Nuclear Medicine Imaging	Definition:	Introduction of radioactive materials into the body for single plane display of images developed from the capture of radioactive emissions
2	Tomographic Nuclear Medicine Imaging	Definition:	Introduction of radioactive materials into the body for three-dimensional display of images developed from the capture of radioactive emissions
3	Positron Emission Tomography	Definition:	Introduction of radioactive materials into the body for three-dimensional display of images developed from the simultaneous capture, 180 degrees apart, of radioactive emissions
4	Non-imaging Nuclear Medicine Uptake	Definition:	Introduction of radioactive materials into the body for measurements of organ function, from the detection of radioactive emissions

	Section D		Radiation Therapy			
0	Beam Radiation	1	Brachytherapy	2	Stereotactic Radiosurgery	Y Other Radiation

	Section F		Physical Rehabilitation and Diagnostic Audiology
0	Speech Assessment	Definition:	Measurement of speech and related functions
1	Motor and/or Nerve Function Assessment	Definition:	Measurements of motor, nerve, and related functions
2	ADL Assessment	Definition:	Measurement of functional level for activities of daily living
3	Hearing Assessment	Definition:	Measurement of hearing and related functions
4	Hearing Aid Assessment	Definition:	Measurement of the appropriateness and/or effectiveness of a hearing device
5	Vestibular Assessment	Definition:	Measurement of the vestibular system and related functions
6	Speech Treatment	Definition:	Application of techniques to improve, augment, or compensate for speech and related functional impairment
7	Motor Treatment	Definition:	Exercise or activities to increase or facilitate motor function

Section F			Physical Rehabilitation and Diagnostic Audiology
8	ADL Treatment	Definition:	Exercise or activities to facilitate functional competence for activities of daily living
9	Hearing Treatment	Definition:	Application of techniques to improve, augment, or compensate for hearing and related functional impairment
B	Hearing Aid Treatment	Definition:	Application of techniques to improve the communication abilities of individuals with cochlear implant
C	Vestibular Treatment	Definition:	Application of techniques to improve, augment, or compensate for vestibular and related functional impairment
D	Device Fitting	Definition:	Fitting of a device designed to facilitate or support achievement of a higher level of function
F	Caregiver Training	Definition:	Training in activities to support patient's optimal level of function

Section G				Mental Health		
1	Psychological Testing	2	Crisis Intervention	5	Individual Psychotherapy
6	Counseling	7	Family Psychotherapy	B	Electroconvulsive Therapy
C	Biofeedback	F	Hypnosis	G	Narcosynthesis
H	Group Therapy	J	Light Therapy		

Section H				Substance Abuse Treatment		
2	Detoxification Services	3	Individual Counseling	4	Group Counseling
5	Individual Psychotherapy	6	Family Counseling	8	Medication Management
9	Pharmacotherapy				

ICD-10-PCS Approaches

Approach	Definition	Access Location	Method	Type of Instrumentation	Example
Open	Cutting through the skin or mucous membrane and any other body layers necessary to expose the site of the procedure	Skin or mucous membrane, any other body layers	Cutting	None	Abdominal hysterectomy
Percutaneous	Entry, by puncture or minor incision, of instrumentation through the skin or mucous membrane and/or any other body layers necessary to reach the site of the procedure	Skin or mucous membrane, any other body layers	Puncture or minor incision	Without visualization	Needle biopsy of liver, Liposuction
Percutaneous endoscopic	Entry, by puncture or minor incision, of instrumentation through the skin or mucous membrane and/or any other body layers necessary to reach and visualize the site of the procedure	Skin or mucous membrane, any other body layers	Puncture or minor incision	With visualization	Arthroscopy, Laparoscopic cholecystectomy
Via natural or artificial opening	Entry of instrumentation through a natural or artificial external opening to reach the site of the procedure	Natural or artificial external opening	Direct entry	Without visualization	Endotracheal tube insertion, Foley catheter placement
Via natural or artificial opening endoscopic	Entry of instrumentation through a natural or artificial external opening to reach and visualize the site of the procedure	Natural or artificial external opening	Direct entry with puncture or minor incision for instrumentation only	With visualization	Sigmoidoscopy, EGD, ERCP
Via natural or artificial opening with percutaneous endoscopic assistance	Entry of instrumentation through a natural or artificial external opening to reach and visualize the site of the procedure, and entry by puncture or minor incision, of instrumentation through the skin or mucous membrane and any other body layers necessary to aid in the performance of the procedure	Skin or mucous membrane, any other body layers	Cutting	With visualization	Laparoscopic-assisted vaginal hysterectomy
External	Procedures performed directly on the skin or mucous membranes and procedure performed indirectly by the application of external force through the skin or mucous membrane	Skin or mucous membrane	Direct or indirect application	None	Closed fracture reduction, Resection of tonsils

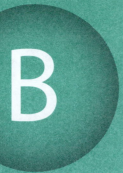
Chapter 1

Check Your Understanding
1. C
3. D
5. A

Code Building

1.

    1.1 Group 1
    1.2 Excision
    1.3 0DB
    1.4 6 for stomach
    1.5 4 for Percutaneous Endoscopic
    1.6 Z and Z for No Device and No Qualifier
    1.7 0DB64ZZ

Section	Body System	Root Operation	Body Part	Approach	Device	Qualifier
Medical and Surgical	Gastrointestinal System	Excision	Stomach	Percutaneous Endoscopic	No Device	No Qualifier
0	D	B	6	4	Z	Z

2.

    2.1 The main term reduction, subterm dislocation states *see* Reposition
    2.2 Upper Joints
    2.3 0RS
    2.4 D for Temporomandibular Joint, Left
    2.5 0 as this is stated to be an open reduction
    2.6 Z and Z for No Device and No Qualifier
    2.7 0RSD0ZZ
    2.8 0RSD04Z

Section	Body System	Root Operation	Body Part	Approach	Device	Qualifier
Medical and Surgical	Upper Joints	Reposition	Temporomandibular Joint, Left	Open	No Device	No Qualifier
0	R	S	D	0	Z	Z

Section	Body System	Root Operation	Body Part	Approach	Device	Qualifier
Medical and Surgical	Upper Joints	Reposition	Temporomandibular Joint, Left	Open	Internal Fixation Device	No Qualifier
0	R	S	D	0	4	Z

3.

3.1 The main term orchiopexy has two cross references, *see* Repair, Male Reproductive System and *see* Reposition Male Reproductive System

3.2 Because the objective of the procedure is to place the undescended testicles into their proper location, the correct root operation Reposition—moving to its normal location, or other suitable location, all or a portion of a body part is selected

3.3 0VS

3.4 C for bilateral as the clinical documentation states testicles

3.5 0 for Open

3.6 Z and Z for No Device and No Qualifier

3.7 0VSC0ZZ

Section	Body System	Root Operation	Body Part	Approach	Device	Qualifier
Medical and Surgical	Male Reproductive System	Reposition	Testis, Bilateral	Open	No Device	No Qualifier
0	V	S	C	0	Z	Z

4.

4.1 *see* Drainage, Anatomical Regions, General

4.2 Drainage-taking or letting out fluids and/or gases from a body part

4.3 0W9

4.4 9 for the pleural cavity on the right side

4.5 3 for percutaneous

4.6 0 for the drainage device and Z for No Qualifier

4.7 0W9930Z

Section	Body System	Root Operation	Body Part	Approach	Device	Qualifier
Medical and Surgical	Upper Joints	Drainage	Pleural Cavity, Right	Percutaneous	Drainage Device	No Qualifier
0	W	9	9	3	0	Z

Chapter 2

Approach Review

1. b
2. c
3. g
4. d
5. a
6. f
7. e

Check Your Understanding

1. c (B5.3a)
3. c (B3.4b)
5. c (A9)
7. b (B3.10c)
9. c (B2.1b)

Case Studies

Case 1

1. a. Resection.
    Rationale: see Guideline B3.8—the entire body part is taken out
    b. 2 the laparoscopic cholecystectomy and the liver biopsy
    c. 0FT44ZZ, 0FB04ZX

Section	Body System	Root Operation	Body Part	Approach	Device	Qualifier
Medical and Surgical	Hepatobiliary System and Pancreas	Resection	Gallbladder	Percutaneous Endoscopic	No Device	No Qualifier
0	F	T	4	4	Z	Z

Section	Body System	Root Operation	Body Part	Approach	Device	Qualifier
Medical and Surgical	Hepatobiliary System and Pancreas	Excision	Liver	Percutaneous Endoscopic	No Device	Diagnostic
0	F	B	0	4	Z	X

Case 3

a. 2
b. 0CBV8ZZ, 0CBT8ZZ
Rationale: See the Index main term Excision, subterms Vocal Cord, Left, Vocal Cord, Right

Section	Body System	Root Operation	Body Part	Approach	Device	Qualifier
Medical and Surgical	Mouth and Throat	Excision	Vocal Cord, Left	Via Natural or Artificial Opening, Endoscopic	No Device	No Qualifier
0	C	B	V	8	Z	Z

Section	Body System	Root Operation	Body Part	Approach	Device	Qualifier
Medical and Surgical	Mouth and Throat	Excision	Vocal Cord, Right	Via Natural or Artificial Opening, Endoscopic	No Device	No Qualifier
0	C	B	T	8	Z	Z

c. B3.2.a—Multiple procedures are coded if the same root operation is performed on different body parts as defined by distinct values of the body part character.
    B3.11a—Inspection of a body part(s) performed in order to achieve the objective of a procedure is not coded separately.

Chapter 3

Check Your Understanding

1. b
3. c
5. b
7. d

1. Root Operation: Resection
   ICD-10-PCS Code: 0FT20ZZ

Section	Body System	Root Operation	Body Part	Approach	Device	Qualifier
Medical and Surgical	Hepatobiliary System and Pancreas	Resection	Liver, Left Lobe	Open	No Device	No Qualifier
0	F	T	2	0	Z	Z

3. Root Operation: Extirpation
   ICD-10-PCS Code: 0TC43ZZ

Section	Body System	Root Operation	Body Part	Approach	Device	Qualifier
Medical and Surgical	Urinary System	Extirpation	Kidney Pelvis, Left	Percutaneous	No Device	No Qualifier
0	T	C	4	3	Z	Z

5. Root Operation: Extraction. See the subterm for Bone Marrow. There are three options, with Iliac being descriptive of the hip bone.
   ICD-10-PCS Code: 07DR3ZX

Section	Body System	Root Operation	Body Part	Approach	Device	Qualifier
Medical and Surgical	Lymphatic and Hemic Systems	Extraction	Bone Marrow, Iliac	Percutaneous	No Device	Diagnostic
0	7	D	R	3	Z	X

7. Root Operation: Destruction
   ICD-10-PCS Code: 015C3ZZ

Section	Body System	Root Operation	Body Part	Approach	Device	Qualifier
Medical and Surgical	Peripheral Nervous System	Destruction	Pudendal Nerve	Percutaneous	No Device	No Qualifier
0	1	5	C	3	Z	Z

9. Root Operation: Fragmentation
   ICD-10-PCS Code: 0TF78ZZ

Section	Body System	Root Operation	Body Part	Approach	Device	Qualifier
Medical and Surgical	Urinary System	Fragmentation	Ureter, Left	Via Natural or Artificial Opening, Endoscopic	No Device	No Qualifier
0	T	F	7	8	Z	Z

11. Root Operation: Extraction
ICD-10-PCS Code: 0KDL0ZZ

Section	Body System	Root Operation	Body Part	Approach	Device	Qualifier
Medical and Surgical	Muscles	Extraction	Abdomen Muscle, Left	Open	No Device	No Qualifier
0	K	D	L	0	Z	Z

Cases

1. The entire adrenal gland on the left side was removed, so Resection is the root operation. Refer to the main term Resection, subterms gland, adrenal, left 0GT2. Consult the 0GT code table to build the code. The approach was laparoscopic, no device, no qualifier. Complete code 0GT24ZZ.

Section	Body System	Root Operation	Body Part	Approach	Device	Qualifier
Medical and Surgical	Endocrine System	Resection	Adrenal Gland, Left	Percutaneous Laparoscopic	No Device	No Qualifier
0	G	T	2	4	Z	Z

Chapter 4

Check Your Understanding

GENERAL QUESTIONS
1. b
3. a
5. c
7. c
9. d

WHICH ROOT OPERATION IS IT?
1. Root Operation: Release
ICD-10-PCS Code: 0RNJ4ZZ

Section	Body System	Root Operation	Body Part	Approach	Device	Qualifier
Medical and Surgical	Upper Joints	Release	Shoulder Joint, Right	Percutaneous Endoscopic	No Device	No Qualifier
0	R	N	J	4	Z	Z

3. Root Operation: Reposition
ICD-10-PCS Code: 0RSJ0ZZ

Section	Body System	Root Operation	Body Part	Approach	Device	Qualifier
Medical and Surgical	Upper Joints	Reposition	Shoulder Joint, Right	Open	No Device	No Qualifier
0	R	S	J	0	Z	Z

5. Root Operation: Transfer
ICD-10-PCS Code: 01X50Z4
The Anterior Interosseous nerve is not listed under the main term Transfer, Nerve. See the Body Part Index and/or the Index under the Anterior Interosseous Nerve, *use* Nerve, Median.

Section	Body System	Root Operation	Body Part	Approach	Device	Qualifier
Medical and Surgical	Peripheral Nervous System	Transfer	Median Nerve	Open	No Device	Ulnar Nerve
0	1	X	5	0	Z	4

7. Root Operation: Division
ICD-10-PCS Code: 01813ZZ

Section	Body System	Root Operation	Body Part	Approach	Device	Qualifier
Medical and Surgical	Peripheral Nervous System	Division	Cervical Nerve	Percutaneous	No Device	No Qualifier
0	1	8	1	3	Z	Z

9. Root Operation: Transplantation
ICD-10-PCS Code: 0TY00Z0

Section	Body System	Root Operation	Body Part	Approach	Device	Qualifier
Medical and Surgical	Urinary System	Transplantation	Kidney, Right	Open	No Device	Allogeneic
0	T	Y	0	0	Z	0

Cases

1. This is a Transfer, as the blood and nerve supply remains intact and the graft is flapped from the forehead to the nose. The flap involved the subcutaneous tissue and skin, so the subcutaneous tissue is the body part, with the skin and subcutaneous tissue as the other layer involved. The approach was via incision. Complete code 0JX10ZB.

Section	Body System	Root Operation	Body Part	Approach	Device	Qualifier
Medical and Surgical	Subcutaneous Tissue and Fascia	Transfer	Subcutaneous Tissue and Fascia, Face	Open	No Device	Skin and Subcutaneous Tissue
0	J	X	1	0	Z	B

Chapter 5

Check Your Understanding

GENERAL QUESTIONS

1. c
3. c

5. b

7. b

1. Root Operation: Removal
    ICD-10-PCS Code: 0QPG05Z
    The device is removed from the right tibia by incision. The Sheffield ring is located in the Device Key with an instruction to use External Fixation Device.

Section	Body System	Root Operation	Body Part	Approach	Device	Qualifier
Medical and Surgical	Lower Bones	Removal	Tibia, Right	Open	External Fixation Device	No Qualifier
0	Q	P	G	0	5	Z

3. Root Operation: Occlusion
    ICD-10-PCS Code: 02L73DK

Section	Body System	Root Operation	Body Part	Approach	Device	Qualifier
Medical and Surgical	Heart and Great Vessels	Occlusion	Atrium, Left	Percutaneous	Intraluminal Device	Left Atrial Appendage
0	2	L	7	3	D	K

5. Root Operation: Replacement
    ICD-10-PCS Code: 0SRC0L9, 0SRD0L9

Section	Body System	Root Operation	Body Part	Approach	Device	Qualifier
Medical and Surgical	Lower Joints	Replacement	Knee Joint, Right	Open	Synthetic Substitute, Unicondylar, Medial	Cemented
0	S	R	C	0	L	9

Section	Body System	Root Operation	Body Part	Approach	Device	Qualifier
Medical and Surgical	Lower Joints	Replacement	Knee Joint, Left	Open	Synthetic Substitute, Unicondylar, Medial	Cemented
0	S	R	D	0	L	9

7. Root Operation: Occlusion
    ICD-10-PCS Code: 02LW3DJ

Section	Body System	Root Operation	Body Part	Approach	Device	Qualifier
Medical and Surgical	Heart and Great Vessels	Occlusion	Thoracic Aorta, Descending	Percutaneous	Intraluminal Device	Temporary
0	2	L	W	3	D	J

9. Root Operation: Replacement, Valvuloplasty, see Replacement Refer to Index under the term Sapien transcatheter aortic valve—use Zooplastic Tissue in Heart and Great Vessels. This reference is also found in the device key.
    ICD-10-PCS Code: 02RF38Z

Section	Body System	Root Operation	Body Part	Approach	Device	Qualifier
Medical and Surgical	Heart and Great Vessels	Replacement	Aortic Valve	Percutaneous	Zooplastic Tissue	No Device
0	2	R	F	3	8	Z

11. a. 5
    b. Bypass and Excision
    c. 02100Z9, 02100AW, 021109W, 03BC4ZZ, 06BQ4ZZ
    LIMA to LAD – 02100Z9

Section	Body System	Root Operation	Body Part	Approach	Device	Qualifier
Medical and Surgical	Heart and Great Vessels	Bypass	Coronary Artery, One Artery	Open	No Device	Internal Mammary, Left
0	2	1	0	0	Z	9

Aorta to PDA via Left Radial artery graft – 02100AW

Section	Body System	Root Operation	Body Part	Approach	Device	Qualifier
Medical and Surgical	Heart and Great Vessels	Bypass	Coronary Artery, One Artery	Open	Autologous Arterial Tissue	Aorta
0	2	1	0	0	A	W

Aorta to diagonal and obtuse marginal via Left saphenous graft – 021109W

Section	Body System	Root Operation	Body Part	Approach	Device	Qualifier
Medical and Surgical	Heart and Great Vessels	Bypass	Coronary Artery, Two Arteries	Open	Autologous Venous Tissue	Aorta
0	2	1	1	0	9	W

Excision of left radial artery – 03BC4ZZ

Section	Body System	Root Operation	Body Part	Approach	Device	Qualifier
Medical and Surgical	Upper Arteries	Excision	Radial Artery, Left	Percutaneous Endoscopic	No Device	No Qualifier
0	3	B	C	4	Z	Z

Excision of left saphenous graft – 06BQ4ZZ

Section	Body System	Root Operation	Body Part	Approach	Device	Qualifier
Medical and Surgical	Lower Veins	Excision	Saphenous Vein, Left	Percutaneous Endoscopic	No Device	No Qualifier
0	6	B	Q	4	Z	Z

Cases

1. There was an open insertion of the dual chamber pacemaker in the subcutaneous pocket of the chest. The cardiac leads were inserted in the right atrium and right ventricle percutaneously.
0JH606Z, 02H63JZ, 02HK3JZ

Section	Body System	Root Operation	Body Part	Approach	Device	Qualifier
Medical and Surgical	Subcutaneous Tissue and Fascia	Insertion	Subcutaneous Tissue and Fascia, Chest	Open	Pacemaker, Dual Chamber	No Qualifier
0	J	H	6	0	6	Z

Section	Body System	Root Operation	Body Part	Approach	Device	Qualifier
Medical and Surgical	Heart and Great Vessels	Insertion	Atrium, Right	Percutaneous	Cardiac Lead, Pacemaker	No Qualifier
0	2	H	6	3	J	Z

Section	Body System	Root Operation	Body Part	Approach	Device	Qualifier
Medical and Surgical	Heart and Great Vessels	Insertion	Ventricle, Right	Percutaneous	Cardiac Lead, Pacemaker	No Qualifier
0	2	H	K	3	J	Z

Chapter 6

Check Your Understanding

GENERAL QUESTIONS
1. c
3. c
5. a
7. c

WHICH ROOT OPERATION IS IT?
1. Root Operation: Repair
   ICD-10-PCS code: 0RQK4ZZ

Section	Body System	Root Operation	Body Part	Approach	Device	Qualifier
Medical and Surgical	Upper Joints	Repair	Shoulder Joint	Percutaneous Endoscopic	No Device	No Qualifier
0	R	Q	K	4	Z	Z

3. Root Operation: Control
   ICD-10-PCS Code: 0W380ZZ

Section	Body System	Root Operation	Body Part	Approach	Device	Qualifier
Medical and Surgical	Anatomical Regions, General	Control	Chest Wall	Open	No Device	No Qualifier
0	W	3	8	0	Z	Z

5. Root Operation: Fusion
   ICD-10-PCS Code: 0SG00K1, 0SG30K1

Section	Body System	Root Operation	Body Part	Approach	Device	Qualifier
Medical and Surgical	Lower Joints	Fusion	Lumbar Vertebral Joint	Open	Nonautologous Tissue Substitute	Posterior Approach, Posterior Column
0	S	G	0	0	K	1

Section	Body System	Root Operation	Body Part	Approach	Device	Qualifier
Medical and Surgical	Lower Joints	Fusion	Lumbosacral Joint	Open	Nonautologous Tissue Substitute	Posterior Approach, Posterior Column
0	S	G	3	0	K	1

7. Root Operation: Creation
   ICD-10-PCS Code: 0W4M0K0

Section	Body System	Root Operation	Body Part	Approach	Device	Qualifier
Medical and Surgical	Anatomical Regions, General	Creation	Perineum, Male	Open	Nonautologous Tissue Substitute	Vagina
0	W	4	M	0	K	0

9. Root Operation: Fusion
   ICD-10-PCS Code: 0RGS04Z

Section	Body System	Root Operation	Body Part	Approach	Device	Qualifier
Medical and Surgical	Upper Joints	Fusion	Carpometatcarpal Joint, Right	Open	Internal Fixation Device	No Qualifier
0	R	G	S	0	4	Z

Cases

1. There are two procedures performed; a hernia repair and an excision of a portion of the small intestine. For the hernia repair see the index main term Repair, Femoral region, Right. Completed by incision. 0YQ70ZZ
   A 3- to 4-inch portion of small intestine was also excised during the procedure. Refer to the index main term Excision, small intestine. Completed by incision. 0DB80ZZ

Section	Body System	Root Operation	Body Part	Approach	Device	Qualifier
Medical and Surgical	Anatomical Regions, Lower Extremities	Repair	Femoral Region, Right	Open	No Device	No Qualifier
0	Y	Q	7	0	Z	Z

Section	Body System	Root Operation	Body Part	Approach	Device	Qualifier
Medical and Surgical	Gastrointestinal System	Excision	Small Intestine	Open	No Device	No Qualifier
0	D	B	8	0	Z	Z

Chapter 7

Code Building Exercises

1.1. Transfemoral, distal femoral diaphysis

1.2. Low. Imagine the femur in thirds. Anywhere in the upper third is high. Anywhere in the middle third is mid, and anywhere in the lower third is low.

1.3. 0Y6C0Z3 – Detachment, Upper leg right, open approach, low

2.1. No

2.2. The Open approach is identified by the word "Incision." The Open approach is supported in the documentation.

2.3. 0Y9B0ZX – Drainage, lower extremity left, open approach, diagnostic

Check Your Understanding

CODING KNOWLEDGE CHECK

1. Answer: upper, scapula, clavicle

    Rationale: The body part value Forequarter describes the entire upper limb plus the scapula and clavicle.

3. Answer: d

    Rationale: This is a complete detachment of the 3rd day, based on the definition of amputation through the tarsometatarsal joint of the foot. This definition is the same as amputation at the most proximal portion of the metatarsal.

5. Answer: False

    Rationale: The body part value assigned is F, Abdominal Wall. Ventral hernias are hernias of the abdomen.

PROCEDURE STATEMENT CODING

1. Root operation: Alteration   Code: 0Y000ZZ

    Root operation: Alteration   Code: 0Y010ZZ

    Rationale: The root operation is Alteration because the procedure is performed for cosmetic reasons. The procedure is coded in the Anatomical Regions, Lower Extremities body system because the procedures are performed on various layers of tissue and in a large area. The body part values are 0 for the right buttock and 1 for the left buttock. No device or qualifier is appropriate.

3. Root operation: Alteration   Code: 0J0M3ZZ

    Root operation: Alteration   Code: 0J0L3ZZ

    Root operation: Alteration   Code: 0W0F0ZZ

    Rationale: These procedures are cosmetic in nature and therefore Alteration is assigned. There are individual body part values for each thigh region (upper leg) within the Subcutaneous Tissue and Fascia body system because liposuction removes subcutaneous tissue. There is a single body part value for the abdominal wall. The liposuction is performed percutaneously, and the abdominoplasty is an open procedure because the incision is below skin level and the operative site is exposed. No devices or qualifiers are appropriate for either procedure.

5. Root operation: Detachment   Code: 0X6W0Z0

Rationale: Because the supernumerary digit contains bone and nail, the root operation Detachment is coded. If the supernumerary digit was composed only of skin, the root operation Excision would be assigned. The qualifier value 0 is for a complete amputation of the little finger of the left hand.

7. Root operation: Repair   Code: 0WQ6XZ2

Rationale: This procedure involves the repair of the neck (Anatomical regions, general), rather than revision of the tracheostomy tube, therefore the root operation is Repair. The approach is X, External and the qualifier is 2, Stoma.

9. Root operation: Creation   Code: 0W4M070

Rationale: The Creation root operation describes the entire process of reassigning the gender from male to female. The body part is M, Perineum, Male in the Anatomical Regions, General body system. The approach is Open. The device value is 7, Autologous Tissue Substitute and the qualifier value is 0, Vagina.

Case Study Coding

1. ICD-10-PCS code: 0W9900Z

Rationale: Insertion of a chest tube is coded to the root operation Drainage, with a device value of 0 for a drainage device. The body part value of 9 is assigned for the pleural cavity on the right side.

3. ICD-10-PCS code: 0YU60JZ

Rationale: The documentation states that mesh was implanted. Therefore, the root operation Supplement is assigned. The left inguinal region is body part value 6 and a device value of J, Synthetic Substitute is assigned. No qualifier is appropriate. The procedure uses an Open approach because an incision is made through the skin and the inguinal canal operative site is exposed.

5. ICD-10-PCS code: 0W33XZZ

Rationale: The root operation Control is coded because the bleeder is the result of a previous procedure. When cautery is used to stop post-op bleeding, Control is the appropriate root operation. The tonsillar area is coded to the body part value of 3, Oral Cavity and Throat. The approach value is X, External.

Chapter 8

Code Building Exercises

1.1. Release the lumbar and sacral nerves. Freeing a body part from an abnormal physical constraint by cutting or the use of force.

1.2. No. These procedures are necessary to complete the release and treat the stenosis. According to coding guideline B3.13 in release procedures the body part value is the body part being freed and not the tissue being manipulated or cut to free the body part.

1.3. 01NB0ZZ – Release, lumbar nerve, open approach

01NR0ZZ – Release, sacral nerve, open approach

2.1. Nerve sheath tumor

2.2. Cranial nerve 8, Acoustic Nerve

2.3. Yes, Supplement, which is putting in or on biologic or synthetic material that physically reinforces and/or augments the function of a portion of a body part.

2.4. K, Nonautologous tissue substitute because Durepair is collagen obtained from bovine tissue. When no zooplastic tissue device option is available, Nonautologous tissue substitute is selected.

2.5. 00BN0ZZ – Excision, acoustic nerve, open approach

00U20KZ – Supplement, dura mater, open approach with nonautologous tissue substitute

See chapter 23 for a discussion of the coding for computer assisted navigation portion of this procedure.

Check Your Understanding

CODING KNOWLEDGE CHECK

1. b

Rationale: Accessing the body part key under cubital nerve directs the coder to Use Nerve, Ulnar. The root operation Repair is used to code procedures involving sutured lacerations. Under Repair, Nerve, Ulnar, the coder is directed to 01Q4. Therefore, the correct option is b.

3. c

Rationale: There are several large cisterns in the brain that may be documented with unique names such as magna, cerebromedullary, pontine, superior or ambient.

5. cerebral, peritoneal

Rationale: The cerebral ventricle is the source of the bypass and the peritoneal cavity is the body part bypassed to, in a ventriculoperitoneostomy, also called a VP shunt procedure.

PROCEDURE STATEMENT CODING

1. Root Operation: Reposition   Code: 01S40ZZ

Rationale: The root operation Reposition is used to code transposition procedures where body parts are moved to a more suitable location. Reposition is assigned because the nerve is moved out of the cubital tunnel groove. The body part value 4, Ulnar Nerve is assigned for this procedure using an Open approach. No device or qualifier values are appropriate for this code.

3. Root Operation: Destruction   Code: 015H3ZZ

Rationale: The root operation Destruction is coded because the nerve is destroyed by the use of a neurolytic agent. The common fibular nerve is part of body part value H, Peroneal Nerve, based on the body part key. The approach is percutaneous.

5. Root Operation: Excision   Code: 00BW3ZX

Rationale: The root operation for the biopsy is Excision. The body part value is W, Cervical spinal cord because the parts of the spine are individually identified in the Excision table. The approach is 3, Percutaneous and the qualifier is X, Diagnostic.

7. Root Operation: Map   Code: 00K83ZZ

Rationale: The root operation Map is coded for this procedure. The basal ganglia, body part value 8, is mapped using a Percutaneous approach.

9. Root Operation: Excision   Code: 00B70ZX

Rationale: The root operation Excision is used to code this procedure. A portion of the parietal lobe of the brain is removed via an Open approach (craniectomy). The index directs the coder to Use Cerebral Hemisphere. This is a biopsy because the pathological identification is not known at the start of the procedure. Therefore, the qualifier X, Diagnostic is assigned.

Case Study Coding

1. ICD-10-PCS code: 0JWS0JZ

Rationale: Because an incision was made, the root operation of Change cannot be coded. The root operation of Revision is used because a portion of a device is repaired or replaced. This portion of the device lives in the subcutaneous layer of the head and neck, which is accessed through an incision into the existing pocket. The device is a synthetic substitute because the valve controls the flow of CSF in a manner similar to the normal anatomy using a synthetic substitute. The device key says that a Holter Valve Ventricular Shunt is coded to "Synthetic Substitute." If the ventricular catheter portion of this device had been revised, it would be code 00W60JZ. If the peritoneal catheter portion of this device had been revised, it would be coded as 0WWG0JZ. This provides three individual codes for the common work of revising a portion of this complicated device, with each being coded in their particular body part location.

3. ICD-10-PCS code: 00C40ZZ

Rationale: The root operation Extirpation is used to code the evacuation of the subdural hematoma. The craniotomy flap was created with multiple burr holes that were connected to remove the bone flap, making this an open procedure. The body part value is 4, Subdural Space, Intracranial because the hematoma was located subdurally. No device value is appropriate because the Jackson-Pratt drain is a short-term, postoperative drain, based on Guideline B6.1b. No qualifier value is appropriate for this code.

5. ICD-10-PCS code: 00B70ZZ, 00U20KZ, 0NR00JZ

Rationale: The root operation for the tumor removal is Excision because the entire cerebral hemisphere is not removed. The tumor is in the frontal, temporal and parietal lobes. The body part key directs the coder to assign body part value 7, Cerebral Hemisphere for these body parts. The approach is open. There is no device or qualifier. The root operation for the use of the DuraGuard bovine pericardial patch is Supplement and the device value is K, Nonautologous Tissue because the zooplastic value is not available in the table. The root operation for the use of the titanium mesh is Replacement. Some of the skull was diseased and required replacement. The body part value is 0, Skull in the Head and Facial Bones body system. The device value is J, Synthetic Substitute and there is no qualifier.

Chapter 9

Code Building Exercises

1.1. Two – The placement of the scleral buckle and the retinopexy

1.2. To allow access to the retina for examination and placement of oil tamponade. The vitrectomy is not the procedure. It is part of the approach to the retina.

1.3. To reinforce the eyeball with a device and to repair the retina using a device. The buckle is a synthetic band that surrounds the eye and keeps the pressure off the retina. The buckle may or may not be removed at a later date. The oil is a synthetic substitute device that holds the retina against the back of the eye while it heals. The oil is not absorbable, and the last line of the report identifies that this is a device and the oil will need to be removed.

1.4. 08U03JZ – Supplement, eye right, percutaneous approach, synthetic substitute

08UE3JZ – Supplement, retina right, percutaneous approach, synthetic substitute

2.1. Three – Removal of polyps from the nasal passages, removal of polyps from the right maxillary sinus, and removal of polyps from the left maxillary sinus

2.2. Excision because the polyps are lesions of a body part that must be removed

2.3. 09BK8ZZ – Excision, nasal mucosa and soft tissue, via natural or artificial opening, endoscopic approach

09BQ8ZZ – Excision, right maxillary sinus, via natural or artificial opening, endoscopic approach

09BR8ZZ – Excision, left maxillary sinus, via natural or artificial opening, endoscopic approach

Check Your Understanding

CODING KNOWLEDGE CHECK

1. c

Rationale: Figure 9.4 shows the eustachian tube from the middle ear to the pharynx.

3. nose, eyes

Rationale: The ethmoid sinus is located in the ethmoid bone, between the nose and the eyes.

5. nose, nasopharynx

Rationale: This airway device is a nasal trumpet or a nasopharyngeal airway between the nose and the nasopharynx.

PROCEDURE STATEMENT CODING

1. Root operation: Replacement   Code: 08RJ3JZ

Root operation: Removal   Code: 08PJ3JZ

Rationale: The root operation for the first procedure performed is Removal of the dislocated lens. The approach is Percutaneous, and the device value is J, Synthetic Substitute. The root operation for the second procedure performed in Replacement for the implant of the new lens. The approach is Percutaneous, and the device value is J, Synthetic Substitute.

3. Root operation: Extirpation   Code: 08C23ZZ

Rationale: The blood clot in the anterior chamber is a foreign body and, therefore, the root operation of Extirpation is assigned. The body part value is 2, Anterior Chamber, Right and the approach is 3, Percutaneous.

5. Root operation: Insertion   Code: 09HE06Z

Root operation: Insertion   Code: 0NH60SZ

Rationale: The root operation Insertion is used to code both procedures. The first procedure is the implantation of the leads into the inner ear. The body part value E, Inner Ear, Left is assigned, along with the device value 6, Multiple Channel Cochlear Prosthesis and no qualifier. The second procedure is the implantation of the external hearing device into the temporal bone. The body part value 6, Temporal Bone is assigned, along with the device value S, Hearing Device and no qualifier. Both procedures are completed using an Open approach.

7. Root operation: Occlusion   Code: 08LY7DZ

Root operation: Occlusion   Code: 08LX7DZ

Rationale: The root operation of Occlusion is assigned. Each lacrimal duct is completely closed with an intraluminal device called a duct plug or punctal plug.

9. Root operation: Bypass   Code: 08133J4

Rationale: The surgeon bypasses the trabecular meshwork of the eye by placing a synthetic shunt from the anterior chamber to the sclera of the eye, relieving intraocular pressure and treating the glaucoma. The root operation is Bypass because the shunt reroutes the fluid around the meshwork from the inside to the outside of the eye. The body part value is 3, Anterior Chamber, Left because that is where the bypass starts and the qualifier is 4, Sclera because that is where the bypass ends. The device value is J, Synthetic Substitute for the synthetic shunt. The device is placed percutaneously through the wall of the eye into the anterior chamber.

Case Study Coding

1. ICD-10-PCS code: 08RK3JZ

Rationale: The root operation Replacement is coded because the intraocular lens is implanted at the same session during which the native lens is removed. The body part value K, Lens, Left is assigned. The approach is percutaneous because the lens is being removed through the small slit in the anterior chamber, not through an open incision. The device value J, Synthetic Substitute is assigned because the device is a manufactured item. No qualifier is appropriate for this code.

3. ICD-10-PCS code: 08R00JZ

Rationale: The root operation Replacement is used to code the total removal of the native eyeball and replacement with a synthetic eyeball. The removal of the native eyeball is included in the replacement procedure. There is no qualifier for this code.

5. ICD-10-PCS code: 08ND3ZZ

Rationale: Synechia is the condition of adhesions between the pupil and the iris. Synechiolysis is the release of those adhesions, coded with the root operation Release. The body part value, D, Iris, Left is assigned because the iris is being released. OS means Oculus Sinister, or the left eye. The approach value is 3, Percutaneous because the spatula was inserted but the anterior chamber was not exposed. No device and qualifier values are appropriate for this code.

Chapter 10

Code Building Exercises

1.1. Folding in and suturing tucks, to tighten weakened or stretched tissue
1.2. J, Synthetic Substitute because Composix E/X mesh is made of polypropylene and polytetrafluoroethylene (PTFE) synthetic materials
1.3. 0BUT4JZ – Supplement, diaphragm, percutaneous endoscopic approach with synthetic substitute
2.1. Two – Drainage of pleural effusion with a drainage device and mechanical pleurodesis
2.2. To destroy the outer layer of pleura with a scratching pad, so that the pleura heal together
2.3. 0W9900Z – Drainage of right pleural cavity, open, with drainage device

   0B5N4ZZ – Destruction of right pleura, percutaneous endoscopic approach

Check Your Understanding

CODING KNOWLEDGE CHECK

1. b

Rationale: A wedge resection procedure involves removing a small, wedge-shaped piece of tissue from the lung, usually for biopsy purposes. Because the entire right upper lobe is not removed, the root operation Excision is coded.

3. base, trachea

Rationale: The carina is the triangular piece of tissue that forms the connection between the trachea and the two bronchial openings that branch off from the trachea.

5. d

Rationale: The root operation Resection is used because the entire body part is removed. A wire snare is appropriate for use as a cutting instrument to perform the resection.

PROCEDURE STATEMENT CODING

1. Root operation: Insertion   Code: 0BHB8GZ

Rationale: The placement of the intraluminal device, endobronchial valve is coded with the root operation of Insertion. Even through the endobronchial valve does restrict airflow somewhat, there is no device value for endobronchial valve in the 0BV table. The root operation Insertion is the only available option and is assigned because the value performs a function. The endobronchial valve is device value G.

3. Root operation: Inspection   Code: 0BJ08ZZ

Rationale: The root operation of Inspection is coded because there are no other procedures identified. The body part value is 0, Tracheobronchial Tree, and the approach is 8, Via Natural or Artificial Opening Endoscopic.

5. Root operation: Inspection   Code: 0WJ94ZZ
   Root operation: Resection   Code: 0BTD0ZZ

Rationale: Two codes are required for this procedure. Because the procedure was discontinued due to the pleural effusion, the root operation Inspection is coded for the initial endoscopic evaluation with a percutaneous endoscopic approach. The root operation Resection is coded for the completed procedure of the open lobectomy of the lung, because the right middle lobe is an entire body part in ICD-10-PCS. Neither code has a device of qualifier value that is appropriate.

7. Root operation: Release, tongue   Code: 0CN7XZZ

Rationale: The frenulum is the small piece of tissue that holds the tongue to the floor of the mouth. Cutting into the frenulum releases the tongue to correct the ankyloglossia (tongue-tie). The root operation Release is coded with a body part value of 7, Tongue. The approach is X, External because the frenulum is visible within the oral cavity. No device or qualifier values are appropriate for this code.

9. Root Operation: Destruction   Code: 0B5B8ZZ

Rationale: The root operation Destruction is coded for the thermoplasty procedure. A thermal wand is delivered via the endoscope to the left lower lobe bronchus where it is activated to destroy excess muscle in the bronchial wall. The approach is 8, Via Natural or Artificial Opening Endoscopic and there is no device or qualifier that is appropriate.

Case Study Coding

1. ICD-10-PCS code: 0CRXXJ1, 0CRWXJ1, 0CDWXZ1, 0CDXXZ1

Rationale: Dental restorations are coded with the root operation Replacement because they replace a portion of the tooth with a synthetic substitute. Tooth numbers 2, 4, 12, and 15 are upper teeth. Tooth numbers 30 and 31 are lower teeth. Both of these codes have the qualifier of 1, Multiple, because multiple upper and lower teeth were replaced. The root operation Extraction is used to code dental extraction because the teeth are being pulled out. Tooth numbers 1 and 16 are upper teeth and tooth numbers 17 and 32 are lower teeth. Both of these codes have the qualifier of 1, Multiple, because multiple upper and lower teeth were extracted. All of the procedures are coded with the approach value of X, External because teeth can be visualized without the use of instruments or incision.

3. ICD-10-PCS codes: 0BBJ8ZX, 0BBH8ZX

   Rationale: The bronchoscopy is the approach to the bronchial tubes. The biopsies are taken of the lung through the bronchial wall. The locations are the left lower lobe and the lingula. The root operation Excision is used to code both biopsies. The approach is 8, Via Natural or Artificial Opening, Endoscopic. There is no device value and both qualifiers are X, Diagnostic to describe the biopsy.

5. ICD-10-PCS codes: 09JH7ZZ, 09JJ7ZZ, 0C5PXZZ, 0C5QXZZ

   Rationale: The examination of the ears under anesthesia is coded separately because a more definitive procedure on the ears is not performed at the same time. The root operation Inspection is used to code this procedure. There is no bilateral body part value; therefore, the procedures on both ears are coded separately. The approach is 7, Via Natural or Artificial Opening. No device or qualifier values are appropriate for these codes. The root operation Destruction is used to code both the coblation of the tonsils and the suction cautery of the adenoids. The approach for both of these procedures is X, External as both body parts can be visualized through the mouth. No device or qualifier values are appropriate for these codes.

Chapter 11

Code Building Exercises

1.1. Replacement because a portion of the aorta is removed and replaced with a dacron graft.
1.2. 04, Lower arteries
1.3. 04R00JZ – Replacement, abdominal aorta, open approach, synthetic substitute
2.1. The clip is placed to restrict the aneurysm back to its normal size.
2.2. 03, Upper Arteries
2.3. G, Intracranial Artery. The PCS system does not specify which artery is involved, only that the artery is intracranial.
2.4. 03VG0CZ – Restriction, intracranial artery, open approach, extraluminal device
3.1. Two – Atherectomy and Percutaneous Transluminal Angioplasty
3.2. A drug-eluting stent (DES) is an expandable scaffold that is placed into a narrowed artery to maintain a dilation and slowly release a drug to inhibit restenosis. A drug-coated balloon (DCB) is a dilation balloon that is coated with a drug that inhibits restenosis. The drug is transferred to the arterial wall during inflation and is slowly released over several months, without placement of a stent. This case uses a drug-coated balloon, not a drug-eluting stent.
3.3. 04CN3ZZ – Extirpation, popliteal artery left, percutaneous approach

   047N3Z1 – Dilation, popliteal artery left, percutaneous approach, drug-coated balloon

Check Your Understanding

CODING KNOWLEDGE CHECK

1. d

   Rationale: Supplement is used because the ring augments the function of the valve and does not reroute the blood flow, dilate the valve, or restrict the valve.

3. Lower arteries

   Rationale: The abdominal aorta is below the level of the diaphragm and is therefore a lower artery.

5. G, Intraluminal Device, Four or More

Rationale: The total number of stents used in all of the arteries treated using the same method is totaled to determine the device value.

PROCEDURE STATEMENT CODING

1. Root operation: Excision   Code: 03B00ZZ

Rationale: The root operation Excision is assigned to the removal of the right internal mammary artery for use as graft material. Resection is not an option in the upper arteries body system. The approach is 0, Open because incisions were made the arterial sites were exposed, and no device or qualifier is appropriate.

3. Root operation: Excision   Code: 03BT0ZX

Rationale: The left temporal artery has a unique body part value of T. The qualifier value of X is assigned because this procedure is a biopsy.

5. Root operation: Extirpation   Code: 03CG3Z7

Rationale: The root operation of Extirpation is used when a vessel is declotted. The Circle of Willis is coded to body part value G, Intracranial Artery, based on the body part key guidance. The approach is Percutaneous because the stent retriever used to remove the clot is delivered by a catheter, and captured in the qualifier value. No device value is coded.

7. Root operation: Bypass, Coronary artery, one artery   Code: 02100Z9

Root operation: Bypass, Coronary artery, one artery   Code: 021009W

Root operation: Excision, Saphenous vein   Code: 06BQ0ZZ

Rationale: See Code Building section of this chapter for a complete discussion of coronary artery bypass coding.

9. Root operation: Excision   Code: 02B70ZK

Rationale: The root operation Excision is assigned to the removal of the left atrial appendage for control of atrial fibrillation, also known as the Maze procedure. The body part value is 7, Atrium, Left and the qualifier value is K, Left Atrial Appendage.

Case Study Coding

1. ICD-10-PCS codes: 041L0JH, 04CK0ZZ

Rationale: The root operation Bypass is used to code the fem-fem bypass procedure. The origin of the bypass is the left common femoral artery (body part value) and the body part bypassed to is the right common femoral artery (qualifier value). An Open approach was used, and a synthetic prosthetic graft was used. In addition, a thrombectomy was performed in the right superficial femoral artery. This is coded with root operation Extirpation with a body part value of K, Femoral Artery, Right. The approach is Open, and no device or qualifier values are appropriate for this code.

3. ICD-10-PCS codes: 02110Z9, 021009W, 06BQ4ZZ

Rationale: This procedure involves the treatment of two coronary arteries with left internal mammary artery bypass grafts and one coronary artery with a saphenous vein graft. The procedures are performed using an Open approach. The LIMA procedure has no device value because the LIMA is not disconnected from the blood source and has body part value 0, because one site is treated with the LIMA. The qualifier is assigned as 9, Internal Mammary, Left. The venous graft has a device value of 9, Autologous

Venous Tissue and a qualifier of W, Aorta as the source of the bypass. The greater saphenous vein is also harvested endoscopically for use as the graft. The root operation Excision is used to code this procedure. The approach is 4, Percutaneous Endoscopic, and no device or qualifier values are appropriate for this code.

5. ICD-10-PCS code: 027034Z

Rationale: The root operation Dilation is used to code this PTCA. The left anterior descending is a coronary artery and one artery was treated. Therefore, the body part value of 0, Coronary Artery, One Artery is assigned. The approach is percutaneous through the femoral artery. The device value is 4, Intraluminal Device, Drug-eluting, and no qualifier value is appropriate for the code.

Chapter 12

Code Building Exercises

1.1. To restrict the flow of gastric juices back into the esophagus by wrapping the fundus of the stomach around the esophagogastric junction

1.2. Restriction

1.3. 0DV44ZZ – Restriction, esophagogastric junction, percutaneous endoscopic approach

2.1. No, because the omentum is not disconnected from the body (harvested). Therefore, it is not a device.

2.2. Repair because the Graham Patch is not a device

2.3. 0DQ64ZZ – Repair, stomach, percutaneous endoscopic approach

Check Your Understanding

CODING KNOWLEDGE CHECK

1. b

Rationale: A scope is used to inspect the intestines. If a definitive procedure is not performed at the same operative session, the root operation Inspection is coded.

3. d

Rationale: An infected suture is a foreign body. Removal of a foreign body is coded to the root operation Extirpation. The approach is Percutaneous Endoscopic or approach value 4. Therefore, the correct option is option d.

5. gallbladder, common bile duct

Rationale: Figure 12.4 displays the cystic duct between the gallbladder and the common bile duct.

PROCEDURE STATEMENT CODING

1. Root operation: Drainage   Code: 0F9440Z

Rationale: The root operation of Drainage is assigned, and the placement of the drainage device is included in character 6 as value 0, Drainage Device. The body part value is 4, Gallbladder.

3. Root operation: Bypass   Code: 0D1M0Z4

Rationale: The creation of a colostomy is the root operation of Bypass. The body part value is M, Descending Colon, and the qualifier is 4, Cutaneous. No device is used.

5. **Root operation: Dilation   Code: 0D770ZZ**

Rationale: The root operation Dilation is coded because the intent of the procedure is to make the opening of a tubular body part larger. This is Dilation because the explanation that accompanies the root operation definition states that dilation is "accomplished by stretching a tubular body part using intraluminal pressure or by cutting part of the orifice or wall of the tubular body part" and this explanation directive must be followed. The pylorus of the stomach has a unique body part value of 7 and the approach is documented as open. There is no appropriate device value or qualifier value.

7. **Root operation: Insertion   Code: 0DHA8UZ**

Rationale: The root operation Insertion is used to code this procedure. The feeding device is placed via a natural orifice using an endoscope. Therefore, the approach value is 8. The body part value is A, Jejunum, and there is no qualifier value.

9. **Root operation: Fragmentation   Code: 0FF9XZZ**

Rationale: The root operation Fragmentation is assigned for the lithotripsy procedure on the common bile duct stone. The approach is X, External because it is extracorporeal lithotripsy.

Case Study Coding

1. **ICD-10-PCS code: 0D774ZZ**

Rationale: The root operation Dilation is used to code the enlargement of the diameter of the pylorus, a tubular body part. The approach is laparoscopic, or approach value 4, Percutaneous Endoscopic. There are no device or qualifier values. Cutting the wall of a tubular body part is one of the ways that dilation can be accomplished based on the explanation that accompanies the root operation definition for Dilation.

3. **ICD-10-PCS codes: 0B110F4, 0DH63UZ, 0BP17DZ**

Rationale: The root operation Bypass is assigned to code the placement of the tracheostomy tube to form a bypass between the trachea and the skin to reroute the air. The body part value is 1, Trachea and the qualifier is value 4, Cutaneous. The tracheostomy is placed using an Open approach because an incision was made to expose the trachea. The root operation Insertion is used to code the insertion of the feeding device into the stomach. This is placed using a percutaneous approach. The device value is U, Feeding Device and there is no qualifier value. The previous endotracheal tube was removed from the trachea. The device value is D, Intraluminal Device.

5. **ICD-10-PCS codes: 0DC38ZZ, 0DB68ZX**

Rationale: The root operation Extirpation is used to code the removal of the foreign body. Even though the foreign body was not removed through the mouth, it was removed from the distal esophagus by sending it through the normal digestive route. The body part value of 3, Esophagus, Lower is assigned. There is no device or qualifier value. The root operation Excision is used to code the stomach biopsy. The body part value 6, Stomach is assigned and the qualifier value of X, Diagnostic is assigned because this was a biopsy. Both procedures are performed using an endoscopic approach through a natural opening, approach value 8.

Chapter 13

Code Building Exercises

1.1. Some of the right upper lobe. There are several segments in each lobe of each lung. Each segment is a discrete anatomical and functional unit, fed by an artery, drained by a vein and separated from the other segments by connective tissue.

1.2. Excision

1.3. 7, Lymphatics, thorax

1.4. 0BBC4ZX – Excision of right upper lung lobe, percutaneous endoscopic, diagnostic

07B74ZX – Excision thorax lymphatic, percutaneous endoscopic, diagnostic

2.1. Root operations that take out some or all of a body part because the lesion is a solid lesion of the spleen. Splenic tissue is being removed.

2.2. Excision because the core needle cuts a small tube of tissue for analysis

2.3. 3, Percutaneous approach

2.4. 07BP3ZX – Excision, spleen, percutaneous approach, diagnostic

Check Your Understanding

CODING KNOWLEDGE CHECK

1. thorax

   Rationale: The body part key tells the coder that the body part is Lymphatic, Thorax.

3. b

   Rationale: The root operation Release is used to code adhesiolysis. The body part being freed from an abnormal physical constraint is the spleen, body part value P.

5. glomera

   Rationale: The section of this chapter on the organization of the Endocrine system lists the synonyms for the structures of the endocrine system. The para-aortic body is also called the corpus glomera aortica.

PROCEDURE STATEMENT CODING

1. Root operation: Resection   Code: 0GTG0ZZ

   Rationale: The root operation Resection is assigned when the entire body part is removed. The body part value for the left lobe of the thyroid gland is G. The approach is Open and there are no device or qualifier values.

3. Root operation: Drainage   Code: 0G9G00Z

   Rationale: The root operation Drainage is assigned for the drainage of the thyroid cyst and the placement of the drain. The body part value is G, Thyroid Gland Lobe, Left and the approach is 0, Open. The device value is 0, Drainage Device.

5. Root operation: Excision   Code: 0GB10ZZ

   Rationale: Only a portion of the pineal body is removed; therefore, the root operation Excision is assigned. Craniectomy indicates that the approach is open because a portion of the skull is removed to expose the brain. There are no device or qualifier values.

7. Root operation: Resection   Code: 07T50ZZ

   Rationale: Even though the procedure description states Excision, the root operation Resection is assigned when an entire lymph node chain is removed. The approach is open and there are no device or qualifier values.

9. Root operation: Reposition   Code: 0GSN0ZZ

   Rationale: The root operation of Reposition is assigned for the procedure of autotransplantation, which means moving within the body. The body part value is N, Inferior parathyroid gland, right, and the approach is 0, Open. This procedure is commonly performed along with the thyroidectomy to salvage the parathyroid gland(s) by moving them to another location within the body.

Case Study Coding

1. ICD-10-PCS codes: 0GBG0ZX, 0GTG0ZZ

   Rationale: Based on Guideline B3.4 both the biopsy and the subsequent resection are coded, both of the same body part value, G, Thyroid Gland Lobe, Left. The procedures are performed with an Open approach because the previous incision was reopened to expose the thyroid. The excision has a qualifier value of X, Diagnostic and the resection has no qualifier.

3. ICD-10-PCS code: 07DR3ZX

   Rationale: Bone marrow biopsies are not coded to the root operation Excision. They are coded to the root operation Extraction. Aspiration procedures are performed percutaneously. The body part value in this case is R, Bone Marrow, Iliac. Bone marrow aspirations are biopsies and are coded with the qualifier X, Diagnostic.

5. ICD-10-PCS code: 07TP4ZZ

   Rationale: The spleen is completely removed from this patient. This is coded with the root operation Resection. The approach is percutaneous endoscopic for the laparoscopy. There was no device or qualifier.

Chapter 14

Code Building Exercises

1.1. Yes. Guideline B3.5, Overlapping Layers
1.2. Subcutaneous tissue and fascia. The necrotic body part is identified as fascia.
1.3. 0JB80ZZ – Excision, abdominal subcutaneous tissue and fascia, open approach
2.1. Two, because excision of skin to be replaced is not coded.
2.2. The definition of the root operation Excision and Guideline B3.9, Excision for Graft
2.3. 0HRMX74 – Replacement, skin right foot, autologous tissue substitute, partial thickness
     0HBHXZZ – Excision, skin right upper leg (for the harvesting)

Check Your Understanding

CODING KNOWLEDGE CHECK

1. b

   Rationale: The right wrist is part of the right lower arm, based guideline B4.6. When a laceration extends through overlapping layers, the body part value for the deepest structure is coded, based on guideline B3.5. This procedure is coded as 0JQG0ZZ.

3. c

   Rationale: Reattachment is not an available root operation for the subcutaneous layer, only the skin. In ICD-10-PCS, the subcutaneous layer has separate body part values. Therefore, the default root operation of Repair must be used. This procedure is coded as 0JQ00ZZ.

5. b

   Rationale: The toenail is a body part that is partially removed with a surgical scissors. This meets the definition of the root operation Excision.

1. **Root operation: Destruction   Code: 0H5AXZD**

    Rationale: The root operation Destruction is assigned for the cryocautery of the lesions. The body part value is A, Skin, Inguinal. The approach is X, External and the qualifier is D, Multiple because five lesions were destroyed.

3. **Root operation: Repair   Code: 0JQR0ZZ**

    Rationale: The root operation Repair is used to code repair of lacerations. The body part value of R is assigned for the left foot subcutaneous tissue and fascia laceration. The approach is Open because the subcutaneous layer was sutured. This means the subcutaneous layer was exposed. No device value or qualifier value is appropriate.

5. **Root operation: Extirpation   Code: 0HCQXZZ**

    Rationale: The root operation Extirpation is used to code the evacuation of the hematoma from under the fingernail. The approach is X, External. No device value or qualifier value is appropriate.

7. **Root operation: Excision   Code: 0JBG0ZZ**

    Root operation: Transfer   Code: 0JXG0ZB

    Rationale: The root operation Transfer is coded for the advancement flap, and the body part is coded to the deepest layer transferred. The qualifier describes all of the layers that were transferred. The root operation Transfer does not include the excision of the scar. The eschar removal is coded with the root operation Excision. This is coded to the subcutaneous tissue and fascia because a 3rd degree burn goes through the depth of the subcutaneous layer.

9. **Root operation: Release   Code: 0HNDXZZ**

    Rationale: The root operation Release is assigned when the scar is incised. The elbow is being constrained by the tight skin. Therefore, the body part value is D, Skin, Lower Arm. Guideline B4.6 says that the elbow is considered part of the lower arm. The approach is X, External.

Case Study Coding

1. **ICD-10-PCS Codes: 0HR8X74, 0HRHX74, 0HRJX74**

    Rationale: The root operation Replacement is used to code these free skin grafts. The grafts are placed on the buttocks, body part value 8; on the right upper leg, body part value H; and on the left upper leg, body part value J. The approach is X, External. The device value is 7, Autologous Tissue Substitute and the qualifier value is 4, Partial Thickness because the epidermal graft is only a partial thickness of the skin. There is no excision code for the graft because the donor skin was excised previously and sent to the laboratory for culturing. See the section on Devices and Qualifiers in this chapter for further details on tissue culturing.

3. **ICD-10-PCS Codes: 06H033Z, 0JHM3XZ**

    Rationale: The root operation Insertion is coded for both procedures. The body part value 0, Inferior Vena Cava is assigned for the insertion of the infusion device, as the point where the tip rests. The approach is 3, Percutaneous and the device value is 3, Infusion Device. No qualifier value is appropriate for this code. The body part value M, Subcutaneous Tissue and Fascia, Left Upper Leg is assigned for the location of the tunnel. The approach value is 3, Percutaneous and the device value is X, Vascular Access Device, Tunneled. No qualifier value is appropriate for this code.

5. ICD-10-PCS Codes: 0JH60WZ, 02HV33Z

Rationale: The venous access port is placed in a subcutaneous pocket in the chest wall. The root operation Insertion is used to code this procedure. The body part value 6, Subcutaneous Tissue and Fascia, Chest is assigned. The approach is Open and the device value W, Vascular Access Device, Totally Implantable is assigned. There is no qualifier. The infusion device is inserted into the superior vena cava and is coded with the root operation Insertion. The body part value V, Superior Vena Cava is assigned. This approach is 3, Percutaneous because the site of the procedure is not visualized. There is no qualifier. See chapter 11 for additional explanation.

Chapter 15

Code Building Exercises

1.1. To replace the anterior cruciate ligament with a graft

1.2. No, because the plugs are used to attach the tendon graft into the tibia and femur. They are integral to the process of attaching the graft. Regular sutures cannot be used on bone; therefore, bone plugs are left attached and anchored to the recipient bone.

1.3. Yes, because the procedure was started with one approach and completed through a different approach. See guideline B3.2d.

1.4. Yes, the harvest of the tendon used for the graft. See guideline B3.9.

1.5. 0MRN07Z – Replacement, knee ligament right, open approach, autologous tissue substitute

0LBQ0ZZ – Excision, knee tendon right, open approach

0SJC4ZZ – Inspection, knee joint right, percutaneous endoscopic approach

2.1. Reattachment, defined as putting back in or on all or a portion of a separated body part to its normal location or other suitable location.

2.2. Knee tendon

2.3. 0LMQ0ZZ – Reattachment, knee tendon, right, open approach

Check Your Understanding

CODING KNOWLEDGE CHECK

1. d

Rationale: Based on guideline B4.7, the structures of the fingers are coded the hand when no specific body part value is available.

3. b

Rationale: A biceps tenodesis procedure moves the biceps tendon to the humerus. Therefore, the root operation Reposition is assigned.

5. bursa

Rationale: A bursa is the structure between a bone and tendon that forms a cushion.

PROCEDURE STATEMENT CODING

1. Root operation: Drainage   Code: 0M910ZZ

Rationale: Incision and drainage is the root operation Drainage. The body part value 1 for shoulder bursa is assigned. Incision indicates that the approach is Open. No device value or qualifier value is appropriate for this code.

3. **Root operation: Repair   Code: 0KQ50ZZ**

Rationale: The root operation Repair is assigned for the repair of the ruptured muscle. The body part value is 5, Shoulder Muscle, Right. The index directs the coder to use the muscle of the shoulder as the body part. The approach is 0, Open. No device or qualifier is appropriate.

5. **Root operation: Release   Code: 0LNV3ZZ**

Rationale: The root operation Release is assigned when the tendon sheath is incised to release the extensor digitorum brevis tendon of the right foot. The body part value is V, Foot Tendon, Right. The index directs the coder to use the foot tendon body part. The approach is 3, Percutaneous. No device or qualifier is appropriate.

7. **Root operation: Excision   Code: 0KBS3ZX**

Rationale: The index directs the coder to use the lower leg muscle body part. The root operation Excision is used to code a biopsy. The approach is 3, Percutaneous. The qualifier value X, Diagnostic is assigned for a biopsy.

9. **Root operation: Excision   Code: 0LBN0ZZ**

Rationale: The root operation Excision is used to code this procedure. The body part value N is assigned for the Lower Leg Tendon, Right. The approach is Open and no device value or qualifier value is appropriate for this code.

Case Study Coding

1. **ICD-10-PCS codes: 0RQX0ZZ, 0LQ80ZZ, 0MQ80ZZ**

Rationale: The root operation Repair is used to code all three procedures—the repair of the joint capsule, the tendon, and the ligament. The body part value X is assigned for the left finger phalangeal joint. The body part value 8 is assigned for the left hand tendon and the left hand bursa and ligament. All procedures used an Open approach because the wounds were already open, and no device value or qualifier value is appropriate for any of these codes.

3. **ICD-10-PCS codes: 0PTN0ZZ, 0LX60ZZ**

Rationale: The root operation Resection is used to code the complete removal of the trapezium bone, a carpal bone, body part value N. The root operation Transfer is used to code the transfer of the flexor carpi radialis tendon, which is a lower arm and wrist tendon. Both procedures are performed with an Open approach because an incision was made to expose the bone. No device value or qualifier value is appropriate for this code.

5. **ICD-10-PCS codes: 0PSR04Z, 0LQ70ZZ**

Rationale: The root operation Reposition is used to code the fracture reduction. The body part value R, Thumb Phalanx, Right is assigned. The approach is Open because the wound was already open and no device value or qualifier value is appropriate for this code. The root operation Repair is used to code the restoration of the extensor pollicus longus tendon, body part value 7. The approach is Open and no device value or qualifier value is appropriate for this code. The removal of the bone fragments is not coded separately because the removal is integral to the procedure of repositioning the fractured bone.

Chapter 16

Code Building Exercises

1.1. To remove the infected joint prosthesis and perform a temporary replacement

1.2. Articulating spacer

1.3. Replacement

1.4. 9, Hip joint, right

1.5. 0SP90JZ – Removal, Hip joint right, open approach, synthetic substitute

0SR90EZ– Replacement, Hip joint right, open approach, articulating spacer

0SB90ZX – Excision, Hip joint right, open approach, diagnostic

2.1. Fusion of vertebral joints at L4-L5 and L5-S1

2.2. Qualifier J for Posterior Approach to the Anterior Column (incision made in the patient's back to reach the anterior interbody joint)

Qualifier 1 for Posterior Approach to the Posterior Column (incision made in the patient's back to reach the posterior facet joints)

2.3. 0, Lumbar vertebral joint and 3, Lumbosacral joint

2.4. Guideline B3.10c. The first bullet identifies that A, Interbody Fusion Device will be assigned for the anterior fusion. The third bullet identifies that the posterior bone graft will be coded as 7, Autologous Tissue Substitute.

2.5. No. These procedures are necessary to treat the stenosis and prepare the joint space for Fusion.

2.6. For Dura Mater, Spinal, the body part key states Use: Spinal Meninges

2.7. 0SG00AJ – Fusion, Lumbar vertebral joint, Open approach, Interbody fusion device, Posterior Approach to the Anterior Column

0SG30AJ – Fusion, Lumbosacral joint, Open approach, Interbody fusion device, Posterior Approach to the Anterior Column

0SG0071 – Fusion, Lumbar vertebral joint, Open approach, Autologous tissue substitute, Posterior Approach to the Posterior Column

0SG3071 – Fusion, Lumbosacral joint, Open approach, Autologous tissue substitute, Posterior Approach to the Posterior Column

00QT0ZZ – Repair, Spinal meninges, Open approach

3.1. 1, Shoulder tendon, right because four tendons make up the rotator cuff. The muscles (Teres minor, supraspinatus, subscapularis, infraspinatus) that they attach to bone are classified as shoulder muscles. Therefore, the tendons are shoulder tendons.

3.2. Subacromial decompression is the Release of the shoulder joint. The word "decompression" is frequently associated with the concept of Release.

3.3. 0LQ14ZZ – Repair, shoulder tendon right, percutaneous endoscopic approach

0RNJ4ZZ – Release, shoulder joint right, percutaneous endoscopic approach

Check Your Understanding

CODING KNOWLEDGE CHECK

1. M

Rationale: Bone growth stimulator is device value M.

3. d

Rationale: The body of the vertebra is supplemented with glue, to reinforce the broken vertebra.

5. b.

> Rationale: T1 means the vertebra itself. Corpectomy is the only procedure that is performed on the vertebra itself. Discectomy and fusion are performed on the space, such as T1-T2. Alteration is not an option because alteration is only done to improve the appearance of a body part.

Procedure Statement Coding

1. Root operation: Reposition   Code: 0PSM0ZZ

> Rationale: Repair of a displaced fracture is the root operation of Reposition. The right pisiform bone is one of the carpal bones. No device is used and no qualifier is appropriate.

3. Root operation: Replacement   Code: 0RRK00Z

> Rationale: The left shoulder joint is replaced with a reverse prosthesis (ball on glenoid and socket on humerus) or device value 0, Synthetic Substitute, Reverse Ball, and Socket. The removal of the native shoulder joint is included in the replacement procedure and not coded separately. The approach is Open because the Open approach is the only approach available for shoulder replacement surgery.

5. Root operation: Excision   Code: 0SBD4ZZ

> Rationale: The root operation Excision is assigned because only part of the meniscus is removed. The body part value is D, Knee Joint, Left because the meniscus is a knee joint structure. The approach is 4, Percutaneous Endoscopic because this was done through an arthroscope. No device or qualifier is appropriate.

7. Root operation: Removal   Code: 0PPG35Z

> Rationale: The root operation Removal is assigned to procedures that remove devices from body parts. The body part value is G, Humeral Shaft, Left. The approach is 3, Percutaneous and the device value is 5, External Fixation Device.

9. Root operation: Drainage   Code: 0R9W00Z

> Rationale: Incision and drainage is the root operation Drainage using an Open approach. A drainage device was left in place and coded with the device value of 0.

Case Study Coding

1. ICD-10-PCS code: 0SRR019

> Rationale: Replacement of the femoral surface of the right hip is body part value R. The prosthesis is a metal synthetic substitute, 0, and the qualifier is value 9 for Cemented. The removal of the native femoral head is included in the replacement procedure and not coded separately.

3. ICD-10-PCS code: 0S9C00Z

> Rationale: The root operation is Drainage. The body part value is C, Knee Joint, Right because the incision is made into the joint capsule. A hemovac drain is placed for the device value of 0. The irrigation is not coded separately as this is integral to effectively draining the joint.

5. ICD-10-PCS code: 0RG10A0

> Rationale: The nerve root at C5-C6 is released by the removal of some of the intervertebral disc but is not coded separately when a fusion is performed. Fusion is the final objective of the procedure. Fusion of a vertebral joint using an interbody fusion device and packed with allograft bone is coded to the device Interbody Fusion Device. The spinal approach used is qualifier value 0 for Anterior Approach of the body and Anterior Approach to the spinal column.

Chapter 17

Check Your Understanding

1.1. Three, dilation of bladder neck, dilation of the left ureter and fragmentation of ureteral calculus

1.2. Dilation of bladder neck and left ureter – Root operations that alter the diameter or route of a tubular body part. Remember that cutting the wall of a tubular body part is performed with the intent of dilating the body part.

Fragmentation of ureteral calculus – Root operations that take out solids/liquids/gases from a body part

1.3. Dilation of bladder neck and ureter – Dilation

Fragmentation of ureteral calculus – Fragmentation

1.4. No, the stent is represented in the 6th character for the device. The stent maintains the dilation of the left ureter to allow for passage of the fragmented ureteral stone.

1.5. 0T778DZ Dilation of the left ureter with intraluminal device, via natural or artificial opening, endoscopic

0T7C8ZZ Dilation of the bladder neck, via natural or artificial opening, endoscopic

0TF7XZZ Fragmentation of the left ureter, external approach

See chapter 24 on Imaging for the discussion on fluoroscopy coding.

2.1. Guideline B5.2, Open approach with percutaneous endoscopic assistance.

2.2. 0TT00ZZ – Resection, right kidney, open approach

See chapter 23 for information on coding the robotic assistance procedure.

Check Your Understanding

1. a

Rationale: Ablation destroys the tissue and therefore, Destruction is the appropriate root operation.

3. c

Rationale: Both the ileal conduit bypass and the laser destruction are coded.

5. 3, Percutaneous

Rationale: The needle is placed into the bladder through the skin above the pubic bone.

1. Root operation: Occlusion   Code: 0TL70ZZ

Rationale: The only root operation performed is Occlusion, the surgical ligation of the ureter to prevent further hemorrhage. The approach is 0, Open based on the description of exploratory laparotomy.

3. Root operation: Fragmentation   Code: 0TFBXZZ

Rationale: The root operation Fragmentation is assigned for the lithotripsy procedure. The body part value is B, Bladder. The approach is X, External because extracorporeal shock wave lithotripsy is done from the outside of the body. No device or qualifier is appropriate.

5.   Root operation: Repair   Code: 0TQB0ZZ

Rationale: The root operation Repair is assigned for the suturing of the bladder, body part value B, Bladder. The approach is 0, Open as this is the only approach option and no device or qualifier is appropriate.

7.   Root operation: Change   Code: 0T29X0Z

Rationale: The root operation Change is used to replace a ureterostomy tube because a device is removed, and an identical device is placed in the body part without cutting or puncturing the skin. The approach is X, External because the skin is not opened.

9.   Root operation: Insertion   Code: 0THC0LZ

Rationale: The root operation Insertion is used because a non-biological appliance is inserted to help the muscles of the bladder neck maintain urinary continence. The device value is L, Artificial Sphincter. The Open approach is specified.

Case Study Coding

1.   ICD-10-PCS code: 0TSD0ZZ

Rationale: This procedure is performed on the urethra and not on the glans penis. The intent of the procedure is to reposition the urethra to the correct location in the tip of the glans penis and therefore the root operation Reposition is coded. An Open approach is used because an incision was made to expose the urethra as it was moved.

3.   ICD-10-PCS code: 0TCB0ZZ

Rationale: The root operation Extirpation is used to describe the removal of the stone from the bladder. The Open approach is used to remove the stone with an incision in a suprapubic fashion. The Jackson-Pratt drain is not coded, as the drain is relatively temporary.

5.   ICD-10-PCS codes: 0TV78ZZ, 0TV68ZZ

Rationale: The Deflux injection is used to restrict the ureteral opening and prevent reflux of the urine up the ureters. The Deflux is a substance and not a device. This procedure is performed bilaterally; however, the root operation Restriction does not have a body part value defined for bilateral ureters. Two procedure codes are required to describe the procedures performed, one for each ureter. Approach value 8, Via Natural or Artificial Opening Endoscopic, is used for both procedures.

Chapter 18

Code Building Exercises

1.1.   To remove the necrotic testicle that could not be saved

1.2.   No, the exploration is integral because a definitive procedure was ultimately performed at the same body site.

1.3.   0VT90ZZ – Resection, testicle right, open approach

2.1.   Two, to treat the phimosis and dilate the urethra

2.2.   The penis is being released. Release is freeing a body part from an abnormal physical constraint by cutting or by use of force. The penis was constricted by the foreskin, which was cut, but the body part that was being released was the penis.

2.3.   In this case, the Foley is not a drainage device. It was placed to maintain the dilation of the urethra while it heals. This is device value, D, Intraluminal Device.

2.4. 0VNSXZZ – Release, penis, external approach

0T7D7DZ – Dilation, urethra with intraluminal device, via natural or artificial opening

Check Your Understanding

CODING KNOWLEDGE CHECK

1. c

Rationale: The seminal vesicle is found where the vas deferens enters the prostate and is not part of the spermatic cord. The Dartos fascia surrounds the testicles and the spermatic cords within the scrotum. The epididymis is found at the top of the testicle and is not part of the spermatic cord. The vas deferens is found within the spermatic cord.

3. Destruction

Rationale: Destruction is the physical eradication of all or a portion of a body part by the direct use of energy, force or a destructive agent. The laser is an energy source.

5. T or prepuce

Rationale: The prepuce surrounds and protects the head of the penis and is removed during the circumcision procedure.

PROCEDURE STATEMENT CODING

1. Root operation: Resection   Code: 0VT00ZZ

Rationale: The root operation Resection is used to code this procedure because the term prostatectomy typically describes the removal of the entire prostate. The retropubic approach is an Open approach as described in the approach section of this chapter. No device value or qualifier value is appropriate for this code.

3. Root operation: Removal   Code: 0VPS0JZ

Root operation: Supplement   Code: 0VUS0JZ

Rationale: The root operation Removal is used to code the removal of the original prosthesis. The insertion of the new prosthesis is coded to the root operation Supplement because the prosthesis augments the function of the body part. The approach for both procedures is open. The device value for both procedures is J, Synthetic Substitute. No qualifier is appropriate for either code.

5. Root operation: Excision   Code: 0VB90ZX

Rationale: The root operation Excision is used for the biopsy of the right testes, body part value 9. The approach is 0, Open and the qualifier is X, Diagnostic for the biopsy.

7. Root operation: Extirpation   Code: 0VC50ZZ

Rationale: The root operation Extirpation is used to code the removal of the foreign body from the scrotum. The approach is Open and no device or qualifier value is appropriate for this code.

9. Root operation: Resection   Code: 0VTK0ZZ

Rationale: The root operation Resection is assigned for the surgical removal of the left epididymis, body part value K because the epididymis is an individually named body part. The approach is 0, Open. No device or qualifier is appropriate.

Case Study Coding

1. ICD-10-PCS code: 0VLQ0ZZ

   Rationale: The root operation Occlusion is used to code the intent of the procedure. The intent is to occlude the bilateral vas deferens regardless of whether a small piece is removed or the ends are cauterized. Male sterilization is occlusion of the vas deferens bilaterally. The body part value Q describes the bilateral vas deferens. The approach is open because an incision was made, and the vas was exposed through the incision and no device value or qualifier value is appropriate for the code.

3. ICD-10-PCS code: 0VTC0ZZ

   Rationale: The root operation Resection is used to code the orchiectomy. The body part value C, Testes bilateral is assigned. The approach is Open because an incision was made into the scrotum to resect the testes and no device or qualifier value is appropriate for this code.

5. ICD-10-PCS code: 0VTTXZZ

   Rationale: The root operation Resection is used to code the complete removal of the prepuce. The approach is X, External because the procedure is performed on the skin. No device or qualifier value is appropriate for this code.

Chapter 19

Code Building Exercises

1.1. Revision because the device is malfunctioning.
1.2. G, Vagina
1.3. 0UWH0JZ – Revision, vagina and cul-de-sac, synthetic substitute, open approach

    0UQG0ZZ – Repair, vagina, open approach
2.1. Two, vaginal suspension using a device and rectocele repair using a device
2.2. Supplement is assigned for both procedures because a device is used to accomplish both. In the vaginal suspension, the device augments the function and in the rectocele repair, the defect is repaired with a device. If a device had not been used, the root operation would have been Reposition. But, when a device is used to accomplish the procedure, Supplement is selected.
2.3. K, Nonautologous because it is made of porcine material and no zooplastic option is available.
2.4. 0UUG0KZ – Supplement, vagina, nonautologous tissue substitute, open approach

    0JUC0KZ – Supplement, subcutaneous tissue and fascia, pelvic region, nonautologous tissue substitute, open approach

Check Your Understanding

CODING KNOWLEDGE CHECK

1. False

   Rationale: The vulva is a combination of external female genitalia.

3. c

   Rationale: The term "subtotal hysterectomy," also called a supracervical hysterectomy, means that only the uterus is removed and the cervix remains intact.

5. d

Rationale: Body part values for combined structures, such as vagina and cul-de-sac, are available for use in coding the root operations that involve devices or inspection (Change, Insertion, Inspection, Removal, and Revision). The body part values for combined structures are not available for use with any other root operations used in this system.

PROCEDURE STATEMENT CODING

1. Root operation: Excision   Code: 0UBMXZX

Rationale: The root operation Excision is coded to describe the vulvar biopsy. The approach is X, External because the excision takes place directly on the skin or mucous membranes. The qualifier X, Diagnostic is assigned for this biopsy.

3. Root operation: Extraction Code: 0UDN3ZZ

Rationale: The harvesting of ova is the root operation of Extraction because the ova are pulled out of the ovary. The body part value is N, Ova and the approach is 3, Percutaneous. No device or qualifier is appropriate.

5. Root operation: Occlusion Code: 0ULG7ZZ

Rationale: Colpocleisis is a procedure performed to secure the vaginal walls together internally and obliterate the vaginal opening using a vaginal approach. This procedure is performed without endoscopic assistance, directly on the vaginal mucosa. Sutures are used; therefore, no device or qualifier are appropriate.

7. Root operation: Destruction   Code: 0U5B7ZZ

Rationale: The root operation Destruction is assigned because the ablation process destroys the lining of the uterus, with the body part value of B, Endometrium. The approach is 7, Via Natural or Artificial Opening because no scope is used with the heat wand that does the destruction. No device or qualifier is appropriate.

9. Root operation: Drainage   Code: 0U9L0ZZ

Rationale: The root operation Drainage is coded. To access the body part in the index, see Drainage, Gland, Vestibular. The approach is open because surgical drainage means the site was surgically opened. The documentation states that no drainage device is used. No qualifier is appropriate as the documentation does not state that this was a biopsy.

Case Study Coding

1. ICD-10-PCS codes: 0UT94ZZ, 0UT24ZZ, 0UT74ZZ

Rationale: The root operation of Resection is assigned to the cutting out of uterus (including cervix), bilateral fallopian tubes and bilateral ovaries. The procedure was performed with a percutaneous endoscopic approach. This is a laparoscopic hysterectomy because all of the organs were disconnected using the laparoscope tools. The disconnection with the laparoscope tools is the determining factor. The location from which the organs are removed from the body does not determine the type of hysterectomy that was performed. No device or qualifier values apply for either code.

3. ICD-10-PCS code: 0UVC0CZ

Rationale: The root operation Restriction is used to code the cerclage procedure. The approach is an abdominal approach, or an approach value of 0, Open. An extraluminal device is used to restrict the cervix, for a device value of C, Extraluminal Device. No qualifier value is appropriate for this code.

5. ICD-10-PCS codes: 0UT9FZZ, 0UT2FZZ, 0UT7FZZ, 0UTC7ZZ

Rationale: Three codes are required to describe the laparoscopic resections completed in the hysterectomy with bilateral salpingo-oophorectomy, each with the approach value of F, Via Natural or Artificial Opening with Percutaneous Endoscopic Assistance. The approach value of F is assigned because the resection is performed via the endoscope, using the Endostapler attachment that staples and cuts at the same time. The body parts are removed through the natural opening, but were resected using the endoscope. An additional code is required to describe the resection of the cervix, done through a vaginal approach without the use of the endoscope must also be assigned. This is coded with approach value 7, Via Natural or Artificial Opening. No device values or qualifier values are appropriate for any of the procedures.

Chapter 20

Code Building Exercises

1.1. Extraction

1.2. The surgeon described the incision as a low transverse incision, which is classified to qualifier value of 1, Low.

1.3. Control, because this was postoperative hemorrhage that was not controlled by a definitive procedure. Therefore, Control should be coded.

1.4. 10D00Z1 Extraction of products of conception, low cervical, open approach

0W3R7ZZ Control, genitourinary tract, via natural or artificial opening

2.1. 0, High

2.2. Abdominal wall. F, Abdominal wall in the Anatomical Regions, General

2.3. 10D00Z0 – Extraction, products of conception, high, open approach

0UT90ZZ – Resection, uterus, open approach

0UT20ZZ – Resection, ovaries, bilateral, open approach

0UT70ZZ – Resection, fallopian tubes, bilateral, open approach

0WBF0ZZ – Excision, abdominal wall, open approach

Check Your Understanding

CODING KNOWLEDGE CHECK

1. a

Rationale: The 7th character value of 0 describes a high incision.

3. False

Rationale: These qualifier values describe the body systems of the products of conception, not the pregnant female.

5. False

Rationale: Delivery of all products of conception using the same method and approach are coded with one code.

PROCEDURE STATEMENT CODING

1. Root operation: Extraction, retained products of conception Code: 10D17ZZ

Rationale: The use of a curette indicates that the root operation Extraction is coded. Retained placental fragments are Products of Conception, Retained. No device or qualifier is appropriate for the code.

3. **Root operation: Reposition Code: 10S0XZZ**

Rationale: An external version procedure was performed, which is coded with the root operation Reposition. An external approach is used, as indicated in the procedure name. No device or qualifier are appropriate for this code.

5. **Root operation: Extraction Code: 10D07Z7**

Rationale: The root operation Extraction is used to code this procedure because a form of instrumentation was used to extract the products of conception. The approach value of 7 is assigned because it was a vaginal delivery, through a natural opening. The qualifier value of 7 is assigned for internal version.

7. **Root operation: Extraction Code: 10D07Z3**

Root operation: Division   Code: 0W8NXZZ

Rationale: The use of forceps determines that this is the root operation Extraction. The qualifier value of 3, Low Forceps, is assigned. The episiotomy is coded to the root operation Division. The body part value is N, Perineum, Female in the Anatomical Regions, General body system and the approach is External. The episiotomy repair is not coded because closure of an operative incision is included in the procedure.

9. **Root operation: Delivery   Code: 10E0XZZ**

Root operation: Division   Code: 0W8NXZZ

Rationale: Spontaneous vaginal deliveries are coded with only one code in ICD-10-PCS. The root operation Delivery is used to code this case. The episiotomy is coded to the root operation Division. The body part value is N, Perineum, female in the Anatomical Regions, General body system, and the approach is external. The episiotomy repair is not coded because closure of an operative incision is included in the procedure.

11. **Root operation: Change   Code: 102073Z**

Rationale: The root operation Change is assigned because the monitoring electrode is removed and reinserted without cutting. The body part value is 0, Product of Conception, and the approach is 7, Via Natural or Artificial Opening. The device value is 3, Monitoring Electrode. No qualifier is appropriate.

Case Study Coding

1. **ICD-10-PCS code: 10D00Z1**

Rationale: The root operation Extraction is used to code cesarean section deliveries. The approach is Open, and the qualifier identifies the uterine approach as low cervical in this case.

3. **ICD-10-PCS code: 10E0XZZ**

Rationale: Delivery was accomplished without the assistance of instruments; therefore, the root operation Delivery is coded. The root operation Delivery always uses an external approach. No device value or qualifier value applies to this code.

5. **ICD-10-PCS codes: 10D00Z0, 10907ZC**

Rationale: The root operation Extraction is coded for the cesarean section. The approach is Open, and the qualifier is 0 for a classical incision. Artificial rupture of membranes is coded as drainage of amniotic fluid, with a code being provided by the Index.

Chapter 21

Check Your Understanding

1. Peritoneal dialysis

Rationale: The root operation is Irrigation in the Administration Section of ICD-10-PCS. The main term in the index is Irrigation with a sub-term of Peritoneal cavity and the substance is Dialysate.

3. b

Rationale: The interrogation of the pacemaker is the root operation Measurement. The function/device value is S, Pacemaker. There is no qualifier.

5. Measurement, 4A0D7BZ

Rationale: Urinary manometry is measuring the pressure within an organ, in this case the urinary bladder. The root operation is Measurement and the code is 4A0D7BZ. The entire 7 characters of the code are provided in the Index.

1. Root operation: Introduction   Code: 3E0U33Z

Rationale: The root operation Introduction is used to code the administration of the anti-inflammatory into a joint of the spine.

3. Root operation: Introduction   Code: 3E0234Z

Rationale: The root operation Introduction is used to code the administration of the serum, toxoid, or vaccine. The injection location is intramuscular, and the approach is percutaneous. The substance value is 4, Serum, Toxoid, or Vaccine, and there is no qualifier.

5. Root operation: Drainage   Code: 009700Z

Root operation: Monitoring   Code: 4A100BZ

Root operation: Excision   Code: 0JBM0ZZ

Root operation: Replacement   Code: 0NR007Z

Rationale: The root operation Drainage is used to code the procedure to drain the intracranial abscess, body part value 7, Cerebral Hemisphere. The approach is open through the craniectomy. The device value is 0, Drainage Device, and there is no qualifier value for this code. The root operation Monitoring is used to code the placement of the intracranial pressure device and the monitoring. The approach is Open. The function/device value is B, Pressure, and there is no qualifier for this code. The root operation Excision is used to code the harvesting of the fascia graft from the patient's upper leg using an Open approach. The root operation Replacement is used to temporarily replace the skull. The device value is 7, Autologous Tissue Substitute. No qualifier value is appropriate for this code.

Case Study Coding

1. ICD-10-PCS code: 3E0G8GC

Rationale: Achalasia is a disorder in which peristalsis in the esophagus is reduced. This can be treated by Botox injection, coded with the root operation Introduction. This section of ICD-10-PCS does not provide specific body part values and therefore G, Upper GI is coded for this injection into the esophagus.

The approach value is 8, Via Natural or Artificial Opening, Endoscopic. The substance value is G, Other Therapeutic Substance and the qualifier is C, Other Substance. See Coding Tip in this chapter on Botox.

3. ICD-10-PCS codes: 3E0R33Z and 3E0R3BZ

Rationale: The root operation Introduction is used to code this injection. This is an epidural injection of steroid, mixed with local anesthetic for pain control. This is coded to the substance value 3, Anti-inflammatory. The approach is percutaneous. The Marcaine and Fentanyl are regional anesthetics that ease the pain along the region of the epidural space being injected and are coded separately as substance value B, Anesthetic Agent.

5. ICD-10-PCS codes: 3E04305, 3E043GC

Rationale: The root operation Introduction is used to code the introduction of the chemotherapy and the introduction of the antiemetic (Ondansetron). All substances are introduced through a central vein. The chemotherapy has a substance value of 0, Antineoplastic and a qualifier value of 5, Other Antineoplastic. The antiemetic has a substance value of G, Other Therapeutic Substance and a qualifier value of C, Other Substance.

Chapter 22

Check Your Understanding

CODING KNOWLEDGE CHECK

1. Cardiac assistance using an implanted impeller pump

Rationale: This procedure is the root operation Assistance of the cardiac system. The qualifier value of D is an impeller pump.

3. c

Rationale: ECMO is coded to the root operation Performance because it takes over the entire function of circulatory function and provided oxygenation at the membrane level. Peripheral veno-venous ECMO is coded with the qualifier of H.

5. True

Rationale: Mechanical ventilation uses equipment. Mouth-to-mouth resuscitation is a nonmechanical method for performing ventilation.

PROCEDURE STATEMENT CODING

1. Root operation: Assistance   Code: 5A09357

Rationale: The root operation Assistance is used to code this procedure because the patient can breathe independently but needs assistance with breathing in enough oxygen. The body system value is 9, Respiratory. The duration value is 3, Less than 24 Consecutive Hours and the function is 5, Ventilation. The qualifier value is 7, Continuous Positive Airway Pressure.

3. Root operation: Performance   Code: 5A1D80Z

Rationale: The root operation Performance is used to code this procedure. Hemodialysis performs the function of filtration of urine from the body when the kidney can no longer filter and make urine. The duration value is 8 is for prolonged intermittent dialysis. There is no qualifier for this code.

5. Root operation: Transplantation   Code: 0BYM0Z0

Root operation: Perfusion   Code: 6ABB0BZ

Rationale: The root operation Transplantation is used to code the successful bilateral lung transplant. The body part value is M, Lungs Bilateral. The approach is Open, and the lungs are from an unrelated donor for a qualifier of 0, Allogeneic. The root operation of Perfusion is assigned because the lungs were perfused by extracorporeal means in preparation for the transplant, which was successful.

7. Root operation: Shockwave Therapy   Code: 6A930ZZ

Rationale: The root operation Shockwave Therapy is used to code this single session of therapy to the musculoskeletal system. Shockwave therapy is used to treat calcifications of the tendons.

9. Root operation: Performance   Code: 5A1955Z

Rationale: The root operation Performance is used to code the mechanical ventilation for greater than 96 hours. The function value is 5, Ventilation. There is no qualifier for this code.

Case Study Coding

1. ICD-10-PCS code: 5A02210

Rationale: The root operation Assistance is used to code the use of the IABP because it assists the cardiac output that is insufficient without the pump. The duration value is 2, Continuous, because the patient will continue on the balloon pump either permanently or until the heart has sufficiently healed to allow the removal. The insertion of the balloon pump is not coded as it is not considered a device in ICD-10-PCS.

3. ICD-10-PCS codes: 02100Z9, 021109W, 02110A9, 06BP4ZZ, 5A1221Z

Rationale: The root operation Bypass is used to code the bypass from two coronary arteries from the aorta using the autologous venous free graft from the right saphenous vein. The root operation Bypass is used to code the bypass from the left internal mammary artery which was anastomosed to one coronary artery. There is no device value for this code because the LIMA is not a free graft. The LIMA is the source of the bypass. Bypass is also coded for the T-graft made of autologous arterial tissue from the right internal mammary artery. In addition, the root operation Excision is used to the code harvesting of the saphenous vein for the graft, using a percutaneous endoscopic approach. The bypass procedure used an Open approach because CP bypass was used. The CP bypass is coded with root operation Performance. The cardioplegia, or the introduction of cold solution into the heart to protect it during the period of ischemia on CP bypass, is not coded separately because this is integral to the CP bypass procedure. The harvesting of the right internal mammary is not coded separately because it was performed through the same incision.

5. ICD-10-PCS codes: 021009W, 02100Z9, 06BP0ZZ, 5A1221Z

Rationale: The root operation Bypass is used to code the bypass from 1 coronary artery site from the aorta using the autologous venous free graft from the right saphenous vein (obtuse marginal from the aorta). The root operation Bypass is used to code the bypass from the left internal mammary artery, which was anastomosed to one coronary artery site (anterior descending). There is no device value for this code because the LIMA is not a free graft. The LIMA is the source of the bypass. In addition, the root operation Excision is used to the code harvesting of the saphenous vein for the graft, using an Open approach. The bypass procedure used an Open approach because CP bypass was used. The CP bypass is coded with the root operation Performance. The cardioplegia, or the introduction of cold solution into the heart to protect it during the period of ischemia on CP bypass is not coded separately because this is integral to the CP bypass procedure.

Chapter 23

Check Your Understanding

CODING KNOWLEDGE CHECK

1. Isolation

    Rationale: The qualifier value 6 in Section 8, Other Procedures means Isolation.

3. g

5. b

7. a

PROCEDURE STATEMENT CODING

1. Root operation: Chiropractic Manipulation   Code: 9WB1XHZ

    Root: Chiropractic Manipulation   Code: 9WB2XHZ

    Rationale: The root operation is Manipulation. The body region values are 1, Cervical and 2, Thoracic. The approach is always X, External. The method is H, Short Lever Specific Contact, and there is no qualifier.

3. Root operation: Chiropractic Manipulation   Code: 9WB2XKZ

    Rationale: The main index term is Chiropractic Manipulation. The body region value is 2, Thoracic, and the method value is K, Mechanically Assisted. The approach is always X, External. There is no qualifier for this code.

5. Root operation: Osteopathic Treatment   Code: 7W05X4Z

    Rationale: The root operation is Treatment, found in the index under Osteopathic Treatment. The body region value is 5, Pelvis. The approach is X, External. The method value is 4, Indirect, and there is no qualifier.

7. Method: Near Infrared Spectroscopy   Code: 8E023DZ

    Rationale: The main index term is Near Infrared Spectroscopy and the body region is 2, Circulatory System even though the location is the head. The vessels are being evaluated, not the head. The approach is Percutaneous and there is no qualifier.

9. Root operation: Excision   Code: 00B70ZZ

    Method: Computer assisted   Code: 8E09XBZ

    Rationale: The root operation Excision is used to code the excision of the lesion within the cerebral hemisphere. The approach is open (craniotomy) and there is no device value or qualifier appropriate for this code. An additional code is required for the computer-assisted procedure method. The main term in the index is Computer Assisted. The body region is 9, Head and Neck Region. The approach is X, External. There is no qualifier for this code.

11. Root operation: Excision   Code: 0GB10ZZ

    Root operation: Computer assisted procedure   Code: 8E09XBG

    Rationale: The root operation Excision is used to describe the partial removal of the pineal gland, also called the pineal body. The approach is Open, and there no device value or qualifier value appropriate for this code. An additional code is required for the computer assisted portion of the procedure. The main term in the index is Computer assisted procedure. The body region value is 9, Head and Neck Region. The approach is X, External. The method value is B, Computer Assisted Procedure, and the qualifier value is G, With Computerized Tomography.

Case Study Coding

1. ICD-10-PCS code: 8E0H30Z

Rationale: Acupuncture only has two codes in ICD-10-PCS. When the procedure is therapeutic and not for anesthesia, the only code provided in the index is 8E0H30Z.

3. ICD-10-PCS codes: 0SRC0J9, 8E0YXBZ

Rationale: The root operation Replacement is used to code these procedures. The right knee was replaced with a synthetic substitute, device value J. The approach is open and the qualifier value is 9, Cemented. The removal of the native joint is not coded separately. The computer-assisted navigation should be coded separately. The main index term is Computer assisted procedure, and the body region value is Y, Lower Extremity. The approach is X, External. The method value is B, Computer Assisted Procedure, and the qualifier value is Z, No Qualifier.

Chapter 24

Check Your Understanding

CODING KNOWLEDGE CHECK

1. Plain Radiography

Rationale: The ICD-10-PCS index directs the coder to use the root type Plain Radiography to code this procedure.

3. c

Rationale: Positron Emission Tomography is a root type in the Nuclear Medicine section of ICD-10-PCS.

5. True

Rationale: The Imaging section is organized in a manner similar to the Medical and Surgical section of ICD-10-PCS with the tables for one body system together and the tables for the root types in the same order under each body system.

Case Study Coding

1. ICD-10-PCS codes: 04793ZZ, B418ZZZ

Rationale: The angioplasty is coded with the root operation Dilation of the lower arteries and the body part 9, Renal Artery, Right. The approach is 3, Percutaneous and there is no device or qualifier value. The angiograms are coded with the root operation Fluoroscopy of the lower arteries and the body part value 8, Renal Arteries, Bilateral. The last 3 characters of the code are Z, None.

3. ICD-10-PCS codes: 4A023N7, B2111ZZ, B2151ZZ, 02703ZZ, 3E07317

Rationale: The root operation Measurement is used to code the left ventricular pressures. The coronary angiography in multiple locations is coded with the root operation Fluoroscopy using low osmolar contrast material. The left ventriculogram is coded with the root operation Fluoroscopy of the heart, also using low osmolar contrast material. The PTCA was performed, although unsuccessful, and coded with the root operation Dilation of a coronary artery. No device value or qualifier value is appropriate for this code. The thrombolytic therapy (heparin) is coded with the root operation Introduction into a coronary artery. The substance value is 1, Thrombolytic and the qualifier value is 7, Other Thrombolytic.

Chapter 25

Check Your Understanding

CODING KNOWLEDGE CHECK

1. B, Cochlear Implant Treatment

   Rationale: The definition of the cochlear implant treatment root type is "application of techniques to improve the communication abilities of individuals with cochlear implant."

3. c

5. g

7. b

9. Replacement.

   Rationale: This special valve deployment method meets the definition of Replacement.

PROCEDURE STATEMENT CODING

1. Root operation: Electroconvulsive Therapy   Code: GZB2ZZZ

   Rationale: The root type is electroconvulsive therapy. The index has a cross reference from electroshock therapy to electroconvulsive therapy. This is a bilateral-single seizure treatment and the index provides the entire 7-character code.

3. Root operation: Detoxification Services   Code: HZ2ZZZZ

   Rationale: The root type Detoxification Services is used to code this procedure. The index provides all 7 characters for this code.

5. Root operation: Reposition   Code: XNS4032

   Rationale: The growth rods reposition the thoracic spine. These magnetically controlled rods are in New Technology Group 2.

7. Root operation: Intellectual and Psychoeducational test   Code: GZ12ZZZ

   Rationale: WAIS testing is the Wechsler Adult Intelligence Scale test (from the examples of psychological tests in this chapter), an intellectual and psychoeducational test in the Mental Health Section. This service is root type 1 and this test is type qualifier 2. All mental health codes end in ZZZ.

9. Root operation: Motor Treatment   Code: F07Z8FZ

   Rationale: The root type is 7, Motor Treatment and the type qualifier is 8, Transfer Training. The equipment value is F, Assistive, Adaptive, Supportive, or Protective. The qualifier is Z, None.

Case Study Coding

1. ICD-10-PCS code: XRG10F3

   Rationale: This is a single joint cervical fusion using the new technology of interbody fusion device, radiolucent porous, device value F. The qualifier is 3, New Technology Group 3.

3. ICD-10-PCS codes: X2C0361, 027034Z, 4A023N7, B2151ZZ, B2111ZZ

Rationale: The use of the Diamondback 360 orbital atherectomy catheter to remove plaque from the calcified lesion is coded in the New Technology section with a root operation of Extirpation in the Cardiovascular body system. The left anterior descending coronary artery was then dilated, and a drug eluting stent was placed. This is coded in the Heart and Great Vessels body system. A left heart catheterization (Measurement), left ventriculography, and multiple coronary angiography (Imaging) were also performed.

5. ICD-10-PCS code: XNS4032

Rationale: The magnetically-controlled growing rods and coded in the New Technology section in the Bones body system. The scoliosis is documented as thoracogenic progressive scoliosis of thoracic spine. Therefore, the body part value is 4, Thoracic Vertebra. The rods are anchored in the lumbar spine but not repositioning the lumbar spine. The approach is Open because both ends of the rods must be attached using an open incision.

Exercises and Case Studies

Exercises

1. Root type: Stereotactic radiosurgery   Code: DG20JZZ

   Rationale: The root type Stereotactic Radiosurgery is used to code the destruction of the pituitary tumor using gamma beams. The body part value is 0, Pituitary Gland, and the modality qualifier is J, Stereotactic Gamma Beam Radiosurgery.

3. Root operation: Shock wave therapy   Code: 6A931ZZ

   Rationale: The root operation is Shock Wave Therapy in the Extracorporeal Therapies section of ICD-10-PCS. The body part value is 3, Musculoskeletal and the duration value is 1, Multiple.

5. Root operation: Insertion   Code: 0SH03BZ

   Rationale: The root operation Insertion is used to insert the Spinal Stabilization Device, Interspinous Process, device value B into a lumbar joint. The approach is 3, Percutaneous.

7. Root operation: Measurement   Code: 4A0B7BZ

   Rationale: Manometry is the measurement of pressure within an organ. For this test, a thin catheter is passed through the nose, into the esophagus, and into the stomach. The pressure is measured as the patient swallows. The root operation is Measurement and the body part value is B, Gastrointestinal. The approach is 7, Via Natural or Artificial Opening, and the function/device is B, Pressure. There is no qualifier.

9. Root operation: Insertion   Code: 0QHG08Z

   Root operation: Insertion   Code: 0QHJ08Z

   Rationale: The root operation Insertion is used to place the external fixation device for limb lengthening. The device value, 8, External Fixation Device, limb lengthening is assigned to both.

11. Root operation: Fusion Occipitocervical   Code: 0RG0071

    Root operation: Fusion C1–C4   Code: 0RG2071

    Rationale: The arthrodesis is coded with the root operation Fusion of the Occipitocervical joint (skull to C1) and three cervical joints (C1–C4). The approach is Open, and the device value used to create the fusion was an autograft, 7, Autologous Tissue Substitute. The qualifier value is 1, for posterior approach to the posterior column.

13. Root operation: Beam Radiation   Code: D7031ZZ

Rationale: The root operation Beam Radiation is used to code this procedure. The treatment site is 3, Lymphatics, Neck, and the modality qualifier is 1, Photons 1–10 MeV.

15. Root operation: Fusion   Code: 0SG107J

Root operation: Fusion   Code: 0SG1071

Root operation: Excision   Code: 0PB10ZZ

Rationale: The root operation Fusion is used to code the arthrodesis of two levels (L1–L2 and L2–L3). The device value is 7, Autologous Tissue Substitute. This is a posterior approach to the anterior spine, or qualifier value J. The posterior arthrodesis is performed at two levels using autologous tissue substitute. The autologous bone graft is coded with the root operation Excision and a body part value of 1, Rib, Right.

17. Root operation: Supplement   Code: 0VUS0JZ

Rationale: The root operation Supplement is used to code this procedure because the inflatable prosthesis augments the work of the corpora cavernosa and spongiosum in the erection process. The device value is J, Synthetic Substitute.

19. Root operation: Destruction   Code: 0F520ZZ

Rationale: The root operation of Destruction is used for ablation procedure by any method. The body part value is 2, Liver, Left Lobe. This is an Open approach. No device or qualifier is appropriate for the code.

21. Root operation: Supplement   Code: 0WU84JZ

Rationale: This procedure involves the insertion of a bar under the sternum to expand the chest wall. The bar supplements the chest wall and therefore, the root operation Supplement is coded. The bar is placed percutaneously with the aid of a scope and fixed at either end to the rib cage. The device value J, Synthetic Substitute, is assigned. No qualifier is appropriate for the code.

23. Root type: Psychological tests   Code: GZ10ZZZ

Rationale: The root type is psychological tests, value 1, within the Mental Health section of ICD-10-PCS. The Mullen Scales of Early Learning are a developmental test, type qualifier 0. The remaining values for the code are Z, None.

25. Root operation: Insertion of device into   Code: 0JH00NZ

Rationale: The root operation Insertion is used to place the tissue expander into the subcutaneous tissue of the scalp. The device value is N, Tissue Expander.

27. Root operation: Reposition, pulmonary trunk, open   Code: 02SP0ZZ

Root operation: Reposition, thoracic aorta, open   Code: 02SX0ZZ

Rationale: The Jatene procedure is an arterial switch or the total correction of transposition of great vessels. The arterial switch procedure requires cardiopulmonary bypass and aortic cross clamping. Following aortic cross clamping, the ascending aorta and main pulmonary artery are transected. The left and right coronary artery ostia are visualized and excised from the aortic root with adjacent aortic wall as 'buttons.' The coronary artery buttons are then shifted posteriorly and implanted into the facing sinuses of the main pulmonary artery root. Next, the distal pulmonary artery and its branches are brought forward (LeCompte maneuver), and the distal aorta is moved posteriorly. The distal aorta is now anastomosed to the "new" aortic root. Reconstruction of the pulmonary artery is undertaken next, utilizing a patch of cryopreserved pulmonary artery homograft. Closure of the atrial septal defect completes the arterial switch repair. Transesophageal echocardiography is utilized to help assess adequacy of repair. Delayed sternal closure is sometimes required following surgery (Children's Hospital of Wisconsin 2018). The root operation for this procedure is Reposition. Two codes are required, one for the pulmonary trunk, and one for the thoracic aorta, ascending/arch. Both procedures are performed using an Open approach.

29. Root operation: Removal   Code: 0UPD7HZ

    Rationale: The root operation Removal is used to code removal of the IUD. The body part value is D, Uterus and Cervix and the approach is 7, Via Natural or Artificial Opening. The device value is H, Contraceptive Device.

31. Root operation: Fusion   Code: 0RG6071

    Root operation: Removal   Code: 0RP604Z

    Root operation: Excision   Code: 0QB30ZZ

    Rationale: The main procedure is Fusion. The fusion is accomplished with an autograft into the vertebral joint. In addition, removal of the old hardware is coded with Removal. The autograft harvest is coded with the root operation of Excision. The body part value is 3, Pelvic Bone, Left and this is obtained through an Open approach.

33. Root operation: Destruction   Code: 005K3ZZ

    Rationale: The root operation Destruction is used to code the injection to destroy the trigeminal nerve. The trigeminal nerve is part of the central nervous system and cranial nerves in ICD-10-PCS and is body part value K. The approach is 3, Percutaneous because this was an injection. The use of the Phenol is identified in the root operation Destruction and is not captured in any other way in the code.

35. Root operation: Decompression   Code: 6A150ZZ

    Rationale: HBO is hyperbaric oxygenation. In this case, the HBO is used to treat the carbon monoxide poisoning in the whole body. Therefore, the root operation Decompression is coded. This is a single treatment for the 5th character of 0.

Case Studies

1. ICD-10-PCS codes: 00HU0MZ, 0JH70BZ, BR17ZZZ

    Rationale: One code is assigned for the neurostimulator lead and another for the stimulator generator. The root operation Insertion is coded for both procedures and they both use the Open approach. The device value for the lead is M. The device value for the neurostimulator generator is B, Stimulator Generator, Single Array because a single paddle electrode including 16 leads is inserted. Neither code has a qualifier value. The fluoroscopy guidance is coded using the root type Fluoroscopy of the body part value 7, Thoracic Spine.

3. ICD-10-PCS codes: 041K09N, 06BP0ZZ

    Rationale: The root operation bypass is used to code this procedure. The body part value is K, Femoral Artery, Right. The approach is Open. The device value is 9, Autologous Venous Tissue because the greater saphenous vein was harvested. The qualifier value is N, Posterior Tibial Artery because that is the artery to which the bypass was created. The root operation Excision is used to code the harvesting of the right greater saphenous vein graft. The body part value is P, Saphenous Vein, Right. The approach was Open, and there were no device or qualifier values.

5. ICD-10-PCS code: 04CP0ZZ

    ICD-10-PCS code: 04CR0ZZ

    ICD-10-PCS code: 04UM07Z

    ICD-10-PCS code: 06BQ4ZZ

Rationale: Based on Guideline B4.1c, the embolectomy from the right anterior tibial and right posterior tibial arteries are coded because they are both the furthest anatomical sites from the point of entry, which was the right popliteal artery. Both of the tibial arteries branch independently off of the popliteal artery. The root operation for the embolectomy is Extirpation. The right popliteal artery was patched with an autologous vein patch. The root operation is Supplement. The harvesting of the left saphenous vein is coded with a percutaneous endoscopic approach because it was described as being harvested endoscopically.

7. 0WWG43Z

The peritoneal dialysis catheter is an infusion device that infuses dialysate and retrieves waste products. Coding Clinic, 2nd Quarter 2015 identifies the device value for the catheter as an infusion device. Repositioning of an improperly placed device is coded to the root operation of Revision. The percutaneous endoscopic approach was used.

9. ICD-10-PCS code: 0YU50JZ

Rationale: The root operation Supplement is used to code this procedure because the inguinal hernia repair is completed with the use of Marlex mesh to supplement the inguinal region. The body part value 5, Inguinal Region, Right is assigned. The approach is Open, and the device value is J, Synthetic Substitute. There is no qualifier.

11. ICD-10-PCS codes: 00800ZZ, 8E09XBZ

Rationale: The root operation to disconnect the two halves of the brain at the corpus callosum is Division. The body part key directs the coder to assign the body part as 0, Brain for the corpus callosum. The neuronavigation is coded as a computer assisted procedure. There is no information documented to allow assignment of a qualifier.

13. ICD-10-PCS code: 0D738ZZ

Rationale: The root operation Dilation is used to code the balloon dilation of the lower esophagus, body part value 3, Esophagus, Lower. The approach is 8, Via Natural or Artificial Opening, Endoscopic. There is no device or qualifier value. The upper endoscopy is not coded separately because this was the approach. In addition, the upper endoscopy would be the root operation Inspection, which is not coded if a more definitive procedure is performed at the same time.

15. ICD-10-PCS code: 0B113F4

Rationale: The root operation Bypass is used to code the creation of the new passage between the trachea and the skin using a cricothyroidotomy or cutting into the thyroid cartilage. The body part value is 1, Trachea. The device value is F, Tracheostomy Device, and the qualifier is the location to which the trachea was bypassed, or value 4, Cutaneous.

17. ICD-10-PCS codes: 02U53JZ, 4A023N8

Rationale: The root operation Supplement is used to code the deployment of the Amplatzer device across the atrial septal opening. The approach is 3, Percutaneous. The device value is J, Synthetic Substitute, based on guidance from the Device Key. There is no qualifier. The bilateral heart catheterization procedure is coded as Measurement of the cardiac function with sampling and pressures with a qualifier of 8, Bilateral because pressures were documented from both sides of the heart.

19. ICD-10-PCS codes: 0BBC8ZX, 0BB48ZX, 0BC48ZZ

Rationale: The root operation Excision is used to code the transbronchial biopsy (of the lung). The approach is 8, Via Natural or Artificial Opening, Endoscopic. The qualifier is X, Diagnostic because it is a biopsy. The body part value is C, Upper Lung Lobe, Right. The qualifier is X, Diagnostic because it is a biopsy. The root operation Excision is used to code the endobronchial biopsy of body part value 4, Upper Lobe Bronchus, Right. The approach is 8, Via Natural or Artificial Opening, Endoscopic. The qualifier is X, Diagnostic because it is a biopsy. The root operation Extirpation is used to code the removal of the mucus plug from body part value 4, Upper Lobe Bronchus, Right.

21. ICD-10-PCS code: 8E0H30Z

Rationale: The root operation Other Procedures and a method of Acupuncture are used to code this procedure. The body region is H, Integumentary System and Breast. The approach is 3, Percutaneous. The method is 0, Acupuncture, and there is no qualifier.

23. ICD-10-PCS codes: 02583ZZ, 02K83ZZ, 02703DZ, B2111ZZ

Rationale: Both the ablation and the cardiac map procedures are coded, and both are performed on the conduction mechanism of the heart. The coronary artery dilation and stenting is coded as dilation of one coronary artery with an intraluminal device. The multiple coronary artery angiograms are coded as imaging of multiple coronary arteries using low osmolar contrast material.

25. ICD-10-PCS codes: 00BY0ZZ, 00BT0ZZ, 0RHA04Z, 00JU3ZZ

Rationale: The tumor in this case is described as an intradural mix, intramedullary and extramedullary mass. Both lumbar spinal cord (intramedullary) and spinal meninges (extramedullary) body parts must be assigned. Pedicle screws and rods were used an internal fixation device across the thoracolumbar joint and a lumbar puncture procedure was attempted but was incomplete.

27. ICD-10-PCS codes: 02100Z9, 021009W, 02QL0ZZ, 02UN08Z, 06BQ4ZZ, 5A1221Z

Rationale: The root operation of Bypass is used to code both of the coronary artery grafts. The left internal mammary pedicle graft is not a device, and the left internal mammary is the source of the blood. The saphenous vein is an autologous venous graft with the source of the blood being the aorta. The left ventricular blood supply is improved with transmyocardial revascularization coded as the root operation Repair. The root operation Supplement is assigned for the reconstruction of the pericardium using CorMatrix, a zooplastic product. The root operation of Excision is assigned for the endoscopic harvesting of the left saphenous vein graft. The procedure is performed with the use of the cardiopulmonary bypass machine and code 5A1221Z is assigned for this Performance procedure.

29. ICD-10-PCS codes: 0C5QXZZ, 0C5S7ZZ

Rationale: The root operation Destruction is used to code both the destruction of the adenoids (body part value Q) and lingual tonsil (body part value S, Pharynx based on the body part key). The approach for the adenoidectomy is X, External. The approach for the lingual tonsil is 7, Via Natural or Artificial Opening. No device or qualifier values are appropriate.

31. ICD-10-PCS codes: 0JH608Z, 02H63KZ, 02HK3KZ, B2141ZZ

Rationale: The index directs the coder to use device value 8, Defibrillator Generator for the Implantable Pacing Cardioverter-Defibrillator when inserting it into the Subcutaneous pocket in the chest. The approach is open. The root operation Insertion is used to code the two leads (dual chamber device). The body part values are 6, Atrium, Right and K, Ventricle, Right. The approach is 3, Percutaneous, because they are placed there without visualization of the operative site. The device value is K, Cardiac Lead, Defibrillator. The root operation Fluoroscopy is used to code the fluoroscopic guidance. The body part value is 4, Heart, Right. The contrast value is 1, Low Osmolar. Note: Consult facility policy to determine if a code for intra-operative imaging should be assigned.

33. ICD-10-PCS codes: 03180Z1, 0JH63XZ, 02HV33Z

Rationale: The hemodialysis access is an AV fistula made from the left brachial artery and left cephalic vein above the antecubital fossa (elbow area) in the upper arm. No device is used to make a fistula. A Perm-A-Cath is a tunneled vascular access device, coded with the infusion device in the superior vena cava and the tunnel in the subcutaneous tissue and fascia of the chest.

35. ICD-10-PCS codes: 021209W, 02100Z9, 06BQ0ZZ, 5A1221Z

Rationale: The root operation Bypass is used to code the grafting of the greater saphenous vein to three coronary arteries (body part value 2) and to the aorta (qualifier value W). The root operation Bypass is used to code the bypass to one coronary artery (body part value 0) from the left internal mammary artery (qualifier value 9). There is no device value because the left internal mammary artery remains connected to create the bypass. The root operation Excision is used to code the harvesting of the greater saphenous vein from the left leg via incision. Cardiopulmonary bypass is coded using the root operation Performance.

37. ICD-10-PCS codes: 02Q50ZZ, 02Q90ZZ, 02UG0JZ, 5A1221Z

Rationale: The root operation Repair is used to code the closure of the atrial septal defect using a suture. The root operation Repair is used to code the repair of the chordea tendineae. The root operation Supplement is used to code the reinforcement of the mitral valve with an annuloplasty ring. The device value is J, Synthetic Substitute. Cardiopulmonary bypass is coded using the root operation Performance.

39. ICD-10-PCS code: 0W3R8ZZ

Rationale: The root operation Control is used to fulgurate the bleeders from the previous procedure. The body system is Anatomical Regions, General, and the body part value is R, Genitourinary System because the root operation Control is assigned to large body areas rather than individual body parts. The approach is 8, Via Natural or Artificial Opening, Endoscopic. There is no device value or qualifier value. The removal of the clots is included in the Control procedure and is not coded separately.

41. ICD-10-PCS codes: 0TC40ZZ, 0T770DZ

Rationale: The root operation Extirpation is used to code the removal of the calculus through an open incision. The body part value is 4, Kidney Pelvic, Left. No device or qualifiers values are appropriate. The root operation Dilation is used to code the placement of the stent into the left ureter. The body part value is 7, Ureter, Left. The approach is Open and the device value is D, Intraluminal Device. There is no qualifier.

43. ICD-10-PCS codes: 0TSD0ZZ, 0VNS0ZZ, 0VTTXZZ

Rationale: The root operation Reposition is used to code the relocation of the urethral meatus to the central position in the glans penis. The body part value is D, Urethra. The approach is Open. The root operation Release is used to code the degloving of the penis to release it from the penopubic fat. The body part value being released is S, Penis. The root operation Resection is used to code the complete removal of the pre-puce, body part value T. The approach for the circumcision is X, External.

45. ICD-10-PCS codes: 0UT90ZZ, 0UT70ZZ, 0UT20ZZ

Rationale: Three individual body part values are removed during this procedure (uterus 9, bilateral fallopian tubes 7, and bilateral ovaries 2). The root operation Resection is used to code the complete removal of all these organs. The approach is Open and there are no device or qualifier values.

47. ICD-10-PCS codes: 08BP0ZZ, 08BN0ZZ

Rationale: A medical indication is given for the procedure (interfering with vision), indicating that this is not the root operation Alteration. The root operation Excision is used to code the removal of a piece of levator muscle from each eyelid. The index directs the coder to code the eyelid body part for the levator palpebrae superioris muscle. The body part values are P, Upper Eyelid, Left and N, Upper Eyelid, Right. The approach is Open and no device or qualifier values are appropriate.

49. ICD-10-PCS codes: 0SBD4ZZ, 0MRP07Z

Rationale: The root operation Excision is used to code the meniscectomy of the knee joint (knee cartilage is a knee structure). The approach is 4, Percutaneous Endoscopic. The root operation Replacement is used to code the autologous graft to the anterior cruciate ligament of the knee. The body part value is P, Knee Bursae and Ligament, Left, and the device value is 7, Autologous Tissue Substitute.

References

American Association of Colleges of Osteopathic Medicine (AACOM). 2015a. A Brief Guide to Osteopathic Medicine, for Students, by Students. https://www.aacom.org/news-and-events/publications/a-brief-guide-to-osteopathic -medicine-for-students-by-students.

American Association of Colleges of Osteopathic Medicine (AACOM). 2015b. Introduction to Osteopathic Medicine for Non-DO Faculty: What Makes an Osteopathic Education Different? https://vimeo.com/107184676.

American Chiropractic Association (ACA). 2017. Facts About Chiropractic. Accessed September 14, 2017. https://www .acatoday.org/News-Publications/Newsroom/Facts-About-Chiropractic

American College of Obstetricians and Gynecologists (ACOG). 2015. Practice Bulletin 154: Operative Vaginal Delivery. *Obstetrics and Gynecology* 126(5): 1120–1122.

American Hospital Association (AHA). 2017. Qualifiers for the Root Operation Detachment. *Coding Clinic for ICD-10-CM/PCS*, 2nd Quarter: 3.

American Hospital Association (AHA). 2014. Medical Ventilation. *Coding Clinic for ICD-10-CM and ICD-10-PCS*, 3rd Quarter: 3.

American Hospital Association (AHA). 2012. Ask the Editor—ICD-10-CM/PCS. *Coding Clinic for ICD-9-CM*, 4th Quarter: 104–106.

American Hospital Association (AHA). 2008. Super Saturated Oxygen Therapy. *Coding Clinic for ICD-9-CM*, 4th Quarter: 162.

American Medical Association (AMA). 2018. *CPT 2019: Professional Edition.* Chicago: AMA.

American Rhinologic Society (ARS). 2015. Sinus Anatomy. Accessed July 6, 2018. http://care.american-rhinologic.org /sinus_anatomy.

Applegate, E. J. 2011. *The Anatomy and Physiology Learning System*, 4th ed. St. Louis: Saunders Elsevier.

Aurora Health Care. 2017. Hyperbaric Oxygen Therapy. https://www.aurorahealthcare.org/services/wound-care -hyperbaric-medicine/hyperbaric-oxygen-therapy.

Centers for Medicare and Medicaid Services (CMS). 2019. 2019 ICD-10-PCS. https://www.cms.gov/Medicare/Coding /ICD10/2019-ICD-10-PCS.html.

Centers for Medicare and Medicaid Services (CMS). 2016a. ICD-10 Coordination and Maintenance Committee Meetings. https://www.cms.gov/Medicare/Coding/ICD10/ICD-10-Coordination-and-Maintenance-Committee-Meetings.html.

Centers for Medicare and Medicaid Services (CMS). 2016b. ICD-10-PCS Reference Manual. https://www.cms.gov /Medicare/Coding/ICD10/Downloads/2016-Reference-Manual.zip.

Cespedes R. D., J. C. Winters, and K. H. Ferguson. 2001. Colpocleisis for the treatment of vaginal vault prolapse. Techniques in Urology 7(2):152–60.

Children's Hospital of Wisconsin. 2018. Arterial Switch Procedure for D-transposition of the great arteries. https://www .chw.org/medical-care/herma-heart/for-medical-professionals/pediatric-heart-surgery/arterial-switch-procedure.

Cincinnati Children's Hospital Medical Center. 2018 (February). Craniosynostosis. http://www.cincinnatichildrens.org /health/c/craniosynostosis/.

DeNoon, D. J. 2005. Coblation emerges as tonsillectomy option. WebMD. http://www.webmd.com/children /news/20050923/coblation-emerges-as-tonsillectomy-option.

DiGiovanna, E. L., S. Schiowitz, and D. J. Dowling. 2005. *An Osteopathic Approach to Diagnosis and Treatment,* 3rd ed. Philadelphia: Lippincott, Williams and Wilkins.

Dorland's Illustrated Medical Dictionary, 32nd ed. 2012. Philadelphia: Elsevier Saunders.

Food and Drug Administration (FDA). 2018. Computer-Assisted Surgical Systems. http://www.fda.gov/MedicalDevices /ProductsandMedicalProcedures/SurgeryandLifeSupport/ComputerAssistedSurgicalSystems/default.htm.

Harvey, C. 2018. Cannulation for Neonatal and Pediatric Extracorporeal Membrane Oxygenation for Cardiac Support. *Frontiers in Pediatrics* (6)17. https://www.frontiersin.org/articles/10.3389/fped.2018.00017/full.

Intuitive Surgical, Inc. 2015. The da Vinci Surgical System. http://www.davincisurgery.com/davinci-surgery/davinci -surgical-system/.

Johns Hopkins Medicine. 2018. Intra-aortic balloon pump therapy. https://www.hopkinsmedicine.org/healthlibrary/test_ procedures/cardiovascular/intra-aortic_balloon_pump_therapy_135,341.

Kuehn, L. 2018. *Procedural Coding and Reimbursement for Physician Services.* Chicago: AHIMA.

Kuehn, L. 2015. Single versus multiple array stimulators—Mystery solved! Libman Education. September 4. https://www .libmaneducation.com/single-versus-multiple-array-stimulators-mystery-solved/.

Kuehn, L. 2011. *Psychiatry Services Reported by Physicians.* Distance Education Coding Assessment and Training Solution Course. Chicago: AHIMA.

Linton, D. M. 2005. Special Review—Cuirass Ventilation: A Review and Update. *Critical Care and Resuscitation* 2005(7): 22–28.

Lo, W. M., D. L. Daniels, D. W. Chakeres, F. H. Linthicum, J. L. Ulmer, L. P. Mark, and J. D. Swartz. 1997 (May). Anatomic Moment: The Endolymphatic Duct and Sac. *American Journal of Neuroradiology* 18: 881–887. http://www.ajnr.org /cgi/reprint/18/5/881.pdf.

Massachusetts General Hospital (MGH). 2017. Optical Coherence Tomography (OCT) Registry. Accessed September 14, 2017. http://www.massgeneral.org/heartcenter/research/researchlab.aspx?id=1403.

Mayfield Clinic. 2018. SPECT (single photon emission computed tomography) scan. http://www.mayfieldclinic.com /PE-SPECT.htm.

Mayo Clinic. 2018a. Pyloromyotomy. https://www.mayoclinic.org/diseases-conditions/pyloric-stenosis/multimedia /pyloromyotomy/img-20006399.

Mayo Clinic. 2018b. Right hemicolectomy. https://www.mayoclinic.org/tests-procedures/colectomy/multimedia/right -hemicolectomy/img-20007591.

Mayo Clinic. 2018c. Left hemicolectomy. https://www.mayoclinic.org/tests-procedures/colectomy/multimedia/left -hemicolectomy/img-20007592.

Mayo Clinic. 2015a. Diseases and Conditions: Ectopic Pregnancy. http://www.mayoclinic.org/diseases-conditions/ectopic -pregnancy/basics/definition/CON-20024262.

Mayo Clinic. 2015b. Tests and Procedures: Dilation and Curettage. http://www.mayoclinic.org/tests-procedures/dilation -and-curettage/basics/how-you-prepare/prc-20013836.

McKinley, M. P., V. O'Loughlin, E. E. Pennefather-O'Brien, and R. T. Harris. 2017. *Human Anatomy,* 5th ed. New York: McGraw-Hill.

Medscape. 2018. Decortication Technique. https://emedicine.medscape.com/article/1970123-technique#c2.

Medicine Net. 2016. Laparoscopically Assisted Vaginal Hysterectomy (LAVH). http://www.medicinenet.com /laparoscopically_assisted_vaginal_hysterectomy/article.htm.

Meeker, W. C., and S. Haldeman. 2002. Chiropractic: a profession at the crossroads of mainstream and alternative medicine. *Annals of Internal Medicine* 136(3): 216–227.

Mobile Health News. 2010. CardioMEMS. http://mobihealthnews.com/8793/st-jude-may-acquire-cardiomems-for-375m/.

Mosby's Medical Dictionary, 10th ed. 2017. St Louis: Elsevier.

National Heart, Lung, and Blood Institute (NHLBI). 2011. CPAP. https://www.nhlbi.nih.gov/health-topics/cpap.

National Institute for Physiological Sciences (NIPS). 2010. Hemodynamic responses to the mother's face in infants by near-infrared spectroscopy. http://www.nips.ac.jp/eng/release/2010/12/post_142.html.

National Institutes of Health (NIH). 2017. National Center for Complementary and Alternative Medicine. https://nccih.nih .gov/health/acupuncture/.

National Institutes of Health (NIH). 2011. External Beam Radiation Therapy. http://www.cancer.gov/cancertopics/coping /radiation-therapy-and-you/page3.

National Library of Medicine (NLM). Medline Plus. 2016a. Inflatable artificial sphincter. http://www.nlm.nih.gov /medlineplus/ency/article/003983.htm.

National Library of Medicine (NLM). Medline Plus. 2016b. Cold Knife Cone Biopsy. http://www.nlm.nih.gov/medlineplus/ency/article/003910.htm.

National Library of Medicine (NLM). 2012. Percutaneous transluminal coronary angioplasty (PTCA). https://medlineplus.gov/ency/anatomyvideos/000096.htm.

National Library of Medicine (NLM). Medline Plus. 2011a. Salivary Gland Infections. http://www.nlm.nih.gov/medlineplus/ency/article/001041.htm.

National Library of Medicine (NLM). Medline Plus. 2011b. Bone Marrow Diseases. http://www.nlm.nih.gov/medlineplus/bonemarrowdiseases.html.

Ostrovsky, G. 2010. MedGadget. Under Development: Cavopulmonary Impeller Pump for Fontan Circulation. https://www.medgadget.com/2010/11/under_development_cavopulmonary_impeller_pump_for_fontan_circulation.html.

Pais, V. M., Jr. 2016. Spermatocele Treatment and Management. http://emedicine.medscape.com/article/443432-treatment#a1128.

Purdie, B., A. Harris, and J. J. Beitler. 2009. *Radiation Oncology Concepts.* Victoria: Trafford Publishing.

Rizzo, D. C. 2016. *Fundamentals of Anatomy and Physiology*, 4th Edition. Clifton Park, NY: Delmar, Cengage Learning.

Stedman's Online. 2014. Tooth Numbering Systems. http://www.stedmansonline.com/webFiles/Dict-Dental2/14_med_dent_tooth_numbering.pdf.

The American National Red Cross. 2011. Administering Emergency Oxygen: Airway Adjuncts. https://www.redcross.org/content/dam/redcross/atg/PDF_s/AirwayAdjunctsFactandSkill.pdf.

Ziessman, H. A., and P. Rehm. 2011. *Nuclear Medicine Case Review Series,* 2nd ed. Philadelphia: Elsevier Mosby.

Index

A

abdominal aortic aneurysms, 223
abdominal esophagus, 254
ablation, 81, 107, 163, 223, 383
abortifacient, 400
Abortion root operation
    overview, 400–401
    defined, 400
    devices used with, 384, 400–401
    followed by other procedures, 52, 107, 384, 400–401
abscess, incision and drainage of, 83
accessory pancreatic duct, 252
accessory sinuses, 181, 184
Activities of Daily Living Assessment root type, 482
Activities of Daily Living Treatment root type, 482
Acupuncture method, 450
adenoidectomy, 201
adenoids, 195, 196, 201
adjustable gastric banding, 105–106, 252
Administration section
    overview, 418–422
    approaches used in, 419
    body systems and regions for, 421
    bone marrow and cell transfusion, 42, 96, 272
    case studies, 428–430
    character definition for, 418
    code building cases, 426–427
    description, 5
    qualifiers used in, 422
    root operations used in, 419
    section value for, 423
    substance values for, 419–421
adrenal glands, 267–268, 353–354
airway devices
    for Gastrointestinal system, 256
    for Mouth and Throat, 203
    qualifier values for, 434
    for Respiratory system, 203
    for Sense Organs, 185
Allogenic qualifier, 91, 368, 400–401
Alteration device, 289
Alteration root operation, 132, 142, 182, 287, 289
American Congress of Obstetricians and Gynecologists (ACOG), 404
American Health Information Management Association (AHIMA), 35

American Hospital Association (AHA), 35
amniocentesis, 51, 403
amphiarthroses, 324
ampulla of Vater, 252
amputations. *See* Detachment root operation
anal sphincter, 250–251
anastomosis, 40, 252–253, 329
Anatomical Orifices body system, 417
anatomical regions, 139–157. *See also* general anatomical regions; lower extremities; upper extremities
    Administration section and, 419
    approaches for, 147
    body part values for, 141, 145–147
    body system values for, 139
    case studies, 154–157
    code building cases, 150–151
    code building exercises, 151–152
    Control root operation, 143
    description, 139
    devices common to, 148
    Division root operation, 144
    organization of, 139–143
    Osteopathic section and, 447
    qualifiers used in, 148–149
    root operations used in, 143–144
Ancillary sections. *See* Imaging section; Mental Health section; New Technology section; Nuclear Medicine section; Physical Rehabilitation and Diagnostic Audiology section; Radiation Therapy section; Substance Abuse Treatment section
"and," defined, 38
anesthetic destructive agents, 419
aneurysms, 45, 106, 222–223
angioplasty
    coronary, 48, 224–225
    non-coronary, 228
animal tissue, 96, 111, 222
ankle, 48, 290, 321, 324, 327
annuloplasty ring, 120
anterior chamber of eye, 179–180
anterior colporrhaphy, 383
anterior column (spinal) fusion, 336–337
anterior cruciate ligament (ACL) procedures, 48, 99, 127
anterior lumbar interbody fusion (ALIF), 336
anus, 249–250

aortic body, 267
aortic lymph nodes, 273
aortic valve replacement procedure, 41
aortocoronary bypasses, 42–43, 112, 227
aorto-femoral bypass, 227
appendectomy, 49, 75
appendix, 249–250
approach (character 5)
    overview of guidelines, 49–50
    for Administration procedures, 419
    for anatomical regions procedures, 147
    with changes during procedure, 41
    for Chiropractic section, 453
    for Circulatory system, 232
    CMS file definitions, 22
    code format, 11–14
    decision tree for, 50, 61–62
    definition of, 11
    for Endocrine system, 269
    for Female Reproductive system, 385
    for Gastrointestinal system, 256
    for Hepatobiliary system, 256
    for Lymphatic system, 273
    for Male Reproductive system, 370
    for Measurement and Monitoring root operation, 424
    for Mouth and Throat, 202
    for Nervous system, 166
    for New Technology section, 490
    for Obstetrics section, 403
    through orifices, 12–14, 564. *See also* Via Natural or
        Artificial Opening; Via Natural or Artificial Opening
        Endoscopic; Via Natural or Artificial Opening with
        Percutaneous Endoscopic Assistance
    for Osteopathic section, 448
    for Other Procedures section, 450
    for Placement section, 417
    for Removal root operation, 116
    for Respiratory system, 202
    for Skeletal system, 333–334
    for Sense Organs, 185
    through or on skin or mucous membranes, 11–12. *See also*
        External approach; Open approach; Percutaneous
        approach; Percutaneous Endoscopic approach
    for Urinary System, 357
arteries. *See* coronary arteries; Lower Arteries; Upper Arteries
arteriococcygeal gland (body), 267
artery graft. *See* Autologous Arterial Tissue
arthroplasty, 329
arthroscopy, 48
arthrotomy, 83, 125, 333
articulations. *See* joints
artificial opening approaches. *See* Via Natural or Artificial
        Opening; Via Natural or Artificial Opening Endoscopic;
        Via Natural or Artificial Opening with Percutaneous
        Endoscopic Assistance
artificial respiration, 435
artificial rupture of membrane procedures, 401
ascending colon, 249–250, 254
Assistance root operation, 431–432, 439
atlas, 324
Atmospheric Control root operation, 437

atrial appendage, 106
atrial fibrillation, 106
atrioventricular (AV) canal, 222
auditory canal, 181
auditory ossicle, 181
autografts
    for aortocoronary bypasses, 111
    harvesting guidelines, 43, 74, 112, 132
    for spinal fusion, 338
Autologous Arterial Tissue, 111
Autologous Tissue Substitute, 44, 119, 287–289, 371
Autologous Venous Tissue, 111
autonomic nervous system, 161
AV fistulas and grafts, 229
axiaLIF (axial lumbar interbody fusion), 336
Axial Skeleton body system value, 464
axillo-femoral bypass, 228
axis, 324

B
balanced tension technique, 449
bariatric procedures, 105, 252
Bartholin's glands, 381, 384
Beam Radiation root type, 470
behavioral type qualifier, 486
bilateral body parts. *See* laterality guidelines
bile ducts, 252
bioactive coil, 223
bioactive intraluminal device, 223
Biofeedback root type, 484
biopsy procedures
    bone marrow, 42, 73, 83, 272
    breast, 42, 289
    bronchial, 200
    cervical, 383
    followed by more definitive procedure, 42, 74, 200, 289
    qualifiers for, 42, 73–74
    root operations for, 42, 73, 83, 272, 289
Biphasic Cuirass Ventilation (BCV), 434
bladder
    body part value for, 356
    organization of, 353–354
    procedures, 45, 355, 356–357, 383, 392
bleeding, control of, 43, 66, 127–128, 143–144, 147
blepharoplasty, 132
blood and blood products
    blood cell type qualifier, 439
    Pheresis root operation for, 437, 439
    as substances, 19, 419
    Transfusion root operation for, 419
blood clots, 83, 106
body cavities. *See* general anatomical regions
body part (character 4)
    overview of guidelines, 46–48
    for anatomical regions, 141, 145–147
    bilateralism guidelines, 47, 331, 356
    for bone marrow, 272
    branching of, 47
    for Bypass root operation. *See* Bypass root operation
    for Circulatory system, 42–43, 47–48, 109–110, 229–232
    CMS file definitions, 27

code format, 10
for Control root operation, 128
definition of, 10
demarcation of upper and lower body parts, 39–40,
for Destruction root operation, 83
for ear, 183
for Ear, Nose and Sinus, 183–184
for Endocrine system, 268–269
for Eye, 183
for Female Reproductive system, 384–385
for Gastrointestinal system, 254–255
for gender reassignment, 133
harvesting of, 289
for Hepatobiliary system and pancreas, 254–255
for Imaging section, 465
for Inspection root operation, 45
key for, 10, 23, 47
for lower extremities, 143, 145–147
for Lymphatic system, 272–273
for Male Reproductive system, 369–370
for Mouth and Throat, 201–202
for multiple procedures, 41, 57
for musculoskeletal system, 44, 48, 125, 290, 308–309
for Nervous system, 164–165
for Nuclear Medicine section, 468
for Obstetrics section, 403
for overlapping layers, 42, 74, 73, 93, 121, 290, 308
"peri" prefix for procedure site, guidelines for, 46
for Respiratory system, 75, 201–202
for Sense Organs, 183–184
separating, 43–44, 90
subdivision guidelines, 43, 75
supernumerary digits values, 144
for Transfer root operation, 46
tubular body parts, 45, 105–113, 141
undesignated, 46, 164
for upper extremities, 141, 143
for Urinary system, 356–357
body region (character 4)
    for Chiropractic section, 452
    for Osteopathic section, 448
    for Other Procedures section, 450
    for Placement section, 416–417
body system and region (character 4)
    for Administration section, 419
    for Measurement and Monitoring section, 423–424
    for New Technology section, 489
    for Physical Rehabilitation and Diagnostic Audiology section, 482–483
body system (character 2). See also specific body systems
    overview of guidelines, 39–40
    for Administration section, 419
    for arteries, 213
    body part code format and, 10
    for bones, 321
    for Bursae and Ligaments, 303
    for Central Nervous system and Cranial Nerves, 159
    for Circulatory system, 213
    code format, 5–6
    for Control root operation, 128
    definition of, 5

demarcation of upper and lower body parts, 39
for Detachment root operation, 77
for Ear, Nose, and Sinus, 179
for Endocrine System, 267
for Extracorporeal or Systemic Assistance and
    Performance section, 431–432
for Extracorporeal or Systemic Therapies section, 438
for Eye, 179
for Female Reproductive system, 381
for Gastrointestinal system, 48, 249
general anatomical regions, 139
for Head and Facial Bones, 321
for Heart and Great Vessels, 213
for Hepatobiliary System and Pancreas, 249
for Integumentary system, 285
for joints, 48, 321
for Lower Arteries, 213
for lower extremities, 139
for Lower Veins, 216
for Lymphatic and Hemic system, 267
for Male Reproductive system, 367
for Map root operation, 224
for Measurement and Monitoring section, 423–424
for Mental Health section, 484
for Mouth and Throat, 195
for Muscles, 303
for Nervous system, 159
for Nuclear Medicine section, 467
for Obstetrics, 399
for Peripheral Nervous system, 159
for Physical Rehabilitation and Diagnostic Audiology
    section, 482–483
for Placement section, 415
for Radiation Therapy section, 469
for Respiratory system, 195
for Sense Organs, 179
for Skeletal system, 321
for Skin and Breast, 285
for Subcutaneous Tissue and Fascia, 285
for Substance Abuse Treatment section, 487
for Tendons, 303
for Transfer root operation, 97
for Upper Arteries, 213
for upper extremities, 139
for Upper Veins, 213
for Urinary system, 353
for veins, 213
bone-anchored hearing aid (BAHA), 185
bone cement, 328
bone conduction device, 185
bone grafts, 44, 132, 328, 334–336
bone growth stimulator insertion, 113
bone marrow
    biopsy, 42, 73, 83, 272
    description, 271–272
    transfusion, 96, 271
bones, 321–351
    approaches used for, 333–334
    body system values for, 321
    case studies, 347–351
    code building cases, 341–343

code building exercises, 343–345
devices common to, 334–340
organization of, 321–324
qualifiers used for, 340–341
root operations used for, 324–331
bone ultrasound qualifier, 466
bone x-rays, 465
botulinum toxin, 422
braces, fitting of, 417, 482
Brachytherapy root type, 470
brain, 159–161, 163–164
breast. *See also* Skin and Breast
devices common to, 15, 288–289, 291
organization of, 285
root operations for, 42, 74, 132, 288–289
breast milk, collecting, 450
breech position, 402
bronchial thermoplasty, 200
bronchoalveolar lavage (BAL), 200
bronchoscopy based procedures, 125–126, 199–200
Broviac catheter, 221
B section value, for Imaging, 463
buccal mucosa, 195, 196
Bursae and Ligaments. *See also* Muscular system
body part values, 309
body system value, 303
devices common to, 310
of Female Reproductive system, 381
functions, 303
joints and, 324, 331
organization of, 305
root operations used for, 48, 82, 307–308
button aneurysm, 222
Bypass root operation
aorto-femoral bypass, 227
axillo-femoral bypass, 228
for bleeding control, 143–144
for Central Nervous system, 167
for Circulatory system, 42–43, 109–112, 224–228, 235
coronary artery bypass grafts (CABG), 224–226
of coronary arteries, 42–43 106–108, 224–227, 235
cross-trigonal reimplantation of ureter, 355
defined, 109
discussion, 109–113
femoral-popliteal bypass, 227
for Gastrointestinal system, 252–253
for Male Reproductive system, 371
for Nervous system, 163
of noncoronary arteries, 42–43, 109–110, 227
qualifiers for, 148, 253, 359
for Respiratory system, 203–204
revisions, 118
of Sense Organs, 186
for Urinary system, 355

C

cage style interbody fusion (vertebrae), 335, 337
capsule repair, 331
capsulorrhaphy, 331
capsulotomy, 94
cardiac catheterization, 224, 243, 423, 465

cardiac mapping, 127
cardiac pacing, 432. *See also* pacemakers
cardiopulmonary bypass machine use, 224, 227, 432
cardiovascular system. *See* Circulatory system; Heart and Great Vessels; Lower Arteries; Lower Veins; Upper Veins
Caregiver Training root type, 482
carina, 198
carotid body, 267–269
carotid endarterectomy, 120
carpal tunnel release, 94
cast, application of, 46, 99, 324, 326, 415
cataract surgery, 82, 119
catheterization
Change, root operation for, 118
heart, 223–224, 423, 465
for pulmonary output monitoring, 233
urinary, 356, 358, 415
vascular access device insertion, 16, 219–221, 291
cauterization, 106, 143
cavities. *See* general anatomical regions
cavopulmonary impeller pump device, 435
cecum, 249
cells, transplantation of, 46, 96, 272
cement (bone fixation), 328
Centers for Medicare and Medicaid Services (CMS), 3–4, 33, 465. *See also* CMS file method
Central Nervous System and Cranial Nerves, 159–177
approaches for, 166
body part values for, 164–165
body system values for, 159
case studies, 173–177
code building cases, 168–170
code building exercises, 170–171
devices common to, 167
organization of, 159–160, 267
qualifiers for, 167
root operations used in, 163–164
Transfer root operation, 98
central veno-arterial (VA) ECMO, 435
central venous catheter (CVC), 221
cerclage procedure, 86, 106
cerebral aneurysm, 45, 106, 222–223
cerebral cisterns, 167
cerebral ventricles, 109
cerebrospinal fluid, 109
cervical esophagus, 254
cervix
body part values for, 384
description of, 381
procedures, 85, 106, 384, 386
cesarean deliveries, 386
Cesium-131 collagen implant, 167
Change root operation
approach for, 118
body part value for, 254, 369
defined, 118
of devices, 51, 118, 403
discussion of, 118
Placement section root operation, 415
for Urinary system, 355, 356, 369

characters
    character 1. *See* section
    character 2. *See* body system; section qualifier
    character 3. *See* modality and modality qualifiers; root operation
    character 4. *See* body part; body region; body system and region; treatment site
    character 5. *See* approach; duration value; modality and modality qualifiers; radionuclides
    character 6. *See* device; equipment; function value; isotope values; method; substance
    character 7. *See* qualifier
    code building with. *See* system structure and design
    Conventions guidelines for, 35–39
    overview, 4–5, 71
chest tube drainage, 38, 79, 114, 145
Chiropractic section
    approaches for, 467
    body regions for, 466
    case studies, 470–472
    code building cases, 467–469
    description, 5
    method values for, 467
    procedure types for, 461
    qualifier or, 467
    root operations commonly used in, 466
    section value for, 461, 467
cholecystectomy, 10, 11, 24, 39, 55
choroid, 179
Circulatory system, 213–250. *See also* Heart and Great Vessels; Lower Arteries; Lower Veins; Upper Arteries; Upper Veins
    ablation of cardiac mechanism, 223
    Administration section and, 418, 419
    aneurysm procedures, 222–223
    approaches for, 232
    AV fistulas and grafts, 229
    body part values, 47, 229–232
    body systems of, 5–6, 213
    coronary artery bypass grafting (CABG) procedure, 224–226
    Creation root operation, 222
    devices common to, 232–234
    Drainage root operation, 229
    functions of, 213
    heart catheterization, 223–224, 423, 465
    heart transplantation, 223
    heart valve procedures, 221–222
    Insertion root operation, 219
    laser revascularization, 229
    Map root operation, 223
    organization of, 213–218
    Physical Rehabilitation section and, 482
    PTCA, 224–225
    qualifiers used in, 235–238
    Removal root operation, 221
    Restriction root operation, 222–223
    Revision root operation, 221
    root operations used in, 218–229
circumcision, 371
cisterna chyli (lymph system), 270, 272
cisterns (cerebral), 167

clinical documentation. *See* documentation
clitoris, 381
closed reductions of fractures, 333
closing wedge osteotomy, 328
CMS file method
    application of, 54–55, 59
    body part key, 25, 270
    characters 3–7 definitions, 27
    device key, 25, 27
    front page download, 21
    Index, 20
    navigation, 23–25
    root operation selection, 81
    substance key, 26–27
    tables, 21–22
coagulation, 81, 107
coblation, 81
coccygeal glomus, 267, 268
cochlear implant, 17, 185
Cochlear Implant Treatment root type, 482
code book method, 19, 27–31, 81
code format and building. *See* system structure and design
code tables. *See* tables
coding guidelines. *See* guidelines
coding professional's responsibility
    Conventions guidelines for, 38–39, 86, 96
    querying provider, 37
    terminology selection, 4, 31
cognitive-behavioral techniques, 487
cognitive-behavioral type qualifier, 487
cognitive type qualifier, 486
cold knife cone biopsy, 383
colectomy, 254
collagen implant, 167
Collection method, 229, 450
colon bypass procedures, 253
colonoscopy, 125
colostomy, 105–106
colpocleisis, 383
colpopexy, 383
colporrhaphy, 383
common bile duct, 252
compartment syndrome, 94, 307
complete amputation, 79, 148
Compression root operation, 416
compression stockings, 416
Computer assisted procedure method, 450
Computerized Tomography (CT scan) root type, 464
conception products. *See* Products of Conception
Conduction Mechanism, 216
condyle, 322
congenital anomalies, of heart, 222
conjunctiva, 179
continuous positive airway pressure (CPAP), 433–434
contraceptive devices, 292, 386
contrast material, 419, 465–466
Control root operation
    overview, 127–128
    for bleeding, 43, 127–128, 144
    body system value, for procedures not confined to one body system, 40, 84, 147

defined, 43, 127–128,
   for Ear, Nose and Sinus body system, 143
   for general anatomical regions, 128, 143–144, 147
Conventions (guidelines), 35–39
Coordination and Maintenance Committee Meeting, 3–4, 489
coordination of care for crisis management, 484
cornea, 179
corneal transplant, 96, 183
coronary angiography, 465
coronary arteries
   angioplasty of, 48, 108–109, 224–225
   body part values for, 43, 47–48
   coronary artery bypass grafting (CABG) procedure, 224–226
   Dilation, 107–109
   grafts and, 44, 110–111, 224, 235
   heart catheterization and, 223–224, 423, 465
   for multiple arteries procedures, 42–43, 47–48, 108, 110–111, 224
   qualifier values for, 43
   thrombectomy procedures on, 224
coronary artery bypass grafting (CABG), 224–226
corpus coccygeum, 267
corpus glomera aortica, 267
cosmetic procedures, 132, 144, 182, 287
Counseling root type, 484
counterstrain technique, 449
cranial dura mater, 164
cranial epidural space, 419
Cranial Nerves. See Central Nervous system and Cranial Nerves
craniectomy, 163
craniosynostosis, 163
craniosynostosis surgery, 163
craniotomy, 163
Creation root operation, 133, 144, 222
crest (bone), 322
Crisis Intervention root type, 484, 486
cross-references, in Index, 29
cryotherapy, 81
cul-de-sac, 381, 384–385
curettage, 82. See also dilation and curettage (D&C)
Cutaneous qualifier value
   for Gastrointestinal system, 253

D

Dacron patch, 120
D&C. See dilation and curettage (D&C)
debridement, 42, 74, 83
debriefing treatment, 484
decompression fasciotomy, 307
Decompression root operation, 437
decompression sickness, 437
decompressive laminectomy, 95
defibrillation, 432
defibrillator generator, 219, 289
defusing treatment, 484
Delivery root operation
   overview, 401
   approaches for, 403
   defined, 400–401

   followed by other procedures, 51, 384, 400
   procedures during, 143, 401
   tears and lacerations during, 143–144, 401
densitometry study, 466
depressed skull fractures, 163
dermal layer of skin, 285
descending colon, 249
Destruction root operation
   overview, 83
   with biopsy procedures, 42
   as bleeding control technique, 143
   cauterization and, 143
   for Circulatory system, 223
   defined, 83, 84, 107
   for Female Reproductive system, 383
   for Gastrointestinal system, 253
   for Male Reproductive system, 369
   for Mouth, 201
   terminology for, 83
   thoracoscopy or thoracotomy procedures, 201
Detachment root operation
   overview, 77–83
   approach, 77
   for bleeding control, 143
   body part values, 77, 144–145
   body system values, 40, 77, 85, 144, 147
   defined, 77
   device values, 77–78
   qualifiers, 78–83, 145–146
DETOUR bypass, 228
Detoxification Services root type, 481
developmental test, 485
developmental type qualifier, 487
device (character 6)
   aggregation table for, 23, 27
   for anatomical regions, 148
   for bones and joints, 44–45, 125–128, 334–340
   for Bypass root operation, 43, 48, 227, 230
   for Circulatory system, 219–223, 233
   classification of, 15–19. See also specific devices
   CMS file definitions, 29
   code format, 15–19
   Detachment root operation, 77–78
   Drainage Device, 80
   for Ears, Nose, and Sinus, 185
   for Endocrine system, 270
   for Eye, 185
   for Female Reproductive system, 386
   for Gastrointestinal system, 256–258
   for gender reassignment, 133, 144
   guidelines for, 51
   harvested tissue as, 291
   for Hepatobiliary system, 256–258
   key for, 23, 25–27
   for Lymphatic system, 274
   for Male Reproductive system, 370–371
   for Measurement and Monitoring section, 424–425
   for Mouth and Throat, 203
   for Nervous system, 167
   for New Technology section, 490–491
   for Obstetrics section, 403

for Placement section, 417–418
qualifier values for, 19
for Removal root operation, 116
for Respiratory system, 204
root operations always involving, 113–120, 419. *See also*
    Change root operation; Insertion root operation;
    Removal root operation; Replacement root operation;
    Revision root operation; Supplement root operation
for Sense Organs, 183
for Subcutaneous Tissue and Fascia, 292
for tubular body parts, 105–107
for Urinary system, 358, 369
Device Fitting root type, 417, 481
diagnostic information, affecting coding, 133
diagnostic nuclear medicine, 467
diagnostic sinus endoscopy, 183
dialysate, 419
diaphragm
    description, 197–198
    for upper and lower extremity division, 39–40, 141
diaphragmatic pacemaker leads, 203
diarthroses, 324
Diatrizoate, 465
DIEP free flap, 288
digestive system, 195, 249–251. *See also* Gastrointestinal
    System
dilation and curettage (D&C)
    as Extraction root operation, 84
    section guidelines for, 51, 107, 384, 401
Dilation root operation
    for Circulatory system, 221–225, 228, 235, 465
    defined, 107
    devices for, 235
    discussion of, 107–109
    for Gastrointestinal system, 252, 253
    for Lymphatic system, 271
    for Obstetrics, 401
    for Sense Organs, 182
    of Urinary system, 355
discectomy, 339
discontinued procedure guideline, 41, 143
disc (vertebral), 324
dislocations, 417
displaced fractures, 46, 99, 324, 326, 328, 334
diversion procedures. *See* Bypass root operation
Division root operation
    overview, 94–95
    for anatomical regions, 143–144
    defined, 46, 93, 94–95
    for Integumentary system, 289
    for Muscular system, 311
    for Obstetrics section, 416
DLIF (direct lateral lumbar interbody fusion), 336
documentation. *See also* coding professional's responsibility;
    provider's role in code building
    for biopsies, 73
    Conventions guidelines for, 35
    review for code building, 19, 37–38
    terminology interpretation, 28, 31, 39
dome aneurysm, 222
donor organs, perfusion of, 438

drainage devices
    overview, 51, 84, 147
    Change root operation for, 118
    for Endocrine system, 270
    for Lymphatic system, 274
    Removal root operation for, 116
Drainage root operation
    overview, 83–84
    body system guidelines for, 40, 83, 147
    for Circulatory system, 229
    defined, 83–84, 85, 93
    device values for, 51, 84, 147
    for ear, 183
    for Female Reproductive system, 384
    fluid collection as, 229, 450
    followed by more definitive procedure, 42, 74
    for Obstetrics section, 401
    qualifiers for, 42, 73–74, 83, 84
    for Respiratory system, 200
    for Urinary system, 356
Dressing root operation, 416
drug-coated balloons, 235
drug-eluting intraluminal device, 109, 113, 225, 232–234
dual-chamber cardiac pacemaker, 113
ductus deferens, 367, 368
duodenum, 45, 249, 251–252, 254
dura mater, 159, 161
duration value (character 5)
    for Extracorporeal or Systemic Assistance and
        Performance section, 432–433
    for Extracorporeal or Systemic Therapies, 438

E
Ear, Nose, and Sinus, 179–193
    approaches for, 185
    body part values for, 183–184
    body system value for, 179
    case studies, 190–193
    code building cases, 186–188
    code building exercises, 188–189
    devices common to, 183, 185
    functions of, 179
    organization of, 181–182
    qualifiers used in, 186
    Respiratory system and, 195
    root operations used in, 182–183
ectopic pregnancy, 400
egg (fertilized), 381, 400
EKG measurements, 423
elbow, 48, 290, 324
electrical stimulation, as chiropractic treatment, 454
electricity, measurement and monitoring of, 423–424
electrocautery, 106–107, 143
electrocoagulation, 107
Electroconvulsive Therapy root type, 484
electromagnetic therapy, 437
electronic appliances, defined, 17
embolization, 45, 106, 113, 223, 229
endarterectomy, 86
endobronchial biopsy, 200
endobronchial valve, 15, 200

endocrine gland (generic term), 268
Endocrine system
  approaches for, 269
  body part values for, 268–269
  body system value for, 267
  case studies, 279–283
  code building exercises, 276–277
  devices common to, 270
  functions of, 267
  organization of, 267
  qualifiers for, 270
  root operations used in, 268
Endolymphatic qualifier, 186
endometrium, 81, 81–83, 381, 383–384
endoscopic approaches. *See* Percutaneous Endoscopic
    approach; Via Natural or Artificial Opening Endoscopic;
    Via Natural or Artificial Opening with Percutaneous
    Endoscopic Assistance
endotracheal tube (ET), 11, 203, 434
enterolysis, 254
epicondyle, 322
epidermal layer of skin, 285
epididymis, 367, 368, 369
epidural space, 159, 161, 419
epiglottis, 195
episiorrhaphy, 143–144, 402
episiotomy, 93, 143–144, 402
eponyms, 4
equipment (character 6)
    defined, 17, 19
    for Physical Rehabilitation and Diagnostic Audiology
        section, 483
esophageal airways, 257
esophageal dilations, 107
esophagogastric junction, 11, 249, 251
esophagus, 95, 249, 253–254, 273
ethmoid sinus, 181, 184
eustachian tube, 181
evacuation, of hematomas, 85, 147
Examination method, 451
excisional debridement, 42, 74, 84
Excision root operation
    overview, 72–74
    biopsy procedures and. *See* biopsy procedures
    for bleeding control, 143
    body part subdivision guideline, 43, 75
    in conjunction with separate procedure, 44, 74
    defined, 43, 45, 72, 74, 94, 116
    of diseased body part, 288–289
    for ear, 183
    for Endocrine system, 268
    for Female Reproductive system, 384
    followed by more definitive procedure, 42, 74
    for Gastrointestinal system, 252–253
    harvesting grafts and, 43, 74, 112, 132, 288, 335
    for Male Reproductive system, 369
    for Mouth and Throat, 201
    for overlapping layers, 42, 74, 125, 290, 308
    qualifiers for, 42, 73, 83, 149
    for Respiratory system, 201
    thoracoscopy or thoracotomy procedures, 201

exploratory laparotomy, 126, 357
External approach
    overview, 49–50
    for Administration section, 419
    for bones and joints, 328, 333
    for Chiropractic section, 453
    for Circulatory system, 232
    defined, 13–14
    for Endocrine system, 269
    for indirect application of external force, 49
    for Integumentary system, 291
    for Male Reproductive system, 369
    for Measurement and Monitoring section, 424
    for Mouth and Throat, 202
    for Muscular system, 309
    for New Technology section, 490
    for Obstetrics section, 403
    within orifices, 49
    for Osteopathic treatment, 448
    for Placement section, 417
    for Sense Organs, 185
external cardioversion, 432
external ear, 181
external fixation, 116, 328
external heart assist devices, 220
Extirpation root operation
    overview, 85–86
    for Circulatory system, 225, 228–229, 235
    defined, 118
    for foreign bodies, 86, 200
    for Urinary system, 356
extra-articular manipulation, 453
Extracorporeal or Systemic Assistance and Performance
        section
    body systems for, 432
    case studies, 442–445
    character definition for, 431–436
    code building cases, 439–441
    description, 5
    duration values for, 432–433
    function values for, 433–434
    procedure types included in, 431
    qualifiers for, 434–436
    root operations commonly used in, 431–432
    section value for, 431
Extracorporeal or Systemic Therapies section
    body systems for, 438
    case studies, 442–445
    character definition for, 431–436
    code building cases, 439–441
    description, 5
    duration values for, 438
    qualifier values for, 438–439
    root operations commonly used in, 437
    section value for, 436
extracorporeal membrane oxygenation (ECMO)
coding of, 435–436
description, 435
Extraction root operation
    overview, 82–83
    approaches for, 401

for bleeding control, 144
bone marrow biopsy and, 83, 272
defined, 82–83, 94, 107
for Eye, 182
for Female Reproductive system, 401
followed by more definitive procedure, 42, 74
for liposuction, 287
nonexcisional debridement, 74, 82
for Obstetrics section, 51, 403
qualifiers for, 42, 72, 83
extraluminal device
for aneurysm procedures, 222
for Lymphatic system, 274
with Occlusion root operation, 107
with Restriction root operation, 105
extraocular muscle, 179
Eye, 179–193
approaches for, 185
body part values for, 183–184
body system value for, 179
case studies, 190–193
code building exercises, 188–189
devices common to, 185
functions of, 179
organization of, 179–183
qualifiers used in, 186
root operations used in, 182–183
eyebrow lifts, 132
eyelid, 132, 179

F

face
description, 322
transplantion of, 96, 144
facet, 322
fallopian tubes
body part values for, 47, 384
description of, 381
procedures, 107, 382–383
Falope ring, 107
false joint, 339
Family Counseling root type, 488
Family Psychotherapy root type, 484
fascia. *See* Subcutaneous Tissue and Fascia
fecal incontinence, 257
feeding tube, 118
Female Reproductive system
approaches used in, 385–386
body part values for, 384–385
body system value, 381
case studies, 391–395
code building cases, 387–389
code building exercises, 389–390
devices common to, 386
functions of, 381
organization of, 267, 381–382
qualifiers for, 386–387
root operations used for, 382–384
femoropopliteal bypass procedure, 109, 227
fertilized egg, 381, 400
fetus

description, 381
monitoring of, 403, 423
positioning of, 401–402
fiber-optic bronchoscopy, 45, 126, 201
filtration function values, 434
fine needle aspiration biopsy, 42, 74, 272
fingernails, 287
fingers, 48, 59, 79–80
fissure (bone), 322
fixation procedures (gastrointestinal system), 254
flap procedures, 387–289, 293, 310
flow, measurement of, 424
fluids, collection of, 230, 450. *See also* Drainage root operation
Fluoroscopy root type, 224, 464, 467
foot
amputation levels, 79, 148
rays of, 79, 143, 148–149
toes, 48, 79, 148
foramen, 322
foreign body removal, 86
Forequarter, 141, 145
foreskin transfers, 369
fossa, 322
fovea, 322
fractures
approaches for, 14, 49, 328, 334
cast or splint application, 46, 99, 324, 326, 416
decision making process, 326
root operations for, 45–46, 95, 99, 163, 324–328
Fragmentation root operation
for Circulatory system, 232
defined, 87
guidelines, 87
for Urinary system, 356
free flaps, 288
free grafts, 17, 97, 111, 119, 287, 293
frontal sinus, 181, 185
fulguration, 83
full-thickness procedures, 293
function value (character 6)
for Extracorporeal or Systemic Assistance and Performance section, 433–434
for Measurement and Monitoring section, 424–425
fundoplication procedure, 253
fusiform aneurysm, 222
Fusion root operation
overview, 129–132
defined, 129
device guidelines, 129–130
guidelines for, 44
of joints, 334–338
qualifier guidelines, 129
spinal, 44, 74, 129, 334–338

G

gallbladder, 249, 252
gamma knife, 470
gases. *See* Drainage root operation
gastrectomy, partial, 73
gastric banding, 105, 252
gastric stimulator, 257

gastric tube airways, 257
Gastrointestinal system, 249–266
    approaches for, 256
    body part value for, 48, 254–255
    case studies, 263–266
    code building exercises, 260–262
    contrast media for, 465
    devices common to, 256–258
    functions of, 249
    motility monitoring of, 423
    organization of, 249–252
    qualifiers used in, 258–259
    root operations used in, 252–254
gastrostomy tube (G-tube), 256
gastropexy, 254
gender reassignment, 133, 144
general anatomical regions
    approaches, 50, 147
    body cavities guidelines, 141
    body system values for, 139
    division of upper and lower body parts, 39, 141, 143
    guidelines for use of, 83, 140
    multiple body parts inspection, 45, 126, 145, 357
    for procedures not confined to one body system, 40, 83–84
    root operations for, 143–144
general mobilization, 449
generic body part values, 230, 331
Genitourinary system, for Physical Rehabilitation section, 483
gingiva (upper and lower), 195
G-J tube. See PEG/J tube
glans penis, 368
glenohumeral joint, 334
glomus caroticum, 267
glomus jugulare, 267, 268
gonads, 267
grafts
    autograft. See autografts
    for bones and joints, 44, 132, 328, 334–336
    for Bypass root operation, 44, 110–111, 224–225–227, 229, 235
    for Circulatory system, 224, 232
    defined, 15, 111
    for osteotomies, 328
    for Replacement root operation, 119
    skin grafts, 287
    for Transfer root operation, 97
    for Urinary system, 356
Graham patch, 254
greater saphenous vein, 227
Group Counseling root type, 488
Group Psychotherapy root type, 484
guidelines, 35–67
    for anatomical regions, 39
    application of, 53–61
    for approach, 49–50
    for body part, 46–48
    for body system, 39–40
    Conventions, 35–39
    for device, 51
    for New Technology, 52
    for Obstetrics section, 51

operative report, dissecting, 41, 53–54
overview, 35
for root operations, 40–46
selection of principal procedure, 52–53

H
hand
    Detachment root operation and, 79–80
    finger, body part value guidelines for, 48, 57, 80
    ray of, 80, 141, 143, 148
    Transplantation root operation, 95, 144
Head and Facial Bones, 321–322, 324, 342
Health Care Procedure Coding System (HCPCS), 465
Health Insurance Portability and Accountability Act (HIPAA), 3, 35
Hearing Aid Assessment root type, 482
Hearing Assessment root type, 482
hearing devices, 185, 482
Hearing Treatment root type, 482
Heart and Great Vessels
    aneurysm and, 222–223
    approaches for, 232
    body part values for, 230
    body system value for, 213
    CABG, 224–226
    Destruction root operation, 223
    devices and, 219–221
    functions of, 213
    heart catheterization, 223–224, 423, 465
    heart transplantation, 95–96, 223
    heart valves, 96, 133, 221–222
    laser revascularization, 229
    Map root operation, 223
    organization of, 213–218
    PTCA, 224–225
    qualifiers used in, 235–236
heat as non-manual chiropractic treatment, 453
hematomas, 85, 147
hemiarthroplasty, 330
hemicolectomy, 254
hemic system. See Lymphatic and Hemic systems
hemodialysis, 229, 432
hemorrhaging, control of, 38, 41, 79, 123–125, 139–141, 145
hemorrhoids, 102
hepatic ducts, 254
Hepatobiliary System and Pancreas
    approaches for, 256
    body part values for, 254–255
    devices for, 256–258
    glands of, 267
    organization of, 252
    qualifiers for, 258–259
    transplantations, 95
hernia repair, 120, 126
Hickman catheter, 221
high amputation, qualifier for, 78, 148
high dose rate radiation therapy, 471
high osmolar contrast media, 465
high velocity–low amplitude treatment, 449
Hindquarter, 143, 145
hip

body part value for, 48, 290
   description, 324, 327
   replacement, 119, 329–330
hydrocephalus, 109
hydrosurgery, 82
hymen, 381
hyperbaric oxygen treatment, 434, 437–439
Hyperthermia root operation, 437, 471
Hypnosis root type, 484
hypodermis, 285
hypospadias procedures, 356
hypothalamus, 267
Hypothermia root operation, 437
hysterectomy, 13, 50, 256, 384–385

I

ICD-9-CM system, 3
ICD-10-CM system, 3
ICD-10 Coordination and Maintenance Committee (C&M), 3–4
ICD-10 PCS system
   background and rationale for implementing, 3–4
   guidelines, 35–67. *See also* guidelines
   multiaxial feature of, 4
   overview, 3
   system structure and design, 3–34. *See also* system
      structure and design
   updates, 3–4, 35
ice, as chiropractic treatment, 453
ileocecal junction, 249
ileocecal valve, 249, 251
ileum, 249
iliac artery aneurysm, 222
iliac (bone marrow), 272
Imaging section
   body part values for, 465
   case studies, 475–479
   character definition, 463–466
   code building cases, 472–474
   code format and structure, 5
   contrast values used for, 465–466
   procedure types for, 464
   qualifiers for, 466
   root types used in, 464–465
   section value for, 464
Immobilization root operation, 46, 99, 324, 326, 416, 482
impeller pump, 435
implantable cardioverter-defibrillator, 289
implantable heart assist system, 220
implantable miniature telescope (IMT), 185
implantable pulmonary artery pressure sensor, 233
implants, defined, 15
incision and drainage of abscess, 83
Index
   body part key in, 10, 25, 47, 270
   CMS file method and. *See* CMS file method
   code book method, 19, 27–31, 29–60, 81
   Conventions guidelines for use of, 37
   cross references, 29
   using, 20, 21, 23, 26–29
Indirect method, 449
Individual Counseling root type, 488

Individual Psychotherapy root type, 485, 488
Indwelling device
   Administration root operations for, 418
   body part value, 419
   fluid collection from, 229, 450
   for Other Procedures section, 449
infections, of joint prostheses, 330
inferior parathyroid gland, 268
inferior vena cava (IVC) filter, 60, 220
infusion devices, 116, 270, 274, 292
inguinal region, 140, 143
injection, root operation for, 419
inner ear, 181
Insertion root operation
   overview, 113–115
   of Circulatory system devices, 219–221, 223
   defined, 113
   for endotracheal tube (ET), 434
   for multiple procedures, 113–114
   of obstetric devices, 402–403
   into subcutaneous tissue, 289
   of urinary system devices, 369
Inspection root operation
   overview, 125–126
   for Circulatory system, 232
   defined, 125
   discontinued procedure guideline for, 41, 143
   endoscopic, 126
   for Gastrointestinal system, 256
   as integral part of procedure, 45, 126
   of multiple body parts, 45, 126, 145, 357
   for multiple procedures on same body part, 45, 126
   of overlapping layers, 42, 74, 125, 290, 308
   of Respiratory system, 199, 201
   of sinuses, 183
   of throat, 201
   of Urinary system, 357, 369
Integumentary system, 285–302
   approaches used in, 291
   body part values for, 290–291
   body system value for, 285
   case studies, 298–302
   code building exercises, 296–297
   devices common to, 291–293
   functions of, 285
   organization of, 285–287
   Physical Rehabilitation section and, 482
   qualifiers used in, 293
   root operations used in, 287–288
intellectual and psychoeducational tests, 485
intellectual and psychoeducational type qualifier, 487
interactive type qualifier, 487
Interbody Fusion Device, 44, 130
interbody fusions (vertebrae), 44, 74, 130–132, 335–339
intercarotid body, 267
internal fixation, 116, 324, 328, 334, 339
internal heart assist devices, 220
internal mammary artery bypass, 226–227
internal version procedure, 402
interpersonal type qualifier, 487
interspinous process device (spacer), 336

interstitial brachytherapy, 470
intervertebral space and disc, 324
intestinal adhesion mobilization, 94, 254
intestinal tract, body part values for, 48
intra-aortic balloon pump (IABP), 434
intracardiac pacemaker, 219
intracavitary brachytherapy, 470
intracranial artery, 223
intracranial spaces, 159, 161
intraluminal device
    for aneurysm procedures, 222
    for Bypass root operation, 110
    for esophagus, 257
    for Lymphatic system, 274
    nasal, 185
    for Occlusion root operation, 106–107
    for Restriction root operation, 105
intramedullary fixation device, 328
intraocular lens implant, 82, 119, 183
intraoperative brain mapping, 127
intraoperative electron beam therapy (IOEBT), 472
Intraoperative qualifier value, 19, 51
intrauterine device (IUD), 16, 386
intravascular imaging technique, 465
Introduction root operation, 402, 419
intussusception, 99, 254
in vitro fertilization, 384, 402, 451
iris, 179
Irrigation root operation
    overview, 419
    of devices, 51, 355–356
    of hematomas, 147
    of lungs, 45, 200
    substance values for, 419
Islets of Langerhans, 267
Isolation method, 450, 451
isotope values (character 6), 471–472
Isovue contrast media, 465

J
jejunostomy tube, 256
jejunum, 249, 252, 254
joints, 321–351
    adhesion release on, 95
    approaches used for, 333–334
    body part values for, 48, 333
    body system values for, 321
    case studies, 347–351
    code building cases, 341–343
    code building exercises, 343–345
    description, 303, 324
    devices common to, 334–340
    osteopathic mobilization of, 449
    qualifiers used for, 340–341
    replacement, 329–331
    root operations used for, 324–328
    spinal fusion, 44, 74, 129–132, 334–338
joint spacer, 118

K
kidney
    body part value for, 356–357
    organization of, 353–354
    transplantation, 95, 356, 359
kidney stone, removal of, 49, 51, 86, 358
knee
    body part value for, 48, 289–290
    organization of, 324
    replacement, 329–330
K wires, 334
kyphoplasty, 328

L
labrum, repair of, 331
lacerated tendon, 307
lacerations, 127
lacrimal duct and gland, 179–180, 186
Laminaria, 400
laminectomy, 95, 338
laparoscopic cholecystectomy, 11, 41, 49, 57
laparoscopic procedures
    converted to open procedures, 256
    types of, 14, 49, 50, 256, 386
laparotomy, 55, 126, 253, 329
lap band, 105,
large intestine, 96, 249, 254–255
laryngopharynx (hypopharynx), 196
laryngoscopy, 199
larynx, 195, 196, 197
laser interstitial thermal therapy (LITT), 470
laser prostatectomy, 369
laser revascularization, 229
lateral fluctuation technique, 449
laterality guidelines
    for body parts, 47
    for bones and joints, 331
    for Circulatory system, 224
    for Female Reproductive system, 384
    for Male Reproductive system, 369
    for Muscular system, 308
    for Urinary system, 356–357
latissimus dorsi myocutaneous flap, 289
leads
    Insertion root operation for, 113–114, 203, 220
    of neurostimulators, 17, 163, 167, 289, 292, 358
    Revision root operation, 118
    for temporary devices, 434
left ventriculography, 465
lens, 83, 179, 183
ligaments. *See* Bursae and Ligaments
ligatures, 51
Light Therapy root type, 485
limb-lengthening device, 328
LimFlow, 228
linear accelerators (LINAC radiosurgery), 470
lingual tonsils, 197
liposuction, 82, 287
liquid removal. *See* Drainage root operation
Lisfranc amputation, 79
lithotripsy, 86, 87
liver, 95, 249, 252
living body part transplantation, guidelines for, 46, 95, 272
lobectomy of lung, 43, 75
long lever manipulation, 454

loop electrosurgical excision procedure (LEEP), 383
low amputation, qualifier for, 78, 148
low dose rate radiation therapy, 470
Lower Arteries
    approaches for, 232
    AV fistulas and grafts, 229
    blood collection from, 229, 450
    body part values for, 230
    body system value for, 213
    devices common to, 232, 234
    generic body part values, 230
    organization of, 216
    PTA, 224
    qualifiers used in, 235
    vascular access devices for, 220–221
Lower Bones. *See* bones
lower esophagus, 254
lower extremities
    amputation of. *See* Detachment root operation
    body system value for, 139
    division from upper body parts, 39–40, 143
    organization of, 139
    toes, body part values for, 48, 80, 147
Lower Intestinal Tract, 249, 254
Lower Joints. *See* joints
Lower Veins
    approaches for, 232
    AV fistulas and grafts, 229
    body part values for, 230
    devices common to, 232, 234
    devices for, 220–221
    generic body part values, 230
    Insertion root operation, 220
    organization of, 216
    percutaneous bypasses of, 228
    qualifiers used in, 235
    venipuncture, 229
low osmolar contrast media, 465
low velocity–high amplitude treatment, 449
lumbar puncture (tap), 84, 164
lumpectomy, 288
lung
    body part values for, 201
    description of, 198–199
    irrigation of, 45
    lobectomy, 75
    transplantion of, 95, 201
Lymphatic and Hemic systems
    approaches used in, 273
    body part values for, 272–273
    body system value for, 267
    case studies, 279–283
    code building cases, 274–276
    code building exercises, 276–277
    devices common to, 274
    functions of, 270
    organization of, 270–271
    qualifiers for, 274
    root operations used in, 271–272
lymphatic pump treatment, 449
lymph nodes
    body part value terminology, 272–273
    chain vs. node(s) removal, 76, 271
    description of, 270
    sampling, 42, 74, 288
lymph vessels, 270
lysis of adhesions, 95, 254

M
macular degeneration, 185
Magnetic Resonance Imaging (MRI) root type, 464
magnetic therapy, as non-manual chiropractic treatment, 453
Male Reproductive system, 367–379
    approaches used in, 370
    body part values for, 369–370
    body system value, 367
    case studies, 376–379
    code building cases, 371–373
    code building exercises, 373–375
    devices common to, 370–371
    functions of, 367
    glands of, 267
    organization of, 367–368
    qualifiers for, 371
    root operations used in, 369
malrotation, 254
mammography, 465
Manipulation root operation, 452
manometry of organ, 423
manual traction, 417
Map root operation, 127, 223
massage, 450
mastectomy, 42, 74, 75, 288
mastoid sinus, 182
maxillary sinus, 181
Measurement and Monitoring section
    approaches used for, 424
    body systems for, 423–424
    case studies, 428–430
    character definition for, 423–425
    code building cases, 426–427
    description, 5
    device values for, 278, 424–425
    function values for, 424–425
    for heart catheterization, 225
    procedure types included in, 415
    qualifiers used in, 425
    root operations used in, 423
    section value for, 415
Measurement root operation, 423, 465
meatus, 322
mechanical appliances, defined, 15, 222
mechanical debridement, 82
mechanical traction, 417
mechanical ventilation, 203, 432–433, 435
Medical and Surgical section, 39–51
    anatomical regions guidelines, 39–40. *See also* anatomical regions
    application of guidelines for, 53–61
    approach guidelines, 49–50. *See also* approach (character 5)
    body parts guidelines, 46–48. *See also* body part (character 4)
    body systems guidelines, 5–6, 39–40. *See also* body system (character 2)
    description of, 5, 72

devices guidelines, 51. *See also* device (character 6)
operative report, dissecting, 53, 55
root operations guidelines, 7, 40–46, 53, 541–550.
   See also root operation (character 3)
medication, as substance, 419
Medication Management root type, 485–486, 488
Meditation method, 451
meninges, 161
Mental Health section
   body system value for, 484
   case studies, 494–498
   character definition, 484–487
   code building cases, 491–492
   code format and structure, 5
   procedure types included in, 481
   qualifiers used in, 485–487
   root types commonly used in, 484–485
   section value for, 481
   type qualifiers used in, 484–487
mesentery, 250–251
mesh hernia repair, 120
metal leaflets for heart valves, 222
method (character 6)
   for Chiropractic section, 453–454
   for Osteopathic section, 448–449
   for Other Procedures section, 450–451
microanastomosis, 288
mid amputation, qualifier for, 78, 148
middle ear, 181
middle esophagus, 254
mid-foot amputation, 79
minor cutting, 82
minor salivary gland, 195, 196
miscarriage, 400
mitral valve creation, 133
mitral valve repair, 120
modalities and modality qualifiers (characters 3 & 5),
   for Radiation Therapy, 469–471
monitoring devices, 270, 402, 423–425
Monitoring root operation, 423
monoplanar fixation device, 328
motility, measurement of, 423
Motor and/or Nerve Function Assessment root type, 482
Motor Treatment root type, 482
Mouth and Throat, 195–212
   approaches, 202
   body part value for, 201–202
   body system value for, 195
   case studies, 209–212
   code building cases, 204–205
   code building exercises, 206–207
   devices common to, 203
   Gastrointestinal system and, 249
   organization of, 195–199
   qualifiers used in, 204
   root operations used in, 199–201
mouth-to-mouth resuscitation, 435
mucus plugs, 200
multiplane external fixation device, 328
multiple array stimulator, 292

Muscle energy method, 449
muscle flaps, 310
Muscular system, 303–319
   approaches used for, 309
   body part values for, 308–309
   body systems of, 6, 303
   case studies, 315–319
   code building cases, 311–312
   code building exercises, 313–314
   devices common to, 309–310
   functions of, 303
   organization of, 303–307
   overlapping layers guidelines, 42, 74, 77, 93, 125, 290, 308
   qualifiers used in, 310
   root operations used in, 307–308
musculocutaneous flap transfer, 46, 98
myocutaneous flaps, 310
myringotomy tube placement, 183

N
nails, of fingers and toes, 41, 57, 287
nails (bone fixation), 328
Narcosynthesis root type, 485
Nasal Cavity qualifier, 186
nasal mucosa, 181
nasal septum, 181
nasal trumpet, 185
nasal turbinate, 181
nasopharyngeal airway (NPA), 185
nasopharynx, 181, 196
National Center for Health Statistics (NCHS), 3, 35
natural opening approaches. *See* Via Natural or Artificial
   Opening; Via Natural or Artificial Opening Endoscopic;
   Via Natural or Artificial Opening with Percutaneous
   Endoscopic Assistance
Near infrared spectroscopy (NIRS) method, 451
NEC root operation, 127, 355
needle procedures, approach guidelines, 49, 81–82, 84, 166
nephrostomy, 49, 51, 87, 356, 419
Nervous system, 159–177. *See also* Central Nervous system
   and Cranial Nerves; Peripheral Nervous system
   approaches for, 166
   body part values for, 164–165
   body system values for, 159
   case studies, 173–177
   code building cases, 168–170
   code building exercises, 170–171
   devices common to, 167
   functions of, 159
   organization of, 159–162
   qualifiers used in, 167
   root operations used in, 98, 163–164, 223
neurobehavioral and cognitive status tests, 485
neurobehavioral and cognitive status type qualifier, 487
Neurological system, for Physical Rehabilitation section, 482
neuroplasty, 163
neuropsychological tests, 485
neuropsychological type qualifier, 487
neurorrhaphy, 163
neurostimulator generators and leads, 17, 163, 167, 289, 292, 358

New Technology section
    approach character for, 490
    body systems and regions value for, 489–490
    case studies, 494–498
    character definition for, 489–491
    code building cases, 491–492
    code format and structure, 5
    device/substance/technology character for, 490–491
    guidelines for, 52
    qualifiers for, 491
    root operations for, 489–490
Nissen fundoplication, 253
nodulus caroticus, 267
Nonautologous Tissue Substitute, 167
    for aortocoronary bypasses, 111
    guidelines for, 44–45
    for Male Reproductive System, 369
Non-Axial Skeleton body system value, 463
noncoronary artery bypass procedures, 42–43, 109, 228
nondisplaced fractures, 46, 99, 324, 326, 417
None (body system and regions value), 483
None (type qualifier value), 483
nonexcisional debridement, 82
Nonimaging Nuclear Medicine Probe, 468
Nonimaging Nuclear Medicine Uptake root type, 468
non-manual chiropractic treatments, 453
nonmechanical ventilation, 435
Nose. See Ear, Nose, and Sinus
not elsewhere classified (NEC)
    for devices, 4
    root operation, 127, 355. See also Repair root operation
Nuclear Medicine section
    body part values for, 469
    body system values, 467
    case studies, 475–479
    character definition, 467–469
    code building cases, 472–474
    code format and structure, 5
    procedure types for, 467
    qualifier values for, 469
    radionuclides used in, 469
    root types commonly used in, 467–468
    section value for, 467
nursemaid's elbow, 326
Nuss procedure, 144

O

Obstetrics section, 399–414
    approaches used in, 403
    body part values for, 403
    body system value for, 399
    case studies, 410–414
    code building cases, 405–407
    code building exercises, 407–409
    D&C guidelines, 51, 107, 400
    description, 5
    devices common to, 403
    guidelines for, 51
    Products of Conception, 399–400
    qualifiers for, 403–405

    root operations commonly used in, 400–402
    section value for, 399
obturator airways, 257
Occlusion root operation
    overview, 106–107
    defined, 45, 106
    for embolization, 45, 223, 229
    for Female Reproductive system, 106, 382–383
    for Lymphatic system, 271
    for Male Reproductive system, 106, 369
    for Sense Organs, 182
    for sterilization procedures, 106, 369, 382–383
ocular system. See Eye
Official ICD-10-PCS Guidelines for Coding and Reporting, 3
omental patch, 254
omentum, 250–251
Omnipaque contrast media, 465
online CMS Index file. See CMS file method
Open approach
    overview of guidelines, 49
    for Administration section, 419
    for bones and joints, 333
    for cesarean section deliveries, 403
    for Circulatory system, 219–221, 223, 225–226, 228, 232
    defined, 10, 166
    for Endocrine System, 269
    for Female Reproductive system, 385–386
    for Gastrointestinal system, 256
    for Insertion root operation, 113
    for Integumentary system, 291
    for Measurement and Monitoring section, 424
    for Muscular system, 309
    for New Technology section, 490
    for Obstetrics section, 402
    with percutaneous endoscopic assistance, 49
    for Sense Organs, 185
open heart surgery, 433
opening wedge osteotomy, 336
optical coherence tomography (OCT), 466
optical instrumentation for visualization, 125
Optiray contrast media, 465
oral cavity, 195
orbit, bones of, 322
orchiopexy, 369
organs of Zuckerkandl, 267
orifice approaches. See Via Natural or Artificial Opening; Via Natural or Artificial Opening Endoscopic; Via Natural or Artificial Opening with Percutaneous Endoscopic Assistance
oropharynx, 196
ossicles of ear, 181
Osteopathic section
    approaches used for, 448
    body regions for, 448
    case studies, 457–459
    character definition for, 447–449
    code building cases, 454–455
    description, 5
    method values used for, 448–449
    procedure types for, 447

qualifiers used for, 449
    root operations commonly used in, 447–448
    section value for, 447
ostomy procedures, 148, 253
Other Method (method value), 451
Other Procedures root operation, 449–450
Other Procedures section
    approaches used for, 450
    body regions for, 450
    case studies, 457–459
    character definition, 449–452
    code building cases, 454–455
    description, 5
    for fertilization of eggs, 402
    method values for, 450–451
    procedure types for, 447
    qualifiers for, 451–452
    root operations commonly used in, 449
    section value for, 447
Other Radiation root type, 470
otoplasty, 132
ova, 381
ovary, 267, 381, 384
Oxilan contrast media, 465

P

pacemakers
    function values during procedures, 432
    Insertion root operation for, 113–114, 289
    Removal root operation for, 221
    Revision root operation for, 118
    types of, 219–220
Packing Material, 417
Packing root operation, 416
palate (hard and soft), 195, 196, 249
palatine bone, 322
palatine tonsils, 196
Palladium seeds, 470
Pancreas. *See* Hepatobiliary System and Pancreas
pancreatic duct, 252
pancreatic islet cells, 272
para-aortic body, 267, 272
paraganglion extremity, 267, 268
paranasal sinuses, 181–182, 185
parathyroid glands, 267
parotid gland and duct, 195, 196
partial amputation, 79, 149
partial gastrectomy, 73
partial mastectomy, 42, 74, 288, 289
partial thickness of skin, defined, 285
partial-thickness procedure qualifiers, 293
pectus excavatum, 144
pedicle flap, 103, 226, 288–289
PEG/J tube, 257
penis, 120, 367–368
peptic ulcer, 254
percussion, 449
Percutaneous approach
    overview of guidelines, 49
    for abdominal aortic aneurysms, 222

    for Administration Section, 419
    for bones and joints, 333
    for Circulatory system, 232
    decision tree guidelines for, 50
    defined, 10, 147, 166
    for Endocrine system, 269
    for Integumentary system, 291
    for Lymphatic system, 273
    for Measurement and Monitoring section, 424
    for Muscular system, 309
    for New Technology section, 490
    for Obstetrics section, 402
    for Sense Organs, 185
    for Urinary system, 357
percutaneous approaches. *See* Percutaneous approach;
    Percutaneous Endoscopic approach; Via Natural or
    Artificial Opening with Percutaneous Endoscopic
    Assistance
Percutaneous Endoscopic approach
    overview of guidelines, 49–50
    for bones and joints, 333
    decision tree guidelines, 50
    defined, 11, 147
    for Endocrine system, 269
    for Lymphatic system, 273
    for Muscular system, 309
    for New Technology section, 490
    for Obstetrics section, 403
    for Sense Organs, 185
    for Urinary system, 357
percutaneous endoscopic gastrostomy (PEG), 256
percutaneous nephrostomy, 49, 51, 87, 419
percutaneous transluminal angioplasty (non-coronary), 224
percutaneous transluminal coronary angioplasty (PTCA),
    107, 224–225
Performance root operation, 203, 431–432
Perfusion root operation, 437
peri-adrenal lymph nodes, 273
perineal laceration, 144, 385, 402
perineum, 385, 402
peripheral IVs, 220
peripherally inserted central catheter (PICC), 221
Peripheral Nervous system, 159–177
    approaches for, 166
    body part values for, 164–165
    body system values for, 159
    case studies, 173–177
    code building cases, 168–170
    code building exercises, 170–171
    devices common to, 167
    functions of, 159
    organization of, 159–162
    qualifiers used in, 167
    root operations used in, 163–164
    Transfer root operation, 97
peripheral veno-arterial (VA) ECMO, 435
peripheral veno-venous (VV) ECMO, 435
"peri" prefix, for body parts, 46, 357
peri-renal lymph nodes, 273
peritoneal ascites drainage, 85

peritoneal cavity, 109, 140–141

peritoneum, 250

periureteric adhesion release, 357

personality and behavioral tests, 485

personality and behavioral type qualifier, 487

pessary, 15, 386

Pharmacotherapy root type, 488

pharyngeal tonsils, 195, 196

pharynx, 195, 197, 249

Pheresis root operation, 437, 439

Phototherapy, 437

Physical Rehabilitation and Diagnostic Audiology section

    body region values for, 482–483

    body system values for, 482–483

    case studies, 494–498

    character definition for, 481–484

    code building cases, 491–492

    code format and structure, 5

    equipment common to, 483

    fitting of braces and splints, 418, 482

    manual traction, 417

    procedure types included in, 481

    qualifiers used in, 484

    root types commonly used in, 482

    section qualifiers used in, 481–482

    section value for, 481

    type qualifiers common to, 483

Physiological systems and anatomical regions

    Administration root operations for, 419

    body system and regional values for, 419

    for Other Procedures section, 449

Piercing method, 451

pineal body, 267, 268

pituitary gland, 267, 268

Placement section

    approaches used in, 417

    body regions for, 416–417

    body system values for, 415

    case studies, 428–430

    character definition for, 415–418

    code building cases, 426–427

    description, 5

    devices common to, 417–418

    procedure types included in, 415

    qualifiers used in, 418

    root operations used in, 415–416

    section value for, 418

Plain Radiography root type, 464–465

Planar Nuclear Medicine Imaging root type, 468

pleural cavity, 140, 199, 201

pleural effusion, 83

plexus, defined, 161

PLIF (posterior lumbar interbody fusion), 336

polyps, 73

ports, 49, 221

Positron Emission Tomography (PET) root type, 468

posterior colporrhaphy, 383

posterior column fusion (PLF), 337

postoperative hemorrhage, 40, 84, 147

pregnancy. *See* Obstetrics section

pregnancy termination, 400

prepuce, 367, 369

pressure, measurement and monitoring of, 232, 423–424

process (bone), 322, 324

proctopexy, 254

Products of Conception, 51, 399–400

Products of Conception, Ectopic, 400

Products of Conception, Retained, 51, 400

prostatectomy, 369

prostate gland, 366, 367, 368, 369, 470

prostheses

    defined, 15

    for joint replacements, 329–330

    lens, 82, 185

provider's role in code building

    Conventions guidelines for, 37, 81

    terminology selection, 4, 31

psychoanalysis type qualifier, 487

psychodynamic type qualifier, 487

Psychological Testing root type, 485

psychophysiological type qualifier, 487

psychotherapy, 484

pulling veins, 82

pulmonary alveolar proteinosis (PAP), 200

pulsatile compression devices, 434

pyelotomy procedure approaches, 357

pyloromyotomy procedure, 253

pylorus, 249–250

Q

qualifier (character 7)

    for Administration section, 419–421

    for anatomical regions, 148–149

    for biopsy procedures, 42, 73–74, 76, 83–84, 272

    for body layers, 310

    for bones and joints, 44, 340–341

    for Bypass root operation, 42–43, 110, 235–237

    for Chiropractic section, 454

    for Circulatory system, 48, 235–237

    CMS file definitions, 31

    code format, 19

    for Creation root operation, 133, 144

    definition of, 19

    for Detachment root operation, 77–81, 148–149

    for Ear, Nose, and Sinus, 186

    for Endocrine system, 270

    for Extracorporeal or Systemic Assistance and Performance section, 434–436

    for Extracorporeal or Systemic Therapies section, 438–439

    for Extraction root operation, 83

    for Eye, 186

    for Female Reproductive system, 386–387

    for Fusion root operation, 129

    for Gastrointestinal system, 258–259

    for Hepatobiliary System and Pancreas, 258–259

    for Imaging section, 466

    for Integumentary system, 289, 293

    for Lymphatic system, 274

    for Male Reproductive system, 371

    for Measurement and Monitoring section, 425

for Mental Health section, 485–487
for Mouth and Throat, 204
for Nervous system, 167
for New Technology section, 491
for Nuclear Medicine section, 469
for Obstetrics section, 403–405
for Osteopathic section, 449
for Other Procedures section, 451–452
for Physical Rehabilitation and Diagnostic Audiology
    section, 484
for Placement section, 418
for Radiation Therapy, 472
for Resection root operation, 76
for Respiratory system, 204
for Sense Organs, 186
for Substance Abuse Treatment section, 488–489
for Transfer root operation, 46, 97
for Transplantation root operation, 96, 144
for Urinary system, 359
Quinton catheter, 221

R
radial keratotomy, 183
Radiation Therapy section
    body system values for, 469
    case studies, 475–479
    character definition, 469–472
    code building cases, 472–474
    code format and structure, 5
    isotope values for, 471–472
    modalities for, 470–471
    procedure types for, 463
    qualifiers used in, 472
    section value for, 463, 469
    treatment sites for, 470
radical mastectomy, 288
radical resection, 76
radiofrequency ablation, 81, 163
radiofrequency needle ablation, 81
radiological markers, 51
Radionuclides (character 5), 467, 469
realignment of bone, due to deformities, 328
Reattachment root operation
    overview, 97
    defined, 97
    for Integumentary system, 287
    qualifiers, 148
    for Tendons, 307
recalled prosthesis procedures, 330
rectal pull-through, 256
rectocele repair, 383
rectopexy, 99, 254
rectum, 99, 249, 250, 273
reflexology, 450
refusion, 339
rehabilitative exercise, as non-manual chiropractic
    treatment, 453
Release root operation
    overview, 89–91
    body part value for, 45, 94, 254

for bones and joints, 339
defined, 45–46, 94, 307
for Gastrointestinal system, 254
for Muscular system, 307–308
for Nervous system, 163
for Tendons, 307
thoracoscopy or thoracotomy procedures, 201
Removal root operation
    overview, 115–116
    approaches for, 116
    for bones and joints, 330–331
    for Circulatory system, 221, 232
    defined, 115, 119
    of devices, 51, 115–116
    for Gastrointestinal system, 254
    for Male Reproductive system, 369
    for Nervous system, 164
    for Obstetrics section, 402–403
    for Placement section, 415–416
    for unspecified body part, 118
    for Urinary system, 355, 356, 369
renal artery aneurysm, 222
Repair root operation
    overview, 127
    for anatomical regions, 144
    as bleeding control technique, 143–144
    for bones and joints, 331
    for Circulatory system, 229
    defined, 97, 127
    for Female Reproductive system, 383
    for Gastrointestinal system, 254
    for Nervous system, 162
    for Obstetrics section, 143–144, 402
    on overlapping layers, 42, 74, 77, 93, 125, 290, 308
    for Sense Organs, 183
    on tendons, 307
    for Urinary system, 355
Replacement root operation
    for bleeding control, 143
    for bones and joints, 329–331
    for breasts, 288, 289
    defined, 72, 95, 97, 119, 331
    device values for, 119, 289
    free graft and flap procedures, 97, 119, 288, 293
    for Integumentary system, 288, 293
    for Male Reproductive system, 369
    for Sense Organs, 183
Reposition root operation
    overview, 99
    for bleeding control, 143
    for bones and joints, 46, 99, 163, 324–325, 328
    defined, 46, 99
    for Female Reproductive system, 383
    for Gastrointestinal system, 254
    for Integumentary system, 287
    for Male Reproductive system, 369
    for Nervous system, 163
    for Obstetrics section, 403
    for tendons, 307
    for Urinary system, 355

reproductive systems. *See* Female Reproductive system; Male Reproductive system

rerouting procedures. *See* Bypass root operation

Resection root operation
    for biopsies, 42
    for bleeding control, 143
    body part subdivision guideline, 74–76
    for bones and joints, 329
    of bursae, 307
    circumcision as, 369
    defined, 43, 73, 74–76, 116, 126
    for Ear, 183
    for Endocrine system, 268
    for Female Reproductive system, 383, 384
    for Gastrointestinal system, 253
    for Integumentary system, 288, 289
    for Lymphatic system, 271
    for Mouth and Throat, 201
    qualifier for, 76
    of Respiratory system, 201
    thoracoscopy or thoracotomy procedures, 201
    for Urinary system, 356

respiratory assistance, 432

Respiratory system, 195–212
    approaches, 202
    body part values for, 75, 201–202
    body system value for, 195
    case studies, 209–212
    code building cases, 204–205
    code building exercises, 206–207
    devices common to, 203
    functions of, 195
    organization of, 197–199
    for Physical Rehabilitation section, 482
    qualifiers used in, 204
    root operations used in, 199–201

Restoration root operation, 432, 434

Restriction root operation
    for Circulatory system, 45, 222, 223, 229
    defined, 45, 105–107
    discussion of, 105–106
    for Female Reproductive system, 383
    for Gastrointestinal system, 252–253
    for Lymphatic system, 271
    for Sense Organs, 183

restrictive stents, 223

resurfacing of joint surface, 330

retina, 179

Revision root operation
    overview, 118
    for bones and joints, 330
    for Circulatory system, 221, 229
    defined, 118
    for Gastrointestinal system, 254
    guidelines for, 51, 118
    for Male Reproductive system, 369
    of Nervous system, 164
    for Urinary system, 356, 369

rhizotomy, 93

rhythm function values, 434

right lung field, 199

ring fixation device, 328

Robotic assisted procedure method, 451

root operation (character 3)
    overview of guidelines, 40–46
    for Administration section, 418–419
    for anatomical regions, 143–144
    approach change, guidelines for, 41
    for biopsies. *See* biopsy procedures
    for body systems, 20
    for bones and joints, 44–45, 324–331
    case studies, 90–91, 102–104, 123, 135–137
    for Chiropractic section, 452
    for Circulatory system, 218–229
    CMS file definitions, 31
    code format, 6–8
    component guidelines for, 40
    definition of, 6
    description, 71–72
    determination of, 53, 55
    for discontinued procedures, 41, 143
    with Drainage Device, guidelines for, 51
    for Ear, Nose and Sinus, 183–183
    for Endocrine system, 268
    for Extracorporeal or Systemic Assistance and Performance section, 431–432
    for Extracorporeal or Systemic Therapies section, 437,
    for Eye, 182–183
    for Female Reproductive system, 382–384
    fracture treatment guidelines, 46
    fusion procedures guidelines, 44–45
    for Gastrointestinal system, 252–254
    for grafts. *See* grafts
    groups of, 7–8, 53–54. *See also specific groupings*
    for Imaging section, 464–465
    in Lymphatic system, 271–272
    for Male Reproductive system, 369
    for Measurement and Monitoring section, 523
    of Medical and Surgical section, 7, 40–46, 53–54, 541–550
    for Mental Health section, 484–485
    for Mouth and Throat, 199–200
    for multiple procedures, 40–41, 42, 57, 289
    for Nervous system, 163–164
    for New Technology section, 489–490
    for Nuclear Medicine section, 467–468
    for Obstetrics, 400–402
    Obstetrics section, 400–402
    for Osteopathic, 547
    for Other Procedures section, 449
    for overlapping layers, 42, 74, 77, 93, 125, 290, 308
    for Physical Rehabilitation and Diagnostic Audiology, 482
    for Placement section, 415–416
    procedural steps, coding of, 253, 329
    for Radiation Therapy, 548
    for Respiratory system, 199–201
    for Substance Abuse Treatment section, 487–488
    for Urinary system, 355–356

Root Operations Involving Cutting or Separation Only (Group 3), 93–99. *See also* Division root operation; Release root operation

Root Operations that Alter Diameter or Route of a Tubular Body Part (Group 5), 105–113. *See also* Bypass root operation; Dilation root operation; Occlusion root operation; Restriction root operation

Root Operations that Always Involve a Device (Group 6), 113–120. *See also* Change root operation; Insertion root operation; Removal root operation; Replacement root operation; Revision root operation; Supplement root operation

Root Operations that Define Other Objectives (Group 9), 129–133. *See also* Alteration root operation; Creation root operation; Fusion root operation

Root Operations that Define Other Repairs (Group 8), 127–128. *See also* Control root operation; Repair root operation

Root Operations that Involve Examination Only (Group 7), 125–127. *See also* Inspection root operation; Map root operation

Root Operations that Put in or Put Back or Move Some or All of a Body Part (Group 4), 95–99. *See also* Reattachment root operation; Reposition root operation; Transfer root operation; Transplantation root operation

Root Operations that Take Out Solids, Fluids, or Gases from a Body Part (Group 2), 83–88. *See also* Drainage root operation; Extirpation root operation; Fragmentation root operation

Root Operations that Take Out Some or All of a Body Part (Group 1), 72–83. *See also* Destruction root operation; Detachment root operation; Excision root operation; Resection root operation

root type (character 3), for Physical Rehabilitation and Diagnostic Audiology section, 481

Roux-en-Y bariatric procedure, 252

ruptured tendon, 307

S

sacular aneurysm, 222

salivary glands, 195–197, 249

salpingo-oophorectomy, 384

scintigraphy, 467

sclera, 179, 186

scrotum, 367, 369

section (character 1). *See also specific sections*

    Administration section value, 418

    Chiropractic section value, 452

    code format, 5

    definition of, 5

    for dilation and curettage (D&C), 51, 107, 384, 401

    Extracorporeal or Systemic Assistance and Performance section value, 431

    Extracorporeal or Systemic Therapies section value, 431

    Imaging section value, 463

    Measurement and Monitoring section value, 423

    Medical and Surgical section value, 5

    Mental Health section value, 484

    New Technology section value, 489

    Nuclear Medicine section value, 467

    Obstetrics section value, 399

    for Other Procedures section, 449

    Physical Rehabilitation and Diagnostic Audiology section value, 481

    Placement section value, 415

    Radiation Therapy value, 467, 469

    Substance Abuse Treatment section value, 487

section qualifier (character 2), for Physical Rehabilitation and Diagnostic Audiology section, 484

Selection of Principal Procedure, 52

seminal vesicles, 367, 368, 369

Sense Organs, 179–193

    approaches for, 185

    body part values for, 183–184

    body system values for, 179

    case studies, 190–193

    code building cases, 186–188

    code building exercises, 188–189

    devices common to, 185

    functions of, 179

    organization of, 179–182

    qualifiers used in, 186

    root operations used in, 182–183

Sheffield ring external fixator, 118

shockwave lithotripsy, 87

shock wave therapy, 437

short lever manipulation, 454

short-term external heart assist system, 232

shoulder

    body part value for, 48, 290

    organization of, 326

    replacement procedures, 330

shunts, 109, 163

sigmoid bladder procedure, 355

sigmoid colon, 249

sigmoidectomy, 49

simple appliances, defined, 15

simple mastectomy, 288

sinus. *See* Ear, Nose, and Sinus

sinus (bone), 322

sinuses, as generic term, 181

skeletal muscles. *See* Muscular system

skeletal system, 321–351

    approaches used for, 333–334

    body system values for, 321

    case studies, 347–351

    code building cases, 341–343

    code building exercises, 343–345

    devices common to, 334–340

    organization of, 321–324

    qualifiers used for, 340–341

    root operations used for, 324–331

Skene's glands, 381

Skin and Breast

    approaches for, 291

    body system value for, 285

    devices common to, 15, 291–293

    full-thickness procedures, 293

    organization of, 285–287

    partial-thickness procedures, 293

    qualifiers used in, 293

    root operations for, 287–288

    skin and subcutaneous tissue distinction, 285

skin or mucous membranes, approach types through or on, 10–11, 13–14. *See also* External approach; Open

approach; Percutaneous approach; Percutaneous Endoscopic approach
skin pedicle transfer, 97
skull, bones of, 322
skull fractures, 163
sleeve gastrectomy procedure, 252
small intestines, 249
solid matter removal. *See* Extirpation root operation; Fragmentation root operation
somatic nerves, 160–161
spacers, 330
SPECT (single photon emission computed tomography), 467
Speech Assessment root type, 482
Speech Treatment root type, 482
sperm, collecting, 450
spermatic cord, 367, 368, 369
sphenoid sinus, 181
Spinal Canal, 419
spinal cord, 159–161, 163–164
spinal epidural space, 419
spinal fusion, 44, 74, 129–132, 334–338
spinal meninges, 161, 164–165, 167
spine (bone feature), 322
spleen, 249, 270, 272
splints
    application of, 46, 99, 326, 418
    fitting of, 418, 482
standardized psychological testing, 487
stem cells, 271, 272, 419
stenotic pulmonary valve, 107
stents
    for Dilation root operation, 107–109, 113, 355
    for Restriction root operation, 107, 222
Stent Retriever, 86, 235
Stereotactic Radiosurgery root type, 470
sterilization procedures, 369, 383
sternum, 270
stimulator generators, 289
stimulator leads, 310
stomach, 249–250
stoma excision, 148
stones
    bladder, 356
    kidney, 49, 51, 86, 358, 419
stripping veins, 82
subarachnoid space, 159
Subcutaneous Tissue and Fascia
    body part value guidelines for, 48
    body system value for, 285
    devices common to, 292
    organization of, 285, 287, 303
    osteopathic treatment of, 449
    qualifiers used in, 293
    root operations for, 97, 116, 287–289
    skin and subcutaneous tissue distinction, 285
subcutaneous tissue (fat), 285
subdural space, 159
sublingual gland, 195, 196
submaxillary (submandibular) gland, 195, 196
Substance Abuse Treatment section
    body system value, 487

case studies, 494–498
character definition, 487–489
code building cases, 491–492
code format and structure, 5
procedure types included in, 481
qualifier values for, 488–489
root types commonly used in, 487–488
section value for, 481
type qualifiers for, 488
substance (character 6)
    for Administration section, 418
    defined, 17, 418
    key for, 23, 27
    for New Technology section, 503
subtotal hysterectomy, 384
superior parathyroid gland, 268
supernumerary digits, 144
supersaturation (superoxygenation), 435
Supplement root operation
    overview, 120
    for bones and joints, 328
    for Circulatory system, 365
    defined, 115, 123
    device values for, 120
    for Eye, 183
    for Female Reproductive system, 397
    for Gastrointestinal system, 256
    for Male Reproductive system, 369
supportive type qualifier, 487
supracervical hysterectomy, 384
suspension procedure for bladder, 355
Suture Removal method, 451
suture repair
    body system value for, 40, 84, 147
    lacerations, 127
    of nerves, 163
    of tendons, 307
    tubal ligation reversal, 383
sutures, 51
Swan-Ganz catheter, 233
sympathetic nerves, 166
synarthroses, 324
syngeneic qualifier, 96
synovium, 331
synthetic grafts, 222
Systemic Nuclear Medicine Therapy root type, 467
system structure and design, 3–32
    section (character 1), 5. *See also* section
    body systems (character 2), 5–6. *See also* body systems
    root operations (character 3), 6–8. *See also* root operations
    body part (character 4), 10. *See also* body part
    approaches (character 5), 10–14. *See also* approaches
    devices (character 6), 14–19. *See also* devices
    qualifiers (character 7), 19. *See also* qualifier (character 6&7)
    background, 3–4
    clinical documentation and terminology, 31
    CMS file method, 20–27
    code book method, 20
    code building exercises, 32–34
    code building process, 19–30
    code completion, 20–21

code format and structure, 4–19
Conventions guidelines for, 35–39
Index references, other, 29
tables, locating, 20
tables, referencing directly, 30–31

T

tables
Conventions guidelines for use of, 35
location of, 6, 20
online, 24
organization of, 20
referencing directly, 21, 22,
take-down of colostomy or ileostomy, 253
tarsometatarsal joint, 79
technology character, for New Technology section, 489
teeth (upper and lower), 84, 195, 204, 249
temperature, 423, 424, 437
Temporary qualifier, 19, 51
Tendons. *See also* Muscular system
body part values for, 48, 309
body system value for, 303
functions, 303
organization of, 303
root operations for, 303
TENS (transcutaneous electrical nerve stimulation) system, 167
tent (Laminaria), 400
testes, 267, 367, 369
therapeutic fluid, perfusion of, 437
Therapeutic massage method, 447
therapeutic nuclear medicine procedures, 467
thermoplasty, 200
thoracentesis, 83
thoracic duct, 270
thoracic esophagus, 254
thoracoscopy, 201
thoracotomy-based procedures, 201
360-Degree Fusion, 338
Throat. *See* Mouth and Throat
thrombectomy, 39, 224
thumb. *See* fingers
thymus, 270, 272
thyroid, 267, 268
tissue, types of, 201
tissue expanders, 15, 288
tissue rearrangement through flap use, 287
TLIF (transforaminal lumbar interbody fusion), 337
toenails, 41, 57, 287
toes, 48, 79, 148
Tomographic Nuclear Medicine Imaging root type, 467–468
tongue, 195, 249
tonsillectomy, 201
tonsils, 195, 270
TORUS stent graft, 228
total abdominal hysterectomy, 384
total hysterectomy, 384
total joint replacement, 329–331
totally implantable ports (port-A-Cath), 221
total mastectomy, 75, 288
total mechanical ventilation, 432

trachea, 196
tracheobronchial tree, 196
tracheostomy device, 15, 203
Traction root operation
for Placement section, 416–417
transbronchial biopsy, 200
transcatheter valve replacement, 222
Transfer root operation
overview, 97
for flap procedures, 287–289, 293
involving overlapping layers, guidelines for, 97
for Nervous system, 167
qualifiers for, 293, 310
Transfusion root operation
for Administration section, 419
of bone marrow and cells, 46, 96, 270
defined, 46, 96
transmyocardial laser revascularization (TMLR), 229
Transplantation root operation
overview, 95–96
for anatomical regions, 144
of bone marrow cells. *See* Transfusion root operation
of face, 144
for Gastrointestinal system, 252
of heart, 223
for kidney, 356
of living body parts, guidelines for, 46, 95–96, 270
for lung, 204
for Lymphatic system, 270
for ovary, 384
qualifiers for, 95, 356, 404
transurethral resection of the prostate (TURP), 369
transverse colon, 249
transverse position of fetus, turning, 402
transverse rectus abdominis myocutaneous (TRAM) flap, 289
Treatment root operation, 447
treatment site (character 4), 470
tricuspid valves, 133, 213
trocars, 49
trochanter, 322
truncus arteriosus, 222
tubal ligation, 383
tubercle, 322
tuberosity, 322
tubotubal anastomosis, 383
tubular body parts
altering diameter or route of, 105–107. *See also* Bypass root operation; Dilation root operation; Occlusion root operation; Restriction root operation
approaches for, 147
Inspection root operation for multiple parts, 141, 356
values for, 47, 105–107, 141
tumor cells, 470
tumor embolization, 45, 223
tumors, removal of, 73. *See also* Excision root operation
tunica vaginalis, 367, 369
tunneled vascular access devices (VAD), 16, 221, 292
twin deliveries, 401
tympanic membrane, 183
tympanoplasty, 183

tympanostomy tube placement, 183
type qualifier (character)
    for Mental Health section, 484
    for Physical Rehabilitation and Diagnostic Audiology
        section, 481
    for Substance Abuse Treatment section, 487

U
ulcer (gastric) repair, 254
Ultrasonography root type, 464
Ultrasound therapy, 437, 453
Ultraviolet light therapy, 437
Ultravist contrast media, 465
undiversion procedure, 355
unicondylar knee replacement, 329–330
uniplane fixation device, 328
Upper Arteries
    aneurysm procedures, 222
    approaches for, 232
    AV fistulas and grafts, 229
    blood collection from, 229, 450
    body part values for, 229–230
    body system value for, 213
    devices common to, 232–234
    generic body part values, 230
    organization of, 218
    PTA, 224
    qualifiers used in, 235
    vascular access devices for, 220–221
Upper Bones. See bones
upper esophagus, 254
upper extremities
    amputation of. See Detachment root operation
    body system value, 139
    division from lower body parts, 39–40, 141
    fingers, 48, 57, 82
    organization of, 140–141
Upper Intestinal Tract, 254
Upper Joints. See joints
Upper Veins
    approaches for, 232
    AV fistulas and grafts, 229
    body part values for, 230
    body system value for, 213
    devices common to, 232, 234
    generic body part values, 230
    organization of, 216
    qualifiers used in, 235
    vascular access devices for, 220–221
    venipuncture, 229
ureteral stent, 107
ureteroileal conduit procedure, 355
ureterostomy, 355
ureters, 103, 353, 355–357
urethra
    body part value for, 369
    organization of, 353–364, 382
    procedures for, 365, 366
    repair of, 417
urinary catheter, 356, 358, 416

urinary filtration, 430
Urinary system
    approaches used in, 357
    body part values for, 356–357
    body system value, 353
    case studies, 363–366
    code building cases, 359–360
    code building exercises, 360–362
    devices common to, 358
    functions of, 353
    organization of, 353–55
    qualifiers for, 359
    root operations used for, 355–356
urine, formation of, 353
uterine supporting structures, 381
uteropexy, 383
uterus
    body part values for, 384–385
    organization of, 381
    procedures for, 383, 384
uvula, 195

V
vagina, 381, 383, 384–385
valves
    Creation root operation, 133, 222
    procedures involving, 96, 107, 120, 133, 221–223
    types of, 15, 107, 203, 249
varicose vein stripping, 84
vascular access devices, 16, 219–221, 291
vas deferens, 106, 367, 368
vasectomy, 106, 369
vein graft, 111
veins. See Lower Veins; Upper Veins
vein-stripping procedures, 82
venipuncture, 229
ventricular septum repair, 222
ventriculography, 465
ventriculoperitoneal shunt, 109
ventriculoperitoneal (VP) shunt, 164
Versajet, 82
vertebrae and vertebral column
    body part value for, 273
    fractures of, 328
    Fusion root operation, 44, 74, 129, 324–325
    laminectomy, 95
    organization of, 322–324
vertebroplasty, 328
vesicostomy, 355
vessel embolization procedures, 45
Vestibular Assessment root type, 82
vestibular glands, 381
Vestibular Treatment root type, 482
Via Natural or Artificial Opening
    overview, 50
    for Administration Section, 419
    for anatomical regions, 50
    for breast and nipple procedures, 291
    decision tree guidelines, 50
    defined, 11

for Extraction root operation, 403
for Measurement and Monitoring section, 424
for Other Extraction root operation, 403
for Sense Organs, 185
Via Natural or Artificial Opening Endoscopic
overview, 50
for Administration section, 419
for anatomical regions, 147
for breast and nipple procedures, 291
defined, 11–12
for delivery, 403
for Extraction root operation, 403
for Gastrointestinal system, 256
for Male Reproductive system, 369
for Measurement and Monitoring section, 424
for Sense Organs, 185
Via Natural or Artificial Opening with Percutaneous
Endoscopic Assistance, 12–13, 50
visceral manipulation, 453
Visipaque contrast media, 465
vitreous, 179
vocal cord, 195

vocational type qualifier, 487
volvulus of gastrointestinal system, 98, 254
vulva, 381, 382

W
waterjet debridement, 82
wet-to-dry dressing changes, 82
whole-body hyperthermia radiation therapy, 470
whole lung lavage, 200
worn prosthesis procedures, 328
wrist, 48, 290, 322

X
XLIF (extreme lateral interbody fusion), 337

Y
Yoga Therapy method, 451
for anatomical regions, 148
defined, 4
for Endocrine system, 270

Z
zooplastic device, 96, 111, 222